AF616063

ADVANCES IN NEUROLOGY

Volume 91

ADVANCES IN NEUROLOGY

Volume 91

Parkinson's Disease

Editors

Ariel Gordin, M.D., PH.D.
Research Centre
Orion Pharma
Espoo
Finland

Seppo Kaakkola, M.D.
Department of Neurology
University of Helsinki
Helsinki
Finland

Heikki Teräväinen, M.D.
Department of Neurology
University of Helsinki
Helsinki
Finland

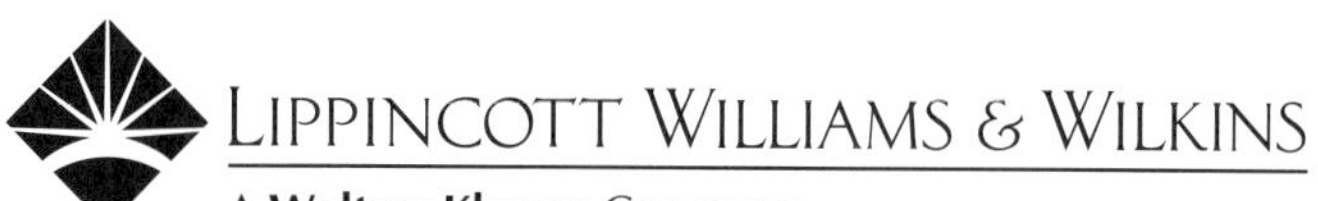

Philadelphia • Baltimore • New York • London
Buenos Aires • Hong Kong • Sydney • Tokyo

Acquisitions Editor: Anne M. Sydor
Developmental Editor: Marc Bendian
Production Editor: Jeff Somers
Manufacturing Manager: Ben Rivera
Cover Designer: Patricia Gast
Compositor: Lippincott Williams & Wilkins Desktop Division
Printer: Maple Press

530 Walnut Street
Philadelphia, PA 19106 USA
LWW.com

Printed in the USA

Library of Congress Cataloging-in-Publication Data

ISBN: 0-7817-4084-3
ISSN: 0091-3952

---

10 9 8 7 6 5 4 3 2 1

Advances in Neurology Series

Vol. 90: Neurological Complications of Pregnancy. Second Edition: *B. Hainline and O. Devinsky, editors.* 368 pp, 2002.
Vol. 89: Myoclonus and Paroxysmal Dyskinesias: *S. Fahn, S.J. Frucht, M. Hallett, D.D. Truon, editors.* 528 pp, 2002.
Vol. 88: Neuromuscular Disorders: *R. Pourmand and Y. Harati, editors.* 368 pp., 2001.
Vol. 87: Gait Disorders: *E. Ruzicka, M. Hallett, and J. Jankovic, editors.* 432 pp., 2001.
Vol. 86: Parkinson's Disease: *D. Calne and S. Calne, editors.* 512 pp., 2001.
Vol. 85: Tourette Syndrome: *D. J. Cohen, C. Goetz, and J. Jankovic, editors.* 432 pp., 2001.
Vol. 84: Neocortical Epilepsies: *P. D. Williamson, A. M. Siegel, D. W. Roberts, V. M. Thadani, and M. S. Gazzaniga, editors.* 688 pp., 2000.
Vol. 83: Functional Imaging in the Epilepsies: *T. R. Henry, J. S. Duncan, and S. F. Berkovic, editors.* 348 pp., 2000.
Vol. 82: Corticobasal Degeneration and Related Disorders: *I. Litvan, C .G. Goetz, and A. E. Lang, editors.* 280 pp., 2000.
Vol. 81: Plasticity and Epilepsy: *H. Stefan, P. Chauvel, F. Anderman, and S.D. Sharvon, editors.* 396 pp., 1999.
Vol. 80: Parkinson's Disease: *Gerald M. Stern, editor.* 704 pp., 1999.
Vol. 79: Jasper's Basic Mechanisms of the Epilepsies. Third Edition: *A. Delgado-Escueta, W. Wilson, R. Olsen, and R. Porter, editors.* 1,132 pp., 1999.
Vol. 78: Dystonia 3:*S. Fahn, C. D. Marsden, and M. R. DeLong, editors.* 374 pp., 1998.
Vol. 77: Consciousness: At the Frontiers of Neuroscience: *H. H. Jasper, L. Descarries, V. F. Castellucci, S. Rossignol, editors.* 300 pp., 1998.
Vol. 76: Antiepileptic Drug Development: *J. A. French, I. E. Leppik, and M.A. Dichter, editors.* 276 pp., 1998.
Vol. 75: Reflex Epilepsies and Reflex Seizures: *B. G. Zifkin, F. Andermann, A. Beaumanoir, and A. J. Rowan, editors.* 310 pp., 1998.
Vol. 74: Basal Ganglia and New Surgical Approaches for Parkinson's Disease: *J. A. Obeso, M. R. DeLong, C. Ohye, and C. D. Marsden, editors.* 286 pp., 1997.
Vol. 73: Brain Plasticity: *H. J. Freund, B. A. Sabel, and O. W. Witte, editors.* 448 pp., 1997.
Vol. 72: Neuronal Regeneration, Reorganization, and Repair: *F. J. Seil, editor.* 416 pp., 1996.
Vol. 71: Cellular and Molecular Mechanisms of Ischemic Brain Damage: *B. K. Siesjö and T. Wieloch, editors.* 560 pp., 1996.
Vol. 70: Supplementary Sensorimotor Area: *H. O. Lüders, editor.* 544 pp., 1996.
Vol. 69: Parkinson's Disease: *L. Battistin, G. Scarlato, T. Caraceni, and S. Ruggieri, editors.* 752 pp., 1996.
Vol. 68: Pathogenesis and Therapy of Amyotrophic Lateral Sclerosis: *G. Serratrice and T. L. Munsat, editors.* 352 pp., 1995.
Vol. 67: Negative Motor Phenomena: *S. Fahn, M. Hallett, H. O. Lüders, and C. D. Marsden, editors.* 416 pp., 1995.
Vol. 66: Epilepsy and the Functional Anatomy of the Frontal Lobe: *H. H. Jasper, S. Riggio, and P. S. Goldman-Rakic, editors.* 400 pp., 1995.
Vol. 65: Behavioral Neurology of Movement Disorders: *W. J. Weiner and A. E. Lang, editors.* 368 pp., 1995.
Vol. 64: Neurological Complications of Pregnancy: *O. Devinsky, E. Feldmann, and B. Hainline, editors.* 288 pp., 1994.
Vol. 63: Electrical and Magnetic Stimulation of the Brain and Spinal Cord: *O. Devinsky, A. Beric, and M. Dogali, editors.* 352 pp., 1993.
Vol. 62: Cerebral Small Artery Disease: *P. M. Pullicino, L. R. Caplan, and M. Hommel, editors.* 256 pp., 1993.
Vol. 61: Inherited Ataxias: *A. E. Harding and T. Deufel, editors.* 240 pp., 1993.
Vol. 60: Parkinson's Disease: From Basic Research to Treatment: *H. Narabayashi, T. Nagatsu, N. Yanagisawa, and Y. Mizuno, editors.* 800 pp., 1993.

Vol. 59: Neural Injury and Regeneration: *F. J. Seil, editor.* 384 pp., 1993.
Vol. 58: Tourette Syndrome: Genetics, Neurobiology, and Treatment: *T. N. Chase, A. J. Friedhoff, and D. J. Cohen, editors.* 400 pp., 1992.
Vol. 57: Frontal Lobe Seizures and Epilepsies: *P. Chauvel, A. V. Delgado-Escueta, E. Halgren, and J. Bancaud, editors.* 752 pp., 1992.
Vol. 56: Amyotrophic Lateral Sclerosis and Other Motor Neuron Diseases: *L. P. Rowland, editor.* 592 pp., 1991.
Vol. 55: Neurobehavioral Problems in Epilepsy: *D. B. Smith, D. Treiman, and M. Trimble, editors.* 512 pp., 1990.
Vol. 54: Magnetoencephalography: *S. Sato, editor.* 284 pp., 1990.
Vol. 53: Parkinson's Disease: Anatomy, Pathology, and Therapy: *M. B. Streifler, A. D. Korczyn, E. Melamed, and M. B. H. Youdim, editors.* 640 p., 1990.
Vol. 52: Brain Edema: Pathogenesis, Imaging, and Therapy: *D. Long, editor.* 640 pp., 1990.
Vol. 51: Alzheimer's Disease: *R. J. Wurtman, S. Corkin, J. H. Growdon, and E. Ritter-Walker, editors.* 308 pp., 1990.
Vol. 50: Dystonia 2: *S. Fahn, C. D. Marsden, and D. B. Calne, editors.* 688 pp., 1988.
Vol. 49: Facial Dyskinesias: *J. Jankovic and E. Tolosa, editors.* 560 pp., 1988.
Vol. 48: Molecular Genetics of Neurological and Neuromuscular Disease: *S. DiDonato, S. DiMauro, A. Mamoli, and L. P. Rowland, editors.* 288 pp., 1987.
Vol. 47: Functional Recovery in Neurological Disease: *S. G. Waxman, editor.* 640 pp., 1987.
Vol. 46: Intensive Neurodiagnostic Monitoring: *R. J. Gumnit, editor.* 336 pp., 1987.
Vol. 45: Parkinson's Disease: *M. D. Yahr and K. J. Bergmann, editors.* 640 pp., 1987.
Vol. 44: Basic Mechanisms of the Epilepsies: Molecular and Cellular Approaches: *A. V. Delgado-Escueta, A. A. Ward, Jr., D. M. Woodbury, and R. J. Porter, editors.* 1,120 pp., 1986.
Vol. 43: Myoclonus: *S. Fahn, C. D. Marsden, and M. H. VanWoert, editors.* 752 pp., 1986.
Vol. 42: Progress in Aphasiology: *F. C. Rose, editor.* 384 pp., 1984.
Vol. 41: The Olivopontocerebellar Atrophies: *R. C. Duvoisin and A. Plaitakis, editors.* 304 pp., 1984.
Vol. 40: Parkinson-Specific Motor and Mental Disorders, Role of Pallidum: Pathophysiological, Biochemical, and Therapeutic Aspects: *R. G. Hassler and J. F. Christ, editors.* 601 pp., 1984.
Vol. 39: Motor Control Mechanisms in Health and Disease: *J. E. Desmedt, editor.* 1,224 pp., 1983.
Vol. 38: The Dementias: *R. Mayeux and W. G. Rosen, editors.* 288 pp., 1983.
Vol. 37: Experimental Therapeutics of Movement Disorders: *S. Fahn, D. B. Calne, and I. Shoulson, editors.* 339 pp., 1983.
Vol. 36: Human Motor Neuron Diseases: *L. P. Rowland, editor.* 592 pp., 1982.
Vol. 35: Gilles de la Tourette Syndrome: *A. J. Friedhoff and T. N. Chase, editors.* 476 pp., 1982.
Vol. 34: Status Epilepticus: Mechanism of Brain Damage and Treatment: *A. V. Delgado-Escueta, C. G. Wasterlain, D. M. Treiman, and R. J. Porter, editors.* 579 pp., 1983.
Vol. 31: Demyelinating Diseases: Basic and Clinical Electrophysiology: *S. Waxman and J. Murdoch Ritchie, editors.* 544 pp., 1981.
Vol. 30: Diagnosis and Treatment of Brain Ischemia: *A. L. Carney and E. M. Anderson, editors.* 424 pp., 1981.
Vol. 29: Neurofibromatosis: *V. M. Riccardi and J. J. Mulvilhill, editors.* 288 pp., 1981.
Vol. 28: Brain Edema: *J. Cervós-Navarro and R. Ferszt, editors.* 539 pp., 1980.
Vol. 27: Antiepileptic Drugs: Mechanisms of Action: *G. H. Glaser, J. K. Penry, and D. M. Woodbury, editors.* 728 pp.,1980.
Vol. 26: Cerebral Hypoxia and Its Consequences: *S. Fahn, J. N. Davis, and L. P. Rowland, editors.* 454 pp., 1979.
Vol. 25: Cerebrovascular Disorders and Stroke: *M. Goldstein, L. Bolis, C. Fieschi, S. Gorini, and C. H. Millikan, editors.* 412 pp., 1979.
Vol. 24: The Extrapyramidal System and Its Disorders: *L. J. Poirier, T. L. Sourkes, and P. Bédard, editors.* 552 pp., 1979.
Vol. 23: Huntington's Chorea: *T. N. Chase, N. S. Wexler, and A. Barbeau, editors.* 864 pp., 1979.
Vol. 22: Complications of Nervous System Trauma: *R. A. Thompson and J. R. Green, editors.* 454 pp., 1979.
Vol. 21: The Inherited Ataxia: Biochemical, Viral, and Pathological Studies: *R. A. Kark, R. Rosenberg, and L. Schut, editors.* 450 pp., 1978.
Vol. 20: Pathology of Cerebrospinal Microcirculation: *J. Cervós-Navarro, E. Betz, G. Ebhardt, R. Ferszt, and R. Wüllenweber, editors.* 636 pp., 1978.

Contents

Epidemiology and Genetics

Imaging in Parkinson's Disease

Medical Treatment of Parkinson's Disease

Contributing Authors

Y. Agid, M.D. *Centre d'Investigation Clinique, Hôpital de la Salpêtrière, 47 boulevard de l'Hôpital, 75013 Paris, France*

Alberto Albanese, M.D. *Istituto Nazionale Neurologico Carlo Besta, Universitá Cattolica del Sacro Cuore, Via G.Celoria, 11, 20133 Milano, Italy*

Christian Andressen, M.D. *Department of Clinical Neurosciences, University Joseph Fourier, INSERM U318, Pavillon B, BP217, F-38043 Grenoble, France; University of Köln, Köln, Germany*

I. Arnulf, M.D. *Hôpital de la Salpêtrière, 47 boulevard de l'Hôpital, 75013 Paris, France*

Ari Barzilai, Ph.D. *Department of Neurobiochemistry, George S. Wise Faculty of Life Sciences, Tel Aviv University, Tel Aviv 69978, Israel*

Paul J. Bédard, M.D. *Neuroscience Research Unit, C.H.U.L. (RC-9800), 2705 Boul. Laurier, Ste-Foy, (Québec) G1V 4G2, Canada*

P. Bejjani, M.D. *Parkinson & Movement Disorders Center, Hôpital Notre Dame des Secours, Beirut, Lebanon*

Alim-Louis Benabid, M.D. *Department of Clinical Neurosciences, University Joseph Fourier, INSERM U318, Pavillon B, BP217, F-38043 Grenoble, France*

Abdelhamid Benazzouz, M.D. *Department of Clinical Neurosciences, University Joseph Fourier, INSERM U318, Pavillon B, BP217, F-38043 Grenoble, France*

Pierre J. Blanchet, M.D., Ph.D. *Experimental Therapeutics Branch, National Institute of Neurological Disorders and Stroke, National Institutes of Health, Bethesda, Maryland; Faculty of Dentistry, University of Montreal, Montreal, Quebec, Canada*

F. Bloch, M.D. *Centre d'Investigation Clinique, Hôpital de la Salpêtrière, 47 boulevard de l'Hôpital, 75013 Paris, France*

A.M. Bonnet, M.D. *Centre d'Investigation Clinique, Hôpital de la Salpêtrière, 47 boulevard de l'Hôpital, 75013 Paris, France*

D. Brandstädter, M.D. *Department of Neurology, Philippe-University Marburg, Germany*

J.M. Brotchie, M.D. *Walton Centre for Neurology and Neurosurgery, Fazakerley, Liverpool, United Kingdom*

Susan M. Calne, CM, R.N. *Pacific Parkinson's Research Centre, University of British Columbia, Purdy Pavilion, University Hospital, 2221 Wesbrook Mall, Vancouver, BC V6T 2B5, Canada*

Donald B. Calne, M.A., B.M., B.Ch., D.M. *Pacific Parkinson's Research Centre, University Hospital, Vancouver, British Columbia V6T 2B5, Canada*

F. Calon, M.D. *Unité de Recherche en Oncologie and Endocrinologie Moléculaire, Centre de Recherche du CHUQ, Quebec, Canada*

Maren Carbon, M.D. *Center for Neurosciences, North Shore-Long Island Jewish Research Institute and Movement Disorders Center, North Shore University Hospital, Manhasset, New York, USA*

Stephan Chabardes, M.D. *Department of Clinical Neurosciences, University Joseph Fourier, INSERM U318, Pavillon B, BP217, F-38043 Grenoble, France*

Thomas N. Chase, M.D. **Experimental Therapeutics Branch, National Institute of Neurological Disorders and Stroke, National Institutes of Health, Bethesda, Maryland*

Dong-Kug Choi, M.D. *Department of Neurology, BB-307, Columbia University, 650 West 168th Street, New York, New York 10032, USA*

Oren Cohen, M.D. *Department of Neurology, BB-307, Columbia University, 650 West 168th Street, New York, New York 10032, USA*

C. Brefel-Courbon, M.D. *Department of Clinical Pharmacology, Faculty of Medicine, INSERM U455, 37 Allees Jules-Guesde, Toulouse France F-31073, France*

Richard Crevenna, M.D. *Department of Neurology, Karl Franzens University, Graz, Austria*

A.R. Crossman, M.D. *Walton Centre for Neurology and Neurosurgery, Fazakerley, Liverpool, United Kingdom*

Dorah Daily, M.D. *Department of Neurobiochemistry, George S. Wise Faculty of Life Sciences, Tel Aviv University, Tel Aviv 69978, Israel*

P. Damier, M.D. *Service de Neurologie, CHU de Nantes, France*

Mahlon R. DeLong,, M.D. *Department of Neurology, Emory University School of Medicine, Suite 6000, Woodruff Memorial Research building, 1659 Pierce Drive, Atlanta, Georgia 30322, USA*

T. Di Paolo, M.D. *Unité de Recherche en Oncologie and Endocrinologie Moléculaire, Centre de Recherche du CHUQ, Quebec, Canada*

Dean E. Dluzen, M.D. *Department of Anatomy, Northeastern Ohio Universities, College of Medicine, Rootstown, Ohio, USA*

B. Dubois, M.D. *INSERM EPI 007, Hôpital de la Salpêtrière, 47 boulevard de l'Hôpital, 75013 Paris, France*

Christine Edwards, M.D. *Center for Neurosciences, North Shore-Long Island Jewish Research Institute and Movement Disorders Center, North Shore University Hospital, Manhasset, New York, USA*

David Eidelberg, M.D. *Center for Neurosciences, North Shore-Long Island Jewish Research Institute and Movement Disorders Center, North Shore University Hospital, Manhasset, New York, USA*

Alicia G. Facca, M.D. *Department of Neurology, University of Miami, School of Medicine, Miami, Florida*

Mathew Farrer, M.D. *Department of Neurology and the Neuroscience Research Laboratory, Mayo Clinic, 4500 San Pablo Road, Jacksonville, Florida 32224, USA*

J. Feger, M.D. *INSERM U289, Department of Experimental Neurology and Therapeutics, Hôpital de la Salpêtrière, 47 Boulevard de l'Hôpital, 75651 PARIS Cedex 13, France*

J. Ferreira, M.D. *Department of Neurology, Egas Moniz Reseacrh Centre, Lisbon University Hospital, Lisbon, Portugal.*

Marie-Jose Fortin, M.D. *McGill Centre for Studies in Ageing, Montreal, Quebec, Canada*

S.H. Fox, M.D. *Motac Neuroscience Ltd., Manchester, United Kingdom*

C. Francois, M.D. *INSERM U289, Department of Experimental Neurology and Therapeutics, Hôpital de la Salpêtrière, 47 Boulevard de l'Hôpital, 75651 PARIS Cedex 13, France*

Raúl de la Fuente-Fernández, M.D. *Pacific Parkinson's Research Centre, Vancouver Hospital and Health Sciences Centre, University of British Columbia, Purdy Pavilion, 2221 Wesbrook Mall, Vancouver, British Columbia V6T 2B5, Canada*

Yoshiaki Furukawa, M.D. *Director, Movement Disorders Research Laboratory (R 211), Centre for Addiction and Mental Health - Clarke Division, 250 College Street, Toronto, Ontario M5T 1R8, Canada*

Thomas Gasser, M.D. *Department of Neurology, Klinikum Großhadern, Ludwig-Maximilians-Universität, Marchioninistr. 15, 81377 München, Germany*

Michèle Gentil, M.D. *Department of Clinical Neurosciences, University Joseph Fourier, INSERM U318, Pavillon B, BP217, F-38043 Grenoble, France*

Manfred Gerlach, M.D. *Department of Clinical Neurochemistry, University Clinic and Health Center for Children and Youth Psychiatry and Psychotherapy, Würzburg, Germany*

Christopher G. Goetz, M.D. *Department of Neurological Sciences, Department of Pharmacology, Rush University/Rush-Presbyterian-St. Luke's Medical Center, Chicago, Illinois, USA*

Lawrence I. Golbe, M.D. *Department of Neurology, University of Medicine and Dentistry of New Jersey, Robert Wood Johnson Medical School, 97 Paterson Street, New Brunswick, New Jersey 08901, USA*

Ariel Gordin, M.D., Ph.D. *Research Centre, Orion Pharma, Orionintie 1, 02100 Espoo, Finland*

Linda Grantier, M.D. *Movement Disorders Clinic, Health Sciences Centre, London, Ontario, Canada*

L. Grégoire, M.D. *Unite de Recherche en Neuroscience, Centre de Recherche du CHUQ, Quebec, Canada*

R. Grondin, M.D. *Unite de Recherche en Neuroscience, Centre de Recherche du CHUQ, Quebec, Canada*

Edna Grünblatt, M.D. *The Bruce Rappaport Faculty of Medicine, Technion - Israel Institute of Technology, P.O.B. 9649, Haifa 31096, Israel; Bayrische Julius-Meximilians-University of Wüzburg, Clinic and Polyclinic of Psychiatry and Psychotherapy, Department of Neurochemistry, Wüzburg, Germany*

Jeanne Hall, M.D. *McGill Centre for Studies in Ageing, Montreal, Quebec, Canada*

Mark Hallett, M.D. *Human Motor Control Section, NINDS, NIH, Building 10, Room 5N226, 10 Center, MSC 1428, Bethesda, Maryland 20892–1428, USA*

E.C. Hirsch, M.D. *INSERM U289, Department of Experimental Neurology and Therapeutics, Hôpital de la Salpêtrière, 47 Boulevard de l'Hôpital, 75651 PARIS Cedex 13, France*

Carl Nikolaus Homann, M.D. *Head of Department and Medical, Superintendent, Klinik Maria Theresia Hospital for Neurological and Orthopedic Rehabilitation, Bad Radkersburg, Austria; Department of Neurology, Karl Franzens University, Graz, Austria*

Martin W.I.M. Horstink, M.D. *Department of Neurology, University Medical Centre, PO Box 9101, 6500 HB Nijmegen, The Netherlands*

J.L. Houeto, M.D. *Centre d'Investigation Clinique, Hôpital de la Salpêtrière, 47 boulevard de l'Hôpital, 75013 Paris, France*

Zhigao Huang, M.D. *Pacific Parkinson's Research Centre, Vancouver Hospital and Health Sciences Centre, University of British Columbia, Purdy Pavilion, 2221 Wesbrook Mall, Vancouver, British Columbia V6T 2B5, Canada*

Mike L. Hutton, M.D. *Department of Neurology and the Neuroscience Research Laboratory, Mayo Clinic, 4500 San Pablo Road, Jacksonville, Florida 32224, USA*

D. Iacono, M.D. *Centre d'Investigation Clinique, Hôpital de la Salpêtrière, 47 boulevard de l'Hôpital, 75013 Paris, France*

Gerd Ivanic, M.D. *Department of Neurology, Karl Franzens University, Graz, Austria*

Vernice Jackson-Lewis, M.D. *Department of Neurology, BB-307, Columbia University, 650 West 168th Street, New York, New York 10032, USA*

Danna Jennings, M.D. *Department of Neurology, The Institute for Neurodegenerative Disorders, 60 Temple St, Suite 8B, New Haven, Connecticut 06510, USA*

Seppo Kaakkola, M.D. *Department of Neurology, University of Helsinki, Helsinki, Finland*

Philippe Kahane, M.D. *Department of Clinical Neurosciences, University Joseph Fourier, INSERM U318, Pavillon B, BP217, F-38043 Grenoble, France*

C. Karachi, M.D. *INSERM U299, Hôpital de la Salpêtrière, 47 boulevard de l'Hôpital, 75013 Paris, France*

Pamela King, M.D. *Movement Disorders Clinic, Glenrose Rehabilitation Hospital, Edmonton, Alberta, Canada*

Stephen Kish, Ph.D. *Human Neurochemical Pathology Section, Centre for Addiction and Mental Health, 250 College Street, Toronto, Ontario M5T 1R8, Canada*

William C. Koller, M.D., Ph.D. *Department of Neurology, University of Miami, School of Medicine, Miami, Florida*

Amos D. Korczyn, M.D., MSc. *Sieratzki Chair of Neurology, Tel-Aviv University Medical School, Ramat-Aviv 69978, Israel*

Adnan Koudsie, M.D. *Department of Clinical Neurosciences, University Joseph Fourier, INSERM U318, Pavillon B, BP217, F-38043 Grenoble, France*

Paul Krack, M.D. *Department of Clinical Neurosciences, University Joseph Fourier, INSERM U318, Pavillon B, BP217, F-38043 Grenoble, France*

Ajit Kumar, M.D. *Pacific Parkinson's Research Centre, Vancouver Hospital and Health Sciences Centre, University of British Columbia, Purdy Pavilion, 2221 Wesbrook Mall, Vancouver, British Columbia V6T 2B5, Canada*

Jan P. Larsen, M.D. *Department of Neurology, Central Hospital of Rogaland, PO Box 8100, N-4068 Stavanger, Norway*

Doris Lenartz, M.D. *Department of Clinical Neurosciences, University Joseph Fourier, INSERM U318, Pavillon B, BP217, F-38043 Grenoble, France; University of Köln, Köln, Germany*

Andres M. Lozano, M.D., Ph.D., FRCSC. *Professor and RR Tasker Chair in Functional Neurosurgery, Toronto Western Hospital, University of Toronto, MC 2-433, 399 Bathurst St., Toronto Ontario M5T 2S8, Canada*

Edwin Mak, M.D. *Pacific Parkinson's Research Centre, University of British Columbia, Purdy Pavilion, University Hospital, 2221 Wesbrook Mall, Vancouver, BC V6T 2B5, Canada*

Silvia Mandel, D.Sc. *Eve Topf and U.S. National Parkinson's Foundation Centers of Excellence for Neurodegenerative Diseases, Bruce Rappaport Family Research Institute and Department of Pharmacology, Faculty of Medicine, Technion, Haifa, Israel*

Kenneth Marek, M.D. *Department of Neurology, The Institute for Neurodegenerative Disorders, 60 Temple St, Suite 8B, New Haven, Connecticut 06510, USA*

Germaine McInnes, M.D. *Movement Disorders Clinic, Glenrose Rehabilitation Hospital, Edmonton, Alberta, Canada*

Eldad Melamed, M.D. *Department of Neurology and Felsenstein Medical Research Institute, Rabin Medical Center, and the Sackler School of Medicine, Tel Aviv University, Tel Aviv, Israe*

V. Mesnage, M.D. *Centre d'Investigation Clinique, Hôpital de la Salpêtrière, 47 boulevard de l'Hôpital, 75013 Paris, France*

O. Messouak, M.D. *Centre d'Investigation Clinique, Hôpital de la Salpêtrière, 47 boulevard de l'Hôpital, 75013 Paris, France*

Leo Verhagen Metman, M.D. *Experimental Therapeutics Branch, National Institute of Neurological Disorders and Stroke, National Institutes of Health, Bethesda, Maryland; Department of Neurology, Rush-Presbytarian-St. Luke's Medical Center, Chicago, Illinois*

Lorella Minotti, M.D. *Department of Clinical Neurosciences, University Joseph Fourier, INSERM U318, Pavillon B, BP217, F-38043 Grenoble, France*

M-P Muriel, M.D. *INSERM U289, Department of Experimental Neurology and Therapeutics, Hôpital de la Salpêtrière, 47 Boulevard de l'Hôpital, 75651 PARIS Cedex 13, France*

W.H. Oertel, M.D. *Department of Neurology, Philipps—University of Marburg, Rudolf-Bultmannstr. 8, 35039 Marburg, Germany*

Daniel Offen, M.D. *Department of Neurobiochemistry, George S. Wise Faculty of Life Sciences, Tel Aviv University, Tel Aviv 69978, Israel*

Marco Onofrj, M.D. *Department of Oncology and Neurosciences, University "GD'annunzio," Chieti, Italy*

G. Orieux, M.D. *INSERM U289, Department of Experimental Neurology and Therapeutics, Hôpital de la Salpêtrière, 47 Boulevard de l'Hôpital, 75651 PARIS Cedex 13, France*

Erwin Ott, M.D. *Department of Neurology, Karl Franzens University, Graz, Austria*

P. Payoux, M.D. *Department of Nuclear Medicine, Toulouse University Hospital, Toulouse, France*

Pierre Pollak, M.D. *Department of Clinical Neurosciences, University Joseph Fourier, INSERM U318, Pavillon B, BP217, F-38043 Grenoble, France; University of Köln, Köln, Germany*

Serge Przedborski, *Departments of Neurology and Pathology, BB-307, Columbia University, 650 West 168th Street, New York, New York 10032, USA*

Alex Rajput, M.D. FRCPC *University of Saskatchewan, Division of Neurology, Royal University Hospital, 103 Hospital Drive, Saskatoon, Saskatchewan S7N 0W8, Canada*

Michele Rajput, M.D. *University of Saskatchewan, Division of Neurology, Royal University Hospital, 103 Hospital Drive, Saskatoon, Saskatchewan S7N 0W8, Canada*

Olivier Rascol, M.D., Ph.D. *Department of Clinical Pharmacology, Faculty of Medicine, INSERM U455, 37 Allees Jules-Guesde, Toulouse France F-31073, France*

Peter Riederer, M.D. *Bayrische Julius-Meximilians-University of Wüzburg, Clinic and Polyclinic of Psychiatry and Psychotherapy, Department of Neurochemistry, Wüzburg, Germany*

Seppo Saarikoski, M.D. *Clinical Research Center, Bone and Cartilage Research Unit, University of Kuopio, Kuopio, Finland*

Robert Schlößer, M.D. *Department of Neurochemistry, the Clinic and Polyclinic of Psychiatry and Psychotherapy, Bayerische Julius-Maximilians-University of Würzburg, Würzburg, Germany*

Michael Schulzer, M.D. *Victorian Order of Nurses, St. John's, New Brunswick, Canada*

John Seibyl, M.D. *Department of Neurology, The Institute for Neurodegenerative Disorders, 60 Temple St, Suite 8B, New Haven, Connecticut 06510, USA*

Anat Shirvan, M.D. *Department of Neurobiochemistry, George S. Wise Faculty of Life Sciences, Tel Aviv University, Tel Aviv 69978, Israel*

Monty A. Silverdale, M.D. *Manchester Movement Disorder Laboratory, Division of Neuroscience, School of Biological Sciences, University of Manchester, Oxford Road, Manchester M13 9PT, United Kingdom*

Fabrizio Stocchi, M.D. *Institute of Neurology IRCCS "Neuromed" (Is) and University "La Sapienza," Rome, Italy*

A. Jon Stoessl, *Pacific Parkinsons Research Centre, 2221 Wesbrook Mall, Vancouver, B.C., V6T 2B5, Canada*

Jens Strelau, *Neuroanatomy and Center for Neuroscience, University of Heidelberg, Im Neuenheimer Feld 307, D-69120 Heidelberg, Germany*

Elma Strijks, M.D. *Department of Neurology, University Medical Centre, PO Box 9101, 6500 HB Nijmegen, The Netherlands*

Raimo Sulkava, M.D. *Department of Public Health and General Practice, University of Kuopio, Box 1627, 70211, Kuopio FIN-70211, Finland*

Klaudia Suppan, M.D. *Department of Neurology, Karl Franzens University, Graz, Austria*

A. Hadj Tahar, M.D. *Unite de Recherche en Neuroscience, Centre de Recherche du CHUQ, Quebec, Canada*

Caroline M. Tanner, M.D., Ph.D. *Director, Clinical Research, Parkinson's Institute, 1170 Morse Avenue, Sunnyvale, California 94089–1605, USA*

Peter Teismann, M.D. *Department of Neurology, BB-307, Columbia University, 650 West 168th Street, New York, New York 10032, USA*

Keikki Teräväinen, M.D. *Department of Neurology, University of Helsinki, Helsinki, Finland*

Kim Tieu, M.D. *Department of Neurology, BB-307, Columbia University, 650 West 168th Street, New York, New York 10032, USA*

Sheree Trecartin, M.D. *Movement Disorders Clinic, Health Sciences Centre, London, Ontario, Canada*

Yoshio Tsuboi, M.D. *Department of Neurology, Mayo Clinic, 4500 San Pablo Road, Jacksonville, Florida 32224, USA*

Joseph King Ching Tsui, M.D. *Neurodegenerative Disorders Centre, University of British Columbia, Vancouver, British Columbia, Canada.*

Marjo Tuppurainen, M.D. *Department of Obstetrics and Gynecology, Kuopio University Hospital, FIN-70211 Kuopio, Finland*

Ryan J. Uitti, M.D. *Department of Neurology, Mayo Clinic, 4500 San Pablo Road, Jacksonville, Florida 32224, USA*

Klaus Unsicker, M.D. *Neuroanatomy and Center for Neuroscience, University of Heidelberg, Im Neuenheimer Feld 307, D-69120 Heidelberg, Germany*

Laura Vacca, M.D. *Institute of Neurology IRCCS "Neuromed" (Is) and University "La Sapienza," Rome, Italy*

Laurent Vercueil, M.D. *Department of Clinical Neurosciences, University Joseph Fourier, INSERM U318, Pavillon B, BP217, F-38043 Grenoble, France*

M. Vidailhet, M.D. *Fédération de Neurologie, Hôpital de la Salpêtrière, 47 boulevard de l'Hôpital, 75013 Paris, France*

Miquel Vila, M.D. *Department of Neurology, BB-307, Columbia University, 650 West 168th Street, New York, New York 10032, USA*

M.L. Welter, M.D. *Centre d'Investigation Clinique, Hôpital de la Salpêtrière, 47 boulevard de l'Hôpital, 75013 Paris, France*

Karoline Wenzel, M.D. *Department of Neurology, Karl Franzens University, Graz, Austria*

Thomas Wichmann, M.D. *Department of Neurology, Emory University School of Medicine, Suite 6000, Woodruff Memorial Research Building, 1659 Pierce Drive, Atlanta, Georgia 30322, USA*

Håkan Widner, M.D., Ph.D. *Associate Professor, Department of Clinical Neurosciences, Wallenberg Neuroscience Center, Lund University Hospital, SE-221 85 Lund, Sweden*

Zbigniew K. Wszolek, M.D. *Department of Neurology, Mayo Clinic Jacksonville, 4500 San Pablo Road, Jacksonville, Florida 32224, USA.*

Du Chu Wu, M.D. *Department of Neurology, BB-307, Columbia University, 650 West 168th Street, New York, New York 10032, USA*

J. Yelnik, M.D. *INSERM U299, Hôpital de la Salpêtrière, 47 boulevard de l'Hôpital, 75013 Paris, France*

Moussa B.H. Youdim, M.D. *The Bruce Rappaport Faculty of Medicine, Technion - Israel Institute of Technology, P.O.B. 9649, Haifa 31096, Israel*

Rina Zilkha-Falb, M.D. *Department of Neurobiochemistry, George S. Wise Faculty of Life Sciences, Tel Aviv University, Tel Aviv 69978, Israel*

Ilan Ziv, M.D. *Department of Neurology and Felsenstein Medical Research Institute, Rabin Medical Center, and the Sackler School of Medicine, Tel Aviv University, Tel Aviv, Israel*

Preface

The XIV International Congress on Parkinson's disease (ICPD) took place in Helsinki on July 29 through August 1, 2001. Two associated and comprehensive symposia were held on July 27. These were "40 years of Progress in Movement Disorders based on Human Brain Studies" and "Iron and Oxidative Stress in Neurodegeneration—A tribute to Gerald Cohen." The Congress was organized under the auspices of the World Federation of Neurology Research Committee on Parkinsonism and Related Disorders, and the Finnish Parkinson Association. A small local organizing committee, chaired by Professor Heikki Teräväinen, MD, handled the organizational details of the meeting.

The meeting was held in the Finlandia Hall, designed by the world famous Finnish architect, Alvar Aalto. More than 2300 participants from 55 countries attended the congress. Most of the participants considered the meeting program to be of high quality, according to an on-site survey by an independent Gallup poll organization. Participants also had the opportunity to enjoy the sunny warm weather and the bright Finnish summer evenings.

The present volume of *Advances in Neurology*, based on presentations from the ICPD meeting, follows a long tradition. This book contains manuscripts on papers presented mostly in the plenary lectures, together with a selection of some special papers read in different symposia. These are of high quality and thus give up-to-date knowledge on the topical issues of movement disorders in one volume.

The editorial work has been both stressful and enjoyable. It has indeed been a pleasure and an excellent learning experience for us to have the opportunity to edit the present volume of *Advances in Neurology*, and we want to thank all authors for their contribution. We have in our hands a thorough summary on the latest achievements and knowledge on Parkinson's disease and related disorders.

Professor Melvin Yahr, M.D., the long-standing president of the Extrapyramidal Disease Research Committee on Parkinsonism and Related Disorders of the World Federation of Neurology, describes in the introductory chapter the birth and development of the Committee. After the Congress, he stepped down from this position, to be followed by Professor Donald Calne, MD, from Vancouver, Canada. At the Congress Professor Calne had the honor of giving the second Melvin Yahr Lecture, entitled "Parkinson's Disease Over the Twentieth Century."

The present volume is divided into seven sections. The first section describes the neurobiology of Parkinson's disease. It gives an updated view on the neuroanatomy and pathophysiology of this disease of the basal ganglia and striatum. The knowledge of dopamine receptors is updated, and there are descriptions of possible neurotoxic and neuroprotective mechanisms. The second section deals with epidemiology and genetics. In particular, the understanding of genetics in Parkinson's disease has grown markedly since the last meeting and a record number of papers on this topic were presented at the meeting. The third section describes the state of the art in imaging by PET and SPECT in Parkinson's disease and the fourth section comprehensively reviews medical treatment of both early and late stages of Parkinson's disease. Recent clinical trials are described and the current view regarding positioning of the different medications is discussed. We also attempt a crystal ball approach by looking into the development of emerging dopaminergic and non-dopaminergic medications. The fifth section describes recent developments in the surgical treatment of Parkinson's disease. Again, there is much new material available since the previous meeting in Vancouver in 1999, particularly in the field of deep brain stimulation, which offers much promise to many problematic patients. The sixth section is devoted to comorbid conditions. Sleep disorders, in particular, have attracted much attention recently and the so-called sleep attacks have been a frequent topic both in the scientific and the lay press. Treatment of depression and psychosis in Parkinson's disease are reviewed. The last section discusses parkinsonism and related disorders, such as dementia.

We are confident that this volume, written by internationally recognized medical researchers, will be valuable to those in need of a good comprehensive summary of the central topics in extrapyramidal disease research and in practical patient care.

We thank Ms. Maaret Pekkarinen for her secretarial help in editing this volume and our team at Lippincott Williams & Wilkins, Anne Sydor, Marc Bendian, and Jeff Somers for their contributions to this Work.

Ariel Gordin, MD
Seppo Kaakkola, MD
Heikki Teräväinen, MD

Foreword

On October 10, 1959, the first in this series of Parkinson's symposia was held at the Queen Elizabeth Veteran's Hospital in Montreal, Canada. The Canadian and United States Departments of Veterans Affairs, which were becoming increasingly concerned about the growing numbers of aging survivors of World War I who were exhibiting neurodegenerative disorders, particularly Parkinson's disease (PD), sponsored it. The time and venue of the meeting were not chosen by chance; indeed, it was set so as to coincide with the 25th Anniversary of the Convocation of the Montreal Neurological Institute. In so doing, the organizers felt they could attract attendees with an interest in neurological disorders and, hopefully, some in PD.

This was a necessity at that time, since PD was hardly a high-priority item in the investigative field. In fact, it was very much on the back burner of most neuroscience laboratories. However, there was a growing interest in stereotaxis and its use in neurosurgical procedures as an approach to treatment, particularly thalamotomy and pallidotomy, and it was hoped that these individuals, many attending the Montreal Neurological Institute's Convocation, would form the nucleus for presentations at the symposium. Indeed, this turned out to be the case and most of the meeting dealt with technical aspects of stereotaxis surgery and appropriate target sites. Hence, the scientific scope of that meeting was limited, as was the audience; there were no more than fifty attendees. The chairman of the meeting, Dr. William Middleton stated in his opening remarks that he considered it a means of stimulating interest in the field and attracting new investigators for what he considered an obscure disease of the nervous system. He also hoped that the meeting would open channels for personal interaction in the field among various new disciplines and looked forward to its growth. His hopes have been realized to a considerable extent, as is evident at this XIV International Congress in Helsinki.

We are most grateful and indebted to Professor Heikki Teräväinen, his colleagues, and the Parkinson's Society of Finland who assumed responsibility for organizing this XIV Symposium. The program they have planned follows the tradition of its predecessors and encompasses the recent developments in the field as well as current investigative studies, and addresses the major outstanding issues in PD. Indeed, we are most grateful to them for their efforts in developing this superb program.

In the mid-1960s, Dr. MacDonald Critchley, then president of The World Federation of Neurology (WFN), proposed the formation of a Research Group on Extra-Pyramidal Diseases. It was an area of special interest to him and he recognized it as one that was receiving little attention from the neurological community. He invited me to chair and organize such a group, which would be multidisciplinary, including clinical neurologists, neuropathologists, neurophysiologists, and neurochemists.

There were six members in all in the original group and its charge was to review the present status of the field, set up a mechanism for establishing local registries of Parkinson's patients, document the multitudinous number of factors that might play a role in the etiology of the disease, and then invite in appropriate investigators from other disciplines as was deemed necessary. Under the auspices of the United States' National Institute of Health (NIH), a clinical center for Parkinson's research was set up at Columbia University to implement many of these recommendations. A number of meetings were held on special subjects such as biochemistry and pharmacology of the basal ganglia, structure and function of the thalamus, classification and methods of evaluation of disease severity. A brain bank to collect autopsied brains from Parkinson's patients in both frozen and fixed states was established. Over time, it was apparent that the term "extra-pyramidal" was an anachronism and it was abandoned in favor of Research Committee on Parkinson's Disease and Related Disorders.

Over the years, a number of outstanding investigators became members of the Parkinson's Research Group and have contributed to the success of these programs: André Barbeau, Walter Birkmayer, George Cotzias, David Marsden, Rolf Haessler, Oleh Hornykiewicz, John Gilligham, and Mdme. Fessard, just to name a few. I should also like to pay respect to two stalwart members of this group—Prof. Hiro Narabayashi and Prof. Hans Lakke, both of whom have unfortunately passed away this year. Their guidance and wisdom will be sorely missed. Both were committed researchers in the field and major supporters of the Research Group and the symposia.

The WFN Research Committee on Parkinson's Disease and Related Disorders assumed the responsibility and the sponsorship of the Parkinson's Symposia in 1968. That this was a necessity became evident at the III Parkinson's Disease Symposium organized under the chairmanship of Prof. Gillingham, a neurosurgeon from Edinburgh, Scotland. That meeting highlighted the need for multidisciplinary representation and involvement of scientists from numerous countries. It was the first symposium at which a critical review of the role of catecholamines in PD was held. It heralded a new era in Parkinson's research—the levodopa era. It was an extremely successful meeting, but was open only to invited participants, as was the next meeting being planned by Dr. Jean Siegfried, a neurosurgeon from Zurich, Switzerland. There was, however, neither a formal structure for planning these meetings nor a mechanism for including the growing numbers of investigators entering the field. The Research Committee formulated a plan for future meetings in regard to choice of site, chairman and scientific content. Their major objective was to establish a critical review of new developments in PD: identification of promising areas of research, stimulating investigative studies in areas where interest was lacking but felt to be necessary for orderly progress in the field, and providing a format for an interchange of ideas among scientists.

The symposia also would serve a major teaching role for young investigators interested in the field by sponsoring special seminars on various aspects of the disorder, which would be particularly designed to fulfill this function.

As one looks back over the history of these meetings during the last 42 years, one is impressed by the major presentations given at these symposia. They cover many of the milestones in Parkinson's research and are recorded in the published proceedings of these meetings. They document the steady progress that has been made in understanding both PD and the nervous system in general. They are truly a historical record of the outstanding findings in neuroscience, which have led to the improved treatment of PD and hopefully point the way to our ultimate goal of finding the solution to the riddle of this enigmatic disease. There is, of course, much left to be done. In the interim, we can all be proud that of all the neurodegenerative diseases, none have advanced as much as Parkinson's in symptomatic treatment with improved quality of life and prolonged longevity.

Melvin D. Yahr

Parkinson's Disease: Advances in Neurology, Vol. 91.
Edited by Ariel Gordin, Seppo Kaakkola,
and Heikki Teräväinen
Lippincott Williams & Wilkins, Philadelphia © 2003

Parkinson's Disease Over the Last 100 Years

Donald B. Calne

Pacific Parkinson's Research Centre, University Hospital, Vancouver, British Columbia, Canada

James Parkinson's essay of the shaking palsy (1817), a description of six patients, was followed by further clinical documentation without any significant contributions to pathology, neurochemistry, or etiology. It was not until 1867 that Ordenstein, a pupil of Charcot, described the first effective treatment—hyoscyamine. Almost half a century followed without much progress, until our understanding accelerated with technical and conceptual advances in three major areas: clinical, pharmacological, and pathological.

CLINICAL ADVANCES

Clinical observations have underpinned a series of observations on the heterogeneity of Parkinson's disease (PD). The importance of this heterogeneity is that it raises a fundamentally new idea—that PD is not one nosological entity. If etiology is an essential element in the characterization of a disease, then there are several distinct PDs. More precisely, what we call "Parkinson's disease" is really a syndrome, like peripheral neuropathy or meningitis. As we identify specific causes we will be able to define specific diseases, just as we have defined diabetic neuropathy, or pneumococcal meningitis. In the meantime, it is more correct to use the term "idiopathic parkinsonism," rather than "Parkinson's disease."

The first evidence that parkinsonism could exist in different forms was the recognition that von Economo's encephalitis, which started in Europe in 1919, could evolve into a condition resembling that described by James Parkinson—either immediately, or after a latent period of several years. This postencephalitic parkinsonism differed from idiopathic parkinsonism (IP) because there were often concomitant signs of brainstem damage, such as ocular palsies, and, of course, there was a history of viral encephalitis (1).

Later, in the last century, careful clinical observation led to the recognition of two quite common disorders that often start with symptoms and signs similar to IP—progressive supranuclear palsy (Steele–Richardson–Olszewski syndrome) and multiple system atrophy (Shy–Drager syndrome).

More recently, a wide range of forms of parkinsonism have been associated with particular mutations. Clinical phenotypes virtually identical to IP have been seen in patients with a mutant α-synuclein gene (2), a mutant parkin gene (3), and the spinocerebellar ataxia type 2 mutation (4,5). These correlations between clinical and genetic findings raise, in a more forceful way, the old question of whether most cases of IP derive from an environmental or a genetic cause. Of course, the answer is likely to be a combination of the two, but the question can be rephrased as: Are the predominant risk factors for IP usually environmental or genetic?

Some 15% to 20% of patients with IP have a similarly affected first degree relative (6). Although many have argued that this indicates most patients—the 80% to 85% who do not have a family history—have IP caused by an environmental factor, others hold that these patients have hereditary IP caused by genes with low penetrance. Yet it would be most unusual for causal genes to have such low penetrance, and while there may well be genetic polymorphism, this does not constitute genetic causation. But there is more cogent evidence against the majority of patients having a genetic etiology for IP. Tanner et al. (7) have studied 193 twin pairs in whom at least one twin had IP. An analysis of the concordance rate indicates that among index cases who develop symptoms over the age of 50 years the evidence does not support genetic causation. Since the majority of all patients with IP start to notice their first symptoms after the age of 50 years, we can infer that environmental factors are responsible for most cases of IP. This conclusion is buttressed by case reports (8) and by a recent study of 299 families in whom a parent and child had IP (9). For the genetic hypothesis, one would expect that the risk for the child would correlate inversely with the age at onset of symptoms in the affected parent; however, this was not found. Instead, the younger the child when the parent developed symptoms, the higher the risk for the child; this is exactly what the environmental hypothesis predicts for the younger the child, the closer the shared environment. To provide yet further support for the environmental hypothesis, the risk for the child was higher when the affected relative was the mother—the child's environment is usually shared more closely with the mother.

In a historical context, these findings are not really surprising. In the nineteenth century, many regarded tuberculosis as a genetic disorder because it tended to cluster in families. It is common for people to accept the oversimplification that familial disease is genetic and that sporadic disease is environmental. A closer examination of the facts, however, reveals that families tend to share their environments in addition to their genes, so familial disease is by no means necessarily genetic.

Taking all of this evidence together, we can conclude that

1. IP has several causes.
2. For a minority of patients, the predominant risk is genetic.
3. Correspondingly, for a majority of patients the predominant risk is environmental.
4. The predominance of environmental causations even applies to patients who have an affected first degree relative.

PHARMACOLOGICAL ADVANCES

For patients with IP, the most important advances over the last 100 years have derived from the disciplines of pharmacology and experimental therapeutics. Yet these advances, which now seem so logical and clear, were only achieved in the face of a bitter resistance to new ideas and reluctance to accept irrefutable evidence. The path of enlightenment was not as easy as medical students are taught!

Developments in the pharmacology of IP came in three stages. First, the discovery that dopamine is a neurotransmitter. Second, the discovery that dopamine is depleted in the brains of patients with IP. Third, the discovery that replenishment of dopamine—or administration of a drug that mimics dopamine—leads to a substantial improvement in the symptoms and signs of IP.

The Discovery that Dopamine Is a Neurotransmitter

In 1956, Blaschko, who I remember teaching me pharmacology in Oxford, suggested "the possibility that dopamine has some functions of its own" (10). More importantly, he was joined by Oleh Hornykiewicz, a young pharmacologist from Vienna on a British Council scholarship, (11). The intellectual interaction between these two men was to prove highly fertile and ultimately of great significance for patients with IP. The following year, two articles followed each other in rapid succession in *Nature*. Montague (12) demonstrated the presence of dopamine in the mammalian brain; then Carlsson and his colleagues showed that D,L-dopa reversed the syndrome of immobility induced by reserpine in rabbits and mice (13). Dopamine itself had no effect because it does not cross the blood–brain barrier; in contrast, levodopa can get into the brain, where it is converted to dopamine.

Two years later, Carlsson (14) presented the powerful argument that the antireserpine effect was achieved by dopamine rather than norepinephrine (noradrenaline) because the regional distribution of dopamine was quite different from that of norepinephrine. If dopamine was simply a precursor of norepinephrine, both substances would be expected to be localized in the same subregions of the brain. Subsequently, histofluorescent techniques were developed that allowed direct visualization of dopamine in the neurons of the substantia nigra of the rat, with fibers projecting into the striatum where the axons terminated. Dopamine was present in varicosities distributed along the fibers, and it was concentrated in thousands of arborizing nerve endings deriving from each nigral cell (15). Later, Greengard and his colleagues (16,17) worked out the detailed pharmacological actions of dopamine at the postsynaptic neuron. Two major types of dopamine receptor have been identified—the D1 and the D2 receptors (18)—and these have more recently been separated into five subtypes (19–21).

The Discovery that Dopamine is Depleted in the Brains of Patients with IP

Hornykiewicz (11) began to study dopamine in Blaschko's laboratory, and when he returned home to Vienna, he started a series of experiments on human postmortem brains that would lay the foundation for all the modern forms of treatment for IP. The salient discovery was that the normally high concentration of dopamine in the human striatum was severely depleted in patients with IP (22). Sano published a similar observation in the same year (23). Then Hornykiewicz and his colleagues (24) extended their findings and showed that the substantial depletion of striatal dopamine was always there, and could be regarded as the pharmacological hallmark of IP. Hornykiewicz coined the term "striatal dopamine depletion syndrome," and the key neurochemical change in IP, defined in this way, led to a new era of advances in treatment.

The story of the pivotal significance of the dopaminergic nigrostriatal pathway stands out as a shining example of rational, coherent biomedical research. Yet it was beset with roadblocks thrown up by the very disciplines that had conceived and nurtured it. The great experimental neurologist, Denny-Brown, published a monograph entitled *The Basal Ganglia* in 1964 (25). There was no nigrostriatal projection in his illustration of the complex network of pathways connecting the various components of the basal ganglia, and he went so far as to write, "We have presented reasons against the common assumption that lesions of the substantia nigra are responsible for parkinsonism." In the same vein, as late as 1966, *Pharmacological Reviews* reported the proceedings of the Second Symposium on Catecholamines. The distinguished pharmacologist, Nickerson (26), wrote in the *Summary of Discussion and Commentary*: "...the suffix *ergic* implies "working" or "functioning," and its extension to cover neurons where only "containing" or "bearing" has been proved can be quite misleading. Quotation marks around a word such as "dopaminergic" are an inadequate precaution ...." But, in the words of Oscar Wilde: "If one tells the truth, one is sure, sooner or later, to be found out," and in time, the evidence that dopamine is a neurotransmitter was overwhelming and the depletion of striatal dopamine in IP became the cornerstone for the rational development of treatment.

The Discovery that Replenishment of Dopamine Leads to a Substantial Improvement in IP

As soon as the reduction of striatal dopamine was established in IP, a series of controversial reports appeared claiming that levodopa either did or did not have a beneficial effect on the clinical features of IP. The initial results were inconclusive because levodopa produced prominent side effects such as nausea and hypotension, and these problems overshadowed clinical measurement; they also prevented the normal escalation of dosage that would be undertaken in exploring the possible value of new treatment.

The situation changed entirely following the work of two groups of neurologists in New York. In 1967, Cotzias and his colleagues (27) found that by increasing the dose of levodopa very slowly, they were able to reduce its side effects dramatically. The following year, Yahr and his colleagues (28) reported similar observations. Both groups found that starting with low doses minimized the side effects of levodopa, and a slow increase in intake was tolerated then unequivocal and dramatic benefit was achieved. This was the turning point in treatment for patients with IP.

In later years, peripheral inhibitors of dopa decarboxylase (DDC), such as carbidopa and benserazide, further reduced the nausea associated with levodopa, and a peripheral blocker of dopamine receptors, domperidone, gave added protection. Another useful pharmacokinetic manipulation has been the introduction of inhibitors of catechol-*O*-methyltransferase (COMT), the enzyme responsible for most of the peripheral degradation of levodopa.

With increasing experience, a new problem with levodopa became apparent: induction of choreatic and dystonic movements. Synthetic dopamine agonists, such as bromocriptine, lisuride, pergolide, cabergoline, ropinirole, and pramipexole, have all been found to cause much less of this dyskinesia, though unfortunately these drugs do not achieve the same level of efficacy as levodopa.

PATHOLOGICAL ADVANCES

Although the nineteenth century was the golden age for establishing clinicopathological correlations in the central nervous system, the first important observation on the pathology of IP was not made until 1912. In that year, Franz Lewy described the eosinophilic cytoplasmic inclusion bodies that now bear his name (29). The Lewy body was then found so consistently (initially by those who had apparently consistently failed to see it before) that it became the pathological *sine qua non* for the diagnosis of IP. Indeed, the presence of Lewy bodies in the substantia nigra was soon embedded in the definition of IP, and this has led to many problems in our understanding of what, exactly, constitutes IP.

Because of the central position of the Lewy body in the conceptualization of IP, we must pause to examine what the significance of the Lewy body is, in the light of current attempts to identify its role. The traditional hypothesis proposes that (a) Lewy bodies in the substantia nigra are the hallmark of IP and that (b) Lewy bodies are responsible for neuronal death in IP. Neither of these proposals stands up to critical scrutiny. Let us examine the first proposal, that Lewy bodies in the substantia nigra are the hallmark of IP. Of course, if one defines IP as a neurological disorder with Lewy bodies in the substantia nigra it logically follows that all cases have Lewy bodies in the substantia nigra, but a tautology of this kind is not acceptable in science. Instead, we have to look for evidence that refutes the hypothesis, and such evidence is readily available. In 1989, Rajput and his colleagues (30) reported a group of carefully studied patients who had all the clinical features of IP, including a therapeutic response to levodopa. Pathological examination failed to reveal Lewy bodies. Instead, the substantia nigra contained neurofibrillary tangles. More recently, mutations of the parkin gene have been shown to produce pure progressive parkinsonism that responds to levodopa. Again, pathological examination does not show the presence of Lewy bodies. So, IP can occur without Lewy bodies, and if we broaden the search for Lewy bodies to other parts of the brain and other neurodegenerative conditions, the nonspecific nature of Lewy bodies becomes irrefutable, for they are found in such diverse disorders as dementia (31), Hallervorden-Spatz disease (32), subacute sclerosing panencephalitis (33), multiple system atrophy (31), primary autonomic failure (34), and Down's syndrome (35).

Moving on to examine the second traditional view, that Lewy bodies are responsible for neuronal death in IP, we can return to some of the studies just cited. In the cases of IP described by Rajput and colleagues (30), there was extensive neuronal loss in the substantia nigra without Lewy bodies, and the same is true for the patients with parkinsonism caused by mutation in the parkin gene (Mizuno, personal communication, 2001). To complete the argument against the traditional view, we need evidence that Lewy bodies can occur in the substantia nigra without neuronal death. Here also, the evidence is readily forthcoming. In 1998, van Duinen and his colleagues (36) described a subject with extremely high numbers of Lewy bodies in neurons of the substantia nigra, yet there was no loss of cells, and the subject had no neurological deficits. So IP with nigral cell loss can occur without Lewy bodies, and nigral Lewy bodies can occur without nigral cell loss. We can only conclude that the traditional hypothesis is seriously flawed. Nevertheless, there is no doubt that Lewy bodies are commonly found in IP, so we cannot ignore them.

Causes of Lewy Body Formation

1. Genetic: Mutations in the α-synuclein gene can lead to a phenotype of IP with Lewy bodies in the substantia nigra (2), although this is rare and usually has an earlier onset than most sporadic cases. Recently, a susceptibility locus for later onset IP with Lewy bodies has been reported (37). Furthermore, insertion of a mutant α-synuclein gene results in Lewy body formation in *Drosophila* (38).
2. Infective: Subacute sclerosing panencephalitis is a chronic neurodegenerative disease caused by the measles virus, and there have been several reports of Lewy bodies in this condition (33).
3. Toxic: Rotenone is a naturally occurring toxic agent employed as a pesticide. Experimental administration leads to the formation of Lewy bodies in the rat brain (39). Similarly, chronic administration of methylphenyltetrahydropyridine (MPTP) to mice results in the formation of Lewy bodies (40).

Relation between Lewy Bodies and Neurofibrillary Tangles

Classic neuropathology has taught that Lewy bodies and neurofibrillary tangles are entirely distinct markers of neurodegeneration, the former containing the protein α-synuclein and the latter containing tau protein. The traditional juxtaposing of "synucleinopathies" and "tauopathies" may be an oversimplification, for Lewy bodies and neurofibrillary tangles can coexist in the same brain, and even the same neuron (41).

Causes of Neurofibrillary Tangle Formation

1. Genetic: Several genetic neurodegenerative disorders are characterized by the occurrence of neurofibrillary tangles in the brain. For example, frontotemporal dementia with parkinsonism is caused by mutation N2779K on chromosome 17 (42).
2. Infective: Neurofibrillary tangles are the characteristic finding in parkinsonism consequent upon von Economo's encephalitis (43). Neurofibrillary tangles also occur in subacute sclerosing panencephalitis (33).
3. Toxic: Aluminum intoxication is the best known example of brain damage with formation of neurofibrillary tangles (44). This pathological phenomenon was so striking that when first discovered, aluminum was suggested to be the cause of Alzheimer's disease.
4. Traumatic: Repeated head injury, as experienced by boxers, can lead to neurodegeneration with parkinsonian features and dementia—so-called "pugilist's encephalopathy." This condition can be progressive after the cessation of trauma. Neurofibrillary tangles are commonly found in

the brains of patients with pugilist's encephalopathy (45).

A Unifying Hypothesis

From the studies of Mizuno and colleagues it is clear that high tissue concentrations of α-synuclein are associated with neuronal death in patients with the mutant parkin gene who do not have Lewy bodies. We even know that parkin is an enzyme concerned with protein degradation, and in patients with the mutant parkin gene, this enzyme is decreased, perhaps accounting for the accumulation of α-synuclein in the cytoplasm. From the work of van Duinen and colleagues (36), Lewy bodies can occur without neuronal death. Taken together, these observations raise the possibility that far from being a stage of pathogenesis leading to cell death, the formation of Lewy bodies may represent an attempt to sequester a noxious protein. That toxic aberrant proteins are most lethal when they are free in the cytoplasm, and their incorporation into inclusions may signify a protective effort. The ultimate mechanism of cell destruction may involve one or more of several damaging cascades such as free radical accumulation, atypical inflammatory attack, excitotoxicity, or programmed cell death (46,47).

The risk factors for neurodegeneration with Lewy bodies extend over a wide range, similar to those for neurofibrillary tangles. Trauma has not yet been linked to Lewy bodies, but the newer more sensitive techniques for detecting Lewy bodies have not been applied to patients dying with pugilist's encephalopathy.

Combing all this evidence, we can speculate that certain key features are shared in the most common forms of neurodegeneration—namely, accumulation of a deleterious protein (α-synuclein or tau), and an attempt to limit damage by sequestering the deleterious protein in a cytoplasmic inclusion (Lewy body or neurofibrillary tangle). This hypothesis is summarized in Fig. 1.1.

Finally, if we focus our attention on the most common etiology of IP, the evidence suggests interaction of genetic susceptibility

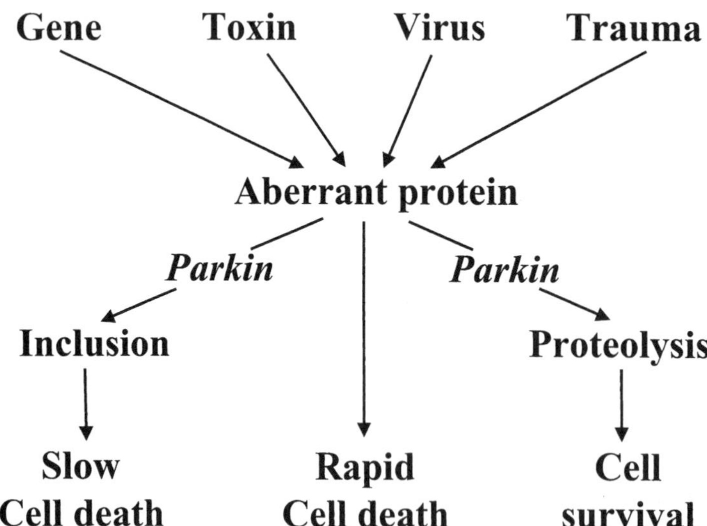

FIGURE 1.1. Diagrammatic representation of the hypothesis presented here for the pathogenesis of neuronal death. The aberrant protein may be α-synuclein (sequestered in Lewy bodies) or tau (sequestered in neurofibrillary tangles).

and environmental risk factors. We are left with one central question: What kind of environmental risk factor would lead to the accumulation of an aberrant protein capable of killing a neuron? Although the traditional view envisions long-term exposure with gradual engagement of all susceptible neurons (the process hypothesis), several clues now suggest that one or a few brief exposures are more likely (the event hypothesis) (48). Are the damaging events likely to be toxic or infective for most patients? Perhaps the next 100 years of research on IP will provide the answer and allow the development of a rational approach to prevention.

REFERENCES

1. Casals J, Elizan TS, Yahr MD. Postencephalitic parkinsonism—a review. *J Neural Transm* 1998;105:645–676.
2. Polymeropoulos MH, Lavedan C, Leroy E, et al. Mutation in the alpha-synuclein gene identified in families with Parkinson's disease. *Science* 1997;276:2045–2047.
3. Kitada T, Asakawa S, Hattori N, et al. Mutations in the Parkin gene cause autosomal recessive juvenile parkinsonism. *Nature* 1998;392:605–608.
4. Furtadao S, Farrer M, Tsuboi Y, et al. Spinocerebellar ataxia type 2 (SCA2) presenting as parkinsonism in an Alberta family: clinical, genetic and PET findings. *Neurology* 2002 In press.
5. Shan DE, Soong BW, Sun CM, Lee SJ, Liao KK, Liu RS. Spinocerebellar ataxia type 2 presenting as familial levodopa-responsive parkinsonism. *Ann Neurol* 2001; 50:812–815.
6. Uitti RJ, Shinotoh H, Hayward M, Schulzer M, Mak E, Calne DB. "Familial Parkinson's disease"—a case-controlled study of families. *Can J Neurol Sci* 1997;24: 127–132.
7. Tanner CM, Ottman R, Goldman SM, et al. Parkinson's disease in twins: an etiologic study. *JAMA* 1999;281: 376–378.
8. Calne S, Schoenberg B, Martin W, Uitti R, Spencer P, Calne DB. Familial Parkinson's disease: possible role of environmental factors. *Can J Neurol Sci* 1987;14: 303–305.
9. de la Fuente-Fernandez R, Calne DB. Evidence for environmental causation of Parkinson's disease. *Parkinsonism and Relat Disord* 2002;8:235–241.
10. Blaschko H. Metabolism and storage of biogenic amines. *Experientia* 1957;13:9–12.
11. Hornykiewicz O. How L-dopa was discovered as a drug for Parkinson's disease 40 years ago. *Wien Klin Wochenschr* 2001;113:855–862.
12. Montague KA. Catechol compounds in rat tissues and in brains of different animals. *Nature* 1957;180: 245–246.
13. Carlsson A, Lindqvist M, Magnusson T. 3,4-Dihydroxyphenylalanine and 5-hydroxytryptophan as reserpine antagonists. *Nature* 1957;180:1200.
14. Carlsson A. The occurrence, distribution and physiological role of catecholamines in the nervous system. *Pharmacol Rev* 1959;11:490–493.
15. Dahlström A, Fuxe K. Further evidence for the existence of monoamine-containing neurons in the central nervous system. *Acta Physiol Scand* 1964;62(Suppl. 232):1–55.
16. Kebabian JW, Petzold GL, Greengard P. Dopamine-sensitive adenylate cyclase in caudate nucleus of rat brain, and its similarity to the "dopamine receptor." *Proc Natl Acad Sci USA* 1972;69:2145–2149.
17. Nishi A, Bibb JA, Snyder GL, et al. Amplification of dopaminergic signaling by a positive feedback loop. *Proc Natl Acad Sci USA* 2000;97:12840–12845.
18. Kebabian JW, Calne DB. Multiple receptor mechanisms for dopamine. *Nature* 1979;227:93–96.
19. Civelli O, Bunzow JR, Grandy DK, et al. Molecular biology of the dopamine receptors. *Eur J Pharmacol* 1991;207:277–286.
20. Sibley DR, Monsma FJJ. Molecular biology of dopamine receptors. *Trends Pharmacol Sci* 1992;131:61–69.
21. Stoof JC. Dopamine receptors in the neostriatum: biochemical and physiological studies. In: Kaiser C, Kebabian JW, eds. *Dopamine receptors*. Washington D.C. American Chemical Society, 2001:117–145.
22. Ehringer H, Hornykiewicz O. Verteilung von Noradrenalin und Dopamin (3-Hydroxytyramin) im Gehirn des Menschen und verhalten bei Erkrankung des Extrapyramidalen Systems. *Klin Wochenschr* 1960;38:1236–1239.
23. Sano I. Biochemistry of the extrapyramidal system. Shinkei Kenkyu No Shipo, *Adv Neurol Sci* 1960;5:42–48.
24. Bernheimer H, Birkmayer W, Hornykiewicz O, Jellinger K, Seitelberger F. Brain dopamine and the syndromes of Parkinson and Huntington: clinical, morphological and neurochemical correlations. *J Neurol Sci* 1973;20: 415–455.
25. Denny-Brown D. *The basal ganglia*. London: Oxford University Press, 1964.
26. Nickerson M. Summary of discussion and commentary. *Pharmacol Rev* 1966;18:801–803.
27. Cotzias GC, van Woert MH, Schiffer LM. Aromatic amino acids and modification of parkinsonism. *New Engl J Med* 1967;276:374–379.
28. Yahr MD, Duvoisin RC, Hoehn MM, Schear MJ, Barrett RE. L-Dopa (L-3,4-dihydroxyphenylalanine)—its clinical effects in parkinsonism. *Trans Amer Neurol Assoc* 1968; 93:56–63.
29. Lewy FH. Paralysis Agitans I. Pathologische Anatomie. In: Lewandowsky M, ed. *Handbüch der Neurologie*. Berlin: Springer, 1912:920–933.
30. Rajput AH, Uitti RJ, Sudhakar S, Rozdilsky B. Parkinsonism and neurofibrillary tangle pathology in pigmented nuclei. *Ann Neurol* 1989;25:602–606.
31. Spillantini MG. Parkinson's disease, dementia with Lewy bodies and multiple system atrophy are α-synucleinopathies. *Parkinsonism Relat Disord* 1999;5: 157–162.
32. Arawaka S, Saito Y, Murayama S, Mori H. Lewy body in neurodegeneration with brain iron accumulation type 1 is immunoreactive for α-synuclein. *Neurology* 1998; 51:887–889.
33. Gibb WR, Scaravilli F, Michund J. Lewy bodies and

subacute sclerosing panencephalitis. *J Neurol Neurosurg Psychiatry* 1990;53:710–711.
34. Kaufmann H, Hague K, Perl D. Accumulation of alpha-synuclein in autonomic nerves in pure autonomic failure. *Neurology* 2001;56:980–981.
35. Raghavan R, Khin-Nu C, Brown A, et al. Detection of Lewy bodies in trisomy 21 (Down's syndrome). *Can J Neurol Sci* 1993;20:48–51.
36. van Duinen SG, Lammers GJ, Maat-Schieman ML, et al. Numerous and widespread α-synuclein–negative Lewy bodies in an asymptomatic patient. *Acta Neuropathol (Berl)* 1999;97:533–539.
37. Hicks A, Pétursson H, Jonsson T, et al. A susceptibility gene for late-onset idiopathic Parkinson's disease successfully mapped. *Am J Hum Gen* 2000;369(Suppl): 200.
38. Feany MB, Bender WW. A Drosophila model of Parkinson's disease. *Nature* 2000; 404:394–398.
39. Betarbet R, Sherer TB, MacKenzie G, et al. Chronic systemic pesticide exposure reproduces features of Parkinson's disease. *Nat Neurosci* 2000;3:1301–1306.
40. Petroske E, Meredith GE, Callen S, et al. Mouse model of parkinsonism: a comparison between subacute MPTP and chronic MPTP/probenecid treatment. *Neuroscience* 2001;106:589–601.
41. Lippa CF, Fujiwara H, Mann DM, et al. Lewy bodies contain altered α-synuclein in brains of many familial Alzheimer's disease patients with mutations in presenilin and amyloid precursor protein genes. *Am J Pathol* 1998;153:1365–1370.
42. Reed LA, Wszolek ZK, Hutton M. Phenotypic correlations in FTDP-17. *Neurobiol Aging* 2001;22:89–107.
43. Josephs KA, Parisi JE, Dickson DW. Postencephalitic parkinsonism of von Economo: tauopathy, synucleinopathy or both? *Neurology* 2001;50 (Suppl 3):A
44. Singer SM, Chambers CB, Newfry GA, Norlund MA, Muma NA. Tau in aluminum-induced neurofibrillary tangles. *Neurotoxicology* 1997;18:63–76.
45. Corsellis JAN, Bruton CJ, Freeman-Browne D. The aftermath of boxing. *Psychol Med* 1973;3:270–303.
46. Jellinger KA. Cell death mechanisms in neurodegeneration. *J Cell Mol Med* 2001;5:313–329.
47. McGeer PL, Yasojima K, McGeer EG. Inflammation in Parkinson's disease. *Adv Neurol* 2001;86:83–89.
48. Calne DB. Is idiopathic parkinsonism a consequence of an event or a process? *Neurology* 1994;44:5–10.

Parkinson's Disease: Advances in Neurology, Vol. 91.
Edited by Ariel Gordin, Seppo Kaakkola,
and Heikki Teräväinen
Lippincott Williams & Wilkins, Philadelphia © 2003

1

Functional Neuroanatomy of the Basal Ganglia in Parkinson's Disease

Thomas Wichmann and Mahlon R. DeLong

Department of Neurology, Emory University School of Medicine, Atlanta, Georgia

Recent neuroscience research has resulted in fresh insights into the structure and function of the basal ganglia and into the pathophysiologic basis of Parkinson's disease (PD) and other movement disorders (1,2). In addition, the renaissance of stereotactic surgery for PD and other movement disorders has provided valuable neuronal and imaging data from human subjects. In this chapter, we focus on the circuitry of the basal ganglia and the proposed circuit models of parkinsonism. A more detailed discussion may be found in the review of Wichmann and DeLong (2).

ANATOMICAL SUBSTRATE FOR CIRCUIT DYSFUNCTION IN PARKINSONISM

To discuss the pathophysiology of parkinsonism, one must consider first in some detail the circuitry, molecular anatomy, and physiology of the basal ganglia and related structures (Fig. 1.1). The basal ganglia include the neostriatum (caudate nucleus and putamen), the ventral striatum, the external and internal pallidal segment (external segment of the globus pallidus [GPe] and the internal segment of the globus pallidus [GPi]), the subthalamic nucleus (STN), and the substantia nigra pars reticulata and pars compacta (SNr and SNc, respectively). The striatum and STN are the main entry points for cortical and thalamic inputs into the basal ganglia. From the input nuclei, information is conveyed over multiple pathways to the principal basal ganglia output nuclei, GPi and SNr. Basal ganglia outflow from GPi and SNr is directed at frontal areas of the cerebral cortex (via the thalamus) and at various brainstem structures (superior colliculus, pedunculopontine nucleus [PPN], and parvicellular reticular formation).

Input to the Basal Ganglia

The most abundant inputs to the basal ganglia arise from the cortex in the form of topographically organized corticostriatal projections (3–5). In primates, projections from the somatosensory, motor, and premotor cortices terminate in the postcommissural putamen, the "motor portion" of the striatum, whereas prefrontal cortical areas project to the caudate nucleus and the precommissural putamen and projections from limbic cortices, the amygdala, and the hippocampus terminate preferentially in the ventral striatum. Cortical projections also terminate in the STN in a topographical manner (6,7). Afferents from the primary motor cortex reach the dorsolateral part of the STN, and afferents from the premotor and supplementary motor areas innervate mainly in the medial third of the nucleus. The prefrontal limbic cortices project to the ventral and most medial portions of the STN.

Topographically organized inputs to the striatum and STN also arise from the intralaminar nuclei of the thalamus, the centro-

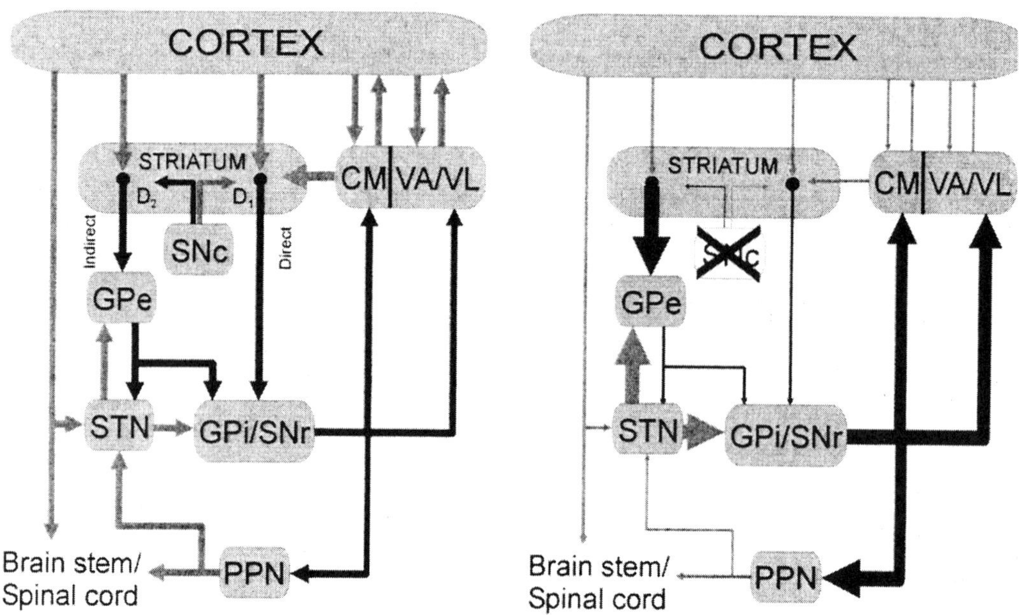

FIGURE 1.1. Simplified schematic diagram of the basal ganglia–thalamocortical circuitry under normal and parkinsonian conditions. Inhibitory connections (*solid arrows*) and excitatory connections (*open arrows*) are shown. The principal input nuclei of the basal ganglia, the striatum, and the subthalamic nucleus are connected to the output nuclei, the internal segment of the globus pallidus and the substantia nigra pars reticulata. Basal ganglia output is directed at several thalamic nuclei (the ventroanterior/ventrolateral nucleus and the centromedian) and at brainstem nuclei (the pedunculopontine nucleus and others). In addition to the changes in the rate of neuronal discharge (shown here as changes in the width of the connecting arrows), there are prominent alterations in discharge patterns. For further explanation of the model, see the text.

median (CM) and parafascicular (Pf) nuclei. In primates, the CM nucleus projects to the motor portions of the putamen and the STN, whereas the Pf nucleus projects to associative and limbic territories (8,9).

Intrinsic Basal Ganglia Connections

Striatal output is directed to the GPi and SNr in a topographical manner that maintains the corticostriatal organization into motor, limbic, associative, and oculomotor territories (3). The connections between the striatum and the output nuclei of the basal ganglia may be viewed as organized into two distinct pathways, the so-called *direct* and *indirect* pathways (1,10). The direct pathway arises from a discrete set of neurons that project monosynaptically to neurons in the GPi and SNr, whereas the indirect pathway arises from a different set of neurons that project to the GPe. Recent evidence indicates that some striatal fugal neurons may collateralize more extensively, reaching the GPe, GPi, and SNr (11). The GPe conveys the information it receives directly and indirectly (via the STN) to the GPi and SNr.

The anatomical relationships between neurons in the GPe, STN, and GPi that constitute the indirect pathway are highly topographical (12,13). Thus, populations of GPe neurons within the sensorimotor, cognitive, or limbic territory are reciprocally connected with populations of neurons in the same functional territories of the STN, and neurons in each of these regions, in turn, innervate the same functional territory of the GPi (12,13). The STN also projects to the striatum, the SNc (14,15), and the pedunculopontine nucleus (14,16).

The population of striatal neurons that gives rise to the direct pathway is further characterized by the presence of the neuropeptides substance P and dynorphin, by the preferential expression of the dopamine D_1 receptors, and by the fact that these neurons (as well as most striatal interneurons) appear to be the targets of thalamic inputs from the intralaminar nuclei of the thalamus (17,18). The population of striatal output neurons that give rise to the indirect pathway preferentially expresses enkephalin and dopamine D_2 receptors (19,20) and may be a major target of cortical inputs (17,18).

Although the segregation of D_1 and D_2 receptors between the direct and indirect pathways is probably not as strict as initially proposed (20,21), it may still serve to explain the apparent differential action of dopamine on striatal output. Striatal dopamine appears to modulate the activity of the basal ganglia output neurons in the GPi and SNr by *facilitation* of transmission over the direct pathway and *inhibition* of transmission over the indirect pathway (22). The net effect of striatal dopamine release appears to be to reduce basal ganglia output to the thalamus and other targets. Dopamine may also more directly influence discharge patterns and rates in the STN and the pallidum via receptors located in these structures.

Output Projections of the Basal Ganglia

The caudoventral motor territory of the GPi projects almost exclusively to the posterior part of the ventrolateral nucleus (VLo in macaques), which sends projections toward the supplementary motor area (SMA) (23–25), the primary motor cortex (M1), and premotor (PM) cortical areas (26). The outflow from pallidal motor areas directed at cortical areas MI, PM, and SMA appears to arise from separate populations of pallidothalamic neurons (26). The more rostromedial associative areas of GPi project preferentially to the parvocellular part of the ventroanterior (VA) and the dorsal VL nucleus (VLc in macaques) (23,27) and may be transmitted, in turn, to prefrontal cortical areas (28,29), as well as motor and supplementary motor regions (25,30).

Other output projections from the GPi arise mostly as collaterals from the pallidothalamic projection. Thus, prominent axon collaterals are sent in a segregated manner to the CM/Pf complex, which project to the cortex and the striatum (see above), constituting one of the many feedback circuits in the basal ganglia–thalamocortical circuitry (23). Additional axon collaterals reach the noncholinergic portion of the PPN (31,32), which, in turn, gives rise to ascending projections to the basal ganglia, the thalamus, and the basal forebrain, as well as to descending projections to the pons, the medulla, and the spinal cord (33).

Although the overlap between motor and nonmotor areas is probably greater in the SNr than in the GPi (34), the SNr can be broadly subdivided into a dorsolateral sensorimotor and a ventromedial associative territory (35). Projections from the medial SNr to the thalamus terminate mostly in the medial magnocellular division of the VA nucleus (VAmc) and the mediodorsal nucleus (MDmc), which, in turn, innervate anterior regions of the frontal lobe including the principal sulcus and the orbital cortex in monkeys (36). Neurons in the lateral SNr project preferentially to the lateral posterior region of the VAmc and to parts of MD nucleus, which are predominately related to posterior regions of the frontal lobe including the frontal eye field and areas of the PM cortex (36). The SNr also sends projections to the noncholinergic neurons of the PPN (32,37). Additional projections reach the parvicellular reticular formation, a region whose neurons are directly connected with orofacial motor nuclei (38), and the superior colliculus, which plays a critical role in the control of saccades (39).

ROLE OF THE BASAL GANGLIA–THALAMOCORTICAL CIRCUITRY IN THE CONTROL OF MOVEMENT

Voluntary movements appear to be initiated at the cortical level of the motor circuit, with output directed to the brainstem and spinal cord, and to multiple subcortical targets including the thalamus, putamen, and STN. Studies of the electrophysiologic properties of corticostriatal projection neurons (arising largely from cortical layer III) have shown that these neurons have slower conduction velocities and lower spontaneous discharge rates and that they respond less frequently to somatosensory input than neighboring corticospinal neurons (40,41).

According to the current model of the function of the basal ganglia–thalamocortical circuitry, activation of striatal neurons that give rise to the direct pathway reduces inhibitory basal ganglia output from targeted neurons with subsequent *disinhibition* of related thalamocortical neurons (42). The net effect of this is increased activity in appropriate cortical neurons, resulting in *facilitation* of the movement. By contrast, activation of the striatal neurons that give rise to the indirect pathway would lead to increased (inhibitory) basal ganglia output on thalamocortical neurons and to *suppression* of movement. Because most of the neurons in the GPi increase their discharge rate with movement, suppression of nonintended movements may be a particularly important role of the basal ganglia.

Clinical and experimental studies suggest that the basal ganglia play a role in specifying the amplitude or velocity of movement (42–44) or in maintaining postural stability during arm movements (42). The combination of information traveling via the direct and the indirect pathways of the motor circuit has been proposed to serve to either "scale" or "focus" movements (45,46), depending on the precise timing and anatomical connectivity. *Scaling* could be achieved by a temporal sequence of activity changes in the basal ganglia. Striatal output, via the direct pathway, would first inhibit specific neuronal populations in the GPi/SNr, thus facilitating movement, followed by disinhibition of the *same* GPi/SNr neuron via inputs over the indirect pathway, leading to inhibition ("braking") of the ongoing movement. In the *focusing* model, by contrast, inhibition of relevant pallidal/nigral neurons via the direct pathway would allow intended movements to proceed, whereas unintended movements would be suppressed by concomitant increased excitatory input via the indirect pathway in *other* GPi/SNr neurons (47,48).

Neither of these models satisfactorily accounts for all experimental findings. Both are at odds with the fact that STN lesions result in spontaneous dyskinesias but do not directly disrupt or alter voluntary movements. In addition, it is difficult to reconcile the focusing model with the fact that basal ganglia neurons become active in the context of movement only after changes in the cortex and thalamus are manifest (47,49,50).

The basal ganglia appear to have multiple functions other than the direct control of ongoing movements. Strong candidates among these are, for instance, a role in movement preparation, self-initiated (internally generated) movements, motor (particularly procedural) learning, and movement sequencing (51–53).

CHANGES IN BASAL GANGLIA CIRCUIT ACTIVITY IN PARKINSONISM

The study of pathophysiological changes in the basal ganglia that result from loss of dopamine transmission in the basal ganglia has been greatly facilitated by the discovery that primates treated with methylphenyltetrahydropyridine (MPTP) develop behavioral and pathological changes that closely mimic the features of PD in humans (54,55).

Changes in the activity over striatopallidal pathways were first suggested by studies in parkinsonian primates, which indicated that metabolic activity (as measured with the 2-deoxyglucose technique) is increased in both pallidal segments (56,57). This was interpreted as evidence for increased activity of the striatum–GPe connection and the STN–GPi pathway, or alternatively, as evidence for increased activity via the projections from the STN to both pallidal segments. Subsequent microelectrode recordings of neuronal activity in the primate MPTP model of parkinsonism showed directly that neuronal discharge is reduced in the GPe and increased in the STN and GPi, compared with normal controls (Fig. 1.2) (58–60). In parkinsonian patients undergoing pallidotomy, it has similarly been shown that the discharge rates in the GPe are significantly lower than those in the GPi (61–63). Recently, we have shown in the MPTP model of parkinsonism that the changes of neuronal activity in the second output nucleus of the basal ganglia, the SNr are qualitatively similar to those occurring in the GPi (64). The changes in discharge rates in the basal ganglia have been interpreted as indicating that striatal dopamine depletion leads to increased activity of striatal neurons of the indirect pathway, resulting in inhibition of the GPe and subsequent disinhibition of the STN and the GPi/SNr. It is likely that other structures and feedback loops, such as those involving the PPN and the CM, aggravate or enhance the abnormalities of discharge in the basal ganglia output nuclei associated with

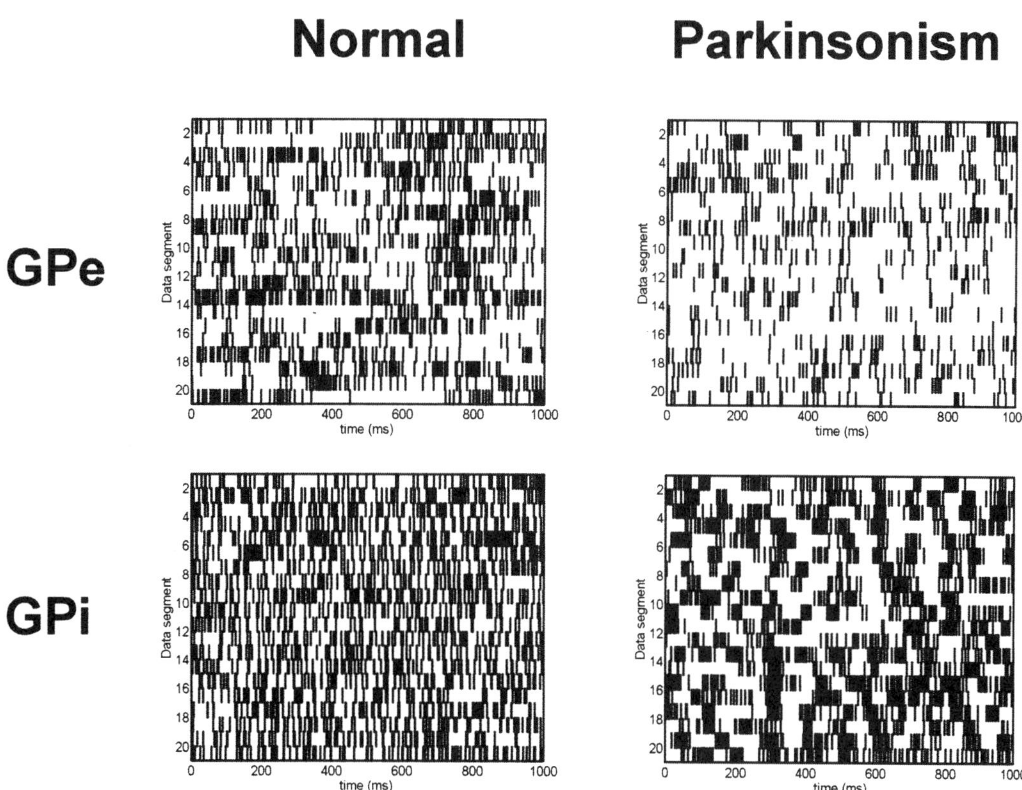

FIGURE 1.2. Raster displays of spontaneous neuronal activity recorded in the external segment of the globus pallidus (GPe) and the internal segment of the globus pallidus (GPi) in normal and parkinsonian primates. The neuronal activity is reduced in the GPe and increased in the GPi. Changes in the subthalamic nucleus and the substantia nigra pars reticulata are qualitatively similar to those seen in the GPi. In addition to the rate changes, there are also obvious changes in the firing patterns of neurons. For further explanations, see the text.

PD (see below). At the cortical level, positron emission tomography (PET) studies in parkinsonian patients have consistently shown reduced activation of motor and premotor areas (65,66).

Brainstem areas such as the PPN may also be directly (i.e., not via feedback interactions) involved in the development of parkinsonian signs. Lesions of this nucleus in normal monkeys can lead to akinesia, possibly by reducing stimulation of SNc neurons by input or by a direct influence on descending pathways (67,68).

A challenge to the proposed pathophysiological model of parkinsonism has arisen from histochemical studies on the amount of messenger RNA (mRNA) for the 67-kD isoform of glutamate decarboxylase (GAD_{67}), which is thought to correlate with the level of activity of GABAergic neurons in the nucleus under study. As predicted, GAD_{67} mRNA activity was found to be increased in GPi neurons in parkinsonian animals (69–71), but unexpectedly, it was unchanged or even increased in the GPe (71–73). These results have been interpreted as evidence that GPe and GPi function may not be tightly linked via the "indirect" pathway and that the observed activity changes in the STN and GPi may primarily be due to altered activity via the cortical subthalamic or CM/Pf subthalamic projection or via dopaminergic inputs to the STN itself. However, the consistent finding of decreased GPe discharge in parkinsonian animals and patients (see above) is difficult to reconcile with this. Conceivably, GAD_{67} mRNA levels may reflect something other than neuronal discharge rates (74,75).

NEUROSURGICAL IMPLICATIONS OF THE PATHOPHYSIOLOGICAL MODELS OF PARKINSONISM

The fact that parkinsonism is a disease affecting a large neuronal network suggests that surgical or pharmacological interventions at various targets within the network could be successful. This concept is supported by the demonstration that lesions of the STN, GPi, or SNr in MPTP-treated primates reverse some or all signs of parkinsonism, presumably by reducing basal ganglia output (76–78). Over the last decade, these results have helped to rekindle interest in functional neurosurgical approaches to the treatment of medically intractable PD. This was first employed in the form of GPi lesions (pallidotomy) (79–82) and more recently with STN lesions (83). In addition, high-frequency deep brain stimulation (DBS) of both the STN and the GPi, whose mechanism of action is still uncertain but appears overall also to inactivate the region stimulated, has been shown to reverse parkinsonian signs (84,85). PET studies in patients who have undergone pallidotomy and in patients with DBS of the STN or GPi have shown that frontal motor areas whose metabolic activity was reduced in the parkinsonian state became again active after the procedure (80,86).

It is clear that the earlier rate-based circuit model of parkinsonism cannot explain many of the clinical and experimental features of the disease. Thus, detailed studies of the results of lesions in human patients with parkinsonism have brought to light several findings that are incompatible with the models. For instance, lesions of the VA/VL nuclei of the thalamus (which completely remove thalamic output) do not lead to parkinsonism and are, in fact, beneficial in the treatment of tremor and rigidity (87,88). Similarly, lesions of the GPi in the setting of parkinsonism improve all aspects of PD without producing dyskinesias or other obvious detrimental effects. In fact, they are highly effective in reducing drug-induced dyskinesias (79,80,89). In contrast to the hypokinetic features of parkinsonism, dyskinesias appear to arise from pathological *reduction* in basal ganglia outflow (90) and, thus, should not respond to, but should be made worse by, further reduction of pallidal outflow (91).

These seemingly paradoxical findings may be explained by the realization that parkinsonism may at least in part result from a combination of problems, including increased discharge rate, altered processing of proprioceptive input, and abnormal timing, patterning, and synchronization of discharge that introduces errors and nonspecific noise into the thalamocortical signal. Altered discharge patterns and synchronization between neighboring neurons have been extensively documented in parkinsonian monkeys and patients. For instance, neuronal responses to passive limb manipulations in the STN, GPi, and thalamus (58–60) have been shown to occur more often, to be more pronounced, and to have widened receptive fields after treatment with MPTP. There is also a marked change in the synchronization of discharge between neurons in the basal ganglia. In contrast to the virtual absence of synchronized discharge of such neurons in normal monkeys (47), a substantial proportion of neighboring neurons in the GP and STN discharge in unison in parkinsonian primates (60). Finally, the proportion of cells in the STN, GPi, and SNr that discharge in oscillatory or nonoscillatory bursts is greatly increased in the parkinsonian state (59,60,92). Oscillatory burst discharge patterns are often seen in conjunction with tremor, which may reflect tremor-related proprioceptive input or a more active participation of basal ganglia in the generation of tremor.

Conceivably, increased phasic activity in the basal ganglia may erroneously signal excessive movement or velocity to precentral motor areas, leading to a slowing or premature arrest of ongoing movements and to greater reliance on external clues during movement. Alternatively, phasic alteration of discharge in the basal ganglia may simply introduce noise into thalamic output to the cortex that is detrimental to cortical operations. Parkinsonian patients have to compensate not only for the loss of basal ganglia contribution to movement, but also for the disruptive influence of the inappropriate basal ganglia output. The therapeutic benefits of GPi and STN lesions suggest that in PD and other movement disorders, the total lack of basal ganglia output is more tolerable than disruptive abnormal output on brainstem and thalamocortical systems. Functional imaging studies have demonstrated that surgical interventions do not necessarily normalize cortical motor mechanisms in parkinsonian subjects but may allow the intact portions of the thalamocortical and brainstem system to more effectively compensate for the loss of the basal ganglia contribution to movement.

CONCLUSIONS

Parkinsonism is clearly associated with increased and disordered discharge and synchronization in motor areas of the basal ganglia–thalamocortical motor loops. Neuronal recording data and the observed effects of pallidal and thalamic lesions suggest that the neuronal basis for the different basal ganglia movement disorders is not just changes in discharge rate, but also altered discharge patterns, abnormal and excessive synchronization of discharge, altered proprioceptive feedback, and the appearance of increased "noise" in the basal ganglia output signal. It is proposed that both ablation and DBS are effective in treating both hypokinetic and hyperkinetic disorders because they remove the abnormal signals directed to the thalamus and brainstem, thus allowing these otherwise intact systems to compensate more effectively for the loss of basal ganglia output.

REFERENCES

1. Albin RL, Young AB, Penney JB. The functional anatomy of basal ganglia disorders. *Trends Neurosci* 1989;12:366–375.
2. Wichmann T, DeLong MR, Davis DL, et al. Neurocircuitry of Parkinson's disease. *Neuropsychopharmacology: the fifth generation of progress.* Philadelphia: Lippincott Williams & Wilkins, 2002:1761–1780.
3. Alexander GE, DeLong MR, Strick PL. Parallel organization of functionally segregated circuits linking basal ganglia and cortex. *Annu Rev Neurosci* 1986;9:357–381.
4. Parent A. Extrinsic connections of the basal ganglia. *Trends Neurosci* 1990;13:254–258.
5. Haber SN, Kunishio K, Mizobuchi M, et al. The orbital and medial prefrontal circuit through the primate basal ganglia. *J Neurosci* 1995;15:4851–4867.
6. Hartmann-von Monakow K, Akert K, Kunzle H. Projections of the precentral motor cortex and other cortical areas of the frontal lobe to the subthalamic nucleus in the monkey. *Exp Brain Res* 1978;33:395–403.
7. Nambu A, Takada M, Inase M, et al. Dual somatotopical representations in the primate subthalamic nucleus:

evidence for ordered but reversed body-map transformations from the primary motor cortex and the supplementary motor area. *J Neurosci* 1996;16:2671–2683.
8. Smith Y, Parent A. Differential connections of caudate nucleus and putamen in the squirrel monkey (Saimiri sciureus). *Neuroscience* 1986;18:347–371.
9. Sadikot AF, Parent A, Smith Y, et al. Efferent connections of the centromedian and parafascicular thalamic nuclei in the squirrel monkey: a light and electron microscopic study of the thalamostriatal projection in relation to striatal heterogeneity. *J Comp Neurol* 1992;320: 228–242.
10. Alexander GE, Crutcher MD. Functional architecture of basal ganglia circuits: neural substrates of parallel processing. *Trends Neurosci* 1990;13:266–271.
11. Parent A, Charara A, Pinault D. Single striatofugal axons arborizing in both pallidal segments and in the substantia nigra in primates. *Brain Res* 1995;698:280–284.
12. Shink E, Bevan MD, Bolam JP, et al. The subthalamic nucleus and the external pallidum: two tightly interconnected structures that control the output of the basal ganglia in the monkey. *Neuroscience* 1996;73:335–357.
13. Smith Y, Bevan MD, Shink E, et al. Microcircuitry of the direct and indirect pathways of the basal ganglia. *Neuroscience* 1998;86:353–387.
14. Kita H, Ki ST. Efferent projections of the subthalamic nucleus in the rat: light and electron microscope analysis with the PHA-L method. *J Comp Neurol* 1987;260: 435–452.
15. Smith Y, Hazrati LN, Parent A. Efferent projections of the subthalamic nucleus in the squirrel monkey as studied by PHA-L anterograde tracing method. *J Comp Neurol* 1990;294:306–323.
16. Hammond C, Rouzaire-Dubois B, Feger J, et al. Anatomical and electrophysiological studies on the reciprocal projections between the subthalamic nucleus and nucleus tegmenti pedunculopontinus in the rat. *Neuroscience* 1983;9:41–52.
17. Sidibe M, Smith Y. Differential synaptic innervation of striatofugal neurones projecting to the internal or external segments of the globus pallidus by thalamic afferents in the squirrel monkey. *J Comp Neurol* 1996;365: 445–465.
18. Parthasarathy HB, Graybiel AM. Cortically driven immediate-early gene expression reflects influence of sensorimotor cortex on identified striatal neurons in the squirrel. *J Neuroscience* 1997;17:2477–2491.
19. Gerfen CR, Engber TM, Mahan LC, et al. D_1 and D_2 dopamine receptor–regulated gene expression of striatonigral and striatopallidal neurons. *Science* 1990;250: 1429–1432.
20. Surmeier DJ, Song WJ, Yan Z. Coordinated expression of dopamine receptors in neostriatal medium spiny neurons. *J Neurosci* 1996;16:6579–6591.
21. Aizman O, Brismar H, Uhlen P, et al. Anatomical and physiological evidence for D_1 and D_2 dopamine receptor colocalization in neostriatal neurons. *Nat Neurosci* 2000;3:226–230.
22. Gerfen CR. Dopamine receptor function in the basal ganglia. *Clin Neuropharmacol* 1995;18:S162–S177.
23. Sidibe M, Bevan MD, Bolam JP, et al. Efferent connections of the internal globus pallidus in the squirrel monkey, I: topography and synaptic organization of the pallidothalamic projection. *J Comp Neurol* 1997;382: 323–347.
24. Schell GR, Strick PL. The origin of thalamic inputs to the arcuate premotor and supplementary motor areas. *J Neurosci* 1984;4:539–560.
25. Inase M, Tanji J. Thalamic distribution of projection neurons to the primary motor cortex relative to afferent terminal fields from the globus pallidus in the macaque monkey. *J Comp Neurol* 1995;353:415–426.
26. Hoover JE, Strick PL. Multiple output channels in the basal ganglia. *Science* 1993;259:819–821.
27. DeVito JL, Anderson ME. An autoradiographic study of efferent connections of the globus pallidus in *Macaca mulatta*. *Exp Brain Res* 1982;46:107–117.
28. Goldman-Rakic PS, Porrino LJ. The primate mediodorsal (MD) nucleus and its projection to the frontal lobe. *J Comp Neurol* 1985;242:535–560.
29. Middleton FA, Strick PL. Anatomical evidence for cerebellar and basal ganglia involvement in higher cognitive function. *Science* 1994;266:458–461.
30. Darian-Smith C, Darian-Smith I, Cheema SS. Thalamic projections to sensorimotor cortex in the macaque monkey: use of multiple retrograde fluorescent tracers. *J Comp Neurol* 1990;299:17–46.
31. Harnois C, Filion M. Pallidofugal projections to thalamus and midbrain: a quantitative antidromic activation study in monkeys and cats. *Exp Brain Res* 1982;47: 277–285.
32. Rye DB, Lee HJ, Saper CB, et al. Medullary and spinal efferents of the pedunculopontine tegmental nucleus and adjacent mesopontine tegmentum in the rat. *J Comp Neurol* 1988;269:315–341.
33. Inglis WL, Winn P. The pedunculopontine tegmental nucleus: where the striatum meets the reticular formation. *Prog Neurobiol* 1995;47:1–29.
34. Hedreen JC, DeLong MR. Organization of striatopallidal, striatonigral and nigrostriatal projections in the macaque. *J Comp Neurol* 1991;304:569–595.
35. Deniau JM, Thierry AM. Anatomical segregation of information processing in the rat substantia nigra pars reticulata. *Adv Neurol* 1997;74:83–96.
36. Ilinsky IA, Jouandet ML, Goldman-Rakic PS. Organization of the nigrothalamocortical system in the rhesus monkey. *J Comp Neurol* 1985;236:315–330.
37. Steininger TL, Rye DB, Wainer BH. Afferent projections to the cholinergic pedunculopontine tegmental nucleus and adjacent midbrain extrapyramidal area in the albino rat, I: retrograde tracing studies. *J Comp Neurol* 1992;321:515–543.
38. von Krosigk M, Smith Y, Bolam JP, et al. Synaptic organization of GABAergic inputs from the striatum and the globus pallidus onto neurons in the substantia nigra and retrorubral field which project to the medullary reticular formation. *Neuroscience* 1993;50: 531–549.
39. Wurtz RH, Hikosaka O. Role of the basal ganglia in the initiation of saccadic eye movements. *Prog Brain Res* 1986;64:175–190.
40. Turner RS, DeLong MR. Corticostriatal activity in primary motor cortex of the macaque. *J Neurosci* 2000;20: 7096–7108.
41. Bauswein E, Fromm C, Preuss A. Corticostriatal cells in comparison with pyramidal tract neurons: contrasting properties in the behaving monkey. *Brain Res* 1989;493: 198–203.
42. Inase M, Buford JA, Anderson ME. Changes in the control of arm position, movement, and thalamic discharge

during local inactivation in the globus pallidus of the monkey. *J Neurophysiol* 1996;75:1087–1104.
43. Georgopoulos AP, DeLong MR, Crutcher MD. Relations between parameters of step-tracking movements and single cell discharge in the globus pallidus and subthalamic nucleus of the behaving monkey. *J Neurosci* 1983;3:1586–1598.
44. Turner RS, Grafton ST, Votaw JR, et al. Motor subcircuits mediating the control of movement velocity: a PET study. *J Neurophysiol* 1998;80:2162–2176.
45. Mink JW, Thach WT. Basal ganglia motor control, III: pallidal ablation: normal reaction time, muscle cocontraction, and slow movement. *J Neurophysiol* 1991;65: 330–351.
46. Nambu A, Tokuno H, Hamada I, et al. Excitatory cortical inputs to pallidal neurons via the subthalamic nucleus in the monkey. *J Neurophysiol* 2000;84:289–300.
47. Wichmann T, Bergman H, DeLong MR. The primate subthalamic nucleus, I: functional properties in intact animals. *J Neurophysiol* 1994;72:494–506.
48. Jaeger D, Gilman S, Aldridge JW. Neuronal activity in the striatum and pallidum of primates related to the execution of externally cued reaching movements. *Brain Res* 1995;694:111–127.
49. DeLong MR. Activity of basal ganglia neurons during movement. *Brain Res* 1972;40:127–135.
50. Turner RS, Anderson ME. Pallidal discharge related to the kinematics of reaching movements in two dimensions. *J Neurophysiol* 1997;77:1051–1074.
51. Wise SP, Murray EA, Gerfen CR. The frontal cortex–basal ganglia system in primates. *Crit Rev Neurobiol* 1996;10:317–356.
52. Graybiel AM. Building action repertoires: memory and learning functions of the basal ganglia. *Curr Opin Neurobiol* 1995;5:733–741.
53. Schultz W. The phasic reward signal of primate dopamine neurons. *Adv Pharmacol* 1998;42:686–690.
54. Burns RS, Chiueh CC, Markey SP, et al. A primate model of parkinsonism: selective destruction of dopaminergic neurons in the pars compacta of the substantia nigra by *N*-methyl-4-phenyl-1,2,3,6-tetrahydropyridine. *Proc Natl Acad Sci USA* 1983;80: 4546–4550.
55. Forno LS, DeLanney LE, Irwin I, et al. Similarities and differences between MPTP-induced parkinsonism and Parkinson's disease. *Adv Neurol* 1993;60:600–608.
56. Crossman AR, Mitchell IJ, Sambrook MA. Regional brain uptake of 2-deoxyglucose in *N*-methyl-4-phenyl-1,2,3,6-tetrahydropyridine (MPTP)–induced parkinsonism in the macaque monkey. *Neuropharmacology* 1985; 24:587–591.
57. Schwartzman RJ, Alexander GM. Changes in the local cerebral metabolic rate for glucose in the 1-methyl-4-phenyl-1,2,3,6-tetrahydropyridine (MPTP) primate model of Parkinson's disease. *Brain Res* 1985;358: 137–143.
58. Filion M, Tremblay L, Bedard PJ. Abnormal influences of passive limb movement on the activity of globus pallidus neurons in parkinsonian monkeys. *Brain Res* 1988;444:165–176.
59. Miller WC, DeLong MR. Altered tonic activity of neurons in the globus pallidus and subthalamic nucleus in the primate MPTP model of parkinsonism. In: Carpenter MB, Jayaraman A, eds. *The basal ganglia II.* New York: Plenum Press, 1987:415–427.
60. Bergman H, Wichmann T, Karmon B, et al. The primate subthalamic nucleus, II: neuronal activity in the MPTP model of parkinsonism. *J Neurophysiol* 1994;72: 507–520.
61. Dogali M, Beric A, Sterio D, et al. Anatomic and physiological considerations in pallidotomy for Parkinson's disease. *Stereotact Funct Neurosurg* 1994;62:53–60.
62. Lozano A, Hutchison W, Kiss Z, et al. Methods for microelectrode-guided posteroventral pallidotomy. *J Neurosurg* 1996;84:194–202.
63. Vitek JL, Kaneoke Y, Turner R, et al. Neuronal activity in the internal (GPi) and external (GPe) segments of the globus pallidus (GP) of parkinsonian patients is similar to that in the MPTP-treated primate model of parkinsonism. *Soc Neurosci* 1993;19:1584(abst).
64. Wichmann T, Bergman H, Starr PA, et al. Comparison of MPTP-induced changes in spontaneous neuronal discharge in the internal pallidal segment and in the substantia nigra pars reticulata in primates. *Exp Brain Res* 1999;125:397–409.
65. Ceballos-Baumann AO, Brooks DJ. Basal ganglia function and dysfunction revealed by PET activation studies. *Adv Neurol* 1997;74:127–139.
66. Eidelberg D, Edwards C. Functional brain imaging of movement disorders. *Neurol Res* 2000;22:305–312.
67. Kojima J, Yamaji Y, Matsumura M, et al. Excitotoxic lesions of the pedunculopontine tegmental nucleus produce contralateral hemiparkinsonism in the monkey. *Neurosci Lett* 1997;226:111–114.
68. Munro-Davies LE, Winter J, Aziz TZ, et al. The role of the pedunculopontine region in basal-ganglia mechanisms of akinesia. *Exp Brain Res* 1999;129:511–517.
69. Soghomonian JJ, Pedneault S, Audet G, et al. Increased glutamate decarboxylase mRNA levels in the striatum and pallidum of MPTP-treated primates. *J Neurosci* 1994;14:6256–6265.
70. Herrero MT, Levy R, Ruberg M, et al. Glutamic acid decarboxylase mRNA expression in medial and lateral pallidal neurons in the MPTP-treated monkeys and patients with Parkinson's disease. *Adv Neurol* 1996;69: 209–216.
71. Herrero MT, Levy R, Ruberg M, et al. Consequence of nigrostriatal denervation and L-dopa therapy on the expression of glutamic acid decarboxylase messenger RNA in the pallidum. *Neurology* 1996;47:219–224.
72. Soghomonian JJ, Chesselet MF. Effects of nigrostriatal lesions on the levels of messenger RNAs encoding two isoforms of glutamate decarboxylase in the globus pallidus and entopeduncular nucleus of the rat. *Synapse* 1992;11:124–133.
73. Chesselet MF, Delfs JM. Basal ganglia and movement disorders: an update. *Trends Neurosci* 1996;19: 417–422.
74. Martin DL, Rimvall K. Regulation of gamma-aminobutyric acid synthesis in the rat brain. *J Neurochem* 1993; 60:395–407.
75. Rimvall K, Martin DL. The level of GAD_{67} protein is highly sensitive to small increases in intraneuronal gamma-aminobutyric acid levels. *J Neurochem* 1994; 62:1375–1381.
76. Bergman H, Wichmann T, DeLong MR. Reversal of experimental parkinsonism by lesions of the subthalamic nucleus. *Science* 1990;249:1436–1438.
77. Wichmann T, Kliem MA, DeLong MR. Antiparkinsonian and behavioral effects of inactivation of the substan-

tia nigra pars reticulata in hemiparkinsonian primates. *Exp Neurol* 2001;167:410–424.
78. Lieberman DM, Corthesy ME, Cummins A, et al. Reversal of experimental parkinsonism by using selective chemical ablation of the medial globus pallidus. *J Neurosurg* 1999;90:928–934.
79. Baron MS, Vitek JL, Bakay RAE, et al. Treatment of advanced Parkinson's disease by GPi pallidotomy: 1 year pilot-study results. *Ann Neurol* 1996;40: 355–366.
80. Dogali M, Fazzini E, Kolodny E, et al. Stereotactic ventral pallidotomy for Parkinson's disease. *Neurology* 1995;45:753–761.
81. Laitinen LV, Bergenheim AT, Hariz MI. Leksell's posteroventral pallidotomy in the treatment of Parkinson's disease. *J Neurosurg* 1992;76:53–61.
82. Lozano AM, Lang AE, Galvez-Jimenez N, et al. Effect of GPi pallidotomy on motor function in Parkinson's disease. *Lancet* 1995;346:1383–1387.
83. Gill SS, Heywood P. Bilateral subthalamic nucleotomy can be accomplished safely. *Mov Disord* 1998;13:201.
84. Limousin-Dowsey P, Pollak P, Van Blercom N, et al. Thalamic, subthalamic nucleus and internal pallidum stimulation in Parkinson's disease. *J Neurol* 1999; 246[Suppl 2]:42–45.
85. Starr PA, Vitek JL, Bakay RA. Deep brain stimulation for movement disorders. *Neurosurg Clin North Am* 1998;9:381–402.
86. Ceballos-Bauman AO, Obeso JA, Vitek JL, et al. Restoration of thalamocortical activity after posteroventrolateral pallidotomy in Parkinson's disease. *Lancet* 1994;344:814.
87. Giller CA, Dewey RB, Ginsburg MI, et al. Stereotactic pallidotomy and thalamotomy using individual variations of anatomic landmarks for localization. *Neurosurgery* 1998;42:56–62.
88. Tasker RR, Lang AE, Lozano AM. Pallidal and thalamic surgery for Parkinson's disease. *Exp Neurol* 1997;144: 35–40.
89. Rabey JM, Orlov E, Spiegelman R. Levodopa-induced dyskinesias are the main feature improved by contralateral pallidotomy in Parkinson's disease. *Neurology* 1995;45:A377.
90. Papa SM, Desimone R, Fiorani M, et al. Internal globus pallidus discharge is nearly suppressed during levodopa-induced dyskinesias. *Ann Neurol* 1999;46: 732–738.
91. Marsden CD, Obeso JA. The functions of the basal ganglia and the paradox of stereotaxic surgery in Parkinson's disease. *Brain* 1994;117:877–897.
92. Filion M, Tremblay L. Abnormal spontaneous activity of globus pallidus neurons in monkeys with MPTP-induced parkinsonism. *Brain Res* 1991;547:142–151.

Parkinson's Disease: Advances in Neurology, Vol. 91.
Edited by Ariel Gordin, Seppo Kaakkola,
and Heikki Teräväinen
Lippincott Williams & Wilkins, Philadelphia © 2003

2

Parkinson Revisited: Pathophysiology of Motor Signs

Mark Hallett

Human Motor Control Section, National Institute of Neurological Disease Center, National Institutes of Health, Bethesda, Maryland

Parkinson's disease (PD) is classically characterized by bradykinesia, rigidity, and tremor at rest. All features seem due to the degeneration of the nigrostriatal pathway, but it has not been possible to define a single underlying pathophysiological mechanism that explains everything. Nevertheless, there are considerable data that give separate understanding to each of the three classic features.

BRADYKINESIA

The most important functional disturbance in patients with PD is a disorder of voluntary movement that is prominently characterized by slowness. This phenomenon is generally called bradykinesia, although it has at least two components, which can be designated as bradykinesia and akinesia (1). Bradykinesia refers to slowness of movement that is ongoing. Akinesia refers to failure of willed movement to occur. There are two possible reasons for the absence of expected movement. One is that the movement is so slow (and small) that it cannot be seen. A second is that the time needed to initiate the movement becomes excessively long.

Although self-paced movements can give information about bradykinesia, the study of reaction-time movements can give information about both akinesia and bradykinesia. In the reaction-time situation, a stimulus is presented to a subject, and the subject must make a movement as rapidly as possible. The time between the stimulus and the start of movement is the *reaction time,* and the time from initiation to completion of movement is the *movement time.* Using this logic, one concludes that prolongation of the reaction time is akinesia and the prolongation of the movement time is bradykinesia. Studies of patients with PD confirm that both the reaction time and the movement time are prolonged. However, the extent of abnormality of one does not necessarily correlate with the extent of abnormality of the other (2). This suggests that they may be impaired by separable physiological mechanisms. In general, prolongation of the movement time (bradykinesia) is better correlated with the clinical impression of slowness than prolongation of the reaction time (akinesia).

Some contributing features of bradykinesia are established. One is that there is a failure to energize muscles up to the level necessary to complete a movement in a standard amount of time. This has been demonstrated clearly with attempted rapid monophasic movements at a single joint (3). In this circumstance, movements of different angular distances are accomplished in approximately the same time by making longer movements faster. The electromyographic (EMG) activity underlying the movement begins with a burst of activity in the agonist muscle of 50 to 100 ms, followed by a burst of activity in the antagonist muscle of 50 to 100 ms, followed variably by a third burst of activity in the agonist. This "triphasic" pattern has relatively fixed timing with movements of different distance, correlating with the fact of similar total times for movements of different distances. Different distances are accomplished by altering the magnitude of the EMG within the fixed duration burst. The pattern is correct in patients with PD, but there is insufficient EMG activity in the burst to accomplish the movement. These patients often must go through two or more cycles of the triphasic pattern to accomplish the movement. Interestingly, such activity looks virtually identical to the tremor at rest seen in these patients. The longer the desired movement, the more likely it is to require additional cycles. These findings were reproduced by Baroni et al. (4), who also showed that levodopa normalized the pattern and reduced the number of bursts.

Berardelli et al. (5) showed that patients with PD could vary the size and duration of the first agonist EMG burst with movement size and added load in the normal way. However, there was a failure to match these parameters appropriately to the size of movement required. This suggests an additional problem in scaling of actual movement to the required movement. A problem in sensory scaling of kinesthesia was demonstrated by Demirci et al. (6). Patients with PD used kinesthetic perception to estimate the amplitude of passive angular displacements of the index finger around the metacarpophalangeal joint and to scale them as a percentage of a reference stimulus. The reference stimulus was either a standard kinesthetic stimulus preceding each test stimulus (task K) or a visual representation of the standard kinesthetic stimulus (task V). The underestimation by the patients with PD of the amplitudes of finger perturbations was significantly greater in task V than in task K. Thus, when kinesthesia is used to match a visual target, distances are perceived to be shorter by the patients with PD. Assuming that visual perception is normal, kinesthesia must be "reduced" in patients with PD. This reduced kinesthesia, when combined with the well-known reduced motor output and probably reduced corollary discharges, implies that the sensorimotor apparatus is "set" smaller in patients with PD than in healthy subjects.

In a slower, multijoint movement task, patients with PD show a reduced rate of rise in muscle activity, which also implies deficient activation (7). On the other hand, Jordan et al. (8) showed that release of force was just as slowed as increase of force, suggesting that slowness to change, and not deficient energy, was the main problem. If termination of activity is an active process, then this finding really does not argue against deficient energy.

A second physiological mechanism of bradykinesia is that there is difficulty with simultaneous and sequential movements (9). That patients with PD have more difficulty with simultaneous movements than with isolated movements was first pointed out by Schwab et al. (10). Quantitative studies show that slowness in accomplishing simultaneous or sequential movements is more than would be predicted from the slowness of each individual movement. With sequential movements, there is another parameter of interest, the time between the two movements, designated the interonset latency (IOL) by Benecke et al. (9). The IOL is also prolonged in patients with PD. This problem, similar to the problem with simple movements, can also be interpreted as insufficient motor energy.

Akinesia would seem to be multifactorial, and a number of contributing factors are already known. As noted, one type of akinesia is the limit of bradykinesia from the point of view of energizing muscles. If the muscle is selected but not energized, there will be no movement. Such phenomena can be recognized on some occasions with EMG studies in which EMG activity will be initiated but will be insufficient to move the body part. Another type of akinesia, again as noted, is prolongation of the reaction time: The patient is preparing to move, but the movement has not yet occurred. Considerable attention has been paid to mechanisms of prolongation of the reaction time. One factor is easily demonstrable in patients with rest tremor, who appear to have to wait to initiate the movement together with a beat of tremor in the agonist muscle of the willed movement (11,12).

Another mechanism of prolongation of the reaction time can be seen in those circumstances in which eye movement must be coordinated with limb movement (13). In this situation, there is a visual target that moves into the periphery of the visual field. Normally, there is a coordinated movement of eyes and limb, the eyes beginning slightly earlier. In PD, some patients do not begin to move the limb until the eye movement is completed. This might be due to a problem with simultaneous movements, as noted already. Alternatively, it might be that patients with PD need to foveate a target before they are able to move to it.

Many studies have evaluated reaction time quantitatively with neuropsychological methods (14). The goal of these studies is to determine the abnormalities in the motor processes that must occur before a movement can be initiated. To understand reaction-time studies, it is useful to consider from a theoretical point of view the tasks that the brain must accomplish. The starting point is the "set" for the movement. This includes the environmental conditions, initial positions of body parts, understanding the nature of the experiment, and in particular some understanding of the expected movement. In some circumstances, the expected movement is described completely, without ambiguity. This is the "simple reaction-time" condition. The movement can be fully planned. It then needs to be held in store until the stimulus comes to initiate the execution of the movement. In other circumstances, the "set" does not include a complete description of the required movement. It is intended that the description be completed at the time of the stimulus that calls for the movement initiation. This is the "choice reaction-time" condition. In this circumstance, the programming of the movement occurs between the stimulus and the response. The choice reaction time is always longer than the simple reaction time, and the time difference is due to this movement programming.

In most studies, the simple reaction time is significantly prolonged in patients with PD compared with healthy subjects (14). On the other hand, patients with PD appear to have normal choice reaction times or the increase in the choice reaction time over the simple reaction time is the same in patients with PD and healthy subjects. Many studies in which cognitive activity was required for a decision on the correct motor response have shown that patients with PD do not have apparent slowing of thinking, called bradyphrenia. We extended the study of choice reaction times by considering three different choice reaction-time tasks that required the same simple movement but differed in the difficulty of the decision of which movement to make (15). Comparing patients with PD with healthy subjects, we found that the patients had a longer reaction time in all three conditions, with the largest difference occurring when the task was the easiest and smallest, not when the task was the most difficult. Thus, the greater the proportion of time there is in the reaction time devoted to motor program selection, the closer to normal are the PD results. Labutta et al. (16) showed that patients with PD have no difficulty holding a motor program in store. Hence, the difficulty must be executing the motor program. Execution of the movement, however, lies at the end of the choice reaction time, just as it does for the simple reaction time. How then can the simple reaction time be abnormal and the choice reaction time be normal? The answer may be that in the choice reaction-time situation, both the motor programming and the motor execution can proceed in parallel.

Transcranial magnetic stimulation (TMS) can be used to study the initiation of execution. With low levels of TMS, it is possible to find a level that will not produce any motor evoked potentials (MEPs) at rest but will produce MEP when there is voluntary activation. Using such a stimulus in a reaction-time situation between the stimulus to move and the response, Starr et al. (17) showed that stimulation close to movement onset would produce a response even though there was still no voluntary EMG activity. A small response first appeared about 80 ms before EMG onset and grew in magnitude closer to onset. This method divides the reaction time into two periods. In the first period, the motor cortex remains "unexcitable." In the second period, the cortex becomes increasingly "excitable" as it prepares to trigger the movement. We found that most of the prolongation of the reaction time was due to prolongation of the later period of rising excitability (18). This result has been confirmed (19). Our finding of prolonged initiation time in patients with PD is supported by studies of motor cortex neuronal activity in reaction-time movements in monkeys rendered parkinsonian with methylphenyltetrahydropyridine (20). In these investigations, there was a prolonged time between initial activation of motor cortex neurons and movement onset.

Thus, an important component of akinesia is the difficulty in initiating a planned movement. This statement would not be a surprise to patients with PD, who often say that they know what they want to do, but they just cannot do it. A major problem in bradykinesia is a deficiency in activation of muscles, whereas the problem in akinesia seems to be a deficiency in activation of the motor cortex. The dopaminergic system apparently provides energy to many different motor tasks, and the deficiency of this system in PD leads to both bradykinesia and akinesia.

Another factor that should be kept in mind is that patients appear to have much more difficulty initiating internally triggered movements than externally triggered movements. This is clear clinically because external clues are often helpful in movement initiation. Examples include improving walking by providing an object to step over or playing marching music. This can also be demonstrated in the laboratory with a variety of paradigms (21,22).

ADDITIONAL HUMAN EVIDENCE FOR DECREASED CORTICAL ACTIVATION IN PD

Rossini et al. (23) showed that the amplitude of the N30 of the median nerve somatosensory evoked potential (SSEP) was diminished in PD. Other peaks of the SSEP were normal and the N30 had normal latency and topography. The origin of the N30 (like most of the waves of the SSEP) is debated, but its decrease does suggest deficient cortical activation.

Studies of movement-related cortical potentials (MRCPs) in patients with PD are controversial, but many studies show a decreased Bereitschafts potential (BP), a slowly rising negativity appearing during the 1 second before self-paced voluntary movements (24–26). In the study by Jahanshahi et al. (26), the BP was deficient with self-paced movements, but not externally triggered movements, suggesting a particular difficulty with internally triggered actions.

Neuroimaging studies show a decreased blood flow response in the supplementary motor area, and sometimes the sensorimotor area, with voluntary movement in patients with PD (26–29). This can be reversed with dopaminergic therapy. In the study by Jahanshahi et al. (26), in which the neuroimaging was done with electroencephalogram (EEG) recording, it was found that there was a deficiency of activation of the supplementary motor area in self-paced movements, but not in externally triggered movement.

The excitability of the motor cortex in patients with PD has been assessed using TMS (30). The threshold for a response was the same in healthy subjects and in patients with PD, there was a trend for the increase in MEP amplitude with stimulus intensity to be greater than normal, but the increase of the MEP amplitude with voluntary contraction was statistically less than normal. These results suggest that control of the excitability of the motor system is abnormal in patients with PD, with enhanced excitability at rest and weak energization during voluntary muscle activation.

There also appears to be slightly less intracortical inhibition in patients with PD. One study found reduced intracortical inhibition (31) while another did not (32). On the other hand, both studies found shortening of the TMS-provoked silent period, which lengthened with dopaminergic treatment.

RIGIDITY

Tone is defined as the resistance to passive stretch. Rigidity is one form of increased tone that is seen in disorders of the basal ganglia ("extrapyramidal disorders") and is particularly prominent in PD. Increased tone can result from changes in (a) muscle properties or joint characteristics, (b) amount of background contraction of the muscle, and (c) magnitude of stretch reflexes. There is evidence for all three of these aspects contributing to rigidity. For quantitative purposes, responses can be measured to controlled stretches delivered by devices that contain torque motors. The stretch can be produced by altering the torque of the motor or by altering the position of the shaft of the motor. The perturbation can be a single step or more complex, such as a sinusoid. The mechanical response of the limb can be measured: The positional change if the motor alters force or the force change if the motor alters position. Such mechanical measurements can directly mimic and quantify the clinical impression (33,34).

There are changes in the passive mechanical properties of muscle in patients with PD. The first suggestion that this might be true came from gait studies that showed reduced dorsiflexion movement of the ankle despite strong tibialis anterior activity and silent triceps surae (35). Subsequently, using a quantitative measure, it was determined that the upper limb of patients with PD was stiffer than that of healthy subjects in the totally relaxed state with no EMG activity present (36). This phenomenon has been called into question by findings of another group that studied the lower leg and found normal contraction parameters (time to peak and half relaxation time), responses to short tetani, and resistance to stretch (37). However, they found an increased resistance to passive stretch under static conditions, presumably elastic in origin. The results may be evidence against a contribution of altered muscle contractile properties to rigidity in PD but still reveal an increased totally passive component.

Patients with PD do not relax well and often have slight contraction at rest. This is a standard clinical and electrophysiological observation, and this mechanism clearly plays a significant part in rigidity.

There are increases in long-latency reflexes in patients with PD. Generally, this is neurophysiologically distinct from the increases in the short-latency reflexes seen in spasticity, an increase in tone of "pyramidal" type. The short-latency reflex is the monosynaptic reflex. Reflexes occurring at a longer latency than this are designated long latency. When a relaxed muscle is stretched, in general, only a short-latency reflex is produced. When a muscle is stretched while it is active, one or more distinct long-latency reflexes are produced after the short-latency reflex and before the time needed to produce a voluntary response to the stretch. These reflexes are recognized as separate because of brief time gaps between them, giving rise to the appearance of distinct "humps" on a rectified EMG trace. Each component reflex, either short or long in latency, has about the same duration, approximately 20 to 40 ms. They appear to be true reflexes because their appearance and magnitude depend primarily on the amount of background force that the muscle was exerting at the time of the stretch and the mechanical parameters of the stretch; they do not vary much with whatever the subject might want to do after experiencing the muscle stretch. By contrast, the voluntary response that occurs after a reaction time from the stretch stimulus is strongly dependent on the will of the subject.

The short-latency stretch reflex can be easily measured with the tendon jerk or H reflex (HR). To obtain a meaningful measure of the response, one must compare the amplitude of the maximal reflex with the amplitude of the EMG in maximum voluntary effort or the amplitude of the EMG produced by supramaximal stimulation of the nerve to that muscle (H/M ratio) (33,34). Unfortunately, large interindividual variability makes the measurement less useful than it might be. The H/M ratio is enhanced in spasticity, but not in parkinsonian rigidity. Another clinically useful test is vibratory inhibition of the HR (38). In healthy subjects, the amplitude of the HR is markedly inhibited by vibration of the muscle. Vibratory inhibition is often dramatically reduced in spasticity, but it is normal in parkinsonian rigidity.

Long-latency reflexes are best brought out with controlled stretches with a device such as a torque motor. Although long-latency reflexes are normally absent at rest, they are prominent in patients with PD (33,34,39,40). Long-latency reflexes are also enhanced in PD with background contraction. Because some long-latency stretch reflexes appear to be mediated by a loop through the sensory and motor cortices, the enhancement of long-latency reflexes has been generally believed to indicate increased excitability of this central loop.

There is some evidence that at least one component of the increased long-latency stretch reflex in PD is a group II–mediated reflex. This suggestion was first made by Berardelli et al. (41) on the basis of physiological features including insensitivity to vibration. It was subsequently supported by the observation that an enhanced late stretch reflex response could not be duplicated with a vibration stimulus (42).

Some studies show a correlation between clinically measured increased tone and the magnitude of long-latency reflexes (41) while others do not (43,44). Long-latency reflexes contribute significantly to rigidity but are apparently not completely responsible for it.

The enhancement of long-latency reflexes can also be brought out by electrical stimulation of a mixed nerve. Such stimulation while the limb is at rest will produce only an M wave and F response in the muscles innervated by that nerve. If a mixed nerve is stimulated while the muscles are active, however, additional responses will be produced (33,34). With mixed nerve stimulation, there is a short-latency response that seems analogous to the HR and one or more long-latency responses (LLRs). One of these LLRs, called LLRII by Deuschl and Lücking (45) may have a transcortical pathway similar to some of the long-latency reflexes to stretch. The LLRI, intermediate in latency between the HR and LLRII, is enhanced in about half of patients with PD.

Some spinal inhibitory reflexes such as reciprocal inhibition and Ib inhibition are deficient, and these mechanisms may also play a role. If inhibition is lacking, there will be excessive activity that could contribute to rigidity or failure to relax.

Reciprocal inhibition is a fundamental mechanism of motor control. There are multiple pathways for reciprocal inhibition, the simplest of which is the disynaptic pathway via the Ia inhibitory interneuron. In the arm, reciprocal inhibition has been studied looking at the effects of radial nerve stimulation on the HR of the flexor carpi radialis (FCR) (46,47). Via various pathways, and therefore at various time intervals after the radial nerve stimulus, the radial afferent traffic can inhibit the motoneuron pools of the FCR. Healthy subjects showed three periods of inhibition, reaching a peak at delays of 0 ms, 10 ms, and 75 ms. The first period of inhibition is caused by disynaptic Ia inhibition, the second period of inhibition is explained as a presynaptic inhibition, and unfortunately, very little is known about the third period of inhibition, but the long latency (75 to 200 ms) appears to be compatible with a polysynaptic pathway. The first relative facilitation (at about a 2-ms delay) is a function of Ib fiber actions, and indirect evidence indicates that the second facilitation (at about a 50-ms delay) can be a function of cutaneous group II action.

Reciprocal inhibition is reduced in patients with dystonia, including those with generalized dystonia, writer's cramp, spasmodic torticollis, and blepharospasm (47,48). Reciprocal inhibition is also abnormally reduced in patients with PD (49). On the other hand, short-latency reciprocal inhibition is increased in the lower extremities, the opposite to what is found in the upper extremities (50).

That Ib inhibition can be found in the human was first demonstrated by the clever experiments of Pierrot-Deseilligny et al. (51). They showed that stimulation of the nerve to the medial head of gastrocnemius provoked short-latency inhibition of the HR in soleus that was most consistent with Ib effects. Presumably this is apparent because there are very few heteronymous Ia projections from the medial head of the gastrocnemius onto soleus motoneurons. In patients with spasticity, Ib inhibition is absent and is replaced by facilitation (52). The explanation for this inversion is not clear. Similarly, Ib inhibition is diminished in PD, and when rigidity is more severe, the inhibition is replaced by facilitation. The authors explain this on the hypothesis of increased activity of the nucleus gigantocellularis of the brainstem.

Reduction of Ib inhibition was confirmed using a different method, electrical stimulation via skin electrodes placed over human tendons, resulting in a reflex inhibition of voluntary activity in the stimulated muscle (53). The threshold of the inhibitory response was significantly increased in PD compared with controls. Also, the latency of the inhibitory wave was increased, and the duration of inhibition was increased in patients.

Inhibitory and excitatory reflex effects from stimulation of cutaneous nerves can be detected by recording changes in levels of tonic voluntary EMG activity of various hand muscles (33,34). These reflexes consist of a series of bursts of EMG activity, separated by periods of inhibition. The first excitatory component is generally agreed to be of spinal origin while there is debate about a supraspinal or even a transcortical loop of the later reflex components. The first inhibitory component is produced by inhibition above the level of the alpha motoneuron, but below the level of the cortex, and is diminished in PD (54).

Recurrent inhibition can be studied using the complicated method developed by Pierrot-Deseilligny et al. (55). While in spasticity some patients show loss of inhibition, there is no loss of inhibition in PD (49).

Delwaide et al. (56) suggested that the magnitude of audiospinal facilitation correlates with rigidity. They compared audiospinal facilitation using the soleus HR in control subjects and patients with PD. In the patients with PD, facilitation was significantly reduced during the 75 to 150 ms after the conditioning stimulation. This reduction was seen bilaterally even in patients with a hemisyndrome. It was corrected by levodopa but not by anticholinergic agents. Facilitation at the 75-ms delay showed an inverse linear correlation with the bradykinesia intensity. The authors explain the results as a reduced excitability of the nucleus reticularis pontis caudalis from which a reticulospinal tract emanates as an effector of audiospinal facilitation.

TREMOR AT REST

The so-called "tremor at rest" is the classic tremor of PD and other parkinsonian states such as those produced by neuroleptics or other dopamine-blocking agents such as prochlorperazine and metoclopramide (34, 57–59). It is present at rest, disappears with action, but may resume with static posture. That the tremor may also be present during postural maintenance is a significant point of confusion with regard to naming this tremor "tremor at rest." It can involve all parts of the body and can be markedly asymmetrical, but it is most typical with a flexion-extension movement at the elbow, pronation and supination of the forearm, and movements of the thumb across the fingers ("pill rolling"). Its frequency is 3 to 7 Hz but is most commonly 4 or 5 Hz, and EMG studies show alternating activity in antagonist muscles. PD is sometimes divided into two types, the akinetic rigid form and the tremor-predominant form; the latter has a better prognosis.

Tremor at rest can also be seen in the parkinsonian-plus disorders, but it is not as common as in PD itself. For example, rest tremor was seen in 29 of 100 patients thought to have multiple system atrophy, but only 9 had a "classic appearance" (60).

Some patients have rest tremor for a number of years without any other evidence of PD, and it has not been clear whether they really have PD. Eleven of these patients underwent fluorine-18 (^{18}F)-dopa positron emission tomography scan studies, and all showed reduced putaminal uptake, an abnormality characteristic of PD (61). This result has been replicated in a double-blind fashion on 5 patients using magnetic resonance imaging. All five showed typical findings of PD, with smudging or decreased distance between the substantia nigra and red nucleus (62) (see Rajput and Rajput in this volume).

The anatomical basis of the tremor at rest may well differ from the classic neuropathology of PD, that of degeneration of the nigrostriatal pathway. For example, ^{18}F-dopa uptake in the caudate and putamen declines with bradykinesia and rigidity but is unassociated with degree of tremor (63). Another point in favor of this idea is that the tremor may be successfully treated with a stereotaxic lesion or deep brain stimulation of the ventral intermediate (VIM) nucleus of the thalamus, a cerebellar relay nucleus (64,65).

In parkinsonian tremor at rest, there may be some mechanical reflex component and some 8- to 12-Hz component, but the most significant component comes from a pathological central oscillator at 3 to 5 Hz. This tremor component is unaffected by loading. Evidence for the central oscillator includes the facts that the accelerometric record and the EMG are not affected by weighting and small mechanical perturbations do not affect it. On the other hand, it can be reset by strong peripheral stimuli such as an electrical stimulus that produces a movement of the body part five times more than the amplitude of the tremor itself (66). Where this strong stimulus acts is not clear, but it does not have to be on the peripheral loop. Additionally, the tremor can be reset by TMS (67,68), presumably indicating a role of the motor cortex in the central processes that generate the tremor. In the studies of Pascual-Leone et al. (68), using a relatively small stimulus, the tremor was reset with TMS, but not with transcranial electrical stimulation. Because TMS affects the intracortical circuitry more, this seems to be further evidence for a role of the motor cortex.

Although cells in the globus pallidus may have oscillatory activity, they are not as well related to the tremor as the cells in the VIM of the thalamus (69,70). Zirh et al. (71) have studied the physiological properties of cells in the VIM in relation to tremor production. They have tried to see if the pattern of spike activity is consistent with specific hypotheses. They examined whether parkinsonian tremor might be produced by the activity of an intrinsic thalamic pacemaker or by the oscillation of an unstable long loop reflex arc. In one study of 42 cells, they found 11 with a sensory feedback pattern, 1 with a pacemaker pattern, 21 with a completely random pattern, and 9 that did not fit any pattern (71). In another study of thalamic neuron activity, some cells with a pacemaker pattern were seen, but these did not participate in the rhythmic activity correlating with tremor (72). These results confirm those of Zirh et al. (71), suggesting that the thalamic cells are not the pacemaker.

Wherever the pacemaker for the tremor, it is important to note that although the tremor is synchronous within a limb, it is not synchronous between limbs (73). Hence, a single pacemaker does not influence the whole body.

There are other types of tremor in PD including an action tremor resembling an essential tremor, but these have not been extensively studied.

REFERENCES

1. Berardelli A, Rothwell J, Thompson PD, et al. Pathophysiology of bradykinesia in Parkinson's disease. *Brain* 2001;124:2131–2146.
2. Evarts EV, Teravainen H, Calne DB. Reaction time in Parkinson's disease. *Brain* 1981;104:167–186.
3. Hallett M, Khoshbin S. A physiological mechanism of bradykinesia. *Brain* 1980;103:301–314.
4. Baroni A, Benvenuti F, Fantini L, et al. Human ballistic arm abduction movements: effects of levodopa treatment in Parkinson's disease. *Neurology* 1984;34: 868–876.
5. Berardelli A, Dick JP, Rothwell JC, et al. Scaling of the size of the first agonist EMG burst during rapid wrist movements in patients with Parkinson's disease. *J Neurol Neurosurg Psychiatry* 1986;49:1273–1279.
6. Demirci M, Grill S, McShane L, et al. A mismatch between kinesthetic and visual perception in Parkinson's disease. *Ann Neurol* 1997;41:781–788.
7. Godaux E, Koulischer D, Jacquy J. Parkinsonian bradykinesia is due to depression in the rate of rise of muscle activity. *Ann Neurol* 1992;31:93–100.
8. Jordan N, Sagar HJ, Cooper JA. A component analysis of the generation and release of isometric force in Parkinson's disease. *J Neurol Neurosurg Psychiatry* 1992;55:572–576.
9. Benecke R, Rothwell JC, Dick JP, et al. Simple and complex movements off and on treatment in patients with Parkinson's disease. *J Neurol Neurosurg Psychiatry* 1987;50:296–303.
10. Schwab RS, Chafetz ME, Walker S. Control of two simultaneous voluntary motor acts in normals and in parkinsonism. *Arch Neurol* 1954;72:591–598.
11. Hallett M, Shahani BT, Young RR. Analysis of stereotyped voluntary movements at the elbow in patients with Parkinson's disease. *J Neurol Neurosurg Psychiatry* 1977;40:1129–1135.
12. Staude G, Wolf W, Ott M, et al. Tremor as a factor in prolonged reaction times of parkinsonian patients. *Mov Disord* 1995;10:153–162.
13. Warabi T, Yanagisawa N, Shindo R. Changes in strategy of aiming tasks in Parkinson's disease. *Brain* 1988;111: 497–505.
14. Hallett M. Clinical neurophysiology of akinesia. *Rev Neurol (Paris)* 1990;146:585–590.
15. Brown VJ, Schwarz U, Bowman EM, et al. Dopamine dependent reaction time deficits in patients with Parkinson's disease are task specific. *Neuropsychologia* 1993; 31:459–469.
16. Labutta RJ, Miles RB, Sanes JN, et al. Motor program memory storage in Parkinson's disease patients tested with a delayed response task. *Mov Disord* 1994;9: 218–222.
17. Starr A, Caramia M, Zarola F, et al. Enhancement of motor cortical excitability in humans by non-invasive electrical stimulation appears prior to voluntary movement. *Electroencephalogr Clin Neurophysiol* 1988;70:26–32.
18. Pascual-Leone A, Valls-Solé J, Brasil-Neto J, et al. Akinesia in Parkinson's disease, I: shortening of simple reaction time with focal, single-pulse transcranial magnetic stimulation. *Neurology* 1994;44:884–891.
19. Chen R, Kumar S, Garg RR, et al. Impairment of motor cortex activation and deactivation in Parkinson's disease. *Clin Neurophysiol* 2001;112:600–607.
20. Watts RL, Mandir AS. The role of motor cortex in the pathophysiology of voluntary movement deficits associated with parkinsonism. *Neurol Clin* 1992;10: 451–469.
21. Majsak MJ, Kaminski T, Gentile AM, et al. The reaching movements of patients with Parkinson's disease under self-determined maximal speed and visually cued conditions. *Brain* 1998;121:755–766.
22. Curra A, Berardelli A, Agostino R, et al. Performance of sequential arm movements with and without advance knowledge of motor pathways in Parkinson's disease. *Mov Disord* 1997;12:646–654.
23. Rossini PM, Babiloni F, Bernardi G, et al. Abnormalities of short-latency somatosensory evoked potentials in parkinsonian patients. *Electroencephalogr Clin Neurophysiol* 1989;74:277–289.
24. Tarkka IM, Reilly JA, Hallett M. Topography of movement-related cortical potentials is abnormal in Parkinson's disease. *Brain Res* 1990;522:172–175.
25. Dick JPR, Rothwell JC, Day BL, et al. The Bereitschafts potential is abnormal in Parkinson's disease. *Brain* 1989;112:233–244.
26. Jahanshahi M, Jenkins IH, Brown RG, et al. Self-initiated versus externally triggered movements, I: An investigation using measurement of regional cerebral blood flow with PET and movement-related potentials in normal and Parkinson's disease subjects. *Brain* 1995; 118:913–933.
27. Playford ED, Jenkins IH, Passingham RE, et al. Impaired mesial frontal and putamen activation in Parkinson's disease: a positron emission tomography study. *Ann Neurol* 1992;32:151–161.
28. Jenkins IH, Fernandez W, Playford ED, et al. Impaired activation of the supplementary motor area in Parkinson's disease is reversed when akinesia is treated with apomorphine. *Ann Neurol* 1992;32:749–757.
29. Rascol O, Sabatini U, Chollet F, et al. Normal activation of the supplementary motor area in patients with Parkinson's disease undergoing long-term treatment with levodopa. *J Neurol Neurosurg Psychiatry* 1994;57: 567–571.
30. Valls-Solé J, Pascual-Leone A, Brasil-Neto J, et al. Abnormal facilitation of the response to transcranial magnetic stimulation in patients with Parkinson's disease. *Neurology* 1994;44:735–741.
31. Ridding MC, Inzelberg R, Rothwell JC. Changes in excitability of motor cortical circuitry in patients with Parkinson's disease. *Ann Neurol* 1995;37:181–188.
32. Berardelli A, Rona S, Inghilleri M, et al. Cortical inhibition in Parkinson's disease. A study with paired magnetic stimulation. *Brain* 1996;119:71–77.
33. Hallett M, Berardelli A, Delwaide P, et al. Central EMG and tests of motor control. Report of an IFCN committee. *Electroencephalogr Clin Neurophysiol* 1994;90: 404–432.
34. Hallett M. Electrophysiologic evaluation of movement disorders. In: Aminoff MJ, ed. *Electrodiagnosis in clinical neurology,* 4th ed. New York: Churchill Livingstone, 1999:365–380.
35. Dietz V, Quintern J, Berger W. Electrophysiological

studies of gait in spasticity and rigidity. Evidence that altered mechanical properties of muscle contribute to hypertonia. *Brain* 1981;104:431–449.
36. Watts RL, Wiegner AW, Young RR. Elastic properties of muscles measured at the elbow in man, II: patients with parkinsonian rigidity. *J Neurol Neurosurg Psychiatry* 1986;49:1177–1181.
37. Hufschmidt A, Stark K, Lucking CH. Contractile properties of lower leg muscles are normal in Parkinson's disease. *J Neurol Neurosurg Psychiatry* 1991;54:457–460.
38. Bour LJ, Ongerboer de Visser BW, Koelman HTM, et al. Soleus H-reflex tests in spasticity and dystonia: a computerized analysis. *J Electromyogr Kinesiol* 1991; 1:9–19.
39. Tatton WG, Bedingham W, Verrier MC, et al. Characteristic alterations in responses to imposed wrist displacements in parkinsonian rigidity and dystonia musculorum deformans. *Can J Neurol Sci* 1984;11:281–287.
40. Rothwell JC, Obeso JA, Traub MM, et al. The behavior of the long-latency stretch reflex in patients with Parkinson's disease. *J Neurol Neurosurg Psychiatry* 1983;46:35–44.
41. Berardelli A, Sabra AF, Hallett M. Physiological mechanisms of rigidity in Parkinson's disease. *J Neurol Neurosurg Psychiatry* 1983;46:45–53.
42. Cody FW, MacDermott N, Matthews PB, et al. Observations on the genesis of the stretch reflex in Parkinson's disease. *Brain* 1986;109:229–249.
43. Meara RJ, Cody FW. Stretch reflexes of individual parkinsonian patients studied during changes in clinical rigidity following medication. *Electroencephalogr Clin Neurophysiol* 1993;89:261–268.
44. Bergui M, Lopiano L, Paglia G, et al. Stretch reflex of quadriceps femoris and its relation to rigidity in Parkinson's disease. *Acta Neurol Scand* 1992;86:226–229.
45. Deuschl G, Lücking CH. Physiology and clinical applications of hand muscle reflexes. *Electroencephalogr Clin Neurophysiol* 1990;[Suppl]41:84–101.
46. Day BL, Marsden CD, Obeso JA, et al. Reciprocal inhibition between the muscles of the human forearm. *J Physiol (London)* 1984;349:519–534.
47. Panizza ME, Hallett M, Nilsson J. Reciprocal inhibition in patients with hand cramps. *Neurology* 1989;39:85–89.
48. Panizza M, Lelli S, Nilsson J, et al. H-reflex recovery curve and reciprocal inhibition of H-reflex in different kinds of dystonia. *Neurology* 1990;40:824–828.
49. Lelli S, Panizza M, Hallett M. Spinal cord inhibitory mechanisms in Parkinson's disease. *Neurology* 1991;41: 553–556.
50. Delwaide PJ, Pepin JL, Maertens de Noordhout A. Parkinsonian rigidity: clinical and physiopathologic aspects. *Rev Neurol* 1990;146:548–554.
51. Pierrot-Deseilligny E, Katz R, Morin C. Evidence of Ib inhibition in human subjects. *Brain Res* 1979;166: 176–179.
52. Delwaide PJ, Pepin JL, Maertens de Noordhout A. Short-latency autogenic inhibition in patients with parkinsonian rigidity. *Ann Neurol* 1991;30:83–89.
53. Burne JA, Lippold OC. Loss of tendon organ inhibition in Parkinson's disease. *Brain* 1996;119:1115–1121.
54. Fuhr P, Zeffiro T, Hallett M. Cutaneous reflexes in Parkinson's disease. *Muscle Nerve* 1992;15:733–739.
55. Rossi A, Mazzocchio R. Presence of homonymous recurrent inhibition in motoneurons supplying different lower limb muscles in humans. *Exp Brain Res* 1991;84: 367–373.
56. Delwaide PJ, Pepin JL, Maertens de Noordhout A. The audiospinal reaction in parkinsonian patients reflects functional changes in reticular nuclei. *Ann Neurol* 1993; 33:63–69.
57. Hallett M. Classification and treatment of tremor. *JAMA* 1991;266:1115–1117.
58. Elble RJ, Koller WC. *Tremor.* Baltimore: Johns Hopkins University Press, 1990.
59. Elble RJ. The pathophysiology of tremor. In: Watts RL, Koller WC, eds. *Movement disorders: neurologic principles and practice.* New York: McGraw-Hill, 1997: 405–417.
60. Wenning GK, Ben Shlomo Y, Magalhaes M, et al. Clinical features and natural history of multiple system atrophy. An analysis of 100 cases. *Brain* 1994;117: 835–845.
61. Brooks DJ, Playford ED, Ibanez V, et al. Isolated tremor and disruption of the nigrostriatal dopaminergic system: an ^{18}F-dopa PET study. *Neurology* 1992;42:1554–1560.
62. Chang MH, Chang TW, Lai PH, et al. Resting tremor only: a variant of Parkinson's disease or of essential tremor. *J Neurol Sci* 1995;130:215–219.
63. Otsuka M, Ichiya Y, Kuwabara Y, et al. Differences in the reduced ^{18}F-Dopa uptakes of the caudate and the putamen in Parkinson's disease: correlations with the three main symptoms. *J Neurol Sci* 1996;136:169–173.
64. Jankovic J, Cardoso F, Grossman RG, et al. Outcome after stereotactic thalamotomy for parkinsonian, essential, and other types of tremor. *Neurosurgery* 1995;37: 680–686.
65. Benabid AL, Pollak P, Gao D, et al. Chronic electrical stimulation of the ventralis intermedius nucleus of the thalamus as a treatment of movement disorders. *J Neurosurg* 1996;84:203–214.
66. Britton TC, Thompson PD, Day BL, et al. Modulation of postural tremors at the wrist by supramaximal electrical median nerve shocks in essential tremor, Parkinson's disease and normal subjects mimicking tremor. *J Neurol Neurosurg Psychiatry* 1993;56:1085–1089.
67. Britton TC, Thompson PD, Day BL, et al. Modulation of postural wrist tremors by magnetic stimulation of the motor cortex in patients with Parkinson's disease or essential tremor and in normal subjects mimicking tremor. *Ann Neurol* 1993;33:473–479.
68. Pascual-Leone A, Valls-Solé J, Toro C, et al. Resetting of essential tremor and postural tremor in Parkinson's disease with transcranial magnetic stimulation. *Muscle Nerve* 1994;17:800–807.
69. Hayase N, Miyashita N, Endo K, et al. Neuronal activity in GP and VIM of parkinsonian patients and clinical changes of tremor through surgical interventions. *Stereotact Funct Neurosurg* 1998;71:20–28.
70. Hurtado JM, Gray CM, Tamas LB, et al. Dynamics of tremor-related oscillations in the human globus pallidus: a single case study. *Proc Natl Acad Sci USA* 1999; 96:1674–1679.
71. Zirh TA, Lenz FA, Reich SG, et al. Patterns of bursting occurring in thalamic cells during parkinsonian tremor. *Neuroscience* 1998;83:107–121.
72. Magnin M, Morel A, Jeanmonod D. Single-unit analysis of the pallidum, thalamus and subthalamic nucleus in parkinsonian patients. *Neuroscience* 2000;96: 549–564.
73. Hurtado JM, Lachaux JP, Beckley DJ, et al. Inter- and intralimb oscillator coupling in parkinsonian tremor. *Mov Disord* 2000;15:683–691.

Parkinson's Disease: Advances in Neurology, Vol. 91.
Edited by Ariel Gordin, Seppo Kaakkola,
and Heikki Teräväinen
Lippincott Williams & Wilkins, Philadelphia © 2003

3

Nondopaminergic Neurons in Parkinson's Disease

E. C. Hirsch, G. Orieux, M-P Muriel, C. Francois, and J. Feger

Inserm U289, Department of Experimental Neurology and Therapeutics, Hôpital de la Salpêtrière, Paris, France

Parkinson's disease (PD) is characterized by a slow and progressive loss of dopaminergic neurons mostly affecting the nigrostriatal pathway. Yet, nondopaminergic neurons are also involved in the pathophysiology of PD. Indeed, neuronal loss has been described in noradrenergic, cholinergic, serotonergic, and even peptidergic neurons in the brain of patients with PD (1). This loss of nondopaminergic neurons most likely participates in the development of the symptoms that do not respond to levodopa therapy. In this context, the loss of norepinephrine-containing neurons in the locus ceruleus and cholinergic neurons in the nucleus basalis of Meynert and the septum participates in the intellectual deterioration observed in some patients with PD. Similarly, the loss of serotonergic neurons in the raphe nuclei may be involved in the depression observed in some patients with PD, although this symptom is difficult to analyze due to possible depressive behavior associated with the disease itself. The distribution of the nondopaminergic lesions has been extensively reviewed and therefore is not addressed in this chapter. In contrast, we discuss the functional alterations in nondopaminergic neurons that occur as a consequence of dopaminergic lesions and the changes observed in nondopaminergic neurons that could account for the absence of efficacy of dopamine-replacement therapy in PD.

FUNCTIONAL CHANGES IN NONDOPAMINERGIC NEURONS ARE A CONSEQUENCE OF DOPAMINE NEURONAL LOSS

Numerous dopaminergic neurons degenerate in the mesencephalon in regions including the substantia nigra pars compacta, the ventral tegmental area, and catecholaminergic cell group A8 (2). This neuronal loss accounts for the reduced dopamine concentrations in the striatum and probably in other basal ganglia areas including the subthalamic nucleus (STN), the pallidal complex, and even in other brain regions such as the cerebral cortex and the thalamus (3–5). The consequence of this altered dopamine concentration is a reduced stimulation of postsynaptic dopamine receptors on nondopaminergic neurons and of auto-receptors located on the dopaminergic neurons themselves. The lack of stimulation of postsynaptic receptors provokes profound changes in the functioning of the basal ganglia circuitry in PD, as discussed below.

According to the model of basal ganglia circuitry proposed in the 1990s (6,7), the input structure of the basal ganglia, the striatum, is connected to the output structures via so-called direct and indirect pathways. In the direct pathway, the striatum is interconnected with the internal segment of the globus pallidus (GPi) and the substantia nigra pars reticulata (SNpr) via a monosynaptic circuit using γ-aminobutyric acid (GABA) as a neurotransmitter. In the indirect pathway, the striatum is also connected to these structures but by three neuronal types in series. This pathway includes successively GABAergic neurons projecting from the external segment of the globus pallidus (GPe) to the STN and glutamatergic neurons projecting from the STN to the GPi and SNpr. Although this is still debated, the striatal GABAergic neurons, which give rise to the direct and indirect pathways, bear different types of dopamine receptors. Dopamine influences the direct pathway via D_1 receptors, which are positively coupled to G proteins, whereas the dopamine effect on the indirect pathway is mediated by D_2 receptors, which are negatively coupled to G proteins. Thus, the reduced expression of striatal dopamine concentrations is thought to provoke hypoactivity of the direct pathway and hyperactivity of the indirect pathway. The hypoactivity of the direct pathway has been confirmed by several experiments showing that the output structure of the basal ganglia circuitry is hyperactive from an electrophysiological, neurochemical, and metabolic point of view (6,8–13). Evidence for the hyperactivity of the indirect pathway is less clear, however, and requires a more careful analysis of the published literature. Indeed, whereas there is no doubt that the STN is hyperactive after nigrostriatal dopaminergic denervation, the origin of its hyperactivity is still debated. According to the model of the basal ganglia circuitry, the hyperactivity of the STN is thought to be due to a decreased inhibition of the afferent fibers originating in the GPe. Yet the origin of the STN hyperactivity is perhaps more complex than that proposed in the model. Electrophysiological recordings in parkinsonian animals have shown that the neurons in the GPe are hypoactive after nigrostriatal degeneration (9,10). Nevertheless, recent studies have questioned this observation (14), as the bursting activity of GPe neurons increased in 1-methyl-4-phenyl-1,2,3,6-tetrahydropyridine (MPTP)-intoxicated animals, and from a biochemical point of view, the hypoactivity of these GABAergic neurons is discussed (15). Indeed, using the expression of the messenger RNA (mRNA) coding for glutamate decarboxylase isoform 67, two independent groups of investigators were unable to detect a decreased expression of this GABAergic marker in GPe neurons (16–19). These studies even reported a nonsignificant increase of this marker in GPe neurons. Analysis of the expression of the mRNA coding for the first subunit of cytochrome oxidase, a metabolic marker that allows measurements of metabolic activity of a cellular resolution, was unable to provide evidence of decreased metabolic activity in the GPe (15,20). Metabolic measurements in the GPe also appear to be contradictory. Indeed, deoxyglucose measurements, which are indicative of the global metabolic activity in the structure, show an increased metabolic activity in the GPe after nigrostriatal denervation (21–23). These results of metabolic measurements should be interpreted with caution because the parameters analyzed by the two methods were different. Thus, deoxyglucose measurements most likely measure the activity in afferent fibers to a given structure (15,24) and take into account the hyperactivity of the striatopallidal terminals. In contrast, cytochrome oxidase mRNA measurements consider the activity of individual intrinsic neurons in a given structure (15). Thus, the latter data suggest that pallidosubthalamic neurons are not hypoactive in parkinsonian syndromes (15,20). The lack of hypoactivity of pallidal neurons in the presence of hyperactive inhibitory terminals in the structure may be explained by other excitatory afferent fibers, which originate in the STN and use glutamate as the neurotransmitter (25). The predominant role assigned to the GPe in the hyperactivity of the STN in parkinsonian syndromes is also called into question by experiments involving electrophysiological recording in rats with a lesion of the substantia nigra or the GP (the equivalent of the GPe in primates) (26). Thus, a unilateral lesion of the substantia nigra results in a major hyperactivity of STN neurons as measured by extracellular recordings. A unilateral lesion of the GP also results in an increased activity in neurons of the STN but this increase is much more moderate. Taken together, these data indicate that the GPe probably participates in the hyperactivity of the STN but that other structures connected to the STN are probably also involved in its hyperactivity.

To identify functional changes in neurons projecting to the STN, combined track tracing experiments and metabolic measurements in rats have been used to analyze the metabolic activity of neuronal cell bodies specifically projecting to the STN. As shown in several species, retrogradely labeled neurons were found in several structures. Cytochrome oxidase mRNA, taken as an index of metabolic activity, was analyzed in these neurons found in the GP, the parafascicular nucleus of the thalamus, the pedunculopontine nucleus, and the cerebral cortex (27). As previously shown, no hypoactivity was detected in the GP (Fig. 3.1). In contrast, the neurons originating in the parafascicular nucleus of the thalamus and in the pedunculopontine nucleus projecting toward the STN were shown to be metabolically hyperactive (Fig. 3.1). Because these neurons use at least in part the excitatory neurotransmitter glutamate, the hyperactivity of these structures may contribute to the hyperactivity of the STN. In contrast, neurons from the cerebral cortex, which were detected in the motor, medial, and lateral (or insular) prefrontal cortical areas and which projected to the STN, were shown to be hypoactive (Fig. 3.1), although this was not pronounced (28). Like the neurons in the thalamic-subthalamic and pedunculopontine-subthalamic pathways, the neurons in the cortical-subthalamic pathway also use glutamate as a neurotransmitter. Taken together, these data suggest that there is a complex regulation of the activity of subthalamic neuronal activity by glutamate afferent fibers, some of which are hy-

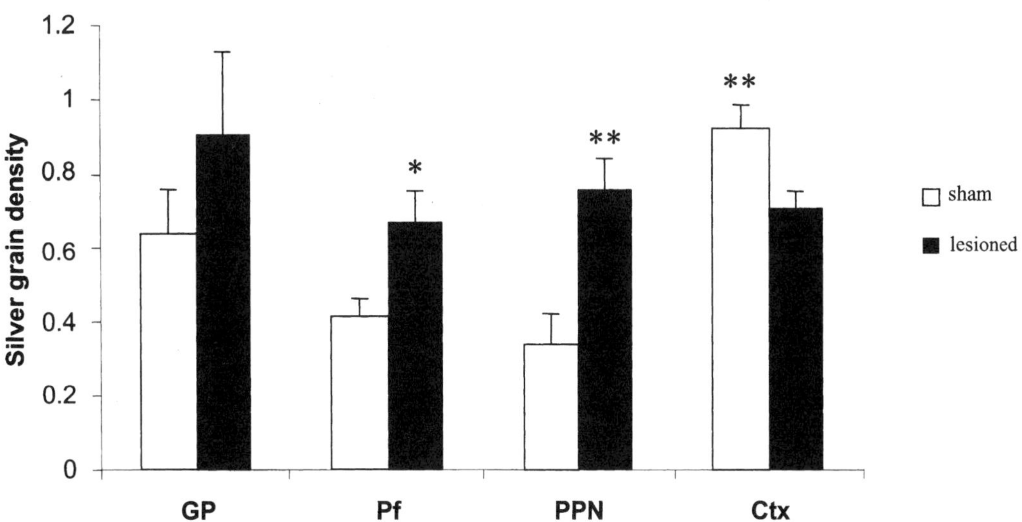

FIGURE 3.1. Levels of cytochrome oxidase first subunit (COI) expression in afferent neurons to the subthalamic nucleus after dopaminergic denervation. COI messenger RNA is estimated by *in situ* hybridization and expressed by silver grain density (grains per micrometer) over neuronal cell bodies. (Ctx, cerebral cortex; GP, globus pallidus; Pf, parafascicular nucleus of the thalamus; PPN, pedunculopontine nucleus. Values represent mean ± SEM; *t* test, $^{*}p < .05$; $^{**}p < .01$.)

peractive and others hypoactive. This complex regulation of STN activity, which also includes the inhibitory afferent fibers arising in the GPe, may account not only for the change in the activity of subthalamic neurons after dopaminergic nigrostriatal pathway degeneration, and in particular for the mean increased firing rate, but also for the changes in the firing pattern of STN neurons (26,29). Indeed, after nigrostriatal denervation, the firing pattern of subthalamic neurons changes from a regular pattern of firing to a bursting activity. In this context, the excitatory influence may account for the bursting activity, whereas the inhibitory influences may account for the pauses. In summary, it is very likely that thalamic and pedunculopontine afferents to the STN play a major role in its hyperactivity. This suggests that a manipulation of glutamate receptors using specific antagonists may represent a therapeutic strategy to alleviate the clinical manifestation of PD. Interestingly, glutamate antagonists acting either on *N*-methyl-D-aspartate (NMDA) receptors (MK-801) or on AMPA receptors (LY 293558) have been shown, when injected systemically, to correct the hyperactivity of STN neurons after dopamine depletion (30). Nevertheless, in these experiments, AMPA receptor antagonists were more potent than NMDA antagonists, suggesting that hyperactive glutamate afferent fibers to STN neurons very likely act on AMPA receptors. Nevertheless, the concept of manipulating AMPA receptors in PD should be treated with caution. AMPA receptors are also expressed in other brain areas and their inhibition may give rise to side effects. Taken as a whole, the data reviewed here indicate that the loss of dopaminergic neurons in the mesencephalon induces profound changes in nondopaminergic neuronal circuits and that these changes definitely play a major role in the symptomatology of the disease. Yet, as discussed in the next paragraph, alterations of nondopaminergic neurons are also involved in the lack of responsiveness to dopamine-replacement therapy in some patients.

NONDOPAMINERGIC NEURONS ARE INVOLVED IN THE LACK OF REACTIVITY TO DOPAMINE-REPLACEMENT THERAPY IN PARKINSONISM

The most commonly used treatment of PD is levodopa, the precursor of dopamine, which restores dopamine concentrations in the brain. More recently, the use of dopamine agonists, which also stimulate dopamine receptors, has been introduced as a therapeutic tool for PD (31). Yet dopamine-replacement therapy is not always effective. In some patients, dopamine-replacement therapy is never effective or loses its efficacy during the course of the disease, whereas other patients are poor responders to this treatment but only during fixed periods each day. In this section, we discuss successively the involvement of nondopaminergic neurons in the long-term and short-term lack of therapeutic reactivity.

Some patients with idiopathic parkinsonism (IP) after a long-term evolution and patients with parkinsonian syndromes such as multiple system atrophy, striatonigral degeneration, and progressive supranuclear palsy respond poorly to dopamine-replacement therapy (32). This lack of long-term efficacy of levodopa or dopamine agonists is very likely due to an alteration of nondopaminergic neurons located downstream to the lesioned dopamine neurons in the neuronal circuitry linking dopaminergic neurons to peripheral effectors of the altered behaviors. Indeed, neuropathological and biochemical studies have reported major lesions of nondopaminergic neurons in parkinsonian syndromes (33,34). For instance, in striatonigral degeneration, GABAergic striatal neurons bearing dopamine receptors degenerate, explaining why dopamine-replacement therapy is not effective in this disease (34). In progressive supranuclear palsy, these striatal GABAergic neurons are relatively preserved, but other striatal neurons degenerate. Indeed, a loss of large cholinergic interneurons bearing D_2 receptors has been reported in the striatum in this disease (35). Furthermore, alterations of neurons located downstream to the striatal neurons in the basal ganglia circuitry have also been reported, because neurofibrillary tangles, the neuropathological hallmark of progressive supranuclear palsy, have been observed in neurons of the STN and the pallidal complex (36). Thus, although the GABAergic neurons bearing dopamine receptors are preserved, dopamine-replacement therapy is not effective because lesions located in series downstream to the dopamine-sensitive neurons are also observed. In this respect, a pharmacological treatment for patients would be extremely difficult to develop. Any such developments would first require careful analysis of the distribution of lesions, then excellent knowledge of the neuronal circuitry, and identification of specific receptors for the neurotransmitter on neurons downstream to the lesions. In the aforementioned diseases, in which lesions are widespread, it seems very unlikely that such specific receptors could be found to develop pharmacological treatments for patients. This probably explains the current lack of effective symptomatic treatment of parkinsonian syndromes displaying a complex distribution of lesions.

The irreversible neuronal lesions mentioned probably account for the long-term absence of effects of dopamine-replacement therapy in some complex forms of parkinsonism. They also account for the progressive loss of effectiveness of dopamine-replacement therapy with the evolution of the disease in IP. Yet, even in patients with IP and with pure dopaminergic lesions, dopamine-replacement therapy is not always effective over time. Indeed, some patients suffer from motor fluctuations with an alternation of "on phases," during which levodopa or dopamine agonists are active and alleviate the clinical manifestation of the disease, and "off phases," during which the treatment is less effective and patients suffer from akinesia and rigidity (37). The pathophysiology of these motor fluctuations is still poorly understood. They may be related to the mode of administration of levodopa, as reported in animal experiments. Thus, Marsden and Obeso (38) showed that fluctuations were less pronounced when levodopa was administered by continuous intracerebral injection than when the medication was given orally. This suggests that on-off phenomena may be the consequence of a lack of constant efficacy of intracerebral dopamine over time. Such a consequence may be the result of variability in striatal dopamine levels when levodopa is administered orally, related in some way to the pharmacokinetics of the compound. However, in some cases, off periods persist despite steady plasma levels of levodopa and dopamine agonists, suggesting a failure in the ability of dopamine receptors to elicit an appropriate motor response when they are stimulated. Furthermore, an alteration of dopamine receptors may also explain the progressive loss of efficacy in levodopa treatment during the evolution of the disease (39).

The receptors for dopamine and other neurotransmitters are generally located predominantly at the surface of the cytoplasmic membrane of postsynaptic neurons. However, recent data demonstrate that *in vivo,* the acute activation of dopamine receptors by direct agonist or endogenously released dopamine provokes a dramatic modification of their subcellular distribution in neurons including internalization in the cytoplasm (40). The modification of the subcellular distribution of the receptors may play a key role in the physiology of striatal nondopaminergic neurons by changing the receptor availability and, thus, neurotransmitter efficiency. In line with this, using a full D_1 agonist, Dumartin et al. (40) showed that the activation of the D_1 receptor evoked its internalization in the striatum. This modified localization of the D_1 receptors was maximal between 20 and 40 minutes after intraperitoneal injection of the D_1 agonist but was still visible 90 minutes later, although it was less pronounced. Four hours after the injection, D_1 receptor localization was identical to that seen in uninjected animals. More recently, using the same D_1 agonist, we showed in rats with a unilateral lesion of the substantia nigra induced by 6-hydroxydopamine that D_1 receptor internalization was not affected

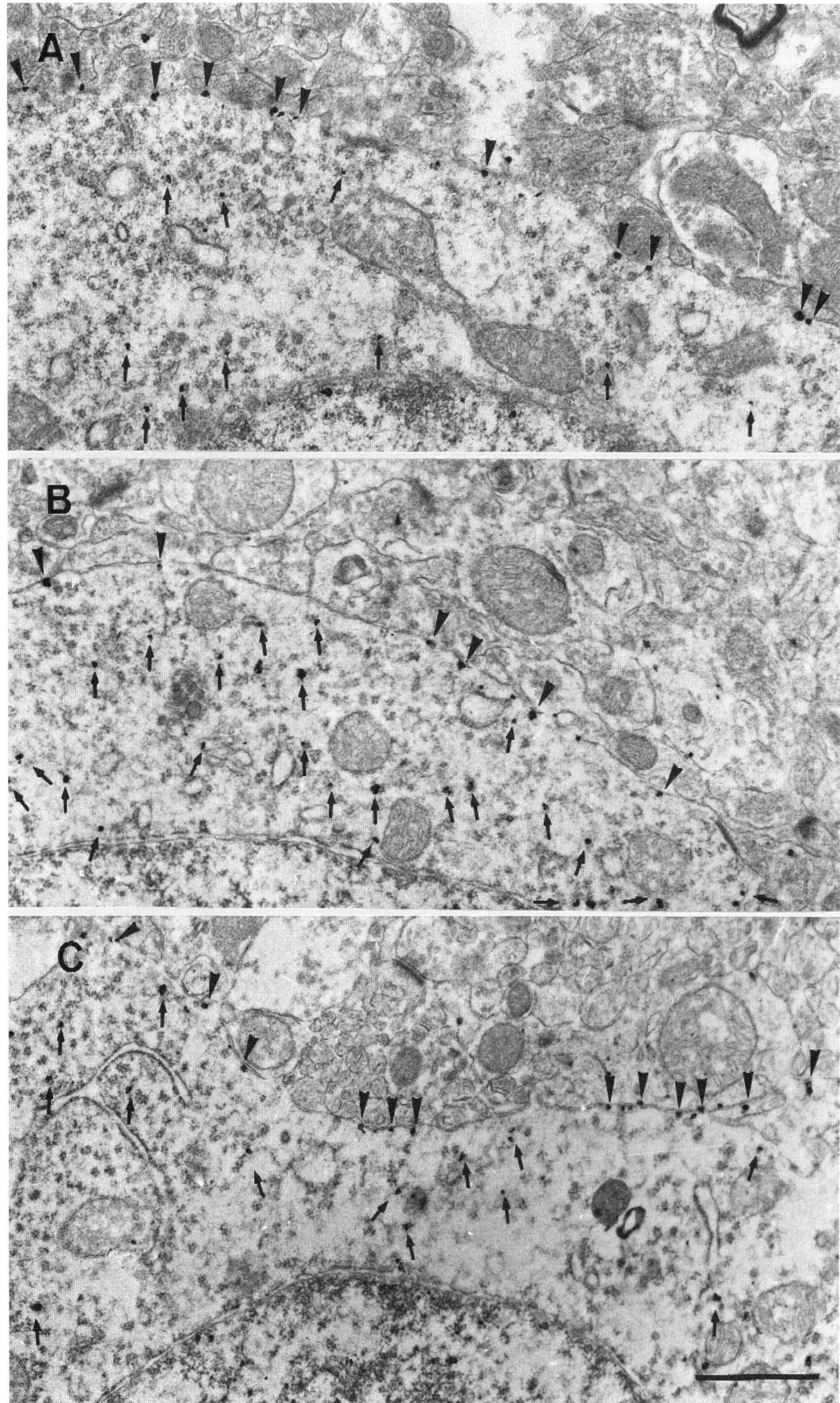

FIGURE 3.2. D_1 dopamine receptor immunoreactivity at the ultrastructural level in striatal neurons of rats treated by a single intraperitoneal injection of saline **(A)**, levodopa **(B)**, or ropinirole **(C)** and sacrificed 40 minutes after this treatment. Shown are staining (*arrowheads*) at the plasma membrane level and staining (*arrows*) in the cytoplasm. Note the concomitant decrease in staining in the cytoplasm seen in the levodopa-treated animals compared with the saline- or ropinirole-treated animals. Bar indicates 1 μm.

by the nigrostriatal denervation (39). As expected from the data obtained in this experimental model of PD, an internalization of D_1 receptors was also observed at postmortem examination in patients with PD treated with levodopa, suggesting that levodopa is also able to elicit D_1 receptor internalization (39). Whether other dopamine agonists such as ropinirole can also induce internalization of D_1 receptors in the striatum has also been analyzed in the same experimental models of the disease. The data show that in contrast to animals receiving levodopa injection, animals treated with ropinirole did not display an internalization of D_1 receptors (Fig. 3.2) (41). This result is likely explained by the fact that ropinirole binds to non-D_1 receptors, whereas levodopa, which increases dopamine levels indirectly, acts on both D_1 and D_2 receptors (43). These data suggest that ropinirole is consequently less likely to desensitize D_1 receptors than levodopa and thus to reduce the efficacy of the treatment. Taken together, these data indicate that changes in dopamine receptor localization on nondopaminergic neurons may be involved in the short-term desensitization and the consequent loss of therapeutic effect over short periods. Various mechanisms have been proposed to try to account for the desensitization of G-protein–coupled receptors. This desensitization involves phosphorylation of the receptors by a member of the G-protein–coupled receptor kinase family, leading to the binding of an arrestig-like protein and ultimately resulting in uncoupling of the receptor from its cognate G protein and decreased functional activity (44,45). The binding of the arrestig molecule also promotes internalization of the receptor through clathrin-coated pits into an endosomal compartment, where it may be dephosphorylated by a G-protein–coupled receptor phosphatase and recycled to the cell surface or degraded via a lysosomal pathway. The whole process of receptor internalization and reintegration into the plasma membrane takes place within a few hours and may thus account for the short-term loss of efficacy of the treatment in PD.

In summary, nondopaminergic neurons are probably involved in both long-term and short-term loss of efficacy of dopamine-replacement therapy. On the one hand, a loss of nondopaminergic neurons in the neuronal circuits linking the postsynaptic neurons bearing dopamine receptors and the effector of the altered behaviors may account for the long-term loss of treatment efficacy. On the other hand, plastic changes involving dopamine receptors and their desensitization may be involved in the short-term loss of treatment efficacy, but other functional changes in the basal ganglia circuitry, mentioned above, may also participate in this phenomenon.

CONCLUSIONS

Nondopaminergic neurons play a major role in the pathophysiology of PD. They are obviously involved in the nondopaminergic responsive symptoms of the disease, which occur at endstage PD. Nevertheless, they also represent potential therapeutic targets because nondopaminergic neurons display activity changes as a consequence of dopaminergic lesions. Restoration of the normal function of nondopaminergic neurons, thus, represents an interesting therapeutic approach. In line with this, one of the most potent therapeutic strategies involving nondopaminergic neurons is deep brain stimulation of the glutamatergic neurons of the STN. A careful analysis of the functional changes induced by the dopamine denervation in as yet unanalyzed brain regions may help to identify new surgical or pharmacological targets for the disease.

REFERENCES

1. Jellinger KA. Post mortem studies in Parkinson's disease—is it possible to detect brain areas for specific symptoms? *J Neural Transm* 1999;56[Suppl]:1–29.
2. Hirsch EC, Graybiel AM, Agid Y. Melanized dopaminergic neurons are differentially susceptible to degeneration in Parkinson's disease. *Nature* 1988;334:345–348.
3. Agid Y, Javoy-Agid F, Ruberg M. Biochemistry of neurotransmitters in Parkinson's disease. In: Marsden CD, Fahn S, eds. *Movement disorders,* 2nd ed. Butterworth, 1987:166–230.
4. Javoy-Agid F, Ruberg M, Taquet H, et al. Biochemical neuropathology of Parkinson's disease. *Adv Neurol* 1984;40:189–198.

5. Agid Y, Cervera P, Hirsch EC, et al. Biochemistry of Parkinson's disease 28 years later: a critical review. *Mov Disord* 1989;4:126–144.
6. Albin RL, Young AB, Penney JB. The functional anatomy of disorders of the basal ganglia. *Trends Neurosci* 1995;18:63–64.
7. Alexander GE, Crutcher MD. Functional architecture of basal ganglia circuits: neural substrates of parallel processing. *Trends Neurosci* 1990;13:266–271.
8. Albin RL, Young AB, Penney JB. The functional anatomy of basal ganglia disorders. *Trends Neurosci* 1989;12:366–375.
9. DeLong MR. Primate models of movement disorders of basal ganglia origin. *Trends Neurosci* 1990;13:281–285.
10. Filion M, Tremblay L. Abnormal spontaneous activity of globus pallidus neurons in monkeys with MPTP-induced parkinsonism. *Brain Res* 1991;547:142–151.
11. Levy R, Hazrati LN, Herrero MT, et al. Re-evaluation of the functional anatomy of the basal ganglia in normal and parkinsonian states. *Neuroscience* 1997;76:335–343.
12. Obeso JA, Rodriguez MC, DeLong MR. Basal ganglia pathophysiology: a critical review. In: Obeso JA, DeLong MR, Ohye C, et al, eds. *The basal ganglia and new surgical approaches for Parkinson's disease.* Philadelphia: Lippincott–Raven Publishers, 1997:3–18.
13. Parent A, Cicchetti F. The current model of basal ganglia organization under scrutiny. *Mov Disord* 1998;13: 199–202.
14. Boraud T, Bezard E, Guehl D, et al. Effects of L-DOPA on neuronal activity of the globus pallidus externalis (GPe) and globus pallidus internalis (GPi) in the MPTP-treated monkey. *Brain Res* 1998;787:157–160.
15. Hirsch EC, Perier C, Orieux G, et al. Metabolic effects of nigrostriatal denervation in basal ganglia. *Trends Neurosci* 2000;23[Suppl]:S78–S85.
16. Herrero MT, Levy R, Ruberg M, et al. Glutamic acid decarboxylase mRNA expression in medial and lateral pallidal neurons in the MPTP-treated monkey and patients with Parkinson's disease. *Adv Neurol* 1996;69: 209–216.
17. Herrero MT, Levy R, Ruberg M, et al. Consequences of nigrostriatal denervation and L-dopa therapy on the expression of the glutamic acid decarboxylase messenger RNA in the pallidum. *Neurology* 1996;47:219–224.
18. Soghomonian JJ, Chesselet MF. Effects of nigrostriatal lesions on the levels of messenger RNAs encoding two isoforms of glutamate decarboxylase in the globus pallidus and entopeduncular nucleus of the rat. *Synapse* 1992;11:124–133.
19. Soghomonian JJ, Pedneault S, Audet G, et al. Increased glutamate decarboxylase mRNA levels in the striatum and pallidum of MPTP-treated primates. *J Neurosci* 1994;14:6256–6265.
20. Vila M, Levy R, Herrero MT, et al. Consequences of nigrostriatal denervation on the functioning of the basal ganglia in human and nonhuman primates: an in situ hybridization study of cytochrome oxidase subunit I mRNA. *J Neurosci* 1997;17:765–773.
21. Mitchell IJ, Clarke CE, Boyce S, et al. Neural mechanisms underlying parkinsonian symptoms based upon regional uptake of 2-deoxyglucose in monkeys exposed to 1-methyl-4 phenyl-1,2,3,6-tetrahydropyridine. *Neuroscience* 1989;32:213–226.
22. Porrino LJ, Burns RS, Crane AM, et al. Changes in local cerebral glucose utilization associated with Parkinson's syndrome induced by 1-methyl-4-phenyl-1,2,3,6-tetrahydropyridine (MPTP) in the primate. *Life Sci* 1987;40:1657–1664.
23. Porrino LJ, Burns RS, Crane AM, et al. Local cerebral metabolic effects of L-dopa therapy in 1-methyl-4-phenyl-1,2,3,6-tetrahydropyridine–induced parkinsonism in monkeys. *Proc Natl Acad Sci USA* 1987;84: 5995–5999.
24. Sokoloff L, Reivich M, Kennedy C, et al. The [^{14}C]deoxyglucose method for the measurement of local cerebral glucose utilization: theory, procedure, and normal values in the conscious and anesthetized albino rat. *J Neurochem* 1977;28:897–916.
25. Nambu A, Tokuno H, Hamada I, et al. Excitatory cortical inputs to pallidal neurons via the subthalamic nucleus in the monkey. *J Neurophysiol* 2000;84: 289–300.
26. Hassani OK, Mouroux M, Féger J. Increased subthalamic neuronal activity after nigral dopaminergic lesion independent of disinhibition via the globus pallidus. *Neuroscience* 1996;72:105–115.
27. Orieux G, Francois C, Féger J, et al. Metabolic activity of excitatory parafascicular and pedunculopontine inputs to the subthalamic nucleus in a rat model of Parkinson's disease. *Neuroscience* 2000;97:79–88.
28. Orieux G, Francois C, Feger J, et al. Activité métabolique de la voie cortico-subthalamique dans un modèle animal de la maladie de Parkinson, provoqué par une lésion unilatérale de la substantia nigra pars compacta chez le rat. 5e Colloque de la Société des Neurosciences, Toulouse, France, 28–31, 2001.
29. Vila M, Perier C, Féger J, et al. Evolution of changes in neuronal activity in the subthalamic nucleus of rats with unilateral lesion of the substantia nigra assessed by metabolic and electrophysiological measurements. *Eur J Neurosci* 2000;12:337–344.
30. Vila M, Marin C, Ruberg M, et al. Systemic administration of NMDA and AMPA receptor antagonists reverses the neurochemical changes induced by nigrostriatal denervation in basal ganglia. *J Neurochem* 1999;73: 344–352.
31. Olanow CW, Jenner P, Brooks D. Dopamine agonists and neuroprotection in Parkinson's disease. *Ann Neurol* 1998;44[Suppl 1]:S167–S174.
32. Agid Y, Graybiel AM, Ruberg M, et al. The efficacy of levodopa treatment declines in the course of Parkinson's disease: do nondopaminergic lesions play a role? *Adv Neurol* 1990;53:83–100.
33. Feany MB, Mattiace LA, Dickson DW. Neuropathologic overlap of progressive supranuclear palsy, Pick's disease and corticobasal degeneration. *J Neuropathol Exp Neurol* 1996;55:53–67.
34. Gibb WR. Neuropathology of Parkinson's disease and related syndromes. *Neurol Clin* 1992;10:361–376.
35. Hirsch EC, Graybiel AM, Hersh LB, et al. Striosomes and extrastriosomal matrix contain different amounts of immunoreactive choline acetyltransferase in the human striatum. *Neurosci Lett* 1989;96:145–150.
36. Hauw JJ, Daniel SE, Dickson D, et al. Preliminary NINDS neuropathologic criteria for Steele–Richardson–Olszewski syndrome (progressive supranuclear palsy). *Neurology* 1994;44:2015–2019.
37. Marsden CD. Problems with long-term levodopa therapy for Parkinson's disease. *Clin Neuropharmacol* 1994;17:S32–S44.

38. Marsden CD, Obeso JA. The functions of the basal ganglia and the paradox of stereotaxic surgery in Parkinson's disease. *Brain* 1994;117:877–897.
39. Muriel MP, Bernard V, Levey AI, et al. L-Dopa induces a cytoplasmic localization of D_1 dopamine receptors in striatal neurons in Parkinson's disease. *Ann Neurol* 1999;46:103–111.
40. Dumartin B, Caille I, Ganon F, et al. Internalization of D_1 dopamine receptor in striatal neurons *in vivo* as evidence of activation by dopamine agonists. *J Neurosci* 1998;18:1650–1661.
41. Muriel MP, Orieux G, Hirsch EC. Levodopa but not ropinirole induces an internalization of D_1 dopamine receptors in parkinsonian rats. *Mov Disord* 2002 (in press).
42. Hassani OK, Mouroux M, Féger J. Increased subthalamic neuronal activity after nigral dopaminergic lesion independent of disinhibition via the globus pallidus. *Neuroscience* 1996;72:105–115.
43. Coldwell MC, Boyfield I, Brown T, et al. Comparison of the functional potencies of ropinirole and other dopamine receptor agonists at human D_2(long), D_3 and D_4 receptors expressed in Chinese hamster ovary cells. *Br J Pharmacol* 1999;127:1696–1702.
44. Pitcher JA, Payne ES, Csortos C, et al. The G-protein–coupled receptor phosphatase: a protein phosphatase type 2A with a distinct subcellular distribution and substrate specificity. *Proc Natl Acad Sci USA* 1995; 92:8343–8347.
45. Gardner B, Liu ZF, Jiang D, et al. The role of phosphorylation/ dephosphorylation in agonist-induced desensitization of D_1 dopamine receptor function: evidence for a novel pathway for receptor dephosphorylation. *Mol Pharmacol* 2001;59:310–321.

Parkinson's Disease: Advances in Neurology, Vol. 91.
Edited by Ariel Gordin, Seppo Kaakkola, and Heikki Teräväinen
Lippincott Williams & Wilkins, Philadelphia © 2003

4

Biochemistry of Parkinson's Disease: Is a Brain Serotonergic Deficiency a Characteristic of Idiopathic Parkinson's Disease?

Stephen J. Kish

Human Neurochemical Pathology Section, Centre for Addiction and Mental Health, Toronto, Ontario, Canada

The major objective of this chapter is to evaluate the strength of the evidence that a brain serotonergic deficiency might be a characteristic of idiopathic Parkinson's disease (PD). The significance of this is related to the possibility that this nondopaminergic change might explain some of the clinically significant disturbances reported in some patients with PD.

COULD A BRAIN SEROTONERGIC DEFICIENCY EXPLAIN SOME OF THE NONMOTOR DISTURBANCES IN PD?

The observations in PD showing that degeneration of brain dopaminergic neurons is the fundamental characteristic of both PD (1,2) and parkinsonism caused by a dopaminergic neurotoxin methylphenyltetrahydropyridine (MPTP) (3) and that human parkinsonism can be reversed by levodopa (2,4) have established unequivocally the role of nigrostriatal dopamine in this movement disorder.

However, in addition to the classic signs of the parkinsonian motor abnormalities (e.g., bradykinesia, rigidity, tremor, and postural instability), it is now recognized that some patients with this condition suffer from various nonmotor difficulties, including depression and cognitive impairment (5–7). Furthermore, it is now argued that for many patients, these nonmotor problems can have a much greater negative impact on quality of life than the motor impairment. Thus, Schrag et al. (8) confirmed the general impression of many neurologists by demonstrating that in addition to postural instability, two nonmotor problems, namely depression and cognitive impairment, appeared to have the greatest impact on quality of life in patients with PD. Significantly, the strongest predictor of quality of life in patients with PD was not the motor disability, but the presence of depression (8), which is assumed to be present in approximately 40% of patients with PD (7).

In principle, the nonmotor difficulties in PD could be explained by the primary dopaminergic disturbance. Because the caudate nucleus and the nucleus accumbens/ventral striatum, by virtue of their anatomical connections to specific cerebral cortical subdivisions, are considered to subserve aspects of cognition and mood, respectively (9,10), the memory and mood abnormalities in some patients with PD could be explained by degeneration of dopaminergic neurons to these brain areas.

However, the lack of correlation between depression and the severity of the motor disturbances, as well as the unresolved issue of the ability of dopaminergic therapy to ameliorate depression in PD (7), suggests that parkinsonian depression might not be simply an expected reaction to a chronic brain disorder and is not explained by the primary striatal dopamine deficiency. Similarly, the failure of dopaminergic therapy to completely normalize cognition in early PD (11) suggests that part of the cognitive difficulties in PD might have a nondopaminergic basis. As discussed below, an unproven hypothesis is that these "secondary" disturbances could be consequent to a brain serotonergic deficiency.

In human brain, serotonergic neurons originate in the lower brainstem in raphe nuclei, including the dorsal and median nuclei, and project to all regions of the brain (12). Pharmacological studies in humans have suggested a biological role for the brain serotonin system in regulation of such biological processes as mood, cognition, sleep, and appetite (13). However, despite much investigation, no human behavioral disorder has yet been described in which the etiological involvement of the brain serotonin system is established. To date, damage to serotonergic neurons has been reported in the brains of some patients with Alzheimer's disease (14–17) and in some chronic users of alcohol (18,19)—two disorders characterized by regionally widespread brain pathology. The objective here is to assess the strength of the evidence, involving examination of postmortem and living brain, that PD represents a state of decreased brain serotonergic neuron concentration.

REVIEW OF DATA ON SEROTONIN AND PD

Neuropathological and neurochemical studies suggest degeneration of entire brain serotonergic neurons in at least a subgroup of patients with clinically advanced PD. The finding of a decreased number of brain dopaminergic neurons in PD has been convincingly established by neuropathological procedures, involving measurement of concentration of cell bodies of dopaminergic neurons in the substantia nigra and by biochemical procedures in postmortem and living brain employing neurochemical "markers" of neuronal integrity at nerve terminal areas in the striatum (caudate, putamen, nucleus accumbens). These neurochemical markers include dopamine itself, its biosynthetic enzymes tyrosine hydroxylase, dopa decarboxylase, and the dopamine transporter. Although the status of the brain serotonin system in PD has been much less intensively studied, compared with that of the dopamine system, the available data, primarily derived from postmortem brain findings, strongly suggest that a moderate (approximately 40%) loss of serotonergic neurons originating in the raphe area of the lower brainstem occurs in at least a subgroup of patients with the advanced disorder.

Postmortem Brain Biochemical Data

In 1961, Bernheimer et al. (20) first reported a moderate reduction in brain serotonin (44% to 63%) in autopsied brain of patients with PD. Since then, postmortem neurochemical studies of patients with PD have employed three serotonergic markers to assess the integrity of the brain serotonin system in this disorder: serotonin (20–26), the rate-limiting biosynthetic enzyme tryptophan hydroxylase (27), and the serotonin transporter (SERT) as assessed by radioligand binding (24,25,28). As shown in Table 4.1, the results of the biochemical postmortem studies of serotonin markers in PD are, in general, consistent with the early study by Bernheimer et al. (20). Thus, levels of all the serotonergic markers are generally moderately reduced (i.e., not as severe as the striatal dopamine reduction) and with a sufficient variation in the magnitude of the reduction, so many patients with PD fall within the normal control range. This is in contrast with the dopamine reduction in PD, in which no overlap exists between the range of dopamine values in the putamen of patients with PD versus that of healthy subjects (26,29).

Examination of the postmortem neurochemical data of Wilson et al. (26) revealed that in the caudate of patients with PD, mean serotonin and dopamine levels were similarly

TABLE 4.1. *Neurochemical postmortem studies of brain serotonin markers in patients with idiopathic Parkinson's disease*

Reference	No. of patients	Brain areas	Serotonergic marker	Mean % change vs. controls	Comments
Bernheimer et al., 1961 (20)	4–6	Striatum, diencephalon, substantia nigra	Serotonin	44–63%	
Fahn et al., 1971 (21)	2	Five striatal subdivisions	Serotonin	9–85%	
Rinne et al., 1974 (22)	3–5	Striatum, hypothalamus, substantia nigra, cerebral cortex	Serotonin	No change in L-dopa–treated subjects	Although not explicitly stated, there is probably no statistically significant serotonin reduction in drug-naive patients with PD
Scatton et al., 1983 (23)	10	Caudate, cerebral and hippocampal cortices, hippocampus	Serotonin	5–57%	No L-dopa for at least 4 days before death
Scatton et al., 1983 (23)	9	Same regions	Serotonin	38–51%	L-dopa received 0–24 hr before death
Raisman et al., 1986 (24)	15	Putamen	Serotonin	75%	
D'Amato et al., 1987 (25)	7	Frontal cortex	Serotonin	51%	
Wilson et al., 1996 (26)	12	Caudate, putamen	Serotonin	65% (caudate), 50% (putamen)	Mean dopamine loss in same subjects was 64% (caudate) and 95% (putamen)
Sawada et al., 1985 (27)	1–3	Striatum, diencephalon, substantia nigra, "raphe nucleus"	Tryptophan hydroxylase activity	No change to 78% (thalamus)	Authors acknowledge high variations of enzyme activity in normal human brain
Raisman et al., 1986 (24)	15	Putamen	SERT (^{3}H-imipramine binding; ^{3}H-paroxetine binding)	25%; 30%	
D'Amato et al., 1987 (25)	7	Frontal cortex	SERT (^{3}H-citalopram binding)	37%	
Chinaglia et al., 1993 (28)	4–10	Regionally subdivided striatum, globus pallidus, substantia nigra, cerebral cortex, claustrum	SERT (^{3}H-citalopram binding by autoradiography)	42–75%	Most regionally comprehensive study of SERT in PD
Chinaglia et al., 1993 (28)	2–5	Raphe nuclei	SERT (^{3}H-citalopram binding by autoradiography)	No change	Why is SERT decreased in nerve terminal regions but not in raphe nuclei?

PD, Parkinson's disease; SERT, serotonin transporter.

reduced (64% to 65%), whereas in the putamen, serotonin concentrations were only moderately decreased (50%) and dopamine levels were strikingly reduced by 95%. Nevertheless, a correlational analysis (Pearson) between striatal serotonin and dopamine levels in the patients with PD disclosed a modest positive correlation between levels of the two neurotransmitters, which was statistically significant for the putamen (caudate, $r = 0.48$, $p = .12$; putamen, $r = 0.63$, $p = .03$). Taken together, these neurochemical data suggest that the degeneration of dopaminergic and serotonergic neurons in PD might be, to a limited extent, related.

Interestingly, in an autoradiographic investigation, although SERT levels were found, as expected, to be decreased in most of the examined brain regions of patients with PD, concentrations of the transporter were distinctly normal in the raphe nuclei (28). This suggests either that in the subjects examined in this postmortem investigation, there might have been loss of nerve endings without cell body loss or that cell body loss had occurred but with upregulation of SERT in the remaining cells (30–32).

Postmortem Brain Morphological Data

To date, the integrity of raphe cell bodies in PD has been investigated by morphological procedures in some neuropathological studies (25,27,30,31,33–36) in which assessment was made by either qualitative or quantitative cell-counting procedures. Although this information is not available from most of the studies described below, it is reasonable to suggest that most of the examined subjects in the postmortem investigations had clinically advanced and/or endstage PD. As shown in Table 4.2, the extent of raphe cell loss in PD is highly variable among different investigations and, for some of the investigations, within the group of patients with PD.

In terms of the use of a quantitative cell-counting procedure and a representative number of patients examined, the most definitive data are those of two studies by Jellinger (34,36), who provided individual values for both the patients with PD and the control subjects. Examination of these values (see Fig. 3 in reference 34) reveals that on average, the loss of cell bodies in the dorsal raphe, about 40%, is less than that of substantia nigra dopamine cell bodies (see below). Although all of the PD values for dorsal raphe cell number and density fell below the mean value of the controls, about one third of the PD values fell within the control range. This indicates that a below-normal raphe cell number is not a characteristic of all patients with PD, a finding that might explain the failure of some investigators (Table 4.2) to demonstrate raphe cell loss in all patients with PD, particularly when employing a small sample size.

In a follow-up investigation, Paulus and Jellinger (36) provided the first evidence based on direct examination of human brain that depression in PD might be caused by degeneration of raphe serotonergic neurons. Thus, examination of Table 1 in reference 36 reveals that dorsal raphe cell loss in patients with PD who had some history of depression (44%) was more marked than that of patients who did not have a history of depression (24%). In the patients with PD as a group, the magnitude of raphe cell loss was much less than that of dopaminergic medial (60%) or lateral (67%) substantia nigra cell bodies. Although it is reasonable to suggest that brain serotonergic damage should worsen with the progression of the disease, it is an ongoing question whether degeneration of nigral dopamine and raphe serotonin neurons are (e.g., etiologically) related. Using the values in Table 1 in reference 36, comparison of the extent of loss of cell density of dorsal raphe neurons versus cell density of medial and lateral substantia nigra (dopaminergic) neurons in the patients with PD revealed no statistically significant correlation (by either Pearson or Spearman rank) between the serotonergic and dopaminergic indices (range, $r = 0.03$ to 0.21; $p > .05$). This suggests that the time course, and more speculatively etiological process, of serotonergic and dopaminergic damage in PD might be different. The neu-

TABLE 4.2. *Neuropathological postmortem studies of raphe nuclei in patients with idiopathic Parkinson's disease*

Reference	No. of patients	Brain areas	Index	Change in patients with PD vs. controls	Comments
Mann and Yates, 1983 (33)	8	Dorsal raphe	Cell number	"No obvious loss of nerve cells" Occasional cells contained "eosinophilic inclusions similar to Lewy bodies"	Qualitative (vs. quantitative) assessment of neuronal loss
Sawada et al., 1985 (27)	4	Dorsal raphe	Cell number, presence of Lewy bodies	Slight cell loss in one of four patients; Lewy bodies in three of four patients	Semiquantitative
Jellinger, 1986 (34)	28	Dorsal raphe	Cell number, cell density	42% loss (calculated from Fig 4.3)	Quantitative study of largest number of patients with PD
D'Amato et al., 1987 (25)	4	Dorsal and central superior raphe	Cell number	Some neuronal loss	Qualitative
Zweig et al., 1989 (35)	4	Dorsal raphe	Cell number	No cell loss in two patients moderate cell loss in two patients	Semiquantitative
Halliday et al., 1990 (30)	8	Dorsal raphe, median raphe	Density of phenylalanine hydroxylase–positive cells	No cell loss in dorsal raphe; 56% loss in median raphe	Quantitative; dorsal and median raphe data also presented in Halliday et al., 1990 (31)
Halliday et al., 1990 (31)	8	Raphe obscurus (dorsal and medial raphe from above)	Density of phenylalanine hydroxylase–positive cells	44% cell loss; positive for Lewy bodies in dorsal and median raphe and in raphe obscurus	Quantitative
Paulus and Jellinger, 1991 (36)	9 nondepressed 12 depressed	Dorsal raphe	Cell density	24% cell loss in nondepressed patients; 44% cell loss in depressed patients	Quantitative

PD, Parkinson's disease.

ropathological analyses by Jellinger (34) of PD also disclosed a moderate (approximately 35% to 50%) loss of (presumably) cholinergic neurons originating in the nucleus basalis brain area in the nondemented patients with PD. Because the nucleus basalis cholinergic system is considered to subserve aspects of cognition (particularly attention) (37,38), the possibility has to be considered that any cognitive deficits observed in PD could, in principle, be due to dopaminergic, serotonergic, or cholinergic disturbances.

Taken together, the postmortem brain neurochemical and neuropathological data in PD suggest a mild to moderate loss of raphe serotonergic neurons (both cell bodies and axonal endings), at least in patients with endstage PD, but with some patients clearly having levels falling within the range of the controls.

Neuroimaging Data

As shown in Table 4.3, published data on measurement of SERT by neuroimaging in the living brain of patients with PD are limited to four studies employing the radioligand ^{123}I-β-CIT by single-photon emission computed tomography (SPECT) (32,39–41). The advantage of neuroimaging (vs. postmortem) investigations is that measurement of a brain serotonin marker with clinical correlations can easily be made early in the course of the disorder and as the disease progresses. It is reasonable to assume that none of the examined patients with PD in the neuroimaging studies were severely affected by the disorder, as was likely the case in most of the postmortem brain investigations. Excluding the early study in which the extent of the reduction in "hypothalamus midbrain" of the two patients examined was not quantitated (39) and the investigation in which no control group was employed (32), the ^{123}I-β-CIT SPECT data, limited only to early stage PD, suggest that SERT in diencephalon, midbrain, and cerebral cortex is either normal or only slightly reduced in the midbrain/thalamus of patients with PD early in the course of the disorder. The major limitation of the SPECT data, however, is the use of a radioligand (^{123}I-β-CIT) that binds not only to SERT, but also to the dopamine and noradrenaline transporters. This uncertainty regarding the validity of ^{123}I-β-CIT for SERT measurement in human brain is acknowledged by most investigators who employ this nonselective radioligand in SPECT studies (42–46). Because of the lack of selectivity of ^{123}I-β-CIT for SERT, the radioligand is not routinely employed for measurement of SERT in areas of high dopamine transporter concentration such as the dopamine-rich striatum. SPECT data from Pirker et al. (47) show that high doses of the selective serotonin reuptake inhibitor (SSRI) citalopram displace only about 50% of binding of ^{123}I-β-CIT to brainstem and/or thalamus, thereby suggesting that a substantial proportion of ^{123}I-β-CIT is probably binding to non-SERTs and therefore should not be used for measurement of SERT in these brain areas. For similar reasons, it has been suggested that ^{123}I-β-CIT should not be used for measurement of SERT in areas of low SERT density, such as the cerebral cortex, in which the measurement might not be reliable or valid (45,48).

Notwithstanding these important methodological concerns, the findings that ^{123}I-β-CIT binding is either normal or reduced only slightly in the midbrain and/or thalamus of patients with early stage PD (40,41) tentatively suggest that there is likely to be no substantial loss of serotonin neurons early in the course of PD. However, because of the present uncertainty of ^{123}I-β-CIT binding as a valid estimate of SERT in regions in which there exist multiple monoamine neurotransmitter transporters, it would also appear reasonable to consider the results of all investigations employing this procedure to be uncertain.

Assessment of the integrity of raphe neurons in the lower brainstem of patients with PD has also been studied by transcranial sonography, in which echogenicity of raphe neurons (which are normally hyperechogenic) has been reported to be decreased in depressed patients but normal in nondepressed subjects (49). Although the results of this in-

TABLE 4.3. *Brain neuroimaging (SPECT, PET, Ultrasound) studies of serotonergic neurons in living patients with idiopathic Parkinson's disease*

Reference	No. of patients	Brain areas	Procedure	Change in patients with PD vs. controls	Comments
Brücke et al., 1993 (39)	2	Striatum, hypothalamus–midbrain	$^{123}I\beta$-CIT, SPECT	Mild to moderate reduction	Data are qualitative only; no quantitation of time–activity curve $^{123}I\beta$-CIT is not specific for SERT
Kim et al., 1997 (40)	45	Hypothalamus–midbrain	$^{123}I\beta$-CIT, SPECT	Slight, nonsignificant reduction	Abstract presentation Patients are at early stage (Hoehn–Yahr stages 1–3)
Kim et al., 1999 (32)	46	Hypothalamus–midbrain	$^{123}I\beta$-CIT, SPECT	No control group; no correlation with symptom severity	
Haapaniemi et al., 2001 (41)	27	Medial frontal cortex, midbrain, thalamus	$^{123}I\beta$-CIT, SPECT	No change to 9%	Drug-naive, early stage patients (Hoehn–Yahr 1–3)
Becker et al., 1997 (49)	30	"Brainstem raphe"	Transcranial sonography	Normal "raphe echogenicity" in nondepressed PD; decreased in depressed PD	How valid is "raphe echogenicity" as measure of integrity of raphe neurons?

PD, Parkinson's disease; PET, positron emission tomography; SERT, serotonin transporter; SPECT, single-photon emission computed tomography.

vestigation, which employed a novel probe for measurement of serotonin neuron integrity, are consistent with postmortem data, uncertainty regarding the validity of this approach for the accurate assessment of brainstem raphe nuclei and fiber tracts (which should comprise only a very small proportion of the total volume of the structure) makes the interpretation of the results of this interesting investigation somewhat uncertain.

DISCUSSION

A Moderate Brain Serotonin Deficiency Is Probably a Common Feature of Advanced PD

The available postmortem neurochemical and neuropathological brain data suggest that a moderate loss of serotonin neurons is probably a common, but not (unlike the striatal dopamine reduction) an obligatory feature of clinically advanced PD, with some patients having distinctly normal levels. Comparison of two studies (26,36) of the extent of the reduction in striatal raphe cell body number/striatal serotonin concentration versus loss of dopamine and nigral cellularity suggests that the extent of loss of serotonergic neurons in some regions in PD is much less (about one half) than that of dopamine neurons. The findings of no (36) or low (26) correlation between the extent of loss of serotonergic and dopaminergic markers, and particularly the observation that the extent of loss of serotonin (26) in the caudate nucleus and putamen are similar, whereas dopaminergic markers are much more severely decreased in the putamen (26,29), suggest that degeneration of serotonin and dopamine neurons might proceed to a significant extent independently in PD. Insufficient data are available to establish the brain regional extent of the serotonin neuronal loss, whether serotonergic nerve terminal loss precedes cell body degeneration or whether neuronal damage occurs in very early stage PD or is only a late event.

Does the Brain Serotonergic Deficiency in PD Explain any of the Nonmotor Problems in PD?

Because the brain serotonin system is involved in biological processes that are disturbed in some patients with PD (e.g., mood, cognition, sleep), the possibility suggests itself that some of these central nervous system disturbances are explained by degeneration of serotonin neurons in some patients. This issue will certainly be addressed and probably will be resolved to some extent, by measurement in clinically well-characterized patients with early and advanced PD of the status of brain presynaptic serotonergic markers by neuroimaging procedures. Although such studies will be confounded by the presence of a coexisting brain biochemical abnormality (dopaminergic, possibly cholinergic) and in advanced cases exposure to dopaminergic pharmacotherapy, brain serotonergic behavioral correlations in PD might also help to establish more conclusively the extent to which serotonin is involved in normal human behavior. It is also possible that important information on the involvement of the serotonin system in explaining nonmotor abnormalities in PD may be obtained through pharmacological approaches involving serotonergic agents (e.g., SSRIs), but only if these approaches involve a placebo-controlled clinical trial.

Finally, it must be emphasized that despite the quite obvious attraction of a "serotonergic hypothesis of secondary disturbances in PD," we must consider the perhaps more plausible hypothesis that a mild to moderate loss of serotonergic neurons in PD has no functional consequence, with the affective and cognitive disturbances explained entirely by the fundamental and near-total brain dopamine reduction.

Is the Prevalence of Clinically Significant Nonmotor Disturbances in PD Overestimated?

Because emerging data suggest that some nonmotor disturbances in PD, namely depression and cognitive deterioration, might actually affect the quality of life of the patient more than the primary motor disability, it is important to understand the cause of these clinical disturbances. However, it is equally important to establish whether these secondary disturbances are or are not highly prevalent and clinically significant in PD.

In the case of depression in PD, for example, it is generally assumed that approximately 40% of patients suffer from depression (7). Although it is beyond the scope of this chapter to assess the strength of the clinical data that such nonmotor disturbances commonly occur in PD, a reasonable case can be made that at least for "depression" in PD, the prevalence of an affective syndrome in this movement disorder, which would be recognized by a general psychiatrist as being clinically significant, is at least uncertain and may well be much lower than that implied by the literature. For example, in one of the few studies using a psychiatrist-administered Structured Clinical Interview for *Diagnostic and Statistical Manual of Mental Disorders,* fourth edition, a diagnosis of major depression could be made for only 2.7% of the patients with PD (50), leading the investigators to suggest that the prevalence of major depression in PD may be no greater than that in the general elderly population. In striking contrast, in a separate investigation, the prevalence of "moderate to severe depression" in PD, as defined by a score on a self-report depression rating scale (normally used to assist only in diagnosis) and in the absence of a structured interview with a psychiatrist was 19.6% (51). Whereas a *nondepressed* patient with PD will score positively on many items on a depression rating scale because of motor disability, it is probable that the actual severity and "diagnosis" of the PD affective syndrome, as assessed only by a simple depression rating scale (and in the absence of a patient interview), may be incorrect. It is recommended, therefore, that in future studies of brain serotonergic behavioral comparisons in PD, equal emphasis should be given to the reliable and accurate assessment of both behavioral and biochemical measures.

CONCLUSIONS

The basis for some of the secondary disturbances in idiopathic PD involving mood, cognition, and sleep is an area of intense interest; however, the frequency in PD of these abnormalities, particularly depression, is uncertain and controversial. This chapter evaluates the evidence that damage to brain serotonin neurons, which might explain some of these changes, is a common feature of patients with PD. Biochemical studies have confirmed that patients with endstage PD have, on average, moderately decreased brain levels of the neurotransmitter. However, neuropathological investigation of raphe serotonergic cell body number in PD has provided conflicting results, likely related to methodological difficulties, individual patient variation in extent of serotonergic damage, or selective damage to nerve endings but sparing the cell body. No conclusions can yet be drawn from the preliminary neuroimaging investigations of brain serotonin neuron integrity, as inferred from SERT levels, because of uncertainty regarding the validity of the measurements. Thus, the available data suggest that mild to moderate damage to serotonin neurons is a common feature of advanced PD but is probably not observed in all patients. Further investigation is needed to establish whether a brain serotonergic deficiency occurs early or only late in the course of the disorder, represents loss of entire neurons or only nerve endings, or explains any of the secondary disturbances reported in PD.

REFERENCES

1. Ehringer H, Hornykiewicz O. Verteilung von Noradrenalin und Dopamin (3-hydroxytyramin) im Gehirn des Menches und Ihr Ferhalten bei Erkrankungen des Extrapyramidelen Systems. *Klin Wochenschr* 1960;38: 1236–1239.
2. Sano H. Biochemistry of the extrapyramidal system. *Adv Neurol Sci* 1960;5:42–48.
3. Vingerhoets FJ, Snow BJ, Tetrud JW, et al. Positron

emission tomographic evidence for progression of human MPTP-induced dopaminergic lesions. *Ann Neurol* 1994;36:765–770.
4. Birkmayer W, Hornykiewicz O. Der L-3,4-dioxyphenylalanin (DOPA)—Effekt bei der Parkinson Akinese. *Wien Klin Wochenschr* 1961;73:787–788.
5. Brown RG, MacCarthy B. Psychiatric morbidity in patients with Parkinson's disease. *Psychol Med* 1990;20: 77–87.
6. Aarsland D, Larsen JP, Lim NG, et al. Range of neuropsychiatric disturbances in patients with Parkinson's disease. *J Neurol Neurosurg Psychiatry* 1999;67: 492–496.
7. Poewe W, Luginger E. Depression in Parkinson's disease. Impediments to recognition and treatment options. *Neurology* 1999;52[Suppl 3]:S2–S6.
8. Schrag A, Jahanshahi M, Quinn N. What contributes to quality of life in patients with Parkinson's disease? *J Neurol Neurosurg Psychiatry* 2000;69:308–312.
9. Alexander GE, DeLong MR, Strick PL. Parallel organization of functionally segregated circuits linking basal ganglia and cortex. *Ann Rev Neurosci* 1986;9: 357–381.
10. McLeman ER, Warsh JJ, Li PP, et al. The human nucleus accumbens is highly susceptible to G protein downregulation by methamphetamine and heroin. *J Neurochem* 2000;74:2120–2126.
11. Kulisevsky J, Garcia-Sanchez C, Berthier ML, et al. Chronic effects of dopaminergic replacement on cognitive function in Parkinson's disease: a two-year follow-up study of previously untreated patients. *Mov Disord* 2000;15:613–626.
12. Tork I. Anatomy of the serotonergic system. *Ann N Y Acad Sci* 1990;600:9–34.
13. Staley JK, Malison RT, Innis RB. Imaging of the serotonergic system: interactions of neuroanatomical and functional abnormalities of depression. *Biol Psychiatry* 1998;44:534–549.
14. Arai H, Kosaka K, Iizuka R. Changes of biogenic amines and their metabolites in postmortem brains from patients with Alzheimer-type dementia. *J Neurochem* 1984;43:388–393.
15. Burke WJ, Park DH, Chung HD, et al. Evidence for decreased transport of tryptophan hydroxylase in Alzheimer's disease. *Brain Res* 1990;537:83–87.
16. Halliday GM, McCann HL, Pamphlett R, et al. Brain stem serotonin-synthesizing neurons in Alzheimer's disease: a clinicopathological correlation. *Acta Neuropathol (Berlin)* 1992;84:638–650.
17. Tejani-Butt SM, Yang J, Pawlyk AC. Altered serotonin transporter sites in Alzheimer's disease raphe and hippocampus. *Neuroreport* 1995;6:1207–1210.
18. Chen HT, Casanova MF, Kleinman JE, et al. 3H-paroxetine binding in brains of alcoholics. *Psychiatry Res* 1991;38:293–299.
19. Halliday G, Ellis J, Heard R, et al. Brainstem serotonergic neurons in chronic alcoholics with and without the memory impairment of Korsakoff's psychosis. *J Neuropathol Exp Neurol* 1993;52:567–579.
20. Bernheimer H, Birkmayer W, Hornykiewicz O. Verteilung des 5-hydroxytryptamins (Serotonin) im Gehirn des Menschen und sein Verhalten bei Patienten mit Parkinson-syndrom. *Klin Wochenschr* 1961;39: 1056–1059.
21. Fahn S, Libsch LR, Cutler RW. Monoamines in the human neostriatum: topographic distribution in normals and in Parkinson's disease and their role in akinesia, rigidity, chorea, and tremor. *J Neurol Sci* 1971;14: 427–455.
22. Rinne UK, Sonninen V, Riekkinen P, et al. Dopaminergic nervous transmission in Parkinson's disease. *Med Biol* 1974;52:208–217.
23. Scatton B, Javoy-Agid F, Rouquier L, et al. Reduction of cortical dopamine, noradrenaline, serotonin and their metabolites in Parkinson's disease. *Brain Res* 1983;275:321–328.
24. Raisman R, Cash R, Agid Y. Parkinson's disease: decreased density of ^{3}H-imipramine and ^{3}H-paroxetine binding sites in putamen. *Neurology* 1986;36: 556–560.
25. D'Amato RJ, Zweig RM, Whitehouse PJ, et al. Aminergic systems in Alzheimer's disease and Parkinson's disease. *Ann Neurol* 1987;22:229–236.
26. Wilson JM, Levey AI, Rajput A, et al. Differential changes in neurochemical markers of striatal dopamine nerve terminals in idiopathic Parkinson's disease. *Neurology* 1996;47:718–726.
27. Sawada M, Nagatsu T, Nagatsu I, et al. Tryptophan hydroxylase activity in the brains of controls and parkinsonian patients. *J Neural Transm* 1985;62:107–115.
28. Chinaglia G, Landwehrmeyer B, Probst A, et al. Serotonergic terminal transporters are differentially affected in Parkinson's disease and progressive supranuclear palsy: an autoradiographic study with [^{3}H]citalopram. *Neuroscience* 1993;54:691–699.
29. Kish SJ, Shannak K, Hornykiewicz O. Uneven pattern of dopamine loss in the striatum of patients with idiopathic Parkinson's disease: pathophysiologic and clinical implications. *N Engl J Med* 1988;318:876–880.
30. Halliday GM, Blumbergs PC, Cotton RG, et al. Loss of brainstem serotonin- and substance P–containing neurons in Parkinson's disease. *Brain Res* 1990;510: 104–107.
31. Halliday GM, Li YW, Blumbergs PC, et al. Neuropathology of immunohistochemically identified brainstem neurons in Parkinson's disease. *Ann Neurol* 1990;27:373–385.
32. Kim SE, Lee WY, Choe YS, et al. SPECT measurement of iodine-123-β-CIT binding to dopamine and serotonin transporters in Parkinson's disease: correlation with symptom severity. *Neurol Res* 1999;21: 255–261.
33. Mann DM, Yates PO. Pathological basis for neurotransmitter changes in Parkinson's disease. *Neuropathol Appl Neurobiol* 1983;9:3–19.
34. Jellinger K. Overview of morphological changes in Parkinson's disease. *Adv Neurol* 1986;45:1–18.
35. Zweig RM, Jankel WR, Hedreen JC, et al. The pedunculopontine nucleus in Parkinson's disease. *Ann Neurol* 1989;26:41–46.
36. Paulus W, Jellinger K. The neuropathologic basis of different clinical subgroups of Parkinson's disease. *J Neuropathol Exp Neurol* 1991;50:743–755.
37. Kish SJ, Robitaille Y, El-Awar M, et al. Non-Alzheimer's-type pattern of brain choline acetyltransferase reduction in dominantly inherited olivopontocerebellar atrophy. *Ann Neurol* 1989;26:362–367.
38. Kish SJ, El-Awar M, Stuss D, et al. Neuropsychological test performance in patients with dominantly-inherited spinocerebellar atrophy: relationship to ataxia severity. *Neurology* 1994;44:1738–1746.
39. Brücke T, Kornhuber J, Angelberger P, et al. SPECT

imaging of dopamine and serotonin transporters with [123I] β-CIT. Binding kinetics in the human brain. *J Neural Transm Gen Sect* 1993;94:137–146.

40. Kim SE, Choi JY, Choe YS, et al. Serotonin transporters in Parkinson's disease studied with [I-123] β-CIT SPECT. *J Nucl Med* 1997;38:P280.
41. Haapaniemi TH, Ahonen A, Torniainen P, et al. [123I] β-CIT SPECT demonstrates decreased brain dopamine and serotonin transporter levels in untreated Parkinsonian patients. *Mov Disord* 2001;16:124–130.
42. Malison RT, Price LH, Berman R, et al. Reduced brain serotonin transporter availability in major depression as measured by [123I]-2 beta-carbomethoxy-3 beta-(4-iodophenyl)tropane and single photon emission computed tomography. *Biol Psychiatry* 1998;44: 1090–1098.
43. Dahlström M, Ahonen A, Ebeling H, et al. Elevated hypothalamic/midbrain serotonin (monoamine) transporter availability in depressive drug-naive children and adolescents. *Mol Psychiatry* 2000;5:514–522.
44. van Dyck CH, Malison RT, Seibyl JP, et al. Age-related decline in central serotonin transporter availability with [123I]beta-CIT SPECT. *Neurobiol Aging* 2000;21: 497–501.
45. Laruelle M, Abi-Dargham A, van Dyck C, et al. Dopamine and serotonin transporters in patients with schizophrenia: an imaging study with [123I]beta-CIT. *Biol Psychiatry* 2000;47:371–379.
46. Pirker W, Asenbaum S, Hauk M, et al. Imaging serotonin and dopamine transporters with 123I-β-CIT SPECT: Binding kinetics and effects of normal aging. *J Nucl Med* 2000;41:36–44.
47. Pirker W, Asenbaum S, Kasper S, et al. β-CIT SPECT demonstrates blockade of 5-HT-uptake sites by citalopram in the human brain *in vivo*. *J Neural Transm Gen Sect* 1995;100:247–256.
48. Heinz A, Jones DW. Serotonin transporters in ecstasy users. *Br J Psychiatry* 2000;176:193–194.
49. Becker T, Becker G, Seufert J, et al. Parkinson's disease and depression: evidence for an alteration of the basal limbic system detected by transcranial sonography. *J Neurol Neurosurg Psychiatry* 1997;63:590–596.
50. Hantz P, Caradoc-Davies G, Caradoc-Davies T, et al. Depression in Parkinson's disease. *Am J Psychiatry* 1994;151:1010–1014.
51. Schrag A, Jahanshahi M, Quinn NP. What contributes to depression in Parkinson's disease? *Psychol Med* 2001;31:65–73.

Parkinson's Disease: Advances in Neurology, Vol. 91.
Edited by Ariel Gordin, Seppo Kaakkola, and Heikki Teräväinen
Lippincott Williams & Wilkins, Philadelphia © 2003

5

New Insights in Parkinson's Disease Therapy: Can Levodopa-induced Dyskinesia Ever Be Manageable

*‡A. Hadj Tahar, *R. Grondin, *L. Grégoire, †F. Calon, †T. Di Paolo, and *P. J. Bédard

**Unité de Recherche en Neuroscience, Centre de Recherche du CHUQ, Quebec, Canada; †Unité de Recherche en Oncologie and Endocrinologie Moléculaire, Centre de Recherche du CHUQ, Quebec, Canada; and ‡The Institut Universitaire de Gériatrie de Montreal, Montreal, Quebec, Canada*

Parkinson's disease (PD), one of the most common neurological disorders of the elderly, characterized by tremor, rigidity, akinesia, and loss of postural reflexes, still represents a therapeutic challenge. Levodopa, introduced into clinical practice in the late 1960s, remains the cornerstone of PD therapy (1). However, within a few years of initial levodopa treatment, motor fluctuations and dyskinesias occurred in about 50% of treated patients with PD (2,3). Current pharmacological treatment remains disappointing (4). Motor complications tend to become more severe with advancing disease, and the benefits of treatment are ultimately compromised (5). Peak-dose dyskinesia, the most frequent type, occurs typically when antiparkinsonian relief is maximal, and levodopa plasma levels are high or above a critical threshold (6). The exact mechanisms by which levodopa-induced dyskinesia develop are not clearly understood. Monkeys treated with methylphenyltetrahydropyridine (MPTP) are the best current model of PD. MPTP is a neurotoxin discovered by accident in the 1980s, and it is a synthetic derivative of heroin (7). The toxin destroys the dopaminergic neurons of the substantia nigra pars compacta and induces a Parkinson-like syndrome both in humans (7) and in monkeys (8). Moreover, chronic treatment with levodopa causes dyskinesia that is similar to that found in levodopa-treated patients with idiopathic PD in both MPTP-treated monkeys and humans exposed to this toxin (7,9). Here, we summarize our results of experiments performed in a simian model of PD using various therapeutic methods aimed at managing this debilitating adverse effect.

PATHOPHYSIOLOGY OF LEVODOPA-INDUCED DYSKINESIA

Clinical observations and experimental studies suggest that there are at least three risk factors for levodopa-induced dyskinesia. These are (a) chronic exogenous exposure to dopaminergic drugs (mainly when given intermittently); (b) severe dopamine depletion resulting from nigrostriatal denervation (10,11); and (c) the required presence of anatomically intact striatal neurons (12). In fact, functional alterations in glutamatergic neurotransmission within the striatum (i.e., altered signal transduction mechanisms in striatal medium-sized neurons) have been postulated to underlie levodopa-induced dyskinesia (13,14).

Role of Dopaminergic Stimulation

Levodopa treatment consists of providing the natural amino acid precursor of dopamine so, in theory, should not cause serious adverse effects. However, exogenous administration of levodopa does induce significant motor complications when given to patients with PD. Synaptic release of dopamine in the parkinsonian versus the normal brain must be different. Dopamine receptor supersensitivity seen after denervation or chronic levodopa treatment (10) is probably the major contributing factor for the development of levodopa-induced dyskinesia. Dopamine D_1 receptor–mediated mechanisms have traditionally been linked to this phenomenon (15); however, experimental studies using dopamine D_1 receptor selective agonists have shown that these drugs have a less dyskinesiogenic potential than levodopa (16,17). Dopamine D_2 receptor mechanisms have also been implicated. Long-term exposure of the dopamine-depleted putamen to exogenous dopaminergic agents causes (either directly or indirectly) a preferential shift in favor of the striatopallidal pathway (inhibition of the dopaminergic effect), the cell bodies of which bear mainly dopamine D_2 receptors (18,19). Such a shift causes extensive disinhibition of lateral pallidal neurons, which become overactive and depress the subthalamic nucleus (STN), resulting in an excessive inhibition of the output nuclei of the basal ganglia. As a consequence of the disinhibition of the thalamus, the motor cortex is overstimulated, leading to dyskinesia. However, our experience with MPTP-treated cynomolgus monkeys suggests that supersensitivity of D_2 receptor–mediated striatal outflow is sufficient for the induction of levodopa dyskinesia, and that repeated stimulation of short duration is important for the sensitization process (10,20). In fact, the high dyskinesiogenic potential of selective short-acting dopamine D_2 agonists and the favorable outcome on dyskinesia resulting from the continuous stimulation of dopamine D_2 receptors (leading to dopamine D_2 receptor downregulation) are important clues suggesting the primary role of dopamine D_2 receptor–mediated mechanisms in the dyskinesia-priming process (20,21). Nevertheless, data obtained with selective dopamine D_1 or D_2 receptor antagonists, coadministered with levodopa, have shown that drugs that impede dopaminergic transmission improve dyskinesia but not without reappearance of the parkinsonism state (22,23). Thus, selective blockade of dopamine receptors has been shown not to be advantageous in the treatment of levodopa-induced dyskinesia. Moreover, there is no difference in dopamine D_2 or D_1 receptor density between the brain of dyskinetic versus nondyskinetic patients with PD (24). Hence, dyskin esia is unlikely to result from alterations in striatal dopamine receptor binding (25,26).

On the other hand, dopamine receptor stimulation necessary for normal motor function is expected to be tonic in nature, with limited variation (27). Indeed, in the normal state, nigrostriatal projections deliver dopamine to the striatum at a relatively constant rate, maintaining striatal dopamine concentrations at a level from 5 to 10 nM (27,28). In PD, standard dopamine-replacement strategies intermittently provide suprathreshold dopamine concentrations to the synapse. This imposes a pattern of stimulation on the striatal dopamine receptors, which markedly contrasts with the normal nigrostriatal activity described above (29). The striatal cells bearing the dopamine receptors might adapt to this nonphysiological activation for a specific period of time, particularly if there is a minimum number of remaining dopaminergic neurons. However, with progressive neurodegeneration of dopaminergic neurons, the "good" adaptive mechanisms can eventually fail and are replaced by pathological compensatory mechanisms that are unable to preserve homeostasis in the nigrostriatal system. In agreement with this, it has been shown that continuous (more physiological) dopaminergic stimulation counteracts motor fluctuations associated with levodopa therapy in PD. Clinical studies showed that more constant activation of dopamine receptors, through continuous infusion of levodopa or dopamine agonists, counteracts some motor fluctuations in patients with advanced PD, and steady plasma levodopa concentrations have been advocated to prevent or reduce these complications (29). Hence, the pulsatile character of levodopa administration seems to play a major role in dyskinesia induction. Certainly, treatments that permit a continuous, more physiological stimulation of striatal dopamine receptors (i.e., long-acting dopamine receptor agonists) appears to be a useful strategy to control levodopa-induced dyskinesia.

Role of Striatal Dopamine Depletion

Extensive nigral denervation, which is the basic alteration found in PD, appears to be a necessary condition for the appearance of motor complications (30,31). Indeed, long-term administration of levodopa generally does not induce dyskinesia in humans without evidence of PD (32–34). Moreover, dyskinesia induced by dopamine-like agents usually first appears on the most denervated side and is usually more prominent in the more severely affected patients (32). However, it is important to note here that the role of the dopamine denervation in the genesis of dyskinesia was recently questioned by two studies (35,36). Indeed, dyskinesia was induced by levodopa in MPTP-treated monkeys having a weak denervation without obvious signs of parkinsonism (35), and the administration of a strong amount of levodopa could induce dyskinesia in normal marmosets (36). Interestingly, this is associated with some of the typical biochemical alterations that we believe underlie this phenomenon (36).

Role of the Glutamatergic System

The basal ganglia is rich in glutamatergic innervation; in fact, the striatum, and to a lesser degree the STN, receives an important number of glutamatergic projections, particularly from the cortex and the thalamus. The glutamatergic neurons of the STN project to the two segments of the globus pallidus (external and internal) (GPe and GPi, respectively) and to the two parts of the substantia nigra (the pars reticulata and the pars compacta) (37). Thus, it is not surprising that drugs that modify the central glutamatergic neurotransmission can deeply influence motor functions (38). Medium spiny output neurons constitute the main cellular population of the striatum, at least from a quantitative point of view (39). As medium spiny output neurons are the targets of most extrinsic and intrinsic striatal afferents, they serve as the major integrator of information in the striatum and basal ganglia (40). They are also the main group of neurons projecting out of the striatum (40). Anatomical observations and functional studies suggest that dopaminergic and glutamatergic systems interact closely at the level of the medium spiny output neuron dendrites, where both dopamine and glutamate receptors are located (41,42). These interactions are thought to play a crucial role in corticostriatal-mediated synaptic plasticity (43). Indeed, induction of long-term potentiation (LTP) and long-term depression (LTD) in the striatum is regulated by *N*-methyl D-aspartate (NMDA) and acid propionic AMPA (α-amino-3-hydroxy-5-methyl-4-isoxazole) receptor subtypes, as well as dopamine receptors (43). In PD, the nonphysiological replacement of dopamine might alter this fine interaction and induce a pathological form of LTP (43). This provides additional support for the idea that dyskinesia is a consequence of a faulty learning phenomenon that occurs in the striatum (10). The actions of glutamate in the brain are exerted via ionotropic (ionic channels) or metabotropic (coupled to protein G) receptors. NMDA receptors belong to the family of ionotropic receptors, which include AMPA and kainate receptors (44). NMDA receptors are heteromeric complexes comprised of an NR1 subunit (essential for the function of the receptor) and several NR2 subunits (four subtypes exist: NRA, NRB, NRC, and NRD). NR2 confers onto the receptor its pharmacological and biochemical properties (45). In the human, messenger RNAs (mRNAs) for the NR1, NR2B, and to a lesser degree NR2A were detected in the striatum (45,46). Moreover, biochemical studies have shown an upregulation of NMDA receptors in parkinsonian patients and MPTP monkeys treated with levodopa (47,48). This upregulation seems to particularly involve NMDA receptors containing the NR2B subunit (48,49). Moreover, enhanced sensitivity of NMDA receptors, consequent to an alteration in the phosphorylation state of NMDA receptor subunits in medium spiny output neurons, has been observed in a rodent model of PD (14). In agreement with these findings, behavioral studies in MPTP monkeys and clinical trials in patients with PD suggest that blockade of NMDA receptors can prevent or treat levodopa-induced dyskinesia (50,51).

Important alterations in the expression of other genes have also been associated with dyskinesia in MPTP monkeys. For example, it has been reported that preproenkephalin (PPE) mRNA levels are increased in dyskinetic animals (36,52–54). Recently, expression of the adenosine A_{2a} receptor gene was also found to be increased in the striatum of monkeys with levodopa-induced dyskinesia (36). Thus, the development of dyskinesia might be accompanied by a changed pattern of gene expression that could play a causal role. Recent work has extended our knowledge of mechanisms by which gene expression is regulated in striatal neurons. Several cellular components have been identified as being part of potential transcription pathways involved in the pathological response of medium spiny output neurons to chronic perturbation of dopaminergic neurons (55–57). In this respect, chronic *Fos*-related antigens, more specifically delta-*Fos*B isoforms, warrant our attention and are interesting prospects for further research on a molecular basis of dyskinesia (10,58). Finally, inhibition or modification of neuronal activity by deep brain stimulation (DBS) in the STN, a glutamatergic nucleus, markedly reduces dyskinesia in individuals with PD (59). However, lesions of the STN might actually cause or increase dyskinesia (60,61).

MANAGEMENT OF LEVODOPA-INDUCED DYSKINESIA

Once Induced, is Dyskinesia Controllable?

We are forced to agree with a recent report by Ferreira and Rascol (4); although despite the combined efforts of different research teams all over the world, we have yet to find a satisfactory treatment of dyskinesia. Presently, in clinical practice, dyskinesia is attenuated through dose reduction of levodopa, but this often causes an unacceptable aggravation of the parkinsonian state (62). In general, patients choose to endure the dyskinetic over the parkinsonian effects (bradykinesia). A reduction in the dose of levodopa, concomitant with an increase in the dose of a dopamine agonist (63), is another option. This strategy effectively reduces dyskinesia, but often inconsistently. The only drug actually effective in clinics to reduce dyskinesia is amantadine (51,64). This beneficial effect persists even after 1 year of treatment (65). This antidyskinetic action might be related to the antiglutamate properties of amantadine (66). Considering its affinity is relatively higher for the dopamine D_1 and D_4 receptors, versus the D_2 receptors, the effects of clozapine on the dyskinesia were examined (67,68). An improvement of the duration, but not of the severity, of dyskinesia was noted in the first study. Orthostatic hypotension and sedation were common adverse effects. In the second study, low-dose clozapine (50 mg) improved dyskinesia in parkinsonian patients. Although agranulocytosis (potentially fatal) was not observed in these studies, clozapine must be used only to treat severe dyskinesia. Olanzapine, a new atypical antipsychotic that is a clozapine analog that has possibly less risk of agranulocytosis (69), was recently tested in parkinsonian patients. The results showed, however, a decrease in dyskinesia accompanied by a significant reduction of the antiparkinsonian effects of levodopa, even at a low dose of olanzapine (70). Recently, a major step in the treatment of PD was achieved as illustrated by the results of three clinical trials that showed that the early use of dopamine agonists conclusively delayed the occurrence of dyskinesias and motor complications (71–73). These studies showed that dyskinesia was further reduced in patients who were not supplemented with levodopa but were under dopamine agonist monotherapy until the end of the follow-up period (3 to 5 years). However, after the published observations of Frucht et al. (74) of episodic sudden onset of sleep (sleep attacks) in patients with PD on pramipexole and ropinirole, early hopes to delay dyskinesia using dopamine agonists were tempered. Moreover, given the fact that with disease progression, the need for increasing dopamine agonist dosage is compromised by such an undesirable effect, levodopa is often introduced to maximize clinical benefit and may ultimately lead to the emergence of dyskinesia. Hence, there is a pressing need to find alternative strategies to manage motor fluctuations and dyskinesia.

Here, we present the results of two recent studies in MPTP-treated monkeys, using two approaches to attenuate levodopa-induced dyskinesia. In the first experiment (75), we used (*S*)-(–)-3-(3-(methylsulfonyl)phenyl)-1-propylpiperidine (–)-OSU6162), which is a phenylpiperidine derivative exhibiting low affinity for the dopamine D_2 receptor *in vitro* (76). However, *in vivo,* positron emission tomography (PET) scanning studies show that the compound displaces the selective dopamine D_2 receptor antagonist, raclopride (77,78). (–)-OSU6162 increased ^{11}C-SCH 23390 (a dopamine D_1 receptor antagonist) binding, which may indicate a potentiating effect on dopamine D_1 receptor–mediated functions (77,78). Furthermore, (–)-OSU6162 attenuates levodopa- and quinpirole (dopamine D_2 receptor agonist)-induced contraversive circling behavior in unilaterally 6-hydroxydopamine (6-OHDA)–lesioned common marmosets and increases such behavior induced by a dopamine D_1 receptor agonist (78,79). This unique pharmacological profile suggests that (–)-OSU6162 belongs to a new class of functional modulators of dopaminergic systems, having psychomotor state–dependent normalizing properties on D_2 tone (76,80). Hence, we evaluated the effects of (–)-OSU6162 on the antiparkinsonian response and dyskinesia produced by levodopa. Five MPTP-treated cynomolgus monkeys with stable parkinsonian syndromes and reproducible dyskinesias to levodopa were used in this study. The results showed that the coadministration of (–)-OSU6162 with levodopa produced a significant reduction in dyskinesia. This improvement in levodopa-induced dyskinesias occurred mainly at the onset of the levodopa effect, as reflected by an increase in the duration of the "on" state without dyskinesia up to 3.4-fold after (–)-OSU6162 coadministration, as compared with levodopa alone. Our data support the results of Ekesbo et al. (81), who showed that pretreatment with (–)-OSU6162 of MPTP-lesioned common marmosets relieved levodopa-induced dyskinesia. The antidyskinetic effect obtained with (–)-OSU6162 differed considerably from that obtained using classic dopamine D_2 receptor antagonists. In fact, such drugs that impede dopamine transmission improve dyskinesia at the cost of a return to parkinsonism (22,23, 81). It is interesting to note that with (–)-OSU6162 co-treatment, there was no clear dose-dependent effect. This is indeed surprising and not easily explained according to standard pharmacology. One explanation may lie in the observations made by Ekesbo et al. (78) in the primates with a unilateral 6-OHDA lesion of the substantia nigra. They observed that (–)-OSU6162 attenuated rotational behavior induced by apomorphine and the dopamine D_2 receptor agonist quinpirole but increased the rotational response to dopamine D_1 receptor agonists. This is highly unusual for a dopamine antagonist and was described as a "state-dependent effect" of the molecule on dopamine D_1 and D_2 receptor agonist–induced behavior (78). It should be noted here that NMDA receptor antagonists, such as MK-801, have also been shown to accentuate dopamine D_1 receptor responses and to attenuate dopamine D_2 receptor responses (14,38). This demonstrates the close interplay between NMDA- and dopamine-mediated effects in striatofugal projections, and it is possible to target such mechanisms in different ways (78). In the present study, (–)-OSU6162 when combined with levodopa may have exerted opposite effects on dopamine D_1 and D_2 receptors and the resulting motor response may have varied depending on the balance between the modulation of dopamine D_2 receptors (reduction of response) and D_1 receptors (increase of response). This could explain the unusual dose–response curves. In support of its weak dopamine receptor antagonistic effects, (–)-OSU6162 given alone had little effect on motor behavior. Moreover, when given with levodopa, a significant antidyskinetic effect was seen. Hence, the dopamine-antagonizing properties of (–)-OSU6162 are only seen in the dopamine-overactive state and are lost in the case of decreased dopaminergic tone, as in MPTP-lesioned monkeys. Therefore, it is reasonable to assume that (–)-OSU6162 not only shows selectivity for the dopamine D_2 receptor type, but also may have a receptor state–dependent affinity. Furthermore, a more favorable balance of levodopa-induced dopamine D_1/D_2 receptor–mediated output from the striatum may also be a tentative explanation for the antidyskinetic effects of the compound. In addition to its comparatively weak dopamine D_2 receptor antagonistic properties, (–)-OSU6162 increased contraversive circling behavior induced by a dopamine D_1 receptor agonist (78,79). This positive modulation of the activity of striatal output neurons bearing dopamine D_1 receptors (direct pathway) could in part account for its antidyskinetic effects (16). These data suggest that (–)-OSU6162 could be of significant clinical value to reduce levodopa-induced dyskinesia in patients with fluctuating advanced PD (75).

In the second experiment, in the search for an alternative therapy for PD, we attempted to modify the activity of adenosine within the brain. This was achieved using a newly developed selective adenosine A_{2a} receptor antagonist KW-6002 (Ki value of 2.2 nM and about 68-fold selectivity for the A_{2a} receptor over the A_1 receptor) (82). The rationale behind this is based on anatomical, biochemical, and behavioral studies that suggest a possible implication of adenosine A_{2a} receptors in the control of motor activity. In fact, in the striatum, the A_{2a} receptor is coexpressed in the same medium spiny neurons as those bearing dopamine D_2 receptors containing enkephalin and projecting to the GPe (indirect pathway) (83,84). In behavioral studies, nonselective adenosine receptor antagonists, such as caffeine and theophylline, induce motor activation, and this is counteracted by dopamine depletion or dopamine D_1 or D_2 receptor blockade (85,86). Using selective adenosine receptor antagonists, it has been shown that while selective A_1 receptor antagonists potentiate only D_1 agonist–induced motor activation, selective A_{2a} receptor antagonists potentiate both D_1 and D_2 stimulation of motor behavior (87–89). Moreover, the xanthine-selective A_{2a} receptor antagonist KF17837 reverses catalepsy induced by CGS21680, haloperidol, and reserpine in mice (90). Of note, a synergistic effect between levodopa and KF17837 was observed under both dopamine depletion and D_2 receptor blockade (90). KF17837 also antagonizes hypomobility induced by MPTP in mice and reverses the effects of CGS21680 in 6-OHDA–lesioned rats (91). Hence, there is good reason to believe that blockade of the adenosine A_{2a} receptor could help restore the balance of striatal function and could be valuable to the treatment of PD.

In our studies (92,93), monkeys previously rendered parkinsonian by the toxin MPTP and presenting with a stable syndrome for several months were used. All responded readily to levodopa but developed dyskinesia, which manifested with each dose. Both levodopa and KW-6002 were administered orally. KW-6002 increased locomotion and improved parkinsonian symptoms in a significant manner comparable to what was seen with levodopa. Interestingly, despite its ability to reverse motor disability, KW-6002 alone induced little or no dyskinesia. These results fit well with other behavioral studies on 6-OHDA–lesioned rats (86) and MPTP-treated monkeys (94). The mechanism of action of KW-6002 is probably related to adenosine A_{2a} receptor antagonism. Indeed, Svenningsson et al. (95) provided evidence that the stimulatory effects of caffeine are due to inhibition of the tonic stimulatory actions of endogenous adenosine at A_{2a} receptors on striatopallidal GABAergic neurons. In support of this model, it has been shown that caffeine no longer increases spontaneous locomotor activity in A_{2a} receptor knockout mice (96). Furthermore, the γ-aminobutyric acid (GABA)-enkephalin–containing striato-GPe neurons of the indirect pathway are excited by cortical inputs and inhibited by recurrent collaterals (via $GABA_A$ receptors). In PD, the feedback inhibition of the indirect pathway by the recurrent collaterals may be insufficient to control the overactivity of these neurons. It is postulated that A_{2a} receptor stimulation decreases GABA release (97), and consequently, an A_{2a} receptor antagonist, by relieving this antagonism, would enhance recurrent GABA inhibition, thereby reducing the activity of the GABA-containing striatopallidal neurons. In addition, these effects would be expected to occur when the striato-GPe neurons are firing, having relatively little effect when the neurons are inactive. In an electrophysiological study, Mori et al. (98) recently reported that presynaptic A_{2a} receptors localized in collateral axons of striatal GABAergic neurons exert an inhibitory modulation of GABA release in the striatum. Moreover, A_{2a} antagonists of the same family as KW-6002 increase GABA release in the striatum, suggesting that such modulation may be involved in the control of movement. Hence, because inhibition of GABA release onto striatopallidal neurons is likely to increase their activity, antagonists of adenosine A_{2a} receptors should mimic the behavioral effect of a D_2 agonists (99). It should be noted that there is evidence that A_{2a} receptor activation enhanced GABA release in both the striatum and the globus pallidus (100). However, A_{2a} receptor agonists inhibit GABA release from nerve terminals derived from both these areas (97,101).

On the other hand, our results also show that selective blockade of adenosine A_{2a} receptors is less likely to reproduce dyskinesia than levodopa at doses that produce a comparable antiparkinsonian benefit. The reasons for this advantage are not entirely clear. Piccini et al. (102) showed an increase in neuropeptide transmission in the basal ganglia of dyskinetic parkinsonian patients comparative to that seen in those without dyskinesias. Interestingly, after the loss of dopamine or levodopa therapy, the increase in preproenkephalin mRNA requires both A_{2a} and muscarinic acetylcholine receptor activation (103). Prevention of this increase in preproenkephalin expression by A_{2a} receptor blockade is consistent with a reduction in the activity of the striato-GPe neurons that are overactive in an experimental model of PD (104). However, although chronic treatment by caffeine reverses the alterations of enkephalin gene expression in striatopallidal neurons of 6-OHDA–lesioned rats (105), it is not certain that acute treatment by adenosine A_{2a} antagonists can do the same, and long-term studies with KW-6002 are still needed to evaluate such findings. Another explanation is the possibility that adenosine A_{2a} receptors may negatively modulate the activity of striatal glutamate neurotransmission (106), and that this could account for the antidyskinetic effects of KW-6002. These authors have studied in the striatum the interactions between NMDA receptors, adenosine receptors, and the cyclic adenosine monophosphate (cAMP) signaling pathway. Their results demonstrate that both NMDA and the adenosine A_{2a} receptor agonist CPCA increased cAMP levels and that the NMDA-induced increase in cAMP was completely blocked by the NMDA receptor antagonist or the adenosine A_2 receptor antagonist DMPX. These data suggest that striatal NMDA receptors increase cAMP indirectly via stimulation of adenosine A_{2a} receptors. Thus, NMDA receptors and adenosine A_{2a} receptors might share a common signaling pathway within the striatum (106). Alternatively, an increase in GABA-mediated collateral inhibition in the striatum by A_{2a} receptor antagonists could focus the activity of striatal neurons and sharpen the intrastriatal message, resulting in a precise motor command not plagued by dyskinesia (98).

In conclusion, these results show that selective adenosine receptor antagonism improves parkinsonism in MPTP-treated monkeys and lend further support to the view that A_{2a} receptor blockade might be a potential nondopaminergic approach to treat parkinsonian patients, either alone or as an adjunct to levodopa or dopamine agonist therapy.

Once Induced, is Dyskinesia Reversible?

The consensus now is that continuous (more physiological) dopaminergic stimulation is able to counteract or prevent motor fluctuations associated with levodopa therapy in PD (29). Because the dopamine system is thought to be tonically active, oscillations in levodopa concentrations in the brain—caused by diminished capacity of levodopa presynaptic storage as a result of progressive degeneration of nigrostriatal terminals—are believed to be partly responsible for the pathogenesis of dyskinesia (20). Indeed, it has been observed in clinical studies that more constant activation of dopamine receptors, through continuous infusion of levodopa or dopamine agonists, counteracts some motor fluctuations in patients with advanced PD, and steady plasma levodopa concentrations have been advocated to prevent or reduce these complications (29,107,108). However, long-term infusion of levodopa or dopamine agonists, for practical limitations, is difficult to perform in humans and an alternative strategy could be the use of long-acting dopaminomimetic drugs.

Cabergoline is a relatively selective dopamine D_2 agonist that shows prolonged steady binding to the receptor *in vivo* and *in vitro* for at least 72 hours and a long plasma half-life of 65 to 110 hours (109). Therefore, cabergoline represents a useful tool for sustained dopamine D_2 receptor stimulation and for the treatment of PD (110). To evaluate the potential ability of cabergoline to reverse levodopa-induced dyskinesia in a primate model of PD, we compared the effects of levodopa given before and after 6 weeks of administration of cabergoline alone (111). Four MPTP-treated cynomolgus monkeys with a long-standing and stable parkinsonian syndrome, as well as reproducible dyskinesia to levodopa, were used in this study. During cabergoline treatment, the monkeys initially showed marked dyskinesias that were reduced significantly after 4 weeks of treatment without, however, tolerance to its antiparkinsonian effect. Levodopa given 4 days after cabergoline withdrawal produced a significant antiparkinsonian effect, but dyskinesia was dramatically reduced compared with what had been seen before chronic cabergoline treatment. Hence, the major finding of this study is that sustained cabergoline treatment significantly reverses dopaminergic dyskinesias while providing a sustained antiparkinsonian effect. Our results corroborate well with the clinical study of Bejjani et al. (112), which compared the effects of a suprathreshold dose of levodopa (50 mg) given before and after 8 months of continuous bilateral high-frequency stimulation of the STN. This DBS allowed the reduction of the dose of levodopa among these patients. (Levodopa was stopped completely in two of the 12 studied patients.) Their results showed that levodopa given after the 8-month stimulation period induced less dyskinesia. However, the authors did not find a positive correlation between the reduction of the dyskinesia and the duration of STN stimulation or with the percentage of levodopa reduction. In fact, among the two patients for whom levodopa was stopped completely, the improvement of dyskinesia did not differ from that of the other patients. It should be noted that levodopa was maintained, though at a low dose, in most of the patients in this last study. In another study in parkinsonian patients, Baronti et al. (113) showed that a 3-month chronic treatment with the D_2 receptor agonist lisuride failed to improve levodopa-induced dyskinesia. However, the authors (113) reported also that small doses of levodopa were maintained with lisuride (to achieve a good antiparkinsonian response) in their clinical study. Hence, the reversibility of dyskinesia may require a complete and durable "drug holiday" (levodopa withdrawal), sustained dopaminergic stimulation, or DBS of the STN for a longer period (111,112). It is noteworthy that the use of catechol-*O*-methyltransferase (COMT) or monoamine oxidase B (MAO-B) inhibitors with an aim of increasing dopamine stimulation often worsens the dyskinesia (114).

The mechanisms by which continuous selective dopamine D_2 receptor stimulation reduces levodopa- or dopamine D_2 agonist–induced dyskinesia may involve several neurotransmitter systems. Interestingly, MPTP monkeys displaying dyskinesia also had elevated striatal PPE mRNA levels, whereas those with the lowest PPE mRNA expression did not display dyskinesia (53). Similarly, repeated treatment with bromocriptine or lisuride, which induce less dyskinesia, also reduces PPE expression to control the level in 6-OHDA rats (115). Overactive enkephalinergic transmission through reducing GABAergic release in the GPe (116) may play a role in the development of levodopa-induced dyskinesia. Thus, normalization in striatal PPE mRNA levels (increased by denervation and pulsatile repeated levodopa therapy) to a predenervation levels by cabergoline treatment may have played a role in the reduction of levodopa-induced dyskinesia (53). On the other hand, the antidyskinetic effect of cabergoline, which allows continuous, more physiological dopaminergic stimulation, may be related to an NMDA receptor–mediated mechanism. In fact, upregulation of NMDA receptors is seen in PD and their phosphorylation and synthesis are suppressed by tonic D_2 stimulation (117,118). It should be noted also that the increase in PPE mRNA expression (seen after denervation) seems to result from unchecked glutamatergic excitation (119). Blockade of NMDA receptors suppresses the effects of nigrostriatal dopamine deafferentation on striatal PPE mRNA levels and reduces dyskinesia without altering the antiparkinsonian effect (50,120). In conclusion, our data show that reversing the changes in neural function responsible for dyskinesia and "turning back the clock" for the dyskinetic patient is possible. Thus, patients with PD can benefit from new and better therapeutic strategies, and cabergoline or similar long-acting dopamine D_2 receptor agonist treatment certainly appears a useful strategy for parkinsonian patients with dyskinesias.

Is Dyskinesia Preventable?

One strategy to prevent dyskinesia is to slow down the progression and/or to find a cure for PD, something that is currently impossible. We can, however, better prescribe levodopa therapy, that is, delay its introduction (by using dopamine agonists), decrease its initial dose (by adding a dopamine agonist), or try to administer it in a more constant way (by coadministration of a COMT or an MAO-B inhibitor). For instance, the only proven strategy able to delay the appearance of dyskinesia is the administration of the new generation of dopamine agonists (71–73). In these studies, the maximum follow-up period was 5 years. As Rascol (63) points out, during this period, dyskinesia is not severe in most patients and only a 10-year long-term follow-up or more can definitively answer this question. Moreover, these new agonists also have their own side effect, known as sleep attacks (74). It should be noted, however, that sleep attacks seem to be a common characteristic to all the dopaminergic agents including levodopa (63). Thus, the scenario is not likely to change and stopping the use of levodopa does not seem to be imminent. In the search for rational, improved, or alternative therapies to prevent dyskinesia, one possibility that recently has become apparent is to modify the activity of glutamate within the brain.

Several lines of evidence have recently indicated that alteration of the NMDA receptors' function as a consequence of chronic intermittent levodopa therapy may play an important role in the pathophysiology of levodopa-induced dyskinesia (see previous discussion). In a recent study, using MPTP monkeys, we investigated whether selective NMDA receptor antagonism could prevent the appearance of dyskinesia (121). We compared the induction of dyskinesia in eight drug-naive parkinsonian monkeys divided in two groups. One group received levodopa alone and the other one received levodopa plus a selective antagonist of NMDA receptors containing the NR2B subunit. CI-1041, a substitute of piperidine related to ifenprodil, is more than 1,000-fold selective for NR1A/2B-cloned NMDA receptors (122). It acts at an allosteric modulation site as a novel NMDA antagonist that blocks NR2B-containing NMDA receptors with a nanomolar affinity (24 nM) (122). Both levodopa (100 mg) and CI-1041 (10 mg/kg) were given orally. After 4 weeks of treatment with levodopa alone, all four animals developed moderate dyskinesia either choreic or dystonic in nature. CI-1041 co-treatment completely prevented the induction of dyskinesia in three animals and only one monkey developed mild dyskinesia at the end of the fourth week of treatment in the levodopa plus CI-1041 group. The magnitude and duration of the antiparkinsonian action of levodopa was similar in both groups. The exact mechanism by which CI-1041 prevented levodopa-induced dyskinesia is not completely clear. Chronic pulsatile levodopa administration profoundly affects striatal NMDA receptor subunits, particularly NR2B and its tyrosine-phosphorylation state, which affects ultimately their function (47–49,123,124). Hence, the administration of CI-1041 with levodopa might prevent the changes in NMDA receptor function, which could prevent the appearance of side effects (14). In accordance with this idea, long-term activity-dependent changes in the efficacy of glutamatergic synaptic transmission, which reflects synaptic plasticity, have been described in the striatum, and dopamine and glutamate interaction is thought to play a crucial role in their induction (43). The nonphysiological replacement of dopamine causes a hyperactivity of the NMDA receptor function and favors the induction of a pathological form of LTP (43). This pathological form of LTP, in striatal spiny neurons, might represent the cellular substrate underlying the dyskinetic symptoms that complicate chronic levodopa treatment in many patients (125). This provides additional support for the idea that dyskinesia is the consequence of a faulty learning phenomenon that takes place in the striatum (10,126). The activation of glutamate NMDA receptors is a crucial condition for the induction of this "pathological" corticostriatal LTP. Thus, it is possible that CI-1041 co-treatment, by blocking NMDA receptor hyperactivity, blocked the induction of LTP and prevented the appearence of levodopa-induced dyskinesia.

In conclusion, our data show that co-treatment with CI-1041 prevented dyskinesia, a finding that conclusively shows the contribution of NMDA receptor–mediated mechanisms in levodopa-induced dyskinesia genesis and gives further evidence that prevention of this disabling side effect is possible. In the clinic, the initial use of amantadine in PD could have a dopa-sparing effect. Can amantadine then prevent dyskinesia? Our results using an NMDA receptor antagonist, which was able to prevent dyskinesia in MPTP-treated monkeys, suggest that this is probably possible in patients with PD (121).

CONCLUSIONS

The findings summarized in this review have led us to hypothesize that alterations of glutamatergic neurotransmission in the striatum, subsequent to pulsatile levodopa administration, play a pivotal role in dyskinesia genesis. Indeed, the beneficial effects of symptomatic treatment of dyskinesia with KW-6002 may pass through modulation of striatal glutamatergic function (106). Similarly, the reversibility of dyskinesia may also be related to a glutamatergic mechanism. Cabergoline might, via its tonic D_2, have corrected the alterations in both phosphorylation and synthesis of NMDA receptors responsible for dyskinesia (111). Finally, the prevention of dyskinesia seen in MPTP monkeys by a selective blockade of NMDA receptors containing the NR2B subunit removes any doubt of their link with this debilitating side effect. At the molecular level, alterations in striatal glutamate receptor function may induce gene expression in the medium spiny output neurons and trigger a cascade of other interrelated changes in peptide- and/or *Fos*-related antigens, which are responsible for the abnormal response to dopamine-like agents that in primates and humans translates into the emergence of dyskinesia (10,127).

ACKNOWLEDGMENTS

We wish to thank Steve Brochu for his excellent technical assistance. A. Hadj Tahar holds a fellowship from EJLB Foundation (Institut de Gériatrie de Montreal). This work was supported by a grant from the Canadian Institutes of Health Research and the Parkinson Foundation of Canada (PJB and TDP).

REFERENCES

1. Jankovic J. Parkinson disease: a half century of progress. *Neurology* 2001;57[Suppl 3]:S1–S3.
2. Grandas F, Galiano ML, Tabernero C. Risk factors for levodopa-induced dyskinesias in Parkinson's disease. *J Neurol* 1999;246:1127–1133.
3. Obeso JA, Rodriguez-Oroz MC, Chana P, et al. The evolution and origin of motor complications in Parkinson's disease. *Neurology* 2000;55:S13–S20.
4. Ferreira JJ, Rascol O. Prevention and therapeutic strategies for levodopa-induced dyskinesias in Parkinson's disease. *Curr Opin Neurol* 2000;13:431–436.
5. Marsden CD. Problems with long-term levodopa therapy for Parkinson's disease. *Clin Neuropharmacol* 1994;17:S32–S44.
6. Muenter MD, Sharpless NS, Tyce GM, et al. Patterns of dystonia ("I-D-I" and "D-I-D-") in response to levodopa therapy for Parkinson's disease. *Mayo Clin Proc* 1977;52:163–174.
7. Langston JW, Ballard PA. Parkinsonism induced by 1-methyl-4-phenyl-1,2,3,6-tetrahydropyridine: implication for treatment and the pathophysiology of Parkinson's disease. *Can J Neurol Sci* 1984;11:160–165.
8. Burns RS, Chiueh CC, Markey SP, et al. A primate model of parkinsonism: selective destruction of dopaminergic neurons in pars compacta of the substantia nigra by 1-methyl-4-phenyl-1,2,3,6-tetrahydropyridine. *Proc Natl Acad Sci USA* 1983;80: 4546–4550.
9. Bédard PJ, Di Paolo T, Falardeau P, et al. Chronic treatment with levodopa, but not bromocriptine, induces dyskinesia in MPTP-parkinsonian monkeys. Correlation with (3H) spiperone binding. *Brain Res* 1986;379:294–299.
10. Bédard PJ, Blanchet PJ, Lévesque D, et al. Pathophysiology of levodopa-induced dyskinesias. *Mov Disord* 1999;14:S4–S8.
11. Bezard E, Brotchie JM, Gross CE. Pathophysiology of levodopa-induced dyskinesia: potential for new therapies. *Nat Rev Neurosci* 2001;2:577–588.
12. Blanchet PJ, Gomez-Mancilla B, Di Paolo T, et al. Is striatal dopaminergic receptor imbalance responsible for levodopa-induced dyskinesias? *Fundam Clin Pharmacol* 1995;9:434–442.
13. Verhagen Metman L, Locatelli ER, Bravi D, et al. Apomorphine responses in Parkinson's disease and the pathogenesis of motor complications. *Neurology* 1997;48:369–372.
14. Chase TN, Oh JD. Striatal dopamine- and glutamate-mediated dysregulation in experimental parkinsonism. *Trends Neurosci* 2000;23:S86–S91.
15. Blanchet PJ, Gomez-Mancilla B, Bédard PJ. DOPA-induced "peak dose" dyskinesias: clues implicating D_2 receptor–mediated mechanisms using dopaminergic agonists in MPTP monkeys. *J Neural Transm* 1995;45: 103–112.
16. Grondin R, Bedard PJ, Britton DR, et al. Potential therapeutic use of selective dopamine D_1 receptor agonist, A-86929: an acute study in parkinsonian levodopa-primed monkeys. *Neurology* 1997;49:421–426.
17. Rascol O, Blin O, Thalamas C, et al. ABT-431, a D_1 receptor agonist prodrug, has efficacy in Parkinson's disease. *Ann Neurol* 1999;45:736–741.
18. Tedroff J, Pedersen M, Aquilonius SM, et al. Levodopa-induced changes in synaptic dopamine in patients with Parkinson's disease as measured by [^{11}C]raclopride displacement and PET. *Neurology* 1996;46:1430–1436.
19. Crossman AR. Functional anatomy of movement disorders. *J Anat* 2000;196:519–525.
20. Blanchet PJ, Calon F, Martel JC, et al. Continuous administration decreases and pulsatile administration increases behavioral sensitivity to a novel dopamine D_2 agonist (U-91356A) in MPTP-exposed monkeys. *J Pharmacol Exp Ther* 1995;272:854–859.
21. Grondin R, Goulet M, Di Paolo T, et al. Cabergoline, a long-acting dopamine D_2-like receptor agonist, produces a sustained antiparkinsonian effect with transient dyskinesias in parkinsonian drug-naive primates. *Brain Res* 1996;735:298–306.
22. Klawans HL, Weiner WJ. Attempted use of haloperidol in the treatment of levodopa-induced dyskinesias. *J Neurol Neurosurg Psychiatry* 1974;37:427–430.
23. Grondin R, Doan VD, Gregoire L, et al. D_1 receptor blockade improves levodopa-induced dyskinesia but worsens parkinsonism in MPTP monkeys. *Neurology* 1999;52:771–777.
24. Turjanski N, Lees AJ, Brooks DJ. *In vivo* studies on striatal dopamine D_1 and D_2 site binding in levodopa-treated Parkinson's disease patients with and without dyskinesias. *Neurology* 1997;49:717–723.
25. Calon F, Hadj Tahar A, Blanchet PJ, et al. Dopamine-receptor stimulation: biobehavioral and biochemical consequences. *Trends Neurosci* 2000;23:S92–S100.
26. Blanchet PJ, Calon F, Morissette M, et al. Regulation of dopamine receptors and motor behavior following pulsatile and continuous dopaminergic replacement

strategies in the MPTP primate model. In: Calne DB, Calne SM, eds. *Advances in Neurology,* 86th ed. Philadelphia: Lippincott Williams & Wilkins, 2001: 337–345.
27. Schultz W. Predictive reward signal of dopamine neurons. *J Neurophysiol* 1998;80:1–27.
28. Metman LV, Konitsiotis S, Chase TN. Pathophysiology of motor response complications in Parkinson's disease: hypotheses on the why, where, and what. *Mov Disord* 2000;15:3–8.
29. Chase TN. Levodopa therapy: consequences of the nonphysiologic replacement of dopamine. *Neurology* 1998;50:S17–S25.
30. Nutt JG, Holford NH. The response to levodopa in Parkinson's disease: imposing pharmacological law and order. *Ann Neurol* 1996;39:561–573.
31. Langston JW, Quik M, Petzinger G, et al. Investigating levodopa-induced dyskinesias in the parkinsonian primate. *Ann Neurol* 2000;47[Suppl 1]:S79–S89.
32. Mones RJ. Analysis of levodopa induced dyskinesias in 51 patients with parkinsonism. *J Neurol Neurosurg Psychiatry* 1971;34:668–673.
33. Nutt JG. Levodopa-induced dyskinesia: review, observations, and speculations. *Neurology* 1990;40: 340–345.
34. Rajput AH, Fenton M, Birdi S, et al. Is levodopa toxic to human substantia nigra? *Mov Disord* 1997;12: 634–638.
35. Di Monte DA, McCormack A, Petzinger G, et al. Relationship among nigrostriatal denervation, parkinsonism, and dyskinesias in the MPTP primate model. *Mov Disord* 2000;15:459–466.
36. Zeng BY, Pearce RK, MacKenzie GM, et al. Alterations in preproenkephalin and adenosine-2a receptor mRNA, but not preprotachykinin mRNA correlate with occurrence of dyskinesia in normal monkeys chronically treated with levodopa. *Eur J Neurosci* 2000;12:1096–1104.
37. Rodriguez MC, Obeso JA, Olanow CW. Subthalamic nucleus-mediated excitotoxicity in Parkinson's disease: a target for neuroprotection. *Ann Neurol* 1998; 44[Suppl 3]:S175–S188.
38. Starr MS. Glutamate/dopamine D_1/D_2 balance in the basal ganglia and its relevance to Parkinson's disease. *Synapse* 1995;19:264–293.
39. Kita H, Kitai ST. Glutamate decarboxylase immunoreactive neurons in rat neostriatum: their morphological types and populations. *Brain Res* 1988;447:346–352.
40. Parent A, Harzati LN. Functional anatomy of the basal ganglia. I. The cortico-basal ganglia–thalamo–cortical loop. *Brain Res* 1995;20:91–127.
41. Cepeda C, Buchwald NA, Levine MS. Neuromodulatory actions of dopamine in the neostriatum are dependent upon the excitatory amino acid receptor subtypes activated. *Proc Natl Acad Sci USA* 1993;90:9576–9580.
42. Kotter R. Postsynaptic integration of glutamatergic and dopaminergic signals in the striatum. *Prog Neurobiol* 1994;44:163–196.
43. Calabresi P, Giacomini P, Centonze D, et al. Levodopa-induced dyskinesia: a pathological form of striatal synaptic plasticity? *Ann Neurol* 2000;47:S60–S68.
44. Dingledine R, Borges K, Bowie D, et al. The glutamate receptor ion channels. *Pharmacol Rev* 1999;51:7–61.
45. Ravenscroft P, Brotchie J. NMDA receptors in the basal ganglia. *J Anat* 2000;196:577–585.
46. Kosinski CM, Standaert DG, Counihan TJ, et al. Statement of *N*-methyl D-aspartate receptor subunit mRNAs in the human brain: striatum and globus pallidus. *J Comp Neurol* 1998;390:63–74.
47. Ulas J, Weihmüller FB, Brunner LC, et al. Selective increase of NMDA-sensitive glutamate binding in the striatum of Parkinson's disease, Alzheimer's disease, and mixed Parkinson's disease/Alzheimer's disease patients: an autoradiographic study. *J Neurosci* 1994;14: 6317–6324.
48. Calon F, Morissette M, Ghribi O, et al. Alteration of glutamate receptors in the striatum of dyskinetic 1-methyl-4-phenyl-1,2,3,6-tetrahydropyridine–treated monkeys following dopamine agonist treatment. *Prog Neuropsychopharmacol Biol Psychiatry* 2002;26: 127–138.
49. Ravenscroft P, Brotchie J. Alterations in striatal NR1 and NR2B NMDA receptor subunit expression in the 6-OHDA–lesioned rat model of levodopa-induced dyskinesia. *Parkinsonism Related Disord* 1999; 5[Suppl]:S42.
50. Papa SM, Chase TN. Levodopa-induced dyskinesias improved by a glutamate antagonist in parkinsonian monkeys. *Ann Neurol* 1996;39:574–578.
51. Blanchet PJ, Konitsiotis S, Chase TN. Amantadine reduces levodopa-induced dyskinesias in parkinsonian monkeys. *Mov Disord* 1998;13:798–802.
52. Herrero MT, Augood SJ, Hirsch EC, et al. Effects of L-dopa on preproenkephalin and preprotachykinin gene expression in the MPTP-treated monkey striatum. *Neuroscience* 1995;68:1189–1198.
53. Morissette M, Grondin R, Goulet M, et al. Differential regulation of striatal preproenkephalin and preprotachykinin mRNA levels in MPTP-lesioned monkeys chronically treated with dopamine D_1 or D_2 receptor agonists. *J Neurochem* 1999;72:682–692.
54. Calon F, Birdi S, Hornykiewicz O, et al. Increase of preproenkephalin mRNA statement in the putamen of Parkinson's disease patients with levodopa-induced dyskinesias. *J Neuropathol Exp Neurol* 2002;61: 186–196.
55. Doucet JP, Nakabeppu Y, Bédard PJ, et al. Chronic alterations in dopaminergic neurotransmission produce a persistent elevation of ΔFosB-like proteins(s) in both the rodent and primate striatum. *Eur J Neurosci* 1996; 8:365–381.
56. Nestler EJ, Kelz MB, Chen J. Delta FosB: a molecular mediator of long-term neural and behavioral plasticity. *Brain Res* 1999;835:10–17
57. Gerfen CR. Molecular effects of dopamine on striatal-projection pathways. *Trends Neurosci* 2000;23[Suppl]: S64–S70.
58. Tekumalla PK, Calon F, Rahman Z, et al. Elevated levels of delta FosB and RGS9 in striatum in Parkinson's disease. *Biol Psychiatry* 2001;50:813–816.
59. Benabid AL, Krack PP, Benazzouz A, et al. Deep brain stimulation of the subthalamic nucleus for Parkinson's disease: methodologic aspects and clinical criteria. *Neurology* 2000;55[Suppl 6]:S40–S44.
60. Guridi J, Herrero MT, Luquin MR. Subthalamotomy in parkinsonian monkeys. Behavioural and biochemical analysis. *Brain* 1996;119:1717–1727.
61. Krack P, Pollak P, Limousin P, et al. From off-period dystonia to peak-dose chorea. The clinical spectrum of varying subthalamic nucleus activity. *Brain* 1999;122: 1133–1146.

62. Metman LV, van den Munckhof P, Klaassen AA, et al. Effects of supra-threshold levodopa doses on dyskinesias in advanced Parkinson's disease. *Neurology* 1997; 49:711–713.
63. Rascol O. Medical treatment of levodopa-induced dyskinesias. *Ann Neurol* 2000;47[Suppl 1]: S179–S188.
64. Rajput AH, Rajput A, Lang AE, et al. New use for an old drug: amantadine benefits levodopa-induced dyskinesia. *Mov Disord* 1998;13:851.
65. Metman LV, Del Dotto P, LePoole K, et al. Amantadine for levodopa-induced dyskinesias: a 1-year follow-up study. *Arch Neurol* 1999;56:1383–1386.
66. Danysz W, Parsons CG, Kornhuber J, et al. Aminoadamantines as NMDA receptor antagonists and antiparkinsonian agents—preclinical studies. *Neurosci Biobehav Rev* 1997;21:455–468.
67. Bennett JP Jr, Landow ER, Schuh LA. Suppression of dyskinesias in advanced Parkinson's disease, II: increasing daily clozapine doses suppress dyskinesias and improve parkinsonism symptoms. *Neurology* 1993;43:1551–1555.
68. Durif F, Vidailhet M, Assal F, et al. Low-dose of clozapine improves dyskinesias in Parkinson's disease. *Neurology* 1997;48:658–662.
69. Moore NA, Tye NC, Axton MS, et al. The behavioral pharmacology of olanzapine, a novel 'atypical' antipsychotic agent. *J Pharmacol Exp Ther* 1992;262: 545–551.
70. Manson AJ, Schrag A, Lees AJ. Low-dose olanzapine for levodopa induced dyskinesias. *Neurology* 2000;55: 795–799.
71. Rinne UK, Bracco F, Chouza C, et al. Early treatment of Parkinson's disease with cabergoline delays the onset of motor complications. Results of a double-blind levodopa controlled trial. *Drugs* 1998;55[Suppl 1]: 23–30.
72. Parkinson Study Group. Pramipexole vs levodopa as initial treatment for Parkinson disease: a randomized controlled trial. *JAMA* 2000;284:1931–1938.
73. Rascol O, Brooks DJ, Korczyn AD, et al. A five-year study of the incidence of dyskinesia in patients with early Parkinson's disease who were treated with ropinirole or levodopa. *N Engl J Med* 2000;342:1484–1491.
74. Frucht S, Rogers JD, Greene PE, et al. Falling asleep at the wheel: motor vehicle mishaps in persons taking pramipexole and ropinirole. *Neurology* 1999;52: 1908–1910.
75. Hadj Tahar A, Ekesbo A, Grégoire L, et al. Effects of acute and repeated treatment with a novel dopamine D_2 receptor ligand on levodopa-induced dyskinesias in MPTP monkeys. *Eur J Pharmacol* 2001;412:247–254.
76. Sonesson C, Lin C-H, Hansson LO, et al. Substituted (*S*)-phenylpiperidines and rigid congeners as preferential dopamine autoreceptor antagonists: synthesis and structure-activity relationships. *J Med Chem* 1994;37: 2735–2753.
77. Ekesbo A, Torstenson R, Harvig P, et al. Effects of the substituted (*S*)-3-phenylpiperidine (–)-OSU6162 on PET measurements of [^{11}C]SCH23390 and [^{11}C]raclopride binding in primate brain. *Neuropharmacology* 1999;38:331–338.
78. Ekesbo A, Andren PE, Gunne LM, et al. Motor effects of (–)-OSU6162 in primates with unilateral 6-hydroxydopamine lesions. *Eur J Pharmacol* 2000;389: 193–199.
79. Tedroff J, Sonesson C, Waters N, et al. Are dyskinesias and motor fluctuations in Parkinson's disease due to a shift in the 'energy landscape' for the D_2 receptor? *Mov Disord* 1997;12[Suppl 1]:S112.
80. Tedroff J, Torstenson R, Hartvig P, et al. Effects of the substituted (*S*)-3-phenylpiperidine (–)-OSU6162 on PET measurements in subhuman primates: evidence for tone-dependent normalization of striatal dopaminergic activity. *Synapse* 1998;28:280–287.
81. Ekesbo A, Andren PE, Gunne LM, et al. (–)-OSU6162 inhibits levodopa-induced dyskinesias in a monkey model of Parkinson's disease. *NeuroReport* 1997;8: 2567–2570.
82. Nonaka H, Saki M, Ichimura M, et al. Novel potent adenosine A_{2a} receptor antagonists. *Mov Disord* 1997; 12[Suppl 1]:120.
83. Fink JS, Weaver DR, Rivkees SA, et al. Molecular cloning of the rat A_2 adenosine receptor: selective coexpression with D_2 dopamine receptors in rat striatum. *Mol Brain Res* 1992;14:186–195.
84. Pollack AE, Harrison MB, Wooten FG, et al. Differential localization of A_{2a} adenosine receptor mRNA with D_1 and D_2 dopamine receptor mRNA in striatal output pathways following a selective lesion of striatonigral neurons. *Brain Res* 1993;631:161–166.
85. Ferré S, Fuxe K, von Euler G, et al. Adenosine-dopamine interactions in the brain. *Neuroscience* 1992;51:501–512.
86. Ferré S, Fredholm BB, Morelli M, et al. Adenosine-dopamine receptor interactions as integrative mechanism in the basal ganglia. *Trends Neurosci* 1997;20: 482–492.
87. Pinna A, Di Chiara G, Wardas J, et al. Blockade of A_{2a} adenosine receptors positively modulates turning behavior and c-*Fos* expression induced by D_1 agonists in dopamine-denervated rats. *Eur J Neurosci* 1996;8: 1176–1181.
88. Popoli P, Gimenez-Llort L, Pezzola A, et al. Adenosine A_1 receptor blockade selectively potentiates the motor effects induced by dopamine D_1 receptor stimulation in rodents. *Neurosci Lett* 1996;218:209–213.
89. Fenu S, Pinna A, Ongini E, et al. Adenosine A_{2a} receptor antagonism potentiates levodopa-induced turning behavior and c-*fos* expression in 6-hydroxydopamine–lesioned rats. *Eur J Pharmacol* 1997;321: 143–147.
90. Kanda T, Shiozaki S, Shimada J, et al. KF17837: a novel selective adenosine A_{2a} receptor antagonist with anticataleptic activity. *Eur J Pharmacol* 1994;256: 263–268.
91. Ongini E, Fredholm BB. Pharmacology of adenosine A_{2a} receptors. *Trends Pharmacol Sci* 1996;17:364–372.
92. Grondin R, Bédard PJ, Hadj Tahar A, et al. Antiparkinsonian effect of a new selective adenosine A_{2a} receptor antagonist in MPTP-treated monkeys. *Neurology* 1999;52:1673–1677.
93. Hadj Tahar A, Grondin R, Grégoire L, et al. Selective adenosine A_{2a} receptor antagonism as an alternative therapy for Parkinson's disease. In: Kase H, Richardson PJ, Jenner P, eds. *Adenosine receptors and Parkinson's disease.* San Diego: Academic Press, 2000: 229–244.
94. Kanda T, Jackson MJ, Smith LA, et al. Adenosine A_{2a} antagonist: a novel antiparkinsonian agent that does not provoke dyskinesia in parkinsonian monkeys. *Ann Neurol* 1998;43:507–513.

95. Svenningsson P, Nomikos GG, Ongini E, et al. Antagonism of adenosine A_{2a} receptors underlies the behavioral activating effect of caffeine and is associated with reduced expression of messenger RNA for NGFI-A and NGFI-B in caudate-putamen and nucleus accumbens. *Neuroscience* 1997;79:753–764.
96. Ledent C, Vaugeois JM, Schiffmann SN, et al. Aggressiveness, hypoalgesia and high blood pressure in mice lacking the adenosine A_{2a} receptor. *Nature* 1997;388: 674–678.
97. Kurokawa M, Kirk IP, Kirkpatrick KA, et al. Inhibition by KF17837 of adenosine A_{2a} receptor–mediated modulation of striatal GABA and ACh release. *Br J Parmacol* 1994;113:43–48.
98. Mori A, Shindou T, Ichimura M, et al. The role of adenosine A_{2a} receptors in the regulating GABAergic synaptic transmission in striatal medium spiny neurons. *J Neurosci* 1996;16:605–611.
99. Richardson PJ, Kase H, Jenner PG. Adenosine receptor antagonists as new agents for the treatment of Parkinson's disease. *Trends Pharmacol Sci* 1997;18: 338–344.
100. Mayfield RD, Larson G, Orona RA, et al. Opposing actions of adenosine A_{2a} and dopamine D_2 receptor activation on GABA release in the basal ganglia: evidence for an A_{2a}/D_2 receptor interactions in globus pallidus. *Synapse* 1996;22:132–138.
101. Kirk IP, Richardson PJ. Adenosine A_{2a} receptor-mediated modulation of striatal [^{3}H]GABA and [^{3}H]acetylcholine release. *J Neurochem* 1994;62:960–966.
102. Piccini P, Weeks RA, Brooks DJ. Alterations in opioid receptor binding in Parkinson's disease patients with levodopa-induced dyskinesias. *Ann Neurol* 1997;42: 720–726.
103. Pollack AE, Wooten GF. D_2 dopaminergic regulation of striatal preproenkephalin mRNA levels is mediated at least in part through cholinergic interneurons. *Brain Res Mol Brain Res* 1992;13:35–41.
104. Henry B, Brotchie JM. Potential of opioid antagonists in the treatment of levodopa-induced dyskinesias in Parkinson's disease. *Drugs Aging* 1996;9:149–158.
105. Schiffmann SN, Vanderhaeghen JJ. Adenosine A_2 receptors regulate the gene expression of striatopallidal and striatonigral neurons. *J Neurosci* 1993;13: 1080–1087.
106. Nash JE, Brotchie JM. A common signaling pathway for striatal NMDA and adenosine A_{2a} receptors: implications for the treatment of Parkinson's disease. *J Neurosci* 2000;20:7782–7789.
107. Quinn N, Parkes D, Marsden D. Control of on/off phenomenon by continuous intravenous infusion of levodopa. *Neurology* 1984;34:1131–1136.
108. Syed N, Murphy J, Zimmerman T Jr, et al. Ten years' experience with enteral levodopa infusions for motor fluctuations in Parkinson's disease. *Mov Disord* 1998; 13:336–338.
109. Fariello RG. Pharmacodynamic and pharmacokinetic features of cabergoline: rationale for use in Parkinson's disease. *Drugs* 1998;55:10–16.
110. Grondin R, Bédard PJ. Cabergoline: a promising agent for the treatment of Parkinson's disease. *CNS Drug Rev* 1996;2:214–225.
111. Hadj Tahar A, Grégoire L, Bangassoro E, et al. Sustained cabergoline treatment reverses levodopa-induced dyskinesias in parkinsonian monkeys. *Clin Neuropharmacol* 2000;23:195–202.
112. Bejjani BP, Arnulf I, Demeret S, et al. Levodopa-induced dyskinesias in Parkinson's disease: is sensitization reversible? *Ann Neurol* 2000;47:655–658.
113. Baronti F, Mouradian MM, Davis TL, et al. Continuous lisuride effects on central dopaminergic mechanisms in Parkinson's disease. *Ann Neurol* 1992;32: 776–781.
114. Olanow CW, Obezo JA. Pulsatile stimulation of dopamine receptors and levodopa-induced motor complications in Parkinson's disease: implications for the early use of COMT inhibitors. *Neurology* 2000;55: S72–S77.
115. Henry B, Crossman AR, Brotchie JM. Characterization of enhanced behavioral responses to L-dopa following repeated administration in the 6-hydroxydopamine-lesioned rat model of Parkinson's disease. *Exp Neurol* 1998;151:334–342.
116. Steiner H, Gerfen CR. Role of dynorphin and enkephalin in the regulation of striatal output pathways and behavior. *Exp Brain Res* 1998;123:60–76.
117. Fitzgerald LW, Deutch AY, Gasic G, et al. Regulation of cortical and subcortical glutamate receptor subunit expression by antipsychotic drugs. *J Neurosci* 1995; 15:2453–2461.
118. Girault JA, Siciliano JC, Robel L, et al. Stimulation of protein-tyrosine phosphorylation in rat striatum after lesion of dopamine neurons or chronic neuroleptic treatment. *Proc Natl Acad Sci USA* 1992;89: 2769–2773.
119. Campbell K, Björklund A. Prefrontal corticostriatal afferents maintain increased enkephalin gene expression in the dopamine-denervated rat striatum. *Eur J Neurosci* 1994;6:1371–1383.
120. Hajji MD, Salin P, Kerkerian-Le Goff L. Chronic dizocilpine maleate (MK-801) treatment suppresses the effects of nigrostriatal dopamine deafferentation on enkephalin but not on substance P expression in the rat striatum. *Eur J Neurosci* 1996;8:917–926.
121. Hadj Tahar A, Grégoire L, Darré A, et al. Prevention of levodopa-induced dyskinesias by a selective NR1A/2B NMDA receptor antagonist in parkinsonian monkeys [Abstract]. *Soc Neurosci* 2001.
122. Whittemore ER, Ilyin VI, Woodward RM. Electrophysiological characterization of CI-1041 on cloned and native NMDA receptors [Abstract]. *Soc Neurosci* 2000.
123. Menegoz M, Lau LF, Herve D, et al. Tyrosine phosphorylation of NMDA receptor in rat striatum: effects of 6-OH-dopamine lesions. *NeuroReport* 1995;7:125–128.
124. Oh JD, Russell DS, Vaughan CL, et al. Enhanced tyrosine phosphorylation of striatal NMDA receptor subunits: effect of dopaminergic denervation and levodopa administration. *Brain Res* 1998;813:150–159.
125. Centonze D, Calabresi P, Giacomini P, et al. Neurophysiology of Parkinson's disease: from basic research to clinical correlates. *Clin Neurophysiol* 1999;110: 2006–2013.
126. Filion M. Physiologic basis of dyskinesia. *Ann Neurol* 2000;47[Suppl 1]:S35–S40.
127. Graybiel AM, Canales JJ, Capper-Loup C. Levodopa-induced dyskinesias and dopamine-dependent stereotypies: a new hypothesis. *Trends Neurosci* 2000;23 [Suppl]:S71–S77.

Parkinson's Disease: Advances in Neurology, Vol. 91.
Edited by Ariel Gordin, Seppo Kaakkola, and Heikki Teräväinen
Lippincott Williams & Wilkins, Philadelphia © 2003

6

Dopamine Receptors in Parkinson's Disease: Imaging Studies

A. Jon Stoessl and Raúl de la Fuente-Fernández

Pacific Parkinson's Research Centre, University of British Columbia, Vancouver, British Columbia, Canada

Although the primary abnormality underlying the manifestations of Parkinson's disease (PD) is a profound loss of dopamine (DA) in the nigrostriatal pathway, there has been longstanding speculation that some complications of long-term therapy may arise from alterations in DA receptors. Postmortem studies have revealed conflicting findings; however, the balance of opinion would suggest that there is an initial increase in D_2 receptor binding as a result of dopaminergic denervation but that levels return to within the reference range after the initiation of levodopa and presumably DA agonist therapy (1). The interpretation of postmortem studies is, however, confounded by numerous factors including difficulties in standardizing the effects of treatment; frequently incomplete clinical data, the effects of other related (e.g., dementia and depression) or unrelated illnesses; and agonal state. These studies will usually be restricted to patients with advanced disease and may not permit the analysis of earlier stages of the illness. In particular, longitudinal analysis is obviously not possible. For all these reasons, great hopes have been pinned on the ability of imaging studies to assess DA receptor function *in vivo.*

DA receptor ligands have been developed for both single-photon emission computed tomography (SPECT) and positron emission tomography (PET). This chapter focuses on PET, which has a number of advantages in terms of resolution and quantitation, but many of the principles and types of studies apply to both. For the purposes of this chapter, studies of postsynaptic receptors and transporters are considered.

Although we focus on studies based on the application of radiolabeled compounds that bind directly to receptors or transporters for DA, it is worth remembering that much useful information can be derived from indirect analysis, in which the effects of dopaminergic stimulation on regional cerebral blood flow (2–4) or local cerebral glucose metabolism (5) are studied.

DOPAMINERGIC RECEPTORS

Although molecular techniques have led to the identification of novel receptors, the original classification of two DA receptor families (6) still applies. The D_1 family of receptors can be labeled for PET using ^{11}C-SCH 23390. Other choices include ^{11}C-SCH 39166 (7) or the ^{11}C-NNC family of compounds (8,9). Although SCH 39166 was expected to be more selective than SCH 23390 (which also binds to 5-hydroxytryptamine$_{2A+C}$ receptors) based on *in vitro* studies, PET studies in humans have revealed a low target-to-background ratio, suggesting that it may be a suboptimal agent. It is not currently possible to selectively image D_5 receptors.

The ligand most widely used for imaging the D_2 family of receptors is ^{11}C-raclopride (RAC). This agent has the advantage of good selectivity for D_2/D_3 receptors and rapid equilibrium. However, the affinity for the D_2 receptor is only moderate (low nanomolar), so it is subject to competition from endogenous DA (10–12). This can be used to assess changes in synaptic levels of DA (see later discussion) but can result in problems of interpretation. If scans are done after a single concentration of ^{11}C-RAC only, it is impossible to determine whether changes in binding reflect alterations in the number of available DA receptors or whether they are due to changes in synaptic DA concentrations. Thus, some investigators prefer to use agents with a higher affinity for the DA receptor, such as ^{11}C- or ^{18}F-labeled spiperone or its derivatives, or ^{18}F-benperidol (13).

Presynaptic DA function can be assessed by labeling the membrane DA transporter (DAT). This is thought to correspond to the density of dopaminergic nerve terminals. Most of the agents used to image the DAT are tropane (cocaine-like) derivatives; these include ^{11}C- (14) and ^{18}F- (15) WIN 35,428, ^{11}C-RTI-32 (16), and various derivatives of β-CIT. Most of these compounds have good selectivity for the DAT compared with other membrane monoamine transporters. However, the kinetic profile of these compounds is such that equilibrium may not be achieved during the scan procedure. An exception is fluoropropyl-β-CIT. This compound is preferable to its ^{11}C-labeled analog because of the longer half-life (108 minutes) of ^{18}F compared with ^{11}C (20 minutes) (17). A 2-hour scan time is sufficient to achieve equilibrium, but sufficient activity would not be detectable using ^{11}C at this late time.

Another option for labeling the DAT is ^{11}C-D-*threo*-methylphenidate, which has been developed by the Brookhaven group (18). This compound has the advantage of excellent selectivity for the DAT, as well as a better kinetic profile than the tropane derivatives.

Although studies of DAT should provide some measure of nerve terminal density, this molecule is subject to pharmacological regulation (19,20). Thus, changes in DAT binding could theoretically arise from medication or compensatory effects, rather than alterations in innervation density. Most investigators have failed to demonstrate an effect of antiparkinsonian treatment on DAT binding *in vivo*. However, a recent report suggests changes after levodopa therapy, whereas the DA agonist pramipexole did not have this effect (21). In contrast, the vesicular monoamine transporter type 2 (VMAT2), which is also expressed by dopaminergic neurons, is not thought to be subject to such regulatory effects. It may therefore be a preferable target for assessing nerve terminal density. However, VMAT2 is expressed by all other monoaminergic neurons as well, although striatal binding is almost entirely to dopaminergic neurons.

CLINICAL STUDIES

Studies of D_2 receptors confirm postmortem findings of increased D_2 binding in early untreated PD. Although increases in ^{11}C-RAC binding could partially reflect reduced receptor occupancy by endogenous DA, rather than a true receptor upregulation, parallel studies using the higher affinity agent ^{11}C-*N*-methylspiperone suggest this is not the case (22). Chronic dopaminergic therapy is associated with a return of D_2 binding to normal, or in more advanced disease, even modestly subnormal levels (23). Increases in D_2 binding are greater in the putamen than in the caudate nucleus (24), and the ratio of putamen-to-caudate ^{11}C-RAC binding remains increased compared with normal subjects, even in patients with advanced disease, on chronic dopaminergic therapy (25). This increase is also seen in patients with familial parkinsonism due to mutations in the gene encoding α-synuclein (25). No consistent changes relating complications of therapy to changes in striatal D_2 binding have been seen (26–28). However, advanced disease may be associated with reduced D_2/D_3 binding in extrastriatal regions, including the medial thalamus and anterior cingulate and dorsolateral prefrontal cortices (29). Not surprisingly, other parkinsonian syndromes characterized by degeneration of striatal and dopaminergic neurons are associated with reduced D_2 binding on PET (30,31).

D_1 receptor binding is normal in PD but reduced in multiple system atrophy (32). Similar to the case for D_2 binding, there is no clear relationship between various complications of treatment and changes in D_1 binding, although a loose inverse correlation between the duration of dyskinesia and D_1 binding has been reported (28).

As is the case for 6-^{18}F-fluorodopa (FD), the uptake of DAT and VMAT2 ligands is reduced in PD. These reductions are asymmetrical (and affect the clinically spared striatum in patients with stage I disease) and affect the putamen more than the caudate (14–16,33). For a given degree of denervation assessed by dihydrotetrabenazine binding, there is a less marked degree of impairment of FD uptake, whereas the reduction of DAT binding is greater than would be predicted (34). This combination of findings would be compatible with compensatory changes designed to maximize the availability of synaptic DA; increased FD uptake may be indicative of increased decarboxylation (i.e., increased DA synthesis), whereas downregulation of the DAT would serve to maintain DA levels within the synapse.

Use of ^{11}C-Raclopride Binding to Estimate Changes in Dopamine Levels

As alluded to earlier in this chapter, ^{11}C-RAC binding to D_2-like receptors is subject to competition from endogenous DA (10–12). Thus, after a challenge with amphetamine, which is known to induce DA release, there is an immediate reduction in RAC (or in the case of SPECT, iodobenzamide) binding, which correlates with increased levels of DA detected by dialysis (35). Amphetamine-induced release of DA estimated by this method is increased in schizophrenic patients (36).

This approach had received relatively little attention in PD. However, it has now been shown that amphetamine-induced release of DA is markedly decreased in PD, with correction after fetal transplantation (37). This correlates with postgraft increases in FD uptake. Furthermore, levodopa results in reduced RAC binding, presumably as a reflection of enhanced availability of DA within the synapse (38). The time course of levodopa-induced changes in RAC binding differs between patients who are prone to medication-associated fluctuations in function (rapid decrease, followed by a rapid return to baseline) and those who maintain a stable response to medication for at least 3 years on chronic levodopa treatment (gradual and sustained decrease in RAC binding) (39) (Fig. 6.1). This suggests that the emergence of motor fluctuations may not be a direct result of levodopa therapy itself, but of the increased turnover of DA in some patients. Strafella et al. (40) recently demonstrated release of DA in the caudate nucleus after transcranial stimulation of the ipsilateral prefrontal cortex in healthy human subjects.

In addition to its important role in motor function, DA is known to be critical for signaling reward (41,42). Koepp et al. (43) showed that monetary rewards derived from playing video games result in increased DA release, assessed by changes in RAC binding. It has not always been clear whether it is the reward itself that results in DA release (or whether the sensation of reward is mediated by DA) or whether the *expectation* of reward may have this effect. It is the expectation of therapeutic benefit that underlies the well-recognized placebo effect. Remarkably, placebo injection itself may result in enhanced DA release throughout the striatum in patients with PD (44) (Fig. 6.2). The magnitude of the response is comparable to that seen in normal subjects after amphetamine administration and is additive to the effects of a short-acting direct DA receptor agonist on RAC binding, with a trend toward a negative interaction (i.e., patients with the greatest placebo response demonstrate less dose–response inhibition of RAC binding after apo-

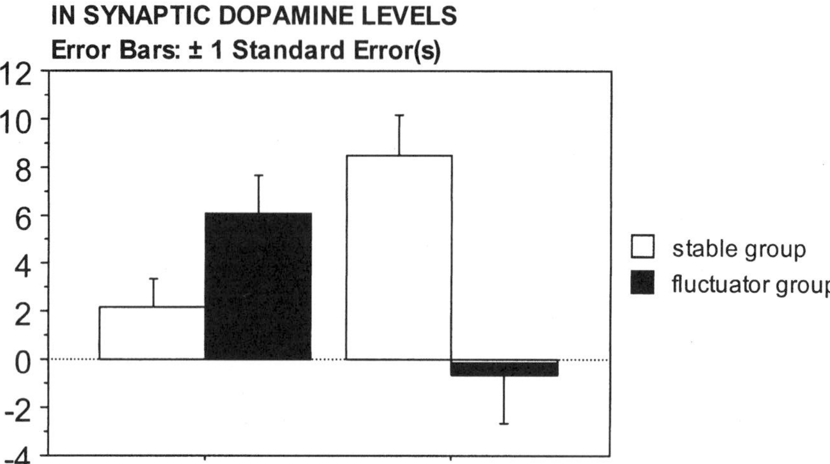

FIGURE 6.1. Estimated levodopa-induced changes in synaptic dopamine concentration. Values are expressed as percent reduction from baseline of ^{11}C-raclopride binding potential in the putamen, both 1 hour and 4 hours after oral administration of 250/25 mg of levodopa/carbidopa. The estimated increase in synaptic dopamine levels 1 hour after levodopa administration was three times higher in patients who developed motor fluctuations during the follow-up period than in stable responders ($p < .05$). By contrast, whereas stable responders maintained increased levels of dopamine 4 hours after levodopa, this level dropped below baseline values (*zero line in the graph*) at the fourth-hour scan in the fluctuation group ($p < .01$). (From de la Fuente-Fernandez R, Lu J-Q, Sossi V, et al. Biochemical variations in the synaptic level of dopamine precede motor fluctuations in Parkinson's disease: PET evidence of increased dopamine turnover. *Ann Neurol* 2001;49:298–303, with permission.)

morphine administration). This finding is the first demonstration of a physicochemical basis for the placebo effect, which has been well demonstrated in PD (45,46) and emphasizes the importance of conducting adequately controlled trials of both medications and surgery in PD. The finding may explain the common observation that medications often seem less impressive when used in routine clinical practice (in which the level of expectation of therapeutic benefit is presumably lower) compared with initial testing in clinical trials (in which the patient derives benefit from both the active drug itself and the high level of expectation associated with participation in the study).

Why have PET Studies of Dopamine Receptors not Been More Informative in PD?

Although a number of changes (as outlined already) have been demonstrated in PD, there has in general been a disappointing paucity of evidence for changes in DA receptor function linked to clinical complications of the disease and its long-term treatment. A number of possible explanations can be advanced for this. Some are technical: Perhaps PET does not have the anatomical resolution or sensitivity to detect relatively subtle changes restricted to discrete brain regions. Newer tomographs with heightened sensitivity and better resolution may detect changes in striatal subregions or in extrastriatal sites that express DA receptors.

Most studies of D_2-like receptors have been performed using ^{11}C-RAC. The relatively low affinity of this compound for the D_2 receptor results in sensitivity to changes in synaptic levels of DA, as discussed earlier in this chapter. It is conceivable that changes in binding resulting from a decline in both the concentration of DA and the number of DA receptors could cancel each other out. Additionally, most studies of both D_1 and D_2 receptors have

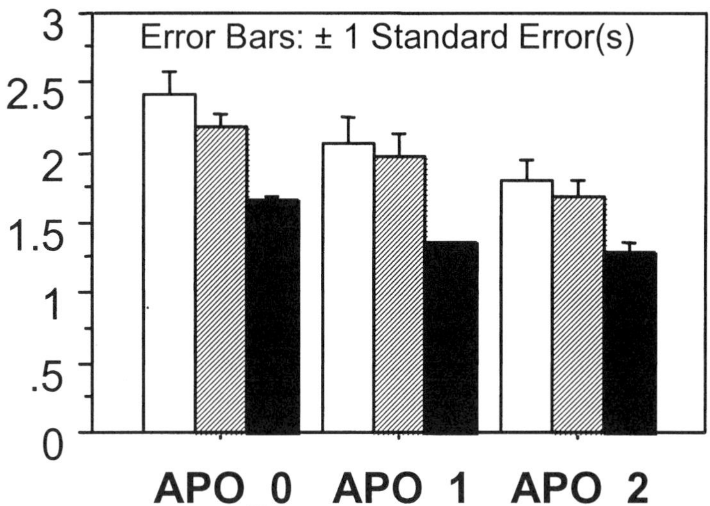

FIGURE 6.2. Effects of apomorphine on ^{11}C-raclopride binding potential in the putamen at baseline *(APO 0)* or after 0.03 *(APO 1)* or 0.06 *(APO 2)* mg/kg of subcutaneous apomorphine. Patients studied in an open fashion (*open bars*) had higher baseline binding than those who received an injection of saline. Additionally, those patients who perceived a placebo effect after the injection of saline (*solid bars*) had much lower levels of binding than those patients who failed to perceive a placebo effect after saline (*hatched bars*). Lower ^{11}C-raclopride binding potential is indicative of striatal dopamine release as a manifestation of the placebo effect. (From de la Fuente-Fernandez R, Ruth TJ, Sossi V, et al. Expectation and dopamine release: mechanism of the placebo effect in Parkinson's disease. *Science* 2001;293:1164–1166, with permission.)

been performed using radiolabeled antagonists, which will bind equally to both high-affinity and low-affinity states of the relevant receptor. Thus, if complications were related to shifts in the affinity state of the receptor, this would probably not be detected. The recent introduction of positron-emitting DA receptor agonists (47,48) may provide interesting new insights, although clinical studies have not yet been reported.

Most likely, however, studies have failed to detect substantial disease-related changes because the available tools do not permit the most important biological questions to be addressed. ^{11}C-RAC binds to D_2 and D_3 receptors, but there are no good positron-emitting tracers for the D_4 receptor. Evidence from animal models suggests that increased expression of the D_3 receptor may play a critical role in the expression of levodopa-induced dyskinesias (49,50); increased D_3 expression would, however, be unlikely to result in altered RAC binding, in view of the relative proportion of D_2 to D_3 receptors in the motor striatum. Thus, until a more D_3-specific positron-emitting ligand becomes available, such changes will not be detected by PET.

Finally, animal studies suggest that the emergence of levodopa-induced complications of therapy may be associated with more impressive changes *downstream* to DA receptors than in the levels of the receptors themselves. These include increased expression of opioid transmitters in the striatonigral and striatopallidal pathways (51–53), as well as increased expression of the immediate early gene *Fos*B (54,55). Piccini et al. (56) reported reduced striatal and thalamic binding of the opioid receptor ligand ^{11}C-diprenorphine in dyskinetic patients with PD, whereas nondyskinetic patients with PD have normal levels of binding. By analogy with DA-related changes in ^{11}C-RAC binding, the reduced levels of binding are thought to reflect increased release of endogenous opioid peptides in the brains of the dyskinetic subjects, in keeping with findings in animal models. Current PET techniques do not permit the detection of changes in the expression of immediate early genes or transcriptional factors. Developments in this arena may prove fruitful in the future.

ACKNOWLEDGMENTS

This work was supported by the Canadian Institutes of Health Research, the National Parkinson Foundation (Miami, Inc.), the British Columbia Health Research Foundation, the Pacific Parkinson's Research Institute, and the Canada Research Chairs Program.

REFERENCES

1. Guttman M, Seeman P, Reynolds GP, et al. Dopamine D_2 receptor density remains constant in treated Parkinson's disease. *Ann Neurol* 1986;19:487–492.
2. Black KJ, Gado MH, Perlmutter JS. PET measurement of dopamine D_2 receptor-mediated changes in striatopallidal function. *J Neurosci* 1997;17:3168–3177.
3. Black KJ, Hershey T, Gado MH, et al. Dopamine D_1 agonist activates temporal lobe structures in primates. *J Neurophysiol* 2000;84:549–557.
4. Jenkins IH, Fernandez W, Playford ED, et al. Impaired activation of the supplementary motor area in Parkinson's disease is reversed when akinesia is treated with apomorphine. *Ann Neurol* 1992;32:749–757.
5. Broussolle E, Cinotti L, Pollak P, et al. Relief of akinesia by apomorphine and cerebral metabolic changes in Parkinson's disease. *Mov Disord* 1993;8:459–462.
6. Kebabian JW, Calne DB. Multiple receptor mechanisms for dopamine. *Nature* 1979;227:93–96.
7. Karlsson P, Sedvall G, Halldin C, et al. Evaluation of SCH 39166 as PET ligand for central D_1 dopamine receptor binding and occupancy in man. *Psychopharmacology (Berlin)* 1995;121:300–308.
8. Halldin C, Foged C, Farde L, et al. [^{11}C]NNC 687 and [^{11}C]NNC 756, dopamine D-1 receptor ligands. Preparation, autoradiography and PET investigation in monkey. *Nucl Med Biol* 1993;20:945–953.
9. Laihinen AO, Rinne JO, Ruottinen HM, et al. PET studies on dopamine D_1 receptors in the human brain with carbon-11-SCH 39166 and carbon-11-NNC 756. *J Nucl Med* 1994;35:1916–1920.
10. Seeman P, Guan HC, Niznik HB. Endogenous dopamine lowers the dopamine D_2 receptor density as measured by ^{3}H raclopride: implications for positron emission tomography of the human brain. *Synapse* 1989;3:96–97.
11. Dewey SL, Smith GS, Logan J, et al. Striatal binding of the PET ligand ^{11}C-raclopride is altered by drugs that modify synaptic dopamine levels. *Synapse* 1993;13:350–356.
12. Volkow ND, Wang G-J, Fowler JS, et al. Imaging endogenous dopamine competition with [^{11}C]raclopride in the human brain. *Synapse* 1994;16:255–262.
13. Moerlein SM, Perlmutter JS, Markham J, et al. *In vivo* kinetics of [^{18}F](*N*-methyl)benperidol: a novel PET tracer for assessment of dopaminergic D_2-like receptor binding. *J Cereb Blood Flow Metab* 1997;17:833–845.
14. Frost JJ, Rosier AJ, Reich SG, et al. Positron emission tomographic imaging of the dopamine transporter with ^{11}C-WIN 35,428 reveals marked declines in mild Parkinson's disease. *Ann Neurol* 1993;34:423–431.
15. Rinne JO, Bergman J, Ruottinen H, et al. Striatal uptake of a novel PET ligand, [^{18}F]beta-CFT, is reduced in early Parkinson's disease. *Synapse* 1999;31:119–124.
16. Guttman M, Burkholder J, Kish SJ, et al. [^{11}C]RTI-32 PET studies of the dopamine transporter in early dopa-naive Parkinson's disease: implications for the symptomatic threshold. *Neurology* 1997;48:1578–1583.
17. Lundkvist C, Halldin C, Ginovart N, et al. [^{18}F]-CIT-FP is superior to [^{11}C]-CIT-FP for quantitation of the dopamine transporter. *Nucl Med Biol* 1997;24:621–627.
18. Volkow ND, Ding Y-S, Fowler JS, et al. A new PET ligand for the dopamine transporter: studies in the human brain. *J Nucl Med* 1995;36:2162–2168.
19. Vanderborght T, Kilbourn M, Desmond T, et al. The vesicular monoamine transporter is not regulated by dopaminergic drug treatments. *Eur J Pharmacol* 1995; 294:577–583.
20. Wilson JM, Kish SJ. The vesicular monoamine transporter, in contrast to the dopamine transporter, is not altered by chronic cocaine self-administration in the rat. *J Neurosci* 1996;16:3507–3510.
21. Guttman M, Stewart D, Hussey D, et al. Influence of L-dopa and pramipexole on striatal dopamine transporter in early PD. *Neurology* 2001;56:1559–1564.
22. Kaasinen V, Ruottinen HM, Nagren K, et al. Upregulation of putaminal dopamine D_2 receptors in early Parkinson's disease: a comparative PET study with [^{11}C]raclopride and [^{11}C]*N*-methylspiperone. *J Nucl Med* 2000;41:65–70.
23. Antonini A, Schwarz J, Oertel WH, et al. Long-term changes of striatal dopamine D_2 receptors in patients with Parkinson's disease: a study with positron emission tomography and [^{11}C]raclopride. *Mov Disord* 1997;12: 33–38.
24. Rinne JO, Laihinen A, Ruottinen H, et al. Increased density of dopamine D_2 receptors in the putamen, but not in the caudate nucleus in early Parkinson's disease: a PET study with [^{11}C]raclopride. *J Neurol Sci* 1995; 132:156–161.
25. Samii A, Markopoulou K, Wszolek ZK, et al. PET studies of parkinsonism associated with mutation in the α-synuclein gene. *Neurology* 1999;53:2097–2102.
26. Kishore A, de la Fuente-Fernandez R, Snow BJ, et al. Levodopa-induced dyskinesias in idiopathic parkinsonism (IP): a simultaneous PET study of dopamine D_1 and D_2 receptors. *Neurology* 1997;48[Suppl 2]:A327.
27. de la Fuente-Fernandez R, Kishore A, Snow BJ, et al. Dopamine D_1 and D_2 receptors and motor fluctuations in idiopathic parkinsonism (IP): a simultaneous PET study. *Neurology* 1997;48[Suppl 2]:A208.
28. Turjanski N, Lees AJ, Brooks DJ. *In vivo* studies on striatal dopamine D_1 and D_2 site binding in L-dopa–treated Parkinson's disease patients with and without dyskinesias. *Neurology* 1997;49:717–723.

29. Kaasinen V, Nagren K, Hietala J, et al. Extrastriatal dopamine D_2 and D_3 receptors in early and advanced Parkinson's disease. *Neurology* 2000;54:1482–1487.
30. Brooks DJ, Ibanez V, Sawle GV, et al. Striatal D_2 receptor status in patients with Parkinson's disease, striatonigral degeneration, and progressive supranuclear palsy, measured with ^{11}C-raclopride and positron emission tomography. *Ann Neurol* 1992;31:184–192.
31. Antonini A, Leenders KL, Vontobel P, et al. Complementary PET studies of striatal neuronal function in the differential diagnosis between multiple system atrophy and Parkinson's disease. *Brain* 1997;120:2187–2195.
32. Shinotoh H, Inoue O, Hirayama K, et al. Dopamine D_1 receptors in Parkinson's disease and striatonigral degeneration: a positron emission tomography study. *J Neurol Neurosurg Psychiatry* 1993;56:467–472.
33. Frey KA, Koeppe RA, Kilbourn MR, et al. Presynaptic monoaminergic vesicles in Parkinson's disease and normal aging. *Ann Neurol* 1996;40:873–884.
34. Lee CS, Samii A, Sossi V, et al. *In vivo* positron emission tomographic evidence for compensatory changes in presynaptic dopaminergic nerve terminals in Parkinson's disease. *Ann Neurol* 2000;47:493–503.
35. Laruelle M, Iyer RN, al-Tikriti MS, et al. Microdialysis and SPECT measurements of amphetamine-induced dopamine release in nonhuman primates. *Synapse* 1997; 25:1–14.
36. Breier A, Su T-P, Saunders R, et al. Schizophrenia is associated with elevated amphetamine-induced synaptic dopamine concentrations: evidence from a novel positron emission tomography method. *Proc Natl Acad Sci USA* 1997;94:2569–2574.
37. Piccini P, Brooks DJ, Björklund A, et al. Dopamine release from nigral transplants visualized *in vivo* in a Parkinson's patient. *Nat Neurosci* 1999;2:1137–1140.
38. Tedroff J, Pedersen M, Aquilonius S-M, et al. Levodopa-induced changes in synaptic dopamine in patients with Parkinson's disease as measured by [^{11}C]raclopride displacement and PET. *Neurology* 1996; 46:1430–1436.
39. de la Fuente-Fernandez R, Lu J-Q, Sossi V, et al. Biochemical variations in the synaptic level of dopamine precede motor fluctuations in Parkinson's disease: PET evidence of increased dopamine turnover. *Ann Neurol* 2001;49:298–303.
40. Strafella AP, Paus T, Barrett J, et al. Repetitive transcranial magnetic stimulation of the human prefrontal cortex induces dopamine release in the caudate nucleus. *J Neurosci* 2001;21:RC157.
41. Phillips AG, Blaha CD, Fibiger HC. Neurochemical correlates of brain-stimulation reward measured by *ex vivo* and *in vivo* analyses. *Neurosci Biobehav Rev* 1989;13:99–104.
42. Schultz W. Reward signaling by dopamine neurons. *Neuroscientist* 2001;7:293–302.
43. Koepp MJ, Gunn RN, Lawrence AD, et al. Evidence for striatal dopamine release during a video game. *Nature* 1998;393:266–268.
44. de la Fuente-Fernandez R, Ruth TJ, Sossi V, et al. Expectation and dopamine release: mechanism of the placebo effect in Parkinson's disease. *Science* 2001;293: 1164–1166.
45. Goetz CG, Leurgans S, Raman R, et al. Objective changes in motor function during placebo treatment in PD. *Neurology* 2000;54:710–714.
46. Shetty N, Friedman JH, Kieburtz K, et al. Parkinson Study Group. The placebo response in Parkinson's disease. *Clin Neuropharmacol* 1999;22:207–212.
47. DaSilva JN, Wilson AA, Nobrega JN, et al. Synthesis and autoradiographic localization of the dopamine D-1 agonists [^{11}C]SKF 75670 and [^{11}C]SKF 82957 as potential PET radioligands. *Appl Radiat Isot* 1996;47: 279–284.
48. Hwang DR, Kegeles LS, Laruelle M. (–)-*N*-[(^{11})C]propyl-norapomorphine: a positron-labeled dopamine agonist for PET imaging of D_2 receptors. *Nucl Med Biol* 2000;27:533–539.
49. Bordet R, Ridray S, Carboni S, et al. Induction of dopamine D_3 receptor expression as a mechanism of behavioral sensitization to levodopa. *Proc Natl Acad Sci USA* 1997;94:3363–3367.
50. Van Kampen JM, Stoessl AJ. Dopamine D_3 receptor antisense attenuates levodopa-induced behavioral sensitization in rats. *Soc Neurosci* 1999;25:336(Abst).
51. Engber TM, Susel Z, Kuo S, et al. Levodopa replacement therapy alters enzyme activities in striatum and neuropeptide content in striatal output regions of 6-hydroxydopamine lesioned rats. *Brain Res* 1991;552: 113–118.
52. Newman DD, Rajakumar N, Flumerfelt BA, et al. A kappa opioid antagonist blocks sensitization in a rodent model of Parkinson's disease. *NeuroReport* 1997;8: 669–672.
53. Henry B, Fox SH, Crossman AR, et al. Mu- and delta-opioid receptor antagonists reduce levodopa-induced dyskinesia in the MPTP-lesioned primate model of Parkinson's disease. *Exp Neurol* 2001;171:139–146.
54. Doucet J-P, Nakabeppu Y, Bedard PJ, et al. Chronic alterations in dopaminergic neurotransmission produce a persistent elevation of *Fos*B-like protein(s) in both the rodent and primate striatum. *Eur J Neurosci* 1997;8: 365–381.
55. Andersson M, Hilbertson A, Cenci MA. Striatal *fos*B expression is causally linked with L-dopa–induced abnormal involuntary movements and the associated upregulation of striatal prodynorphin mRNA in a rat model of Parkinson's disease. *Neurobiol Dis* 1999;6: 461–474.
56. Piccini P, Weeks RA, Brooks DJ. Alterations in opioid receptor binding in Parkinson's disease patients with levodopa-induced dyskinesias. *Ann Neurol* 1997;42: 720–726.

Parkinson's Disease: Advances in Neurology, Vol. 91.
Edited by Ariel Gordin, Seppo Kaakkola, and Heikki Teräväinen
Lippincott Williams & Wilkins, Philadelphia © 2003

7

The Molecular Mechanisms of Dopamine Toxicity

*Ari Barzilai, *Dorah Daily, *Rina Zilkha-Falb, †Ilan Ziv, Daniel Offen, †Eldad Melamed, and Anat Shirvan

**Department of Neurobiochemistry, George S. Wise Faculty of Life Sciences, Tel Aviv University, Tel Aviv, Israel; and †Department of Neurology and Felsenstein Medical Research Institute, Rabin Medical Center, and the Sackler School of Medicine, Tel Aviv University, Tel Aviv, Israel*

Parkinson's disease (PD) is a severe and progressive motor disorder of the central nervous system. The primary pathological change in the parkinsonian brain is the degeneration of the dopaminergic neurons of the *substantia nigra pars compacta* (SNpc) in the ventral midbrain. Although the pathological changes and motor dysfunction characterizing this disease are well documented, the mechanism responsible for the death of these neurons has not been established. Extensive postmortem studies have provided evidence supporting the notion that oxidative stress is involved in the pathogenesis of PD. The SNpc is a dopamine (DA)-rich brain region that contains neuromelanin and exhibits a high tissue iron content. DA, iron, and to some extent neuromelanin can induce oxidative stress. It is possible that each factor by itself or interactions between them are involved in the pathological mechanism that underlies the relatively specific neurodegeneration seen in PD.

Traces of these factors are evident in the substantia nigra of patients with PD. They include alterations in iron content; impaired mitochondrial function; alterations in the antioxidant protective systems (most notably superoxide dismutase and reduced glutathione [GSH]); and oxidative damage to lipids, proteins, and DNA (1–3).

DA exerts its toxic effects through its oxidative metabolites. It generates free radicals either through autooxidation or through metabolic conversion by monoamine oxidase (MAO). During autooxidation, DA is converted to semiquinone and superoxide anion, which, in turn, react with another DA molecule to generate semiquinone and hydrogen peroxide, which is a relatively stable radical with mild toxicity. During normal metabolism, DA is converted by MAO-B to 3,4-dihyroxyphenyl-acetaldehyde and to 3,4-dihydroxyphenylacetic acid. Hydrogen peroxide is produced during that reaction and can be neutralized by glutathione peroxidase or catalase, or in the presence of iron, generates the highly toxic hydroxyl radicals.

Numerous studies have shown that the introduction of DA results in cell death, both *in vivo* and in cell cultures. Administration of DA into the *striatum* (4) resulted in presynaptic and postsynaptic damage, while intraventricular injection of DA to rats resulted in dose-dependent death of the animal (5). Furthermore, toxins that caused extensive release of DA also caused degeneration of dopaminergic neurons (6–8). Several studies demonstrated DA-dependent cell death in mesencephalic, cerebellar, striatal, and cortical primary neuron cultures (9–13). DA toxicity is suggested to be mediated extraneuronally (transport independent) or interneuronally (transport dependent) (13–15). DA toxicity has been attributed to several mechanisms, including the formation of highly reactive oxygen species (ROS), quinones and semiquinones generated by DA autooxidation, and its enzymatic metabolism by MAO-B, which leads to a state of oxidative stress (4,9,16–19).

DA was also shown to induce apoptosis (Fig. 7.1) in chick sympathetic neurons (20–22); in the human neuroblastoma (NMB) cell line (16,23); and in nonneuronal cells (24). Indeed, several groups identified nuclear apoptotic processes in PD substantia nigra tissue (25–27). DA-induced apoptosis was suggested to be linked to the p53 gene (28), and cell death could be partially suppressed by overexpression of the protooncogene Bcl-2 (29,30).

DA is also capable of attenuating the mitochondrial respiratory chain. The finding by Ben-Shachar et al. (5) that DA can inhibit complex I activity was taken further by Cohen et al. (31), who suggested that the inhibition may be via an indirect mechanism involving MAO activity. In support of this hypothesis is a selective decrease of approximately 40% in complex I activity in the substantia nigra, platelets, and skeletal muscles of parkinsonian patients (32–35). Significantly reduced activity of mitochondrial complex I in the rat brain followed chronic administration of levodopa, which is associated with elevated DA concentrations in the brain (36). An increase in dopaminergic activity after D-methamphetamine treatment was associated with a significant decrease in striatal adenosine triphosphate concentrations (37), which also indicates mitochondrial malfunction. Taken

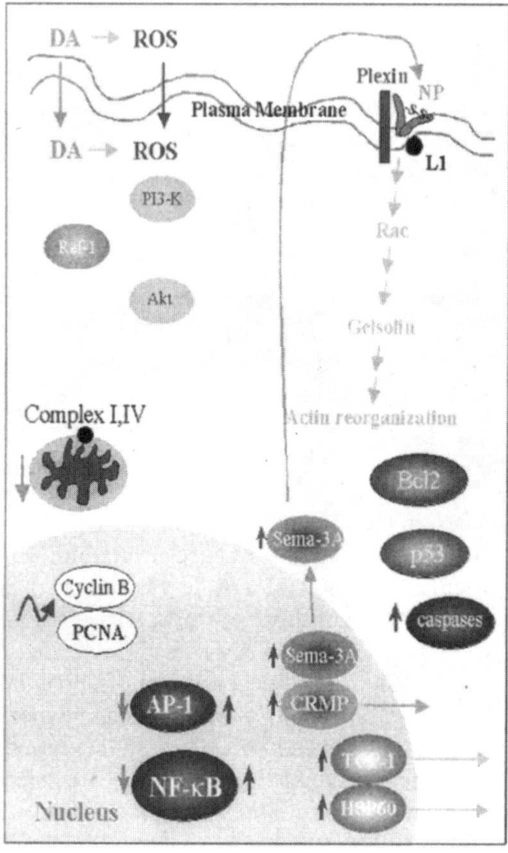

FIGURE 7.1. Schematic of dopamine (DA)-induced apoptosis. DA-induced apoptosis is mediated through its oxidative metabolites, which can be formed by autooxidation or intracellularly by monoamine oxidase B–dependent DA oxidation. The DA oxidative metabolites, quinones and hydrogen peroxide, can generate a vast array of responses as depicted in this cartoon. DA-induced apoptosis is dependent on caspase activation and can be inhibited by Bcl-2 overexpression. Inhibition of mitochondrial complex I activity plays a role in DA toxicity. DA alters the activities of at least two signal transduction pathways, phosphoinositide-3-kinase/Akt and JNK/AP-1. DA administration leads to alterations in gene expression that can be classified as follows: (a) alterations in cell-cycle–related genes; (b) induction of stress proteins T-complex protein 1 (TCP1) and heat shock protein 60 (HSP60); (c) activation of AP-1 and depending on the cell system, changes in nuclear factor B activation; and (d) sharp induction of collapsin response mediator protein and semaphorin IIIA; the latter is a secreted protein that binds to the neuropilin-plexin-L1 receptor complex and activates the death process.

together, these findings indicate that DA can induce cellular death in *in vivo* and *in vitro* models by the activation of several cellular mechanisms.

DOPAMINE-INDUCED APOPTOSIS IS MEDIATED THROUGH ALTERATIONS IN GENE EXPRESSION

T-complex Protein 1δ

DA toxicity is associated with the induction of T-complex protein 1δ (TCP-1δ). Chaperonin-containing TCP-1, a large multisubunit complex of 800 to 900 kd, is a protein complex considered to be the cytosolic homolog of mitochondrial heart shock protein 60 (Hsp60). These two complexes have a characteristic oligomeric structure consisting of two heptameric rings stacked one on top of the other to form a large double-ring complex. The complexes recognize proteins in nonnative conformation, preventing premature folding and aggregation, and mediate the acquisition of the native structure (38). The process of protein folding and oligomeric assembly of newly synthesized is critically important for cellular viability. The Hsp were considered part of the defense mechanism against different kinds of stress stimuli (39,40). However, Zilkha-Falb et al. (41) found that overexpression of the chick homolog to TCP-1δ, a member of the molecular chaperone family of proteins, accelerated DA-induced apoptosis in sympathetic neurons; inhibition of TCP-1δ expression in these neurons using antisense technology significantly reduced DA-induced neuronal death. These findings suggest a functional role for TCP-1δ as a positive mediator of DA-induced neuronal apoptosis. These results are consistent with recent reports that some of the Hsp may contribute to enhancing apoptotic cell death. Such a role is further supported by studies of Xanthoudakis et al. (42), showing that Hsp60 accelerated the maturation of pro–caspase-3 by upstream activator proteases during camptothecin-induced apoptosis in the Jurkat cells. Roperch et al. (43) demonstrated upregulation of a complementary DNA fragment corresponding to the TCP-1 chaperonin subunit as a result of various apoptotic stimuli.

THE ROLE OF SEMAPHORINS IN DOPAMINE-INDUCED APOPTOSIS

Exposure of sympathetic neurons to DA for 6 hours resulted in a sharp induction of collapsin response mediator protein (CRMP) and semaphorin IIIA (SemaIIIA), evidenced by differential display methodology (44). CRMP and SemaIIIA take part in the intricate processes of wiring the nervous system. They belong to a large family of axonal guidance molecules that can confer attractive or repulsive cues (45–49). The secreted and highly conserved axon guidance molecule SemaIIIA isolated from chick brain (50) acts as a repulsive cue in axonal pathway formation during neuronal development (51,52). SemaIIIA belongs to the semaphorin family of proteins suggested to have a functional role in neuronal development by inhibiting growth cone extension in unwanted directions in a receptor-mediated process (46,47,52). Several distinct members of the semaphorin family exist within the same organism and display differential distribution in specific areas of the developing nervous system (47,48,52–55). All members of this family (both within and between species) share a highly conserved sema domain. In particular, there was 93% amino acid homology in the sema domain between the chick collapsin-1 and its human paralog SemaIIIA. A family of receptors (or components of receptors) for semaphorins, the neuropilins, were recently described (56–58). These receptors are differentially expressed during development and were suggested to interact with various collapsins through two independent binding sites: one that signals the biological response and one that potentiates the response (59). Whereas neuropilins bind the ligand plexin, and L1 regulates the binding specificity of the receptor to various semaphorins (49,58,60), a role for semaphorins in neuronal cell death has not yet been suggested.

When Shirvan et al. (44) tested whether semaphorins are involved in neuronal death, they found that antibodies directed against SemaIIIA provided marked and prolonged protection of several neuronal cell types from DA-induced apoptosis. Moreover, neuronal apoptosis was inhibited by antibodies against neuropilin-1, a putative component of the SemaIIIA/collapsin-1 receptor. Induction of neuronal apoptosis was also caused by exposure of neurons to SemaIIIA-AP secreted from 293EBNA cells. Antibodies to collapsin-1 were effective in blocking the SemaIIIA-induced death process (61). These findings were the first to show a linkage between axonal guidance molecules that led to growth cone collapse during development and neuronal death. Similarly, exposure of nerve growth factor–dependent sensory neurons, or Dev cells (undifferentiated cell line derived from a cerebellar primitive neuroectodermal tumor (PNET) to SemaIIIA resulted in cell death with apoptotic characteristics (62,97). A growing body of evidence links semaphorins to neurodegenerative processes. An altered pattern of SemaIV staining was observed in three patients with Alzheimer's disease compared with healthy individuals (63). Deteriorated migration and axonal pathfinding and brain wiring is a main neuropathological feature of Down's syndrome. Proteomics analysis to detect differences in protein expression between control, Down's syndrome, and Alzheimer's disease brains revealed a deterioration in repulsive guidance molecules such as DRP-2 and semaphorins, suggesting a role for these molecules in brain disease (64). Furthermore, injection of anti-SemaIIIA antibodies into rat eyes significantly inhibited axotomy-induced neuronal death (A. Shirvan, *unpublished data, 2002*). CRMP is thought to mediate semaphorin-induced growth cone collapse through a signal transduction cascade involving G protein (65). However, recent studies indicate that CRMP may also be involved in the process of neurodegeneration. Highly phosphorylated forms of CRMP were shown to be associated with neurofibrillary tangles in Alzheimer's disease brains (66,67). Overexpression of CRMP in mouse NMB cell lines resulted in cytoplasm blebbing and apoptosis. CRMP was found to be associated with microtubules, suggesting that CRMP functions by regulating the dynamics of microtubules (68). Taken together, these results show that DA induces the expression of genes that are active during early development, leading to axonal collapse and under certain circumstances neuronal death. Moreover, neuronal apoptosis is similar to other forms of injury and degenerative processes that are mediated through the activation of CRMP and SemaIIIA.

GLUTAREDOXIN PROTECTS NEURONAL CELLS FROM DOPAMINE-INDUCED DEATH THROUGH NF-B ACTIVATION

In our quest for protective agents against DA toxicity, we examined whether glutaredoxin (Grx), a member of the thiol transferase family of proteins, was capable of attenuating DA apoptotic potential. Grx proteins are generally 10-kd proteins that catalyze GSH disulfide oxidoreductions via two redox-active cysteine residues. The active site sequence (Cys-Pro-Tyr-Cys) is conserved in a variety of species (69–76). Daily et al. (77,78) showed that only the active form of Grx could protect cerebellar granule neurons against DA toxicity. However, the mechanism by which Grx confers its protection is not clear.

We found that Grx is capable of penetrating into neuronal cells by a mechanism that is not dependent on coated pits. It is likely that Grx exerts its protective effects through the reduction of specific intracellular proteins, although our results cannot rule out the possibility that Grx activates intracellular processes through specific receptor activation. Analyzing the signal transduction pathways activated by Grx revealed a multistep activation of at least two central signaling pathways: the Ras-phosphoinositide-3-kinase (PI-3K) and the Jun *N*-terminal kinase-AP-1 pathways. Whereas DA downregulated the activity of PI-3K and Akt (an important antiapoptotic kinase), Grx activated these proteins, probably through Ras activation. Furthermore, Grx significantly increased the expression levels of redox factor 1 (Ref-1), which is a multifunctional protein that stimulates the DNA binding activity of numerous transcription factors. Ref-1 also possesses apurinic/apyrimidinic endonuclease DNA repair activity against DNA damage caused by ROS, ultraviolet, and ionizing radiation. DA on the other hand, blocks the expression of Ref-1. The activation of both pathways, Ras-PI-3K-Akt and JNK-AP-1, culminated in the activation of nuclear factor-κB (NF-κB), which is an essential survival factor for cerebellar granule neurons. In contrast, DA downregulated these pathways and consequently blocked NF-κB. Ref-1 affected both the AP-1 and NF-κB signaling pathways, as AP-1 and NF-κB binding activities were attenuated by the introduction of Ref-1 antisense. This accords with previous studies showing the involvement of Ref-1 in the redox regulation of AP-1 and NF-κB (42,79,80). The position of Ref-1 in the signaling cascade is most likely downstream of PI-3K but upstream of Akt. Interestingly, Akt activation is dependent on newly synthesized Ref-1. In the presence of Ref-1 antisense, which inhibits Ref-1 transcription and translation, Grx2 could not stimulate Akt activity. This finding demonstrates that activation of the Ras/PI-3 kinase/Akt pathway is dependent on alterations in gene expression.

DOPAMINE CAUSES DNA DAMAGE AND P53 ACTIVATION

Neurotoxins, which exert their toxicity by generating ROS, are dependent on p53 activation to execute the death process. DA is among these toxins. Its autooxidation forms DA quinone, a reactive molecule that spontaneously decomposes to generate additional reactive species that can modify cellular macromolecules such as proteins, lipids, and DNA. Increased levels of 8-hydroxyguanine, the major product of DNA oxidation, were observed in the presence of levodopa, DA, and 6-hydroxydopamine and were dependent on the presence of copper ions (81). The conversion of DA to reactive DA quinone was accelerated by tyrosinase. Tyrosinase increased DA-induced DNA modification by two orders of magnitude. Antioxidants markedly reduced these DNA modifications (82). Miura et al. (83) reported that catecholamine-induced DNA strand breaks are due to ferryl species and 8-hydroxyguanine formation and are mediated through hydroxyl radicals. It is known that DNA damage increases p53 levels, triggering either repair or apoptosis in response to moderate or severe damage, respectively (84,85). Human NMB cells express an active and inducible form of p53, making them suitable for analysis of the role of this gene in DA-induced apoptosis and differentiation. Indeed, Porat and Simantov (86) exposed these cells to different concentrations of DA and found that low DA concentration induced differentiation while high concentrations induced apoptosis. Treatment with high concentrations led to increased expression of p53 that peaked 3 to 6 hours from the challenge but before cell death. Thus, treatment with a high DA concentration may result in oxidation products and/or free radicals that heavily damage DNA, thereby increasing p53 levels and initiating a cascade of events that lead to apoptosis. Lower concentrations of DA apparently exert milder damage on the DNA and induce growth arrest and differentiation. Somewhat different results were obtained by Daily et al. (28). Exposure of mouse cerebellar granule neurons to DA resulted in increased p53 phosphorylation, rather than elevation of protein levels. Using a temperature-sensitive p53 activation system in leukemia LTR6 cells, p53 inactivation dramatically attenuated DA toxicity, indicating that DA exerts its toxic effects through activation of p53. 6-Hydroxydopamine-induced apoptosis in PC12 cells was also shown to be mediated by the activation of p53 and Bax: Upregulation of p53 was demonstrated 4 hours after exposure to 6-hydroxydopamine and preceded the morphological changes associated with the death process (87). Similar to 6-hydroxydopamine, treatment of human NMB cells with 1-methyl-4-phenylpyridine can generate the expression of p53 (88). Taken together, these results show that neurotoxins, which exert their toxicity by generating ROS, are dependent on p53 activation to execute the death process.

THE ROLE OF THE BCL-2 SYSTEM IN DOPAMINE-INDUCED APOPTOSIS

The Bcl-2 family is a group of proteins that act as a major control system of apoptosis. The family consists of several structurally related proteins, several of which function as potent inhibitors of the death program (e.g., Bcl-2, Bclx-L); others function as inducers of apoptosis (e.g., Bax, Bak). Several of these proteins are localized to the outer mitochondrial membrane. They can act as multifunctional proteins: They are capable of forming pores within the mitochondrial membrane, and they govern mitochondrial permeability transition pores, which are mega channels that play an important role in the apoptotic cascade. In addition, members of the Bcl-2 family serve as docking proteins regulating cytosolic levels of downstream mediators of apoptosis (89). We found that overexpression of Bcl-2 in PC12 cells effectively inhibited DA toxicity (29), and that neuronal cells from Bcl-2–deficient mice are more susceptible to DA-induced apoptosis (90). These results demonstrate the strategic role of the Bcl-2 system in regulation of the cellular response to the apoptosis-triggering effect of the endogenous neurotransmitter.

CASPASES AND DOPAMINE-INDUCED APOPTOSIS

Caspases (aspartate-specific cysteine proteases) in general, and caspase-3 in particular, are central effectors of neuronal apoptosis. Significantly higher levels of activated caspase-3 were observed in dopaminergic neurons of patients with PD compared with age-matched controls (91). DA-induced apoptosis is also caspase dependent. Marked protection against DA-induced death was conferred on the sympathetic neurons by the universal caspase inhibitor BAF (Boc-Asp-FMK). The same caspase inhibitor (BAF) was highly effective in protecting the sympathetic neurons from SemaIIIA and SemaIIIA-derived peptide (amino acid position 363-380)-induced death (61). Caspase-1 and caspase-3 inhibitors (YVAD-CHO and DEVD-CHO, respectively) were also effective in protecting PC12 against DA-induced apoptosis (98). These results indicate that the death process induced either by DA or by SemaIIIA is mediated by caspase activation.

CELL-CYCLE–RELATED GENES

Recently, some similarities were drawn between cell division and apoptosis. It was hypothesized that neuronal cell death is linked to inappropriate induction of several cell-cycle regulators (92–94). A loss of tight cell-cycle control was suggested to drive postmitotic neurons into an abortive cell cycle, leading to their inevitable self-destruction program. To detect genes whose expression is transcriptionally regulated during the early stages of DA-triggered apoptosis, Shirvan et al. (95) applied the differential display method to cultured sympathetic neurons. One of the upregulated genes was identified as cyclin B2, which exhibited two waves of induction and destruction, at both the messenger RNA and the protein level, resembling the sequential oscillations typical of two successive mitotic events in proliferating cells. The time window between the two waves was characterized by a change in expression of other cell-cycle-stage–specific genes, and oscillations in proliferating cell nuclear antigen and alterations in cyclin A were observed. Cyclin D1 and cyclin-dependent kinases were not detected and there was no sign of active DNA synthesis, indicating that activation of cell-cycle components is incomplete. Compared with a normal cell cycle, the temporal expression profile of these mediators was unsynchronized. Whereas the first wave of cell-cycle changes occurred before the commitment of the cells to the death process and could be tolerated by the cells, the second wave of changes coincided with the death commitment point. CDK5, one of the cyclin-dependent kinases usually found in neurons, was found to alter its expression pattern as a result of DA exposure. Induction of CDK5 protein coincided with the time when neurons were irreversibly committed to die (95,96).

CONCLUSIONS

Most of the studies show that DA exerts it toxic effects through its oxidative metabolites. Even though cells are equipped with very elaborate antioxidative mechanisms, overwhelming levels of oxidants can generate a situation known as oxidative stress, which leads to cellular demise. It is tempting to speculate that DA exerts its toxic effects through oxidative damage to macromolecules such as DNA, protein, and lipid processes, which are sufficient to induce and execute the death. Some of the more recent research argues against this assumption and points to a different picture. It seems that DA oxidative metabolites do not function as the executioners of the death process, but as signal molecules. A number of observations support this idea: (a) DA-induced apoptosis is mediated through p53 activation, and cells that do not express p53 exhibit no sensitivity to DA, even though DA undergoes autooxidation and generates free radicals and (b) the fact that TCP-1δ antisense treatment or anti-SemaIIIA antibodies can protect neurons against DA toxicity not by their ability to act as an antioxidant but specifically may indicate that DA-generated free radicals are not sufficient to induce cell death. DA-generated free radicals can act as signal molecules that activate an intricate web of signals, leading to the gene expression required to set in motion the apoptotic machinery.

In summary, two major events are necessary for DA-induced apoptosis: the generation of free radicals and the activation of specific target proteins. Two groups of target proteins have been identified. What is needed now is identification of other target proteins that mediate DA-induced apoptosis. Identification of such proteins will enable the development of new therapeutic approaches aimed at antagonizing their activity and antioxidative treatments.

REFERENCES

1. Spencer JPE, Jenner P, Daniel SE, et al. Conjugates of catecholamines with cysteine and GSH in Parkinson's disease: possible mechanisms of formation involving reactive oxygen species. *J Neurochem* 1998;71: 2112–2122.
2. Jenner P, Olanow CW. Oxidative stress and the pathogenesis of Parkinson's disease. *Neurology* 1996;47 [Suppl 3]:S161–S170.
3. Dunnet B, Björklund A. Prospective for new restorative and neuroprotective treatments in Parkinson's disease. *Nature* 1999;399[Suppl]:A32–A39.
4. Fillox F, Townsend JJ. Pre- and postsynaptic neurotoxic effects of dopamine demonstrated by intrastriatal injection. *Exp Neurol* 1993;119:79–88.
5. Ben-Shachar D, Zuk R, Glinka Y. Dopamine neurotoxicity: inhibition of mitochondrial respiration. *J Neurochem* 1995;64:718–723.
6. Sirinathsinghji DJ, Heavens RP, McBribde CS. Dopamine-releasing action of 1-methyl-4-phenyl-1,2,3,6-tetrahydropyridine (MPTP) and 1-methyl-4-phenylpyridine (MPP^+) in the neostriatum of the rat. *Brain Res* 1998;443:101–116.
7. O'Dell SJ, Weihmuller FB, Marshall JF. Methamphetamine-induced dopamine terminals alteration by dopamine D_1 and D_2 antagonists. *J Neurochem* 1993; 60:1792–1799.
8. Gerlach M, Xiao A, Heim C, et al. 1-Trichloromethyl-1,2,3,4-tetrahydro-beta-carboline increases extracellular serotonin and stimulates hydroxyl radical production in rats. *Neurosci Lett* 1998;257:17–20 .
9. Tanaka M, Sotomatsu A, Kanai H, et al. DOPA and dopamine cause cultured neuronal death in the presence of iron. *J Neurochem* 1991;101:198–203.
10. Mytilineou C, Han SK, Cohen G. Toxic and protective effects of L-dopa on mesencephalic cell cultures. *J Neurochem* 1993;61:1470–1478.
11. Rosenberg PA. Catecholamine toxicity in cerebral cortex of dissociated cell culture. *J Neurosci* 1998;8: 2887–2894.
12. Michel PP, Hefti F. Toxicity of 6-hydroxydopamine and dopamine for dopaminergic neurons in culture. *J Neurosci Res* 1990;25:428–435
13. McLaughlin BA, Nelson D, Erecinska M, et al. Toxicity of dopamine to striatal neurons *in vitro* and potentiation of cell death by mitochondrial inhibitor. *J Neurochem* 1998;70:2406–5415.
14. Javitch JA, D'Amato RJ, Strittmatter SM, et al. Parkinsonism-inducing neurotoxin, *N*-methyl-4-phenyl-

1,2,3,6-tetrahydropyridine: uptake of the metabolite *N*-methyl-4-phenylpyridine by dopamine neurons explains selective toxicity. *Proc Natl Acad Sci USA* 1985;82: 2173–2177.

15. Bloom FE, Algeri S, Groppetti A, et al. Lesions of central norepinephrine terminals with 6-OH-dopamine: biochemistry and fine structure. *Science* 1969;166: 1284–1286.
16. Cohen G. Oxidative stress in the nervous system. In: Sies H, ed. *Oxidative stress.* London: Academic Press, 1985:383–401.
17. Fonstedt B. Role of catechol autooxidation in the degeneration of dopamine neurons. *Acta Neurol Scand* 1990;129:12–14.
18. Chiueh CC, Miyake H, Peng MT. Role of dopamine autooxidation, hydroxyl radical generation and calcium overload in underlying mechanisms involved in MPTP-induced parkinsonism. *Adv Neurol* 1993;60:251–258.
19. Hastings TG, Zigmond MJ. Identification of catechol-protein conjugates in neostriatal slices incubated with [^{3}H] dopamine: impact of ascorbic acid and glutathione. *J Neurochem* 1994;63:1126–1132.
20. Ziv I, Melamed E, Nardi N, et al. Dopamine induced apoptosis-like cell death in cultured chick sympathetic neurons—a possible novel pathogenic mechanism in Parkinson's disease. *Neurosci Lett* 1994;170:136–140.
21. Zilkha-Falb R, Ziv I, Nardi N, et al. Monoamine-induced apoptotic neuronal cell death. *Mol Cell Neurobiol* 1997;17:101–118.
22. Masserano JM, Gong L, Kulaga H, et al. Dopamine induces apoptotic cell death of catecholaminergic cell line derived from the central nervous system. *Mol Pharmacol* 1996;50:1309–1315.
23. Gabbay M, Tauber M, Porat S, et al. Selective role of glutathione in protecting human neuronal cells from dopamine-induced apoptosis. *Neuropharmacology* 1996;35:571–578.
24. Offen D, Ziv I, Gorodin S, et al. Dopamine-induced programmed cell death in mouse thymocytes. *Biochim Biophys Acta* 1995;1268:171–177.
25. Tatton NA, Maclean-Fraser A, Tatton WG, et al. A fluorescent double-labeling method to detect and confirm apoptotic nuclei in Parkinson's disease. *Ann Neurol* 1998;44[Suppl 1]:S142–S148.
26. Ruberg M, France-Leonard V, Brugg B, et al., Neuronal death caused by apoptosis in Parkinson's disease. *Rev Neurol* 1997;153:499–508.
27. Anglade P, Vyas S, Javoy-Agid F, et al. Apoptosis and autophagy in nigral neurons of patients with Parkinson's disease. *Histol Histopathol* 1997;12:25–31.
28. Daily D, Barzilai A, Offen D, et al. The involvement of p53 in dopamine-induced apoptosis of cerebellar granule neurons and leukemic cells overexpressing p53. *Cell Mol Neurobiol* 1999;19:261–276.
29. Offen D, Ziv I, Panet H, et al. Dopamine-induced apoptosis is inhibited in PC12 cells expressing Bcl2. *Cell Mol Neurobiol* 1997;17:289–304.
30. Ziv I, Offen D, Haviv R, et al. The proto-oncogene Bcl2 inhibits cellular toxicity of dopamine: possible implications for Parkinson's disease. *Apoptosis* 1997;2: 149–155.
31. Cohen G, Farooqui R, Kesler N. Parkinson's disease: a new link between monoamine oxidase and mitochondrial electron flow. *Proc Natl Acad Sci USA* 1997;94: 4890–4894.
32. Blin O, Desnuelle C, Rascol O, et al. Mitochondrial respiratory failure in skeletal muscle from patient with Parkinson's disease and multiple system atrophy. *J Neurol Sci* 1994;125:95–101.
33. Janetzky B, Hauck S, Youdim MBH, et al. Unaltered aconitase activity but decreased complex I activity in substantia nigra pars compacta of patients with Parkinson's disease. *Neurosci Lett* 1994;169:126–128.
34. Parker WD, Boyson SJ, Parks JK. Abnormalities in electron transport chain in idiopathic Parkinson's disease. *Ann Neurol* 1989;26:719–723.
35. Riederer PE, Sofic W, Rausch D, et al. Transition metals ferritin, glutathione, and ascorbic acid in parkinsonian brains. *J Neurochem* 1989;52:515–520.
36. Przedborski S, Jackson-Lewis V, Muthane U, et al. Chronic levodopa administration alters cerebral mitochondrial respiratory chain activity. *Ann Neurol* 1993; 34:715–723.
37. Chan P, Di Monte DA, Luo JJ, et al. Rapid ATP loss caused by methamphetamine in the mouse striatum: relationship between energy impairment and dopaminergic neurotoxicity. *J Neurochem* 1994;62: 2484–2847.
38. Horwich AL, Willison KR. Protein folding in the cells: function of two families of molecular chaperone Hsp60 and TF-55-TCP-1. *Phil Trans R Soc London Biol Sci* 1993;339:313–326.
39. Freyaldenhoven TE, Ali SF. Heat shock protein protect cultured fibroblast from the cytotoxic effects of MPP^+. *Brain Res* 1996;735:42–49.
40. Creagh EM, Cotter TG. Selective protection by hsp70 against cytotoxic drug—but not Fas-induced T-cell apoptosis. *Immunology* 1999;97:36–44.
41. Zilkha-Falb R, Barzilai A, Djaldeti R, et al. Involvement of T-complex protein-δ in dopamine triggered apoptosis in chick embryo sympathetic neurons. *J Biol Chem* 2000;275:36380–36387.
42. Xanthoudakis S, Miao G, Curran T. The redox and DNA-repair activities of Ref-1 are encoded by nonoverlapping domains. *Proc Natl Acad Sci USA* 1994;91: 23–27.
43. Roperch JP, Lethrone F, Prieur S, et al. SIAH-1 promotes apoptosis and tumor suppression through a network involving the regulation of protein folding, unfolding and trafficking: identification of common effectors with p53 and $p21^{waf1}$. *Proc Natl Acad Sci USA* 1999;96:8070–8073.
44. Shirvan A, Ziv I, Fleminger G, et al. Semaphorins as mediators of neuronal apoptosis. *J Neurochem* 1999;73: 961–971.
45. Goodman CS. The likeness of being: phylogenetically conserved molecular mechanism of growth cone guidance. *Cell* 1994;78:353–356.
46. Goodman CS. Mechanisms and molecules that control growth cone guidance. *Ann Rev Neurosci* 1996;19: 341–377.
47. Kolodkin AL. Growth cones and the cues that repel them. *Trends Neurosci* 1996;19:507–513.
48. Tessier-Lavigne M, Goodman, CS. The molecular biology of axonal guidance. *Science* 1996;274:1123–1131.
49. Song H-J, Poo M-M. The cell biology of neuronal navigation. *Nat Cell Biol* 2001;3:E81–E88.
50. Luo Y, Raible D, Raper JA. Collapsin: a protein in brain that induces the collapse and paralysis of neuronal growth cones. *Cell* 1993;75:217–227.
51. Kolodkin AL, Matthes DJ, Goodman CS. The semaphorin genes encode a family of transmembrane and se-

creted growth guidance molecules. *Cell* 1993;75: 1389–1399.
52. Luo Y, Shepherd I, Li J, et al. A family of molecules related to collapsin in the embryonic chick nervous system. *Neuron* 1995;14:1131–1140.
53. Hamajima N, Natsuda K, Sakata S, et al. A novel gene family defined by human dihydropyrimidinase and three related proteins with differential tissue distribution. *Gene* 1996;180:157–163.
54. Adams RH, Betz H, Puschel AW. A novel class of murine semaphorins with homology to thrombospondin is differentially expressed during early embryogenesis. *Mech Dev* 1996;57:33–45.
55. Puschel AW, Adams RH, Betz H. The sensory innervation of the mouse spinal cord may be patterned by differential expression of and differential responsiveness to semaphorin. *Mol Cell Neurosci* 1996;7:419–431
56. He Z, Tessier-Lavigne M. Neuropilin is a receptor for the axonal chemorepellent semaphorin III. *Cell* 1997; 90:739–751.
57. Kolodkin AL, Levengood DV, Rowe EG, et al. Neuropilin is a semaphorin III receptor. *Cell* 1997;90: 753–762.
58. Chen H, Chedotal A, He Z, et al. Neuropilin-2, a novel member of the neuropilin family, is a high affinity receptor for the semaphorins sema E and sema IV but not sema III. *Neuron* 1997:19:547–559.
59. Koppel AM, Feiner L, Kobayashi H, et al. A 70 amino acid region within the semaphorin domain activates specific cellular response of semaphorin family members. *Neuron* 1997;19:531–537.
60. Feiner L, Koppel AM, Kobayashi H, et al. Secreted chick semaphorins bind recombinant neuropilin with similar affinities but bind different subsets of neurons *in situ*. *Neuron* 1997;19:539–545.
61. Shirvan A, Shina R, Ziv I, et al. Induction of neuronal apoptosis by semaphorin 3A-derived peptide. *Mol Brain Res* 2000;83:81–93.
62. Gagliardini V, Franhauser C. Semaphorin III can induce death in sensory neurons. *Mol Cell Neurosci* 1999;14: 301–316.
63. Hirsch E, Hu LJ, Prignet A, et al. Distribution of semaphorin IV in adult human brain. *Brain Res* 1999;823: 67–79.
64. Lubec G, Nonaka M, Krapfenbauer K, et al. Expression of the dihydropyrimidinase-related protein 2 (DRP-2) in Down syndrome and Alzheimer's disease brain is downregulated at the RNA and dysregulated at the protein level. *J Neural Transm* 1999;57[Suppl]:161–177.
65. Goshima Y, Nakamura F, Strittmatter P, et al. Collapsin-induced growth cone collapse mediated by an intracellular protein related to UNC-33. *Nature* 1995;376: 509–514.
66. Yoshida H, Watanabe A, Ihara Y. Collapsin response mediator protein-2 is associated with neurofibrillary tangles in Alzheimer's disease. *J Biol Chem* 1998;273: 9761–9768.
67. Gu Y, Hamajima N, Ihara Y. Neurofibrillary tangles-associated collapsin response mediator protein-2 (CRMP-2) is highly phosphorylated on Thr-509, Ser-518 and Ser-522. *Biochemistry* 2000;399:4267–4275.
68. Gu Y, Ihara Y. Evidence that collapsin response mediator protein-2 is involved in the dynamics of microtubules. *J Biol Chem* 2000;275:17917–17920.
69. Hoog JO, Jörnvall H, Holmgren A, et al. The primary structure of *Escherichia coli* glutaredoxin. Distant homology with thioredoxins in a superfamily of small proteins with a redox-active cystine disulfide/cysteine dithiol. *Eur J Biochem* 1983;136:223–232.
70. Klintrot IM, Hoog JO, Jörnvall H, et al. The primary structure of calf thymus glutaredoxin. Homology with the corresponding *Escherichia coli* protein but elongation at ends and with an additional half-cysteine/cysteine pair. *Eur J Biochem* 1984;14:417–413.
71. Gan ZR, Wells WW. The primary structure of pig liver thioltransferase. *J Biol Chem* 1987;262:6699–6703.
72. Hopper S, Johnson RS, Biemann K. Glutaredoxin from rabbit bone marrow. Purification, characterization and amino acid sequence determined by tandem mass spectrometry. *J Biol Chem* 1989;264:20438–20447.
73. Gan ZR, Polokoff MA, Jacobs JW, et al. Complete amino acid sequence of yeast thiol transferase (glutaredoxin). *Biochem Biophys Res Commun* 1990;168: 944–951.
74. Ahn BY, Moss B. Glutaredoxin homologue encoded by vaccinia virus is a virion-associated enzyme with thioltransferase and dehydroascorbate reductase activity. *Proc Natl Acad Sci USA* 1992;89:7060–7064.
75. Minakuchi K, Yabushita T, Masumura T, et al. Cloning and sequence analysis of a cDNA encoding rice glutaredoxin. *FEBS Lett* 1994;337:157–160.
76. Padilla CA, Martinez-Galisteo E, Barcenea JA, et al. Purification from placenta, amino acid sequence, structure comparison and cDNA cloning of human glutaredoxin. *Eur J Biochem* 1995;227:27–34.
77. Daily D, Vlamis A, Offen D, et al. Glutaredoxin protects cerebellar granule neurons from dopamine-induced apoptosis via activation of Ref-1 and NF-κB. *J Biol Chem* 2001;276:1335–1344.
78. Daily D, Vlamis A, Offen D, et al. Glutaredoxin protects cerebellar granule neurons from dopamine-induced apoptosis by dual activation of the Ras-phosphoinositide 3 kinase and Jun *N*-terminal kinase pathways. *J Biol Chem* 2001;276:21618–21626.
79. Xanthoudakis S, Miao G, Wang F, et al. Redox activation of Fos-Jun DNA binding activity is mediated by a DNA repair enzyme. *EMBO J* 1992;11:3323–3335.
80. Xanthoudakis S, Curran T. Identification and characterization of Ref-1, a nuclear protein that facilitates AP-1 DNA-binding activity. *EMBO J* 1992;11:653–656.
81. Levay G, Ye Q, Bodell WJ. Formation of DNA adducts and oxidative base damage by copper mediated oxidation of dopamine and 6-hydroxydopamine. *Exp Neurol* 1997;146:570–574.
82. Stokes AH, Brown BG, Lee CK, et al. Tyrosinase enhances the covalent modification of DNA by dopamine. *Brain Res Mol Brain Res* 1996;42:167–170.
83. Miura T, Muraoka S, Fujimoto Y, et al. DNA damage induced by catechol derivatives. *Chem Biol Interact* 2000; 126:125–136.
84. Lakin ND, Jackson SP. Regulation of p53 in response to DNA damage. *Oncogene* 1999;18:7644–7655.
85. Vogt-Sionov R, Haupt Y. The cellular response to p53: the decision between life and death. *Oncogene* 1999;18:6145–6157.
86. Porat S, Simantov R. Bcl-2 and p53: role in dopamine-induced apoptosis and differentiation. *Ann N Y Acad Sci* 1999;893:372–375.
87. Blum D, Wu Y, Nissou MF, et al. p53 and Bax activated by 6-hydroxydopamine–induced apoptosis in PC12 cells. *Brain Res* 1997;751:139–142.
88. Kitamura Y, Kosaka T, Kakimura J-I, et al. Protective ef-

fects of the antiparkinsonian drug talipexole and pramipexole against 1-methyl-4-phenyl-pyridium–induced apoptotic death in human neuroblastoma SH-SY5Y cells. *Mol Pharmacol* 1998;54:1046–1054.
89. Reed JC. Double identity for proteins of the Bcl-2 family. *Nature* 1997;387:773–776.
90. Hochman A, Sternin H, Gorodin S, et al. Enhanced oxidative stress and altered antioxidant in brains of Bcl-2–deficient mice. *J Neurochem* 1998;71:741–748.
91. Hartmann A, Hunot S, Michel PP, et al. Caspase-3: a vulnerability factor and final effector in apoptotic death of dopaminergic neurons in Parkinson's disease. *Proc Natl Acad Sci USA* 2000;97:2875–2880.
92. Herrup K, Busser J. The induction of multiple cell cycle events precede target-related neuronal death. *Development* 1995;121:2385–2395.
93. Bresdesen DJ. Neuronal apoptosis. *Ann Neurol* 1995; 38:839–851.
94. Kranenburg O, Van de Eb AJ, Zantena A. Cyclin D1 is an essential mediator of apoptotic neuronal cell death. *EMBO J* 1996;15:46–54.
95. Shirvan A, Ziv I, Machlin T, et al. Two waves of cyclin B and proliferating cell nuclear antigen (PCNA) expression during dopamine triggered neuronal apoptosis. *J Neurochem* 1997;69:539–549.
96. Shirvan A, Ziv I, Zilkha-Falb R, et al. Expression of cell cycle related genes during neuronal apoptosis: is there a distinct pattern? *Neurochemical Res* 1998;23: 767–777.
97. Bagnard D, Vaillant C, Khuth S-T, et al., Semaphorin 3A-vascular endothelial growth factor-165 balance mediates migration and apoptosis of neuronal progenitor cells by the recruitment of shared receptor. *J Neurosci* 2001;21:3332–3341.
98. Panet H, Barzilai A, Daily D, et al. Activation of nuclear transcription factor kappa B (NF = kappaB) is essential for dopamine-included apoptosis in PC12 cells. *J Neurochem* 2001;77:391–398.

Parkinson's Disease: Advances in Neurology, Vol. 91.
Edited by Ariel Gordin, Seppo Kaakkola, and Heikki Teräväinen
Lippincott Williams & Wilkins, Philadelphia © 2003

8

Free Radical and Nitric Oxide Toxicity in Parkinson's Disease

*†Serge Przedborski, *Vernice Jackson-Lewis, *Miquel Vila, *Du Chu Wu, *Peter Teismann, *Kim Tieu, *Dong-Kug Choi, and *Oren Cohen

*Departments of *Neurology and †Pathology, Columbia University, New York, New York*

Parkinson's disease (PD) is a common neurodegenerative disorder whose cardinal features include tremor, slowness of movement, rigidity, and postural instability (1). Epidemiological data indicate that currently about one million individuals are affected with PD in North America alone and that about 50,000 new cases arise every year (1). Pathologically, PD is characterized primarily by a dramatic degeneration of the nigrostriatal pathway (2). The latter is formed by dopamine-producing neurons whose cell bodies, located in the substantia nigra pars compacta (SNpc), project their axons all the way up to the basal ganglia, where they release dopamine, thereby ensuring dopaminergic neurotransmission. As part of the neurodegeneration of the nigrostriatal pathway, both cell bodies and to an even greater extent striatal nerve terminals degenerate (2). Aside from these prominent features, other aspects of the pathology of PD include the presence of intraneuronal proteinaceous inclusions called Lewy bodies (3). Despite the large body of knowledge about PD, why and how nigrostriatal dopaminergic neurons die in this disease remains an enigma.

Over the years, several pathogenic hypotheses have been proposed in attempts to explain the mechanisms of neuronal loss in PD. Among these, the lion's share has been given to the oxidative stress hypothesis (4), which proposes that the fine-tuned balance between the production and destruction of reactive oxygen species is skewed, resulting in oxidative damage that leads to severe cellular dysfunction and ultimately to cell death. Countless studies have been published in support of this presumed pathogenic scenario (4). Among the plethora of reactive species capable of mediating oxidative damage in PD, mounting evidence points to peroxynitrite as a main culprit (5). Peroxynitrite is a highly reactive, tissue-damaging species that results from the combination of two other reactive species, namely, superoxide and nitric oxide (NO) (Fig. 8.1A). Because of the remarkable reactivity of peroxynitrite, there is very little doubt that it can inflict a variety of oxidative damage such as oxidative modifications of proteins, DNA, and lipids on dopaminergic neurons in the brains of parkinsonian patients.

In this chapter, we summarize the current highlights regarding the potential deleterious role of peroxynitrite in the pathogenesis of PD through the use of the 1-methyl-4-phenyl-1,2,3,6-tetrahydropyridine (MPTP) mouse model, and we review the following points. First, what evidence is there that peroxynitrite is produced in the MPTP mouse model of PD? Second, are both superoxide and NO really required in the proposed deleterious scenario? Third, what is the source of the NO that is involved in the presumed deleterious reaction? And, fourth, does peroxynitrite cause detectable damage after the administration of MPTP?

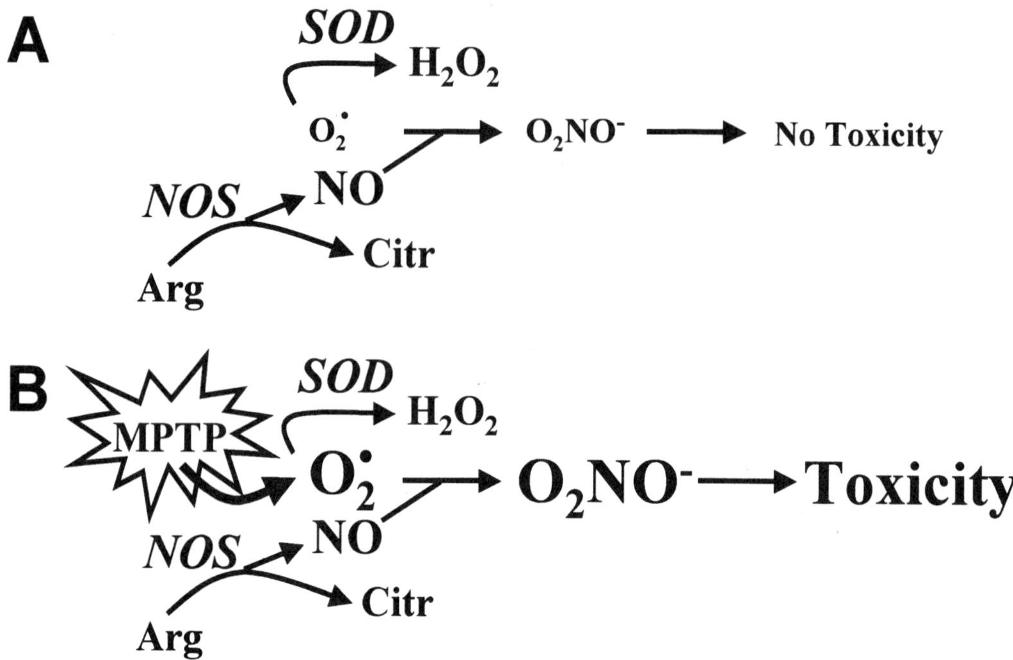

FIGURE 8.1. Superoxide radical ($O_2^{\bullet}$) reacts with nitric oxide (NO) to produce peroxynitrite (O_2NO^-). In normal situations **(A)**, superoxide dismutase detoxifies most of the produced superoxide radicals. On the other hand, NO, which is produced by the oxidation of L-arginine into L-citrulline, is present in high amounts. Because of this, little peroxynitrite is formed, and thus, minimal toxicity is attributable to this reaction. After methylphenyltetrahydropyridine (MPTP) administration **(B)**, the level of $O_2^{\bullet}$ increases dramatically and, thus, more peroxynitrite is produced and significant cytotoxicity now occurs.

MPTP MOUSE MODEL OF PARKINSON'S DISEASE

As a preamble of our discussion, it is worth providing a brief review of the MPTP model (6). That MPTP causes a parkinsonian syndrome was discovered in 1982 when a group of drug addicts in California were rushed to the emergency room with a severe bradykinetic and rigid syndrome (7). Subsequently, it was discovered that this syndrome was induced by the self-administration of street batches of a synthetic meperidine analog, whose synthesis was heavily contaminated by a byproduct, MPTP (8). In the period of a few days after the administration of MPTP, these patients exhibited a severe and irreversible akinetic rigid syndrome akin to PD, and levodopa was tried with great success, relieving the symptoms of these patients. Since the discovery that MPTP causes parkinsonism in human and nonhuman primates, as well as in various other mammalian species, this neurotoxin has been used extensively as a model of PD (6,9,10). For a technical review of MPTP utility and safety, please see Przedborski et al. (11).

In human and nonhuman primates, MPTP produces an irreversible and severe parkinsonian syndrome that replicates almost all of the hallmarks of PD, including tremor, rigidity, slowness of movement, postural instability, and even gait freezing. The responses and the complications to traditional antiparkinsonian therapies are virtually identical to those seen in PD. However, although it is believed that the neurodegenerative process in PD occurs over several years, the most active phase of neuronal death after MPTP administration is presumably completed over a short period of time, producing a clinical condition consistent with "endstage PD" in a few days. Still, brain imaging and neuropathological data suggest that after the acute phase of neuronal death, nigrostriatal dopaminergic neurons continue to succumb at a much lower rate for many years after MPTP exposure (12,13). From a neuropathological standpoint, MPTP administration causes damage to the dopaminergic pathways, which is identical to that seen in PD with a resemblance that goes beyond the degeneration of nigrostriatal dopaminergic neurons. For instance, as in PD, MPTP causes a greater loss of dopaminergic neurons in the SNpc than in the ventral tegmental area (14,15) and a greater degeneration of dopaminergic nerve terminals in the putamen than in the caudate nucleus, at least in monkeys treated with low-dose MPTP (16), but apparently not in acutely intoxicated humans (17). On the other hand, two typical neuropathological features of PD have, until now, been lacking in the MPTP model. First, except for the SNpc, other pigmented nuclei such as the locus ceruleus have been spared, according to most published reports. Second, the eosinophilic intraneuronal inclusions, or Lewy bodies, so characteristic of PD, have thus far not been convincingly observed in MPTP-induced parkinsonism (18). Despite this impressive resemblance between PD and the MPTP model, MPTP has never been recovered from postmortem brain samples or body fluids of parkinsonian patients. Altogether, these findings are consistent with MPTP not causing PD, but being an excellent experimental model of PD. Accordingly, it can be speculated that elucidating the molecular mechanisms of MPTP should lead to important insights into the pathogenesis and treatment of PD.

IS PEROXYNITRITE PRODUCED IN THE MPTP MOUSE MODEL?

Together with its high reactivity, peroxynitrite is known to be very unstable and therefore to have a very short half-life. Consequently, it is virtually impossible to measure the actual content of peroxynitrite in biological samples collected and processed for laboratory measurements. To circumvent this problem, several investigators have exploited the fact that peroxynitrite can induce irreversible amino acid modifications such as the nitration of phenolic groups found in tyrosine residues (19). This example of modification, called tyrosine nitration, can affect tyrosine residues irrespective as to whether they are free or contained within proteins and is regarded as a faithful fingerprint of peroxynitrite involvement in a given pathological process. Over the years, several methods, both chromatographic and immuno-based, have been developed to measure nitrotyrosine content, thanks to the availability of specific antibodies raised against nitrotyrosine (20). To date, there is some evidence that nitrotyrosine formation increases in the brains of parkinsonian patients, particularly wherever Lewy bodies are found (21–23). To examine the question of nitrotyrosine formation in the demise of nigrostriatal dopaminergic neurons in a more dynamic fashion, the MPTP model of PD provides an invaluable tool. High-performance liquid chromatographic (HPLC) studies have shown that nitrotyrosine is increased in selected brain regions after MPTP administration to mice (24). Because of the recent concern regarding the specificity of the molecule detected by HPLC (25), we have used gas chromatography with mass spectroscopy, a method that combines chromatographic ability with the capacity to confirm with certainty the nature of the detected peak (26). Based on this method, we have demonstrated that 24 hours after the last injection of MPTP to mice, the level of nitrotyrosine increases dramatically in the ventral midbrain, the brain region that contains the SNpc, as well as in the striatum (Fig. 8.2) (26). In contrast, at the same time points and in the same animals, we showed that brain regions known *not* to be affected by MPTP (i.e., the cerebellum and the frontal cortex) failed to show any change in the levels of nitrotyrosine (Fig. 8.2) (26). Our data provide compelling evidence

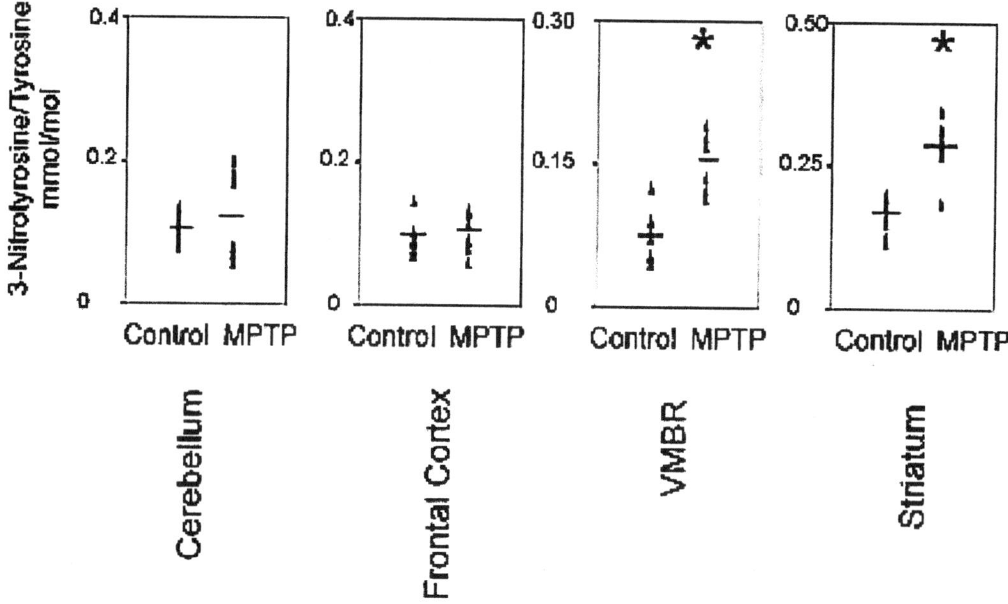

FIGURE 8.2. Gas chromatographic/mass spectroscopic quantification of nitrotyrosine 24 hours after methylphenyltetrahydropyridine (MPTP) administration in cerebellum, frontal cerebral cortex, ventral midbrain (VMBR), and striatum. (*Significantly higher than controls [$p < .05$, Student's t test].) (From Pennathur S, Jackson-Lewis V, Przedborski S, et al. Mass spectrometric quantification of 3-nitrotyrosine, ortho-tyrosine, and o,o'-dityrosine in brain tissue of 1-methyl-4-phenyl-1,2,3,6-tetrahydropyridine–treated mice, a model of oxidative stress in Parkinson's disease. *J Biol Chem* 1999;274:34621–34628, with permission.)

that MPTP does increase nitrotyrosine formation and that these alterations are a reflection of a pathological process specific to MPTP (26). It can also be concluded that these findings strongly support the notion that peroxynitrite is involved in the MPTP-related cascade of deleterious events and possibly in the pathogenesis of PD.

ARE BOTH SUPEROXIDE AND NITRIC OXIDE REQUIRED?

Before embarking on this question, specifically in the MPTP model of PD, it is necessary to remind the reader that peroxynitrite, as stated before, results from the interaction between superoxide and NO (27). In a normal situation, superoxide is constantly produced in a large number of biological reactions within our cells, and its intracellular concentration is maintained at extremely low levels by an abundance of the enzyme superoxide dismutase (SOD), which destroys the superoxide radical (Fig. 8.1A). Conversely, NO is present in abundance, both within cells and in the extracellular space surrounding these cells, due to the production of this reactive species by several isoforms of the NO synthase (NOS) enzyme (Fig. 8.1A). Therefore, because in normal situations the level of superoxide is low, the basal level of peroxynitrite is also low, as is the level of oxidative damage inflicted by peroxynitrite (Fig. 8.1A.). In contrast, in PD as modeled by the MPTP neurotoxin, the level of superoxide increases significantly (Fig. 8.1B), presumably via the blockade of mitochondrial respiration and/or other mechanisms (28). Consequently, the intracellular concentration of superoxide now rises, as does the formation of peroxynitrite and the resulting magnitude of oxidative stress and cytotoxicity (Fig. 8.1B).

In light of this, one might ask whether it is true that superoxide is a rate-limiting factor in this reaction. To address this important question, we have used transgenic mice that express two to three times more SOD in the brain (29) with the prospect that by increasing superoxide detoxification, less superoxide will be available to react with NO, thus less peroxynitrite will be formed and less toxicity will occur (Fig. 8.3A). The results of our study show that MPTP administration causes significant damage to the nigrostriatal pathway in non-transgenic littermates with normal activity of SOD in the brain (30). In contrast, in transgenic animals with increased activity of SOD in the brain, a similar regimen of MPTP causes only minimal damage to the dopaminergic neurons (30). Similar results were observed in transgenic mice expressing manganese SOD, another SOD isoform (31). These findings lead us to conclude that as predicted (Fig. 8.3A), adjusting the amount of superoxide radicals in the brain appears to be a key component in the MPTP neurotoxic process.

The second question regarding MPTP toxic biochemistry is whether there is also a need for NO (Fig. 8.3B). To address this second crucial question, several investigators, including ourselves, have modulated the amount of NO available for this reaction by targeting NOS, the enzyme responsible for NO formation. The use of different NOS antagonists (32–34) has convincingly demonstrated that

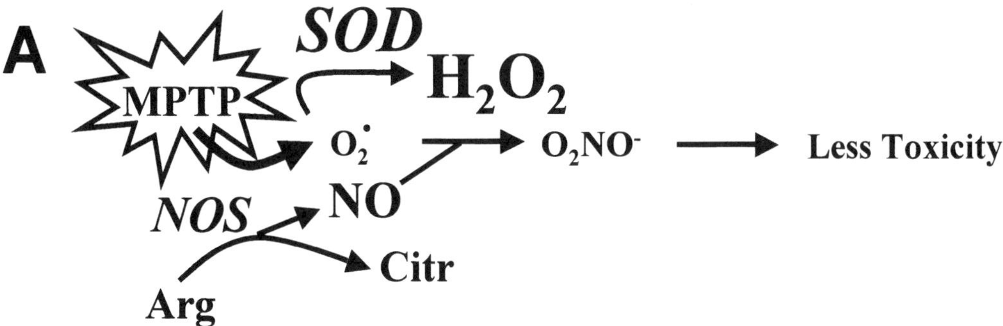

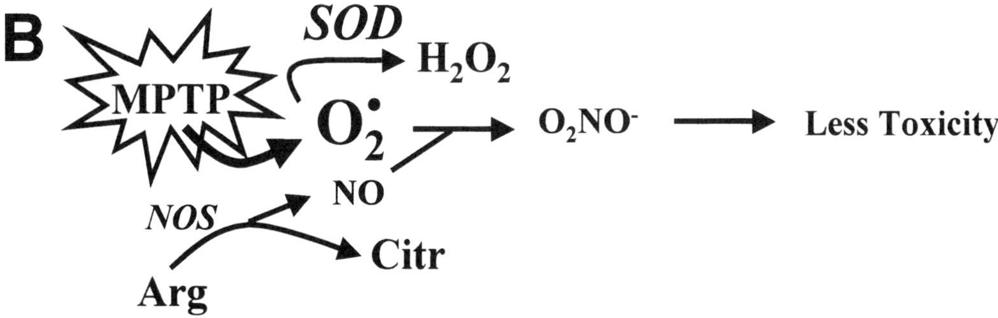

FIGURE 8.3. Effects of genetic interventions on 1-methyl-4-phenyl-1,2,3,6-tetrahydropyridine (MPTP)-related production of peroxynitrite (O_2NO^-) and cytotoxicity. By increasing superoxide dismutase *(SOD)* activity **(A)**, MPTP-related superoxide radical ($O_2^{\bullet}$) production is reduced. Thus, less superoxide radicals are available to react with nitric oxide *(NO)*; consequently, less peroxynitrite is produced, and less cytotoxicity occurs. By blocking nitric oxide synthase *(NOS)* **(B)**, the formation of NO is reduced. Thus, less NO is available to react with superoxide radicals, and consequently, less peroxynitrite is produced and less cytotoxicity occurs.

blockade of NOS, which reduces the production of NO, attenuates significantly MPTP-induced neurotoxicity. Collectively, all of these studies indicate that, as hypothesized, both superoxide and NO are necessary to the deleterious biochemical reaction involved in the MPTP-mediated demise of the nigrostriatal dopaminergic pathway (Fig. 8.3).

WHAT IS THE SOURCE OF NITRIC OXIDE INVOLVED IN MPTP NEUROTOXICITY?

Thus far, three different isoforms of NOS have been cloned and characterized (5). These include neuronal NOS (nNOS), inducible NOS (iNOS), and endothelial NOS (eNOS). All of these isoforms are present in the brain, though in variable abundance. The most abundant isoform nNOS is expressed in several neuronal subtypes, but interestingly, nNOS has not been identified in dopaminergic neurons of the nigrostriatal pathway. Yet, dopaminergic neurons of the nigrostriatal pathway are surrounded by an abundant network of neuronal cell bodies and fibers that contain nNOS (35), suggesting that any NO that will be used by dopaminergic neurons in MPTP neurotoxicity or in the pathogenesis of PD will have to originate from neighboring neurons. In contrast to nNOS, iNOS is normally not expressed in the brain; however, in pathological situations, particularly those associated with gliosis, iNOS can be induced. Consistent with this notion, in the case of PD and in the MPTP model, it has been demonstrated by immunohistochemical methods that glial cells at the level of the SNpc exhibit a robust expression of iNOS (36,37). As for eNOS in the brain, only very discrete populations of neurons seem to express this NOS isoform (38). Otherwise, eNOS is confined to the endothelial cells of blood vessels, which are abundant in all regions of the brain. In regions such as the substantia nigra and the striatum, we found no evidence that eNOS is expressed in neuronal cells (Du Chu Wu and Serge Przedborski, *personal observation, 1999)*. Nevertheless, in these two brain regions, dopaminergic structures entertain a close relationship with blood vessels whose walls exhibit robust eNOS immunoreactivity (Du Chu Wu and Serge Przedborski, *personal observation*). From a pharmacological standpoint, it is important to determine which of these isoforms is responsible for the production of NO in the pathogenesis of PD. Thanks to the development of genetically engineered animals in which the gene for each of the isoforms of NOS has been separately ablated, it became possible to answer this question in a precise fashion. Using mutant mice deficient in nNOS, we were able to demonstrate that ablation of nNOS markedly attenuates MPTP toxicity (32). Indeed, our data on dopamine content in the striatum of these mutant animals show that compared with their wild-type littermates, MPTP inflicts significantly less damage (32). These results indicate that by eliminating nNOS, MPTP neurotoxicity is partially, but not completely, blocked, which suggests that although nNOS plays a significant role in MPTP neurotoxicity, it is probably not the sole isoform of NOS implicated in this process.

Using iNOS knockout mice and their wild-type littermates, both Dehmer et al. (39) and Liberatore et al. (37) showed, first, that not only is there a robust glial reaction after MPTP administration, but also that there is an upregulation of iNOS. More important, these studies demonstrate that the administration of MPTP, through different regimens to iNOS knockout mice and their wild-type littermates, produces significantly less neuronal loss in mutant mice deficient in iNOS compared with their wild-type counterparts (37,39). Again, as for nNOS, toxicity is only attenuated and not prevented in iNOS-deficient mice. As for eNOS, using Western blotting techniques, we have preliminary data showing that the level of expression of eNOS is unaffected by MPTP administration, and more important, that when toxicity to MPTP is assessed in eNOS knockout animals, the ablation of this isoform has no significant impact on the demise of dopaminergic neurons. Collectively, these data suggest that in the

MPTP model, only iNOS and nNOS seem to play a significant role in the neurotoxic process. eNOS, although present, seems not to have a role here. It can also be extrapolated from these data that optimal neuroprotection may be obtained in the MPTP model and possibly in PD, only if both nNOS and iNOS are inhibited.

DOES PEROXYNITRITE CAUSE DETECTABLE DAMAGE AFTER MPTP ADMINISTRATION?

As stated already, peroxynitrite can damage virtually any cellular component, including proteins, lipids, and DNA, as well as dopamine (40). With respect to this chapter, we focus our discussion only on the MPTP-related peroxynitrite effects on proteins. Based on the chromatographic studies mentioned earlier in this chapter, we already know that MPTP causes detectable damage to proteins as a whole, as evidenced by nitrotyrosine levels (Fig. 8.2). This can not only be quantified on Western blot analysis but also visualized. Using this approach, we have demonstrated that after MPTP administration, several proteins with very different molecular masses are indeed nitrated (41). We also show that this phenomenon is time dependent, peaking between 6 and 12 hours after MPTP administration (41). This is not surprising because previously we have reported that MPTP cytotoxicity is also time dependent (42) and that biochemical correlates of MPTP toxicity such as adenosine triphosphate (ATP) depletion can be detected as early as 1 hour after MPTP administration (43). Remarkably, this Western blot study revealed a robust nitration only on some and not all resolved proteins (41), which is an unexpected finding, because virtually all proteins contain at least one tyrosine residue. Therefore, our Western blot data indicate that whereas all proteins *could* potentially be nitrated, only *specific* proteins seem to be nitrated after MPTP administration. To try to identify what specific proteins are nitrated after MPTP administration, we decided to assess the propensity of specific protein candidates to become nitrated after MPTP administration. Herein, we illustrate the case of two such protein candidates: tyrosine hydroxylase (TH), which is the rate-limiting enzyme in dopamine synthesis, and α-synuclein, a small presynaptic protein whose mutations have recently been implicated in the development of a familial form of PD. TH contains 16 tyrosine residues in its primary structure, and most of these are found in the vicinity of its catalytic site. It should also be mentioned that although nitrotyrosine has been presented so far in this chapter as a marker of peroxynitrite, nitrotyrosine can be neurotoxic in its own right. For instance, free nitrotyrosine when injected into the striatum has been shown to cause some nigrostriatal damage (44). In addition, because nitrotyrosine adds negative charges into a protein, which could have an impact on this protein's secondary or tertiary structure, nitrotyrosine could also, in the case of an enzyme, affect its catalytic activity. Relevant to this possibility, we have demonstrated that TH becomes heavily nitrated between 3 and 6 hours after the last injection of MPTP (Fig. 8.4) (41). We have also shown that coinciding with its nitration, TH looses its catalytic activity (Fig. 8.4) (41). Similarly, we have demonstrated that after MPTP administration, α-synuclein becomes heavily nitrated 4 hours after the last MPTP dose (Fig. 8.5.) (45). Interestingly, we found that at the same time point and under the same regimen of MPTP, proteins related to α-synuclein such as β-synuclein or synaptophysin are not nitrated (Fig. 8.5) (45). The possible functional implication of the nitration of α-synuclein is that this small presynaptic protein is known to be quite insoluble, and by perturbing its spatial organization, nitration can conceivably reduce α-synuclein's solubility, thus promoting its precipitation and the formation of aggregates. This view, although difficult to test in the MPTP mouse model, found support in a study performed by Giasson et al. (22), who showed that α-synuclein in the parkinsonian brain is indeed nitrated and that the nitrated form of α-synu-

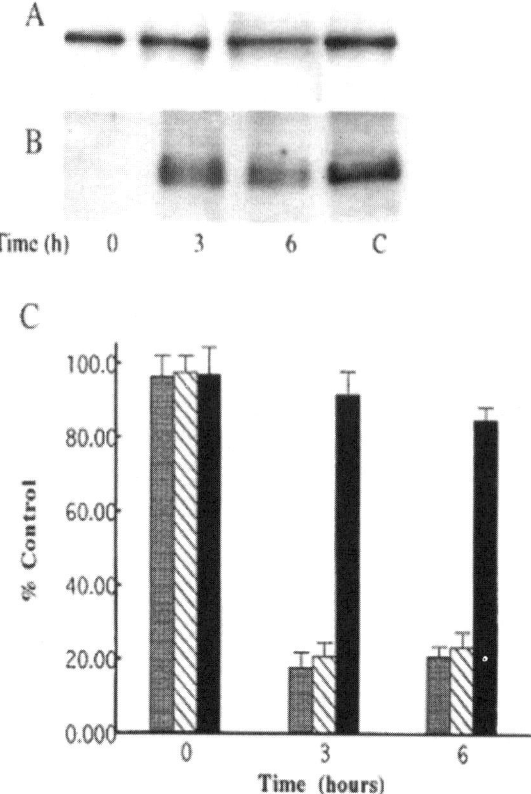

FIGURE 8.4. Inactivation of tyrosine hydroxylase (TH) by tyrosine nitration after 1-methyl-4-phenyl-1,2,3,6-tetrahydropyridine (MPTP) administration. At selected times (0-, 3-, and 6-hour postexposure), TH was immunoprecipitated from the striatum of MPTP-injected mice and then visualized using an anti-TH antibody. **A:** Comparable amounts of immunoprecipitated TH were loaded onto the gel. To assess the presence of tyrosine nitration in immunoprecipitated TH, an anti-nitrotyrosine antibody was used. **B:** TH is markedly nitrated at 3 and 6 hours, but not at 0 hour after MPTP administration. As a positive control **(C)**, TH was immunoprecipitated from peroxynitrite-treated PC12 cells. Paralleling the time course of its nitration, TH enzymatic activity (*hatched bars*), and consequently, production of dopamine (*gray bars*) dropped dramatically at 3 and 6 hours post-MPTP administration **(C)**. Conversely, at those selected times, TH protein contents (*black bars*) did not differ significantly from those of healthy controls, indicating that TH is inactivated as a result of nitration. (From Ara J, Przedborski S, Naini AB, et al. Inactivation of tyrosine hydroxylase by nitration following exposure to peroxynitrite and 1-methyl-4-phenyl-1,2,3,6-tetrahydropyridine (MPTP). *Proc Natl Acad Sci USA* 1998;95:7659–7663, with permission.)

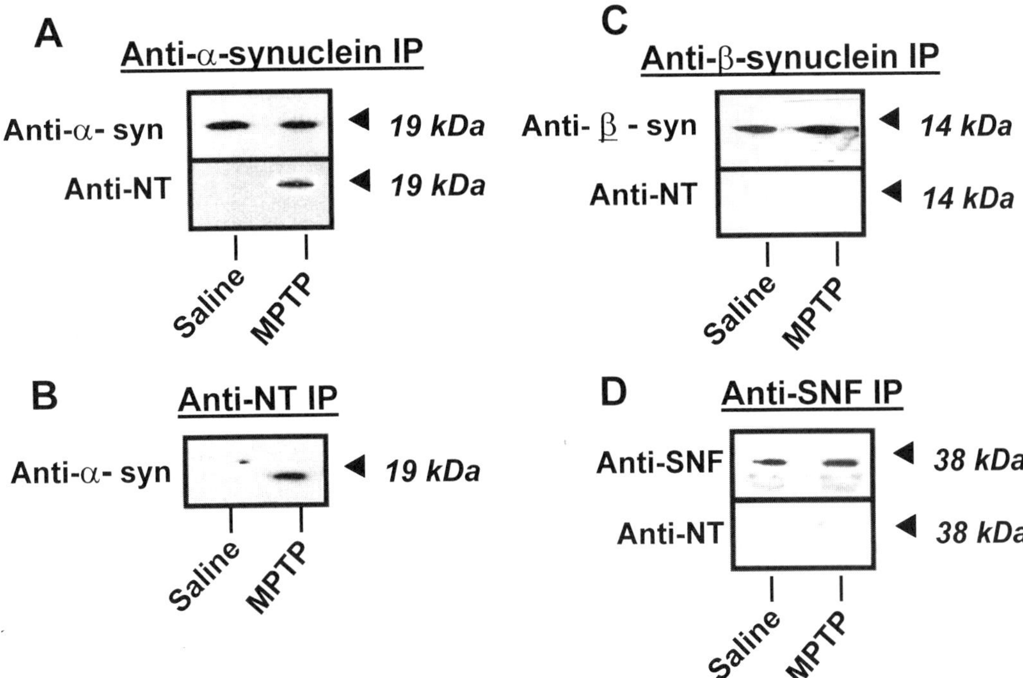

FIGURE 8.5. Tyrosine nitration of striatal α-synuclein, but not of β-synuclein, or synaptophysin, after 1-methyl-4-phenyl-1,2,3,6-tetrahydropyridine (MPTP) injection to mice. After MPTP administration (4 hours after the last injection) or vehicle (saline), striatal proteins were immunoprecipitated using anti-synuclein antibody **(A)**; anti-nitrotyrosine **(B)**; anti-β-synuclein **(C)**; or anti-synaptophysin **(D)**. After having been resolved on gels, proteins were immunostained with anti-nitrotyrosine **(A,C,D [lower panels])**, anti-α-syn **(A [top panel] and B)**, anti-β-syn **(C [top panel])**, and anti-synaptophysin **(D [top panel])**. (From Przedborski S, Chen Q, Vila M, et al. Oxidative post-translational modifications of alpha-synuclein in the 1-methyl-4-phenyl-1,2,3,6-tetrahydropyridine (MPTP) mouse model of Parkinson's disease. *J Neurochem* 2001;76:637–640, with permission.)

clein is preferentially found in dystrophic neurites and Lewy bodies.

CONCLUSIONS

In light of the outlined data, we can propose a pathogenic scenario for PD based on the different steps in the MPTP model (Fig. 8.6). The first step of this scenario relies on the fact that one must agree with the idea that the initiating factor of the deleterious cascade is a molecule that shares similarities with the MPTP active metabolite 1-methyl-4-phenylpyridimium (MPP^+). As such, this putative molecule has to enter dopaminergic neurons via the plasma membrane dopamine transporter (DAT). Once inside dopaminergic neurons, MPP^+ acts on mitochondria, where it blocks mitochondrial respiration. This has two immediate consequences: (a) blockade of the production of ATP, and therefore, an ensuing energy crisis, and (b) an increased production of superoxide. As we indicated already, other mechanisms may also stimulate the production of superoxide after MPTP administration. At the same time, neighboring neurons that contain nNOS produce NO, and later, when gliosis develops, activated glial cells that contain iNOS contribute to the production of NO. NO, known to be quite stable compared to other reactive species, can travel several micrometers away from its site of production. NO, like water, can freely cross the plasma membrane, and thus, after being produced

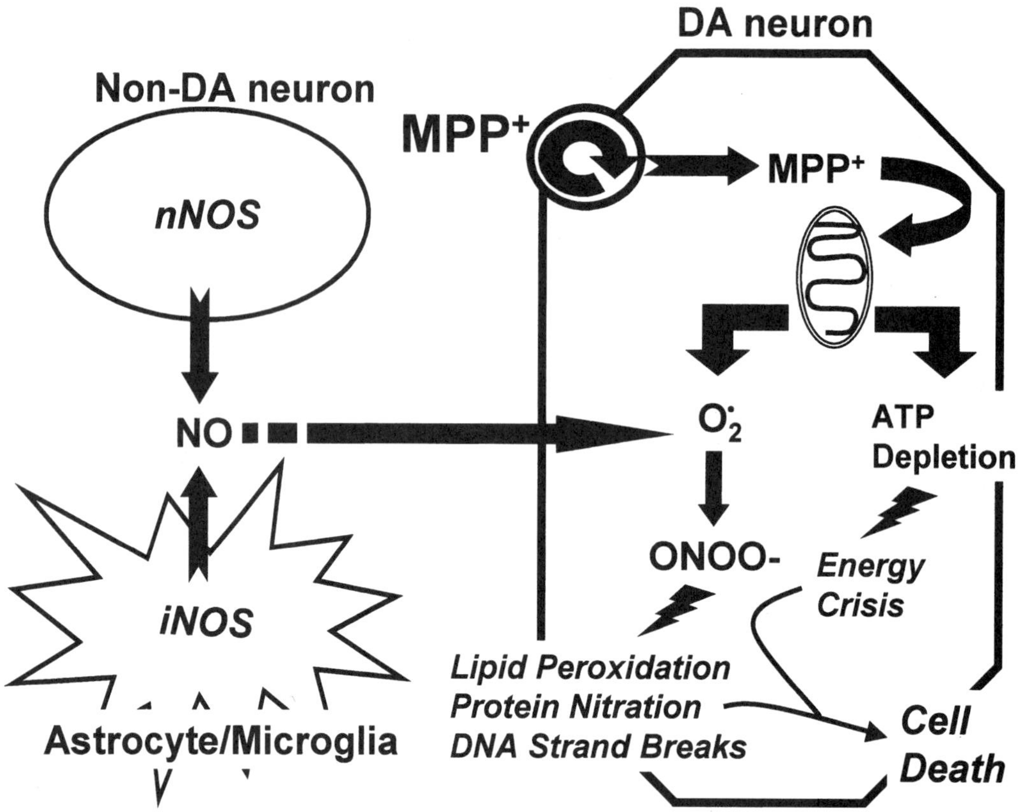

FIGURE 8.6. Proposed scenario of methylphenyltetrahydropyridine neurotoxic process and pathogenesis of Parkinson's disease.

and released extracellularly, NO can easily penetrate dopaminergic neurons (Fig. 8.6). There, NO reacts with superoxide to produce peroxynitrite. Peroxynitrite, in turn, will now inflict severe oxidative damage to lipids, DNA, and proteins such as the nitration of tyrosine residues. Together, oxidative damage and energy crisis lead to cellular dysfunction, which when built up over time can eventually reach a magnitude that is no longer compatible with life, thus neurons die (Fig. 8.6). Although this scenario is primarily relevant to MPTP neurotoxicity, we strongly believe that a similar sequence of events may well underlie the neurodegenerative process in PD.

ACKNOWLEDGMENTS

The authors dedicate this chapter in memory of Dr. Gerald Cohen. The authors' work is supported by the National Institutes of Health/National Institute of Neurological Disorders and Stroke grants R29 NS37345, RO1 NS38586, RO1 NS42269, and P50 NS38370, the US Department of Defense Grant (DAMD 17-99-1-9471), the Lowenstein Foundation, the Lillian Goldman Charitable Trust, the Parkinson's Disease Foundation, the Muscular Dystrophy Association, the ALS Association, and Project-ALS. Peter Teismann is the recipient of a grant from the German Research Foundation (TE 343/1-1).

REFERENCES

1. Fahn S, Przedborski S. Parkinsonism. In: Rowland LP, ed. *Merritt's Neurology.* New York: Lippincott Williams & Wilkins, 2000:679–693.
2. Hornykiewicz O, Kish SJ. Biochemical pathophysiology of Parkinson's disease. In: Yahr M, Bergmann KJ, eds. *Parkinson's disease.* New York: Raven Press, 1987:19–34.

3. Forno LS. Neuropathology of Parkinson's disease. *J Neuropathol Exp Neurol* 1996;55:259–272.
4. Przedborski S, Jackson-Lewis V. ROS and Parkinson's disease: a view to a kill. In: Poli G, Cadenas E, Packer L, eds. *Free radicals in brain pathophysiology.* New York: Marcel Dekker Inc, 2000:273–290.
5. Przedborski S, Dawson TM. The role of nitric oxide in Parkinson's disease. In: Mouradian MM, ed. *Parkinson's disease. Methods and protocols.* New Jersey: Humana Press, 2001:113–136.
6. Pzedborski S, Vila M. MPTP: A review of its mechanisms of neurotoxicity. *Clin Neurosci Res* 2001;1:407–418.
7. Langston JW, Ballard P, Irwin I. Chronic parkinsonism in humans due to a product of meperidine-analog synthesis. *Science* 1983;219:979–980.
8. Langston JW, Irwin I. MPTP: current concepts and controversies. *Clin Neuropharmacol* 1986;9:485–507.
9. Heikkila RE, Sieber BA, Manzino L, et al. Some features of the nigrostriatal dopaminergic neurotoxin 1-methyl-4-phenyl-1,2,3,6-tetrahydropyridine (MPTP) in the mouse. *Mol Chem Neuropathol* 1989;10:171–183.
10. Kopin IJ, Markey SP. MPTP toxicity: implication for research in Parkinson's disease. *Annu Rev Neurosci* 1988; 11:81–96.
11. Przedborski S, Jackson-Lewis V, Naini A, et al. The parkinsonian toxin 1-methyl-4-phenyl-1,2,3,6-tetrahydropyridine (MPTP): a technical review of its utility and safety. *J Neurochem* 2001;76:1265–1274.
12. Vingerhoets FJG, Snow BJ, Tetrud JW, et al. Positron emission tomographic evidence for progression of human MPTP-induced dopaminergic lesions. *Ann Neurol* 1994;36:765–770.
13. Langston JW, Forno LS, Tetrud J, et al. Evidence of active nerve cell degeneration in the substantia nigra of humans years after 1-methyl-4-phenyl-1,2,3,6-tetrahydropyridine exposure. *Ann Neurol* 1999;46:598–605.
14. Seniuk NA, Tatton WG, Greenwood CE. Dose-dependent destruction of the ceruleus-cortical and nigral-striatal projections by MPTP. *Brain Res* 1990;527:7–20.
15. Muthane U, Ramsay KA, Jiang H, et al. Differences in nigral neuron number and sensitivity to 1-methyl-4-phenyl-1,2,3,6-tetrahydropyridine in C57/bl and CD-1 mice. *Exp Neurol* 1994;126:195–204.
16. Moratalla R, Quinn B, DeLanney LE, et al. Differential vulnerability of primate caudate-putamen and striosome-matrix dopamine systems to the neurotoxic effects of 1-methyl-4-phenyl-1,2,3,6-tetrahydropyridine. *Proc Natl Acad Sci USA* 1992;89:3859–3863.
17. Snow BJ, Vingerhoets FJ, Langston JW, et al. Pattern of dopaminergic loss in the striatum of humans with MPTP induced parkinsonism. *J Neurol Neurosurg Psychiatry* 2000;68:313–316.
18. Forno LS, Langston JW, DeLanney LE, et al. Locus ceruleus lesions and eosinophilic inclusions in MPTP-treated monkeys. *Ann Neurol* 1986;20:449–455.
19. Ischiropoulos H. Biological tyrosine nitration: a pathophysiological function of nitric oxide and reactive oxygen species. *Arch Biochem Biophys* 1998;356:1–11.
20. Ye YZ, Strong M, Huang Z-Q, et al. Antibodies that recognize nitrotyrosine. In: Packer L, ed. *Nitric oxide. Physiological and pathological processes.* New York: Academic Press, 1996:201–209.
21. Good PF, Hsu A, Werner P, et al. Protein nitration in Parkinson's disease. *J Neuropathol Exp Neurol* 1998; 57:338–342.
22. Giasson BI, Duda JE, Murray IV, et al. Oxidative damage linked to neurodegeneration by selective alpha-synuclein nitration in synucleinopathy lesions. *Science* 2000;290:985–989.
23. Duda JE, Giasson BI, Chen Q, et al. Widespread nitration of pathological inclusions in neurodegenerative synucleinopathies. *Am J Pathol* 2000;157: 1439–1445.
24. Schulz JB, Matthews RT, Muqit MMK, et al. Inhibition of neuronal nitric oxide synthase by 7-nitroindazole protects against MPTP-induced neurotoxicity in mice. *J Neurochem* 1995;64:936–939.
25. Kaur H, Lyras L, Jenner P, et al. Artifacts in HPLC detection of 3-nitrotyrosine in human brain tissue. *J Neurochem* 1998;70:2220–2223.
26. Pennathur S, Jackson-Lewis V, Przedborski S, et al. Mass spectrometric quantification of 3-nitrotyrosine, ortho-tyrosine, and o,o'-dityrosine in brain tissue of 1-methyl-4-phenyl-1,2,3,6-tetrahydropyridine–treated mice, a model of oxidative stress in Parkinson's disease. *J Biol Chem* 1999;274:34621–34628.
27. Beckman JS, Koppenol WH. Nitric oxide, superoxide, and peroxynitrite: the good, the bad, and the ugly. *Am J Physiol Cell Physiol* 1996;271:C1424–C1437.
28. Lotharius J, O'Malley KL. The parkinsonism-inducing drug 1-methyl-4-phenylpyridinium triggers intracellular dopamine oxidation. A novel mechanism of toxicity. *J Biol Chem* 2000;275:38581–38588.
29. Przedborski S, Jackson-Lewis V, Kostic V, et al. Superoxide dismutase, catalase, and glutathione peroxidase activities in copper/zinc-superoxide dismutase transgenic mice. *J Neurochem* 1992;58:1760–1767.
30. Przedborski S, Kostic V, Jackson-Lewis V, et al. Transgenic mice with increased Cu/Zn-superoxide dismutase activity are resistant to N-methyl-4-phenyl-1,2,3,6-tetrahydropyridine-induced neurotoxicity. *J Neurosci* 1992;12:1658–1667.
31. Klivenyi P, St. Wermer M, Yen HC, et al. Manganese superoxide dismutase overexpression attenuates MPTP toxicity. *Neurobiol Dis* 1998;5:253–258.
32. Przedborski S, Jackson-Lewis V, Yokoyama R, et al. Role of neuronal nitric oxide in MPTP (1-methyl-4-phenyl-1,2,3,6-tetrahydropyridine)-induced dopaminergic neurotoxicity. *Proc Natl Acad Sci USA* 1996;93: 4565–4571.
33. Matthews RT, Yang LC, Beal MF. *S*-methylthiocitrulline, a neuronal nitric oxide synthase inhibitor, protects against malonate and MPTP neurotoxicity. *Exp Neurol* 1997;143:282–286.
34. Schulz JB, Matthews RT, Jenkins B, et al. Blockade of neuronal nitric oxide synthase protects against excitotoxicity *in vivo*. *J Neurosci* 1995;15:8419–8429.
35. Leonard CS, Kerman I, Blaha G, et al. Interdigitation of nitric oxide synthase–, tyrosine hydroxylase–, and serotonin-containing neurons in and around the laterodorsal and pedunculopontine tegmental nuclei of the guinea pig. *J Comp Neurol* 1995;362:411–432.
36. Hunot S, Boissière F, Faucheux B, et al. Nitric oxide synthase and neuronal vulnerability in Parkinson's disease. *Neuroscience* 1996;72:355–363.
37. Liberatore GT, Jackson-Lewis V, Vukosavic S, et al. Inducible nitric oxide synthase stimulates dopaminergic neurodegeneration in the MPTP model of Parkinson disease. *Nature Med* 1999;5:1403–1409.
38. Dinerman JL, Dawson TM, Schell MJ, et al. Endothelial

nitric oxide synthase localized to hippocampal pyramidal cells: implications for synaptic plasticity. *Proc Natl Acad Sci USA* 1994;91:4214–4218.
39. Dehmer T, Lindenau J, Haid S, et al. Deficiency of inducible nitric oxide synthase protects against MPTP toxicity *in vivo*. *J Neurochem* 2000;74:2213–2216.
40. LaVoie MJ, Hastings TG. Peroxynitrite- and nitrite-induced oxidation of dopamine: implications for nitric oxide in dopaminergic cell loss. *J Neurochem* 1999;73: 2546–2554.
41. Ara J, Przedborski S, Naini AB, et al. Inactivation of tyrosine hydroxylase by nitration following exposure to peroxynitrite and 1-methyl-4-phenyl-1,2,3,6-tetrahydropyridine (MPTP). *Proc Natl Acad Sci USA* 1998;95: 7659–7663.
42. Jackson-Lewis V, Jakowec M, Burke RE, et al. Time course and morphology of dopaminergic neuronal death caused by the neurotoxin 1-methyl-4-phenyl-1,2,3,6-tetrahydropyridine. *Neurodegeneration* 1995;4: 257–269.
43. Chan P, DeLanney LE, Irwin I, et al. MPTP-induced ATP loss in mouse brain. *Ann NY Acad Sci* 1992;648:306–308.
44. Mihm MJ, Schanbacher BL, Wallace BL, et al. Free 3-nitrotyrosine causes striatal neurodegeneration *in vivo*. *J Neurosci* 2001;21:RC149:1–5.
45. Przedborski S, Chen Q, Vila M, et al. Oxidative post-translational modifications of alpha-synuclein in the 1-methyl-4-phenyl-1,2,3,6-tetrahydropyridine (MPTP) mouse model of Parkinson's disease. *J Neurochem* 2001;76:637–640.

Parkinson's Disease: Advances in Neurology, Vol. 91.
Edited by Ariel Gordin, Seppo Kaakkola,
and Heikki Teräväinen
Lippincott Williams & Wilkins, Philadelphia © 2003

9
Neuroregeneration

Jens Strelau and Klaus Unsicker

Neuroanatomy and Center for Neurosciences, University of Heidelberg, Heidelberg, Germany

The central nervous system (CNS) and the peripheral nervous system (PNS) of phylogenetic older vertebrates such as teleosts and, in part, amphibians have the capacity to undergo axonal regeneration after injury. Damage of CNS or PNS fiber tracts is followed by an extensive regrowth of axons and the formation of new functional synapses. In contrast, higher vertebrates regenerate PNS axons but fail to regrow CNS fibers. To answer the question about why the mammalian CNS is incapable of overcoming the effects of injuries such as spinal cord trauma and stroke, three hypotheses have been suggested. First, CNS neurons have an intrinsic inability to regenerate. Thus, once neurite growth has stopped at the end of the developmental period, it cannot be reinitiated. Second, the CNS environment is inhibitory to regenerative growth, and regeneration of damaged CNS axons can be induced by replacing an environment that inhibits regeneration with one that encourages it. Third, CNS glia (astrocytes and oligodendrocytes) do not support CNS neurons after injury and extrinsic factors that are required for the growth and survival of the neurons are missing. Understanding the different mechanisms that control regeneration, growth, and survival of neurons is one of the most challenging and important problems addressed by neurobiologists today. This chapter focuses on recent advances concerning the lack of regeneration in the mature mammalian CNS, particularly the knowledge of the intrinsic neuronal state, the environmental myelin-associated inhibitors, and the extrinsic neurotrophic factors.

THE INTRINSIC NEURONAL STATE

The outgrowth, the pathway finding, and the permanent remodeling of axons and synaptic connections are major important processes during the development of the CNS. In the postnatal or mature brain, those adaptive changes are limited. Adult CNS neurons persist in a determined intrinsic state and need to recapitulate at least some of the developmental events for regeneration. Are CNS neurons unable to regenerate because they lose this ability with age? In the PNS, this is clearly not the case. The axonal growth of sensory neurons *in vivo* of about 0.5 mm per day is maintained *in vitro* across a broad range of ages, before and after target innervation (1,2). This was shown also for other types of PNS neurons (2).

Similar studies with CNS neurons are technically more difficult and have not been performed for most types of CNS neurons. However, it has been found that in mammals some retinal ganglion cells (RGCs), a type of CNS neurons, could regenerate their axons through fragments of peripheral nerve grafts (3). These findings provide hope that at least some CNS neurons are able to regenerate. In contrast, experiments with embryonic RGCs showed an age-dependent loss in their ability to regenerate axons out of retinal explants (4), leading some investigators to conclude that the intrinsic state of neurons dictates, in part, the inability to regenerate. If so, what determines the intracellular state of adult CNS neurons and what are the differences to regenerating PNS neurons? Several recent studies have provided convincing evidence that an optimal level of cytosolic cyclic nucleotides is required for axonal growth (5–11). Importantly, Cai et al. (9) reported that preexposure (printing) of neurons to neurotrophins elevates endogenous cyclic adenosine monophosphate (cAMP) and activates protein kinase A (PKA), which blocks inhibition of axonal regeneration. Priming of neurons was required because myelin activates a G_i protein, which blocks increases in cAMP. Consistent with these findings are the results of a more recent study by Cai et al. (11). They reported that the endogenous level of cAMP in RGCs and dorsal root ganglia (DRG) decreases with development and that this downregulation in cAMP coincides with the switch to the inhibition of regeneration. In this study, it has also been shown that an inhibition of signals downstream of cAMP activation (inhibition of PKA) can block early developmental plasticity of spinal tract axons in neonatal rat pups *in vivo.* Thus, intracellular cAMP levels have important effects on axonal regeneration by regulating the influence of inhibitory molecules on growth promotion. However, it is not clear whether this also holds true for all other types of CNS neurons and to what extent the inability of many CNS axons to regenerate is the result of intrinsic factors. A crucial issue for future work is the identification and characterization of factors responsible for cAMP elevation and downstream effector molecules that are involved. One possible candidate responsible for an intrinsic and genetically regulated switch that controls the ability of neurons to extend axons was recently proposed. Chen et al. (12) reported that the protooncogene Bcl-2 plays a key role in this developmental change by promoting the growth and regeneration of retinal axons. Bcl-2 is expressed at high levels by embryonic RGCs and is downregulated during the time in which the neurons lose their regenerative ability (13,14). Using transgenic mice, in which RGCs express Bcl-2 into adulthood, they found that postnatal RGCs retain their regenerative capacity and regenerate into tectal explants. The argument that this effect is not an indirect consequence of the well-known antiapoptotic activity of Bcl-2 was based on control experiments using the caspase inhibitor ZVAD. Caspases are the downstream effectors of apoptosis controlled by Bcl-2, and it was shown that blocking caspases with ZVAD supported neuronal survival but did not promote axon regeneration in culture. This suggests that Bcl-2 may exert its function on axonal growth through a pathway that is independent of the survival-promoting effects. Possibly, this finding may lead to new strategies for the treatment of injuries to the CNS.

THE MYELIN-ASSOCIATED INHIBITORS

Another explanation for the poor regenerative capacity of injured CNS fiber tracts is the existence of inhibitory factors that interfere with axonal growth in the adult CNS. Consistent with this view is the observation that lesioned embryonic spinal cord neurons regenerate within a time that ends at the onset of myelination in the spinal cord (15). Moreover, a number of studies demonstrated the strong inhibitory effect of oligodendrocytes on the outgrowth of neurons in the spinal cord and in the optic nerve (16). Besides oligodendrocytes, subpopulations of astrocytes and activities isolated from glial scar tissue around CNS lesion sites were shown to be inhibitory for neurite growth *in vitro* (17–21). The search for myelin-associated neurite growth inhibitors has lead to the characterization and identification of a large number of molecules such as the myelin-associated glycoprotein (MAG) (22,23), NI35/250/NOGO-A (24–28) and the chondroitin sulfate proteoglycans versican V2 and brevican (29). At present, little is known concerning the functional properties of these molecules, and it should be noted that myelin-associated inhibitory proteins have never been localized in the outer layer of intact myelin membranes. Uninjured myelin does not normally expose inhibitory myelin components to CNS neurons, and it has been shown that adult DRG neurons transplanted into undamaged myelinated areas of adult brain are able to extend axons over significant distances on the surface of intact myelin (1 to 2 mm per day) (30). The question of whether adult CNS neurons will also regenerate their axons through myelinated CNS pathways remains to be answered. CNS neurons could not be similarly transplanted because they would immediately undergo apoptosis. In contrast to the *in vivo* situation, myelin-associated inhibitors are exposed *in vitro.* It may therefore not be surprising that adult DRG neurons cultured on myelin extracts show inhibition of growth (31,32). Together, these findings suggest a scenario involving myelin-associated proteins that after myelin disruption inhibit axon regeneration in the injured CNS.

More recent studies suggest that this view may be an oversimplification of the real situation. Davies et al. (33) showed that DRG neurons are able to extend axons in spinal cord white matter that is undergoing degeneration after spinal cord injury. Similar results were reported by Neumann and Woolf (34). In this study DRG neurons were first axotomized peripherally to enhance their intrinsic growth state. After 1 week, a CNS spinal lesion was performed, and central processes (dorsal column fibers) of preconditioned DRG neurons were shown to grow into and beyond the CNS lesion site. Together, these findings indicate that peripheral DRG neurons are able to grow axons within degenerated or injured CNS pathways, and that inhibitory effects of myelin-associated molecules cannot completely explain the lack of CNS nerve regeneration after spinal cord injury.

In contrast to the above-mentioned inhibitory effects of myelin-associated proteins, it should be noted that myelin could also stimulate axonal growth. This view is supported by studies that show that the same myelin extract that is inhibitory for cultured adult DRG neurons can promote neurite outgrowth in neonatal DRG neurons (32). In addition, it is well documented that embryonic CNS neurons, when cultured on myelin or myelin proteins, such as MAG or myelin-associated oligodendrocyte glycoprotein (MOG), display long-distance growth of processes (35,36). It has also been shown that embryonic CNS neurons transplanted into the adult spinal cord (37) extend axons for long distances through adult white matter pathways (38–40). The molecular mechanisms underlying the switch from promotion to inhibition of axonal growth by myelin during development are unknown.

THE NEUROTROPHIC CONTROL OF AXON REGENERATION IN THE CNS

Transplanted adult DRG neurons survive and regenerate axons in the injured CNS (see previous discussion). Will adult CNS neurons also regenerate if they were able to overcome cell death? One possible strategy to answer this important question could be the investigation of extrinsic factors that control neuron growth and survival. Intact neurons derive neurotrophic support either by means of retrograde transport from the innervated target cell or from anterograde transport to presynaptic terminals, where trophic molecules may be released. Neighboring glial cells, such as Schwann's cells, astrocytes, and oligodendrocytes, do provide neurotrophic factors as well (41). The list of identified neurotrophic factors is long, and it is likely that many peptides with such functions remain to be discovered (42). Neurotrophins comprise a family of neurotrophic molecules that include nerve growth factor (NGF), brain-derived neurotrophic factor, neurotrophin-3 (NT-3), and NT-4/5. There are also members of the transforming growth factor 13 superfamily, insulin-derived growth factors, fibroblast growth factors, and members of the platelet-derived growth factor family that exert trophic functions in the PNS and CNS (43). Together, these neurotrophic peptides elicit diverse important cellular responses such as survival, differentiation, and repair of neurons. Injured CNS neurons may fail to receive and respond to their trophic signals and therefore undergo apoptotic cell death. This raises the possibility that simply promoting the survival of injured or degenerated CNS neurons might be sufficient to allow them to regenerate their axons. But what is essential to promote neuron survival? CNS neurons require simultaneous stimulation by multiple trophic peptides (42,44,45). This view is supported by recent *in vivo* studies that reported that the survival of axotomized RGCs can be promoted only by a coadministration of different factors, together with a cAMP analog (32). In contrast, adult PNS neurons do not die after axotomy, possibly because they do not lose their responsiveness to neurotrophic factors. In addition, several studies have shown that stimulation by a single trophic factor such as NGF or ciliary neurotrophic factor is sufficient to inhibit apoptosis in specific neuron populations of the PNS *in vitro* (46,47). Some PNS neurons may also synthesize their own trophic support, allowing them to remain functional in an autocrine fashion (48).

In the adult PNS, Schwann's cells, the myelin-forming cells of the PNS, survive after nerve axotomy and start to produce neurotrophic factors that strongly promote axonal growth (49,50). Recent studies by Xu et al. (51) have shown that injured CNS fiber tracts were able to regrow through a Schwann's cell–seeded minichannel implanted into a hemisected rat spinal cord. This suggests that the absence of Schwann's cells from the CNS may be one of the reasons that there is no suitable substrate provided for regrowth of CNS neurites. In addition, it is possible that trophic factor secretion by CNS glia (oligodendrocytes and astrocytes) may be regulated differently in the CNS. Immature astrocytes, for example, appear more effective than mature astrocytes in promoting optic nerve axon regrowth when grafted *in vivo* (52), indicating that with age, neurotrophic stimulation is retained in the PNS but is lost in the CNS.

Animal models of different types of brain insults, such as mechanical lesions, hypoxic-ischemic injury, or chemical-induced seizure, have shown that the expression of neurotrophic factors is dynamically regulated by neurons and glial cells (53,54). These changes may represent protective and regenerative mechanisms, and it is likely that neurotrophic factors have specific functions in responses to acute nervous system injury and chronic neurodegenerative diseases. With regard to therapeutic options to inhibit degenerative processes and stimulate regenerative events, neurotrophic factors have been extensively studied, including cell cultures, models for brain diseases, transgenic mice, and genetically modified cells. Thus, the rescuing effect of glial-cell-line–derived neurotrophic factor (GDNF) has been extensively studied using animal models of parkinsonism. Dopaminergic nigrostriatal impairment models such as the mouse methylphenyltetrahydropyridine, the 6-hydroxydopamine, and axotomy models demonstrated that GDNF increases striatal and nigral dopamine levels and protects dopaminergic neurons from degeneration (55,56). However, despite the strong neuroprotective effects of GDNF on nigrostriatal cells, no reports have indicated any significant reinnervation of the lesioned striatum or any signs of functional recovery. These results suggest that the survival-promoting effect alone is not sufficient for a regeneration of nigrostriatal cells, and that additional signals are required.

CONCLUSIONS

Undoubtedly, molecular requirements for axonal regeneration in the CNS are still largely enigmatic. Apparently, neutralization of more than just one axon-inhibitory molecule and application of probably more than a single neuron survival–promoting and axonal regrowth–promoting neurotrophic factor are necessary to make regeneration in the CNS occur. For more detailed insights into the molecular bases of neuron regeneration, it will be necessary to widely apply technologies such as molecular screening by gene chip for examining the effects of neurotrophic and axon-inhibitory molecules on neuronal and glial gene expression. Another important methodical attempt will be the use of genetically modified cells or unmodified progenitor cells that can be transplanted into degenerated brain areas. Moreover, conditional knockouts will help us understand physiological mechanisms underlying neuronal regrowth. Finally, the transfer of new knowledge to the clinic will be an important final step to let patients benefit from benchside advances.

REFERENCES

1. Argiro V, Johnson MI. Patterns and kinetics of neurite extension from sympathetic neurons in culture are age dependent. *J Neurosci* 1982;2:503–512.
2. Davies AM. Intrinsic differences in the growth rate of early nerve fibers related to target distance. *Nature* 1989;337:553–555.
3. David S, Aguayo AJ. Axonal elongation into peripheral nervous system "bridges" after central nervous system injury in adult rats. *Science* 1981;214:931–933.
4. Chen DF, Jhaveri S, Schneider GE. Intrinsic changes in developing retinal neurons result in regenerative failure of their axons. *Proc Natl Acad Sci USA* 1995;92: 7287–7291.
5. Lohof AM, Quillan M, Dan Y, et al. Asymmetric modulation of cytosolic cAMP activity induces growth cone turning. *J Neurosci* 1992;12:1253–1261.
6. Kim YT, Wu CF. Reduced growth cone motility in cultured neurons from *Drosophila* memory mutants with a defective cAMP cascade. *J Neurosci* 1996;16: 5593–5602.
7. Ming GL, Song HJ, Berninger B, et al. cAMP-dependent growth cone guidance by netrin-1. *Neuron* 1997; 19:1225–1235.
8. Song HJ, Ming GL, Poo MM. cAMP-induced switching in turning direction of nerve growth cones. *Nature* 1997;388:275–279.
9. Cai D, Shen Y, De Bellard M, et al. Prior exposure to neurotrophins blocks inhibition of axonal regeneration by MAG and myelin via a cAMP-dependent mechanism. *Neuron* 1999;22:89–101.
10. Goldberg JL, Xu Y, Davidson N, et al. Bcl-2 does not enhance the ability of retinal ganglion cells to extend axons *in vitro*. *Soc Neurosci* 1999;25:496.
11. Cai D, Qiu J, Cao Z, et al. Neuronal cyclic AMP controls the developmental loss in ability of axons to regenerate. *J Neurosci* 2001;21:4731–4739.
12. Chen DF, Schneider GE, Martinou JC, et al. Bcl-2 promotes regeneration of severed axons in mammalian CNS. *Nature* 1997;385:434–439.
13. Castren E, Ohga Y, Berzaghi MP, et al. Bcl-2 messenger RNA is localized in neurons of the developing and adult rat brain. *Neuroscience* 1994;61:165–177.
14. Merry DE, Korsmeyer SJ. Bcl-2 gene family in the nervous system. *Ann Rev Neurosci* 1997;20:245–267.
15. Keirstead HS, Hasan SJ, Muir GD, et al. Suppression of the onset of myelination extends the permissive period for the functional repair of embryonic spinal cord. *Proc Natl Acad Sci USA* 1992;89:11664–11668.
16. Qiu J, Cai D, Filbin MT. Glial inhibition of nerve regeneration in the mature mammalian CNS. *Glia* 2000; 29:166–174.
17. Rudge JS, Silver J. Inhibition of neurite outgrowth on astroglial scars *in vitro*. *J Neurosci* 1990;10:3594–3603.
18. McKeon RJ, Schreiber RC, Rudge JS, et al. Reduction of neurite outgrowth in a model of glial scarring following CNS injury is correlated with the expression of inhibitory molecules on reactive astrocytes. *J Neurosci* 1991;3398–3411.
19. Meiners S, Powell EM, Geller HM. A distinct subset of tenascin/CS-6-PG–rich astrocytes restricts neuronal growth *in vitro*. *J Neurosci* 1995;15:8096–8108.
20. Fitch MT, Silver J. Glial cell extracellular matrix: boundaries for axon growth in development and regeneration. *Cell Tissue Res* 1997;290:379–384.
21. Bovolenta P, Fernaud-Espinosa I, Mendez-Otero R, et al. Neurite outgrowth inhibitor of gliotic brain tissue. Mode of action and cellular localization, studied with specific monoclonal antibodies. *Eur J Neurosci* 1997;9: 977–989.
22. McKerracher L, David S, Jackson DL, et al. Identification of myelin-associated glycoprotein as a major myelin-derived inhibitor of neurite growth. *Neuron* 1994;13:805–811.
23. Mukhopadhyay G, Doherty P, Walsh FS, et al. A novel role for myelin-associated glycoprotein as an inhibitor of axonal regeneration. *Neuron* 1994;13:757–767.
24. Caroni P, Schwab ME. Antibody against myelin-associated inhibitor of neurite growth neutralizes nonpermissive substrate properties of CNS white matter. *Neuron* 1988;1:85–96.
25. Spillmann AA, Amberger VR, Schwab ME. High molecular weight protein of human central nervous system myelin inhibits neurite outgrowth: an effect which can be neutralized by the monoclonal antibody IN-1. *Eur J Neurosci* 1997;9:549–555.
26. Bandtlow CE, Schwab ME. NI-35/250/nogo-a: a neurite growth inhibitor restricting structural plasticity and regeneration of nerve fibers in the adult vertebrate CNS. *Glia* 2000;29:175–181.
27. Goldberg JL, Barres BA. Nogo in nerve regeneration. *Nature* 2000;403:369–370.
28. Chen MS, Huber AB, van der Haar ME, et al. Nogo-A is a myelin-associated neurite outgrowth inhibitor and an antigen for monoclonal antibody IN-1. *Nature* 2000; 403:434–439.
29. Niederost BP, Zimmermann DR, Schwab ME, et al. Bovine CNS myelin contains neurite growth-inhibitory activity associated with chondroitin sulfate proteoglycans. *J Neurosci* 1999;19:8979–8989.
30. Davies SJ, Fitch MT, Memberg SP, et al. Regeneration of adult axons in white matter tracts of the central nervous system. *Nature* 1997;390:680–683.
31. Schwab ME, Kampfhammer JP, Bandtlow CE. Inhibitors of neurite growth. *Ann Rev Neurosci* 1993;16: 565–595
32. Shen YJ, DeBellard ME, Salzer JL, et al. Myelin-associated glycoprotein in myelin and expressed by Schwann cells inhibits axonal regeneration and branching. *Mol Cell Neurosci* 1998;12:79–91.
33. Davies SJ, Goucher DR, Doller C, et al. Robust regeneration of adult sensory axons in degenerating white matter of the adult rat spinal cord. *J Neurosci* 1999;19: 5810–5822.

34. Neumann S, Woolf CJ. Regeneration of dorsal column fibers into and beyond the lesion site following adult spinal cord injury. *Neuron* 1999;23:83–91.
35. Shewan D, Berry M, Cohen J. Extensive regeneration *in vitro* by early embryonic neurons on immature and adult CNS tissue. *J Neurosci* 1995;15:2057–2062.
36. Turnley AM, Bartlett PF. MAG and MOG enhance neurite outgrowth of embryonic mouse spinal cord neurons. *NeuroReport* 1998;9:1987–1990.
37. Li Y, Raisman G. Long axon growth from embryonic neurons transplanted into myelinated tracts of the adult rat spinal cord. *Brain Res* 1993;629:115–127.
38. Davies SJ, Field PM, Raisman G. Long fibre growth of embryonic mouse hippocampal neurons microtransplanted into the adult rat fimbria. *Eur J Neurosci* 1993; 5:95–106.
39. Wictorin K, Björklund A. Axon outgrowth from grafts of human embryonic spinal cord in the lesioned adult rat spinal cord. *NeuroReport* 1992;3:1045–1048.
40. Wictorin K, Brundin P, Gustavii B, et al. Reformation of long axon pathways in adult rat central nervous system by human forebrain neuroblasts. *Nature* 1990;347: 556–558.
41. Goldberg JL, Barres BA. The relationship between neuronal survival and regeneration. *Ann Rev Neurosci* 2000;23:579–612.
42. Meyer-Franke A, Kaplan MR, Pfrieger FW, et al. Characterization of the signaling interactions that promote the survival and growth of developing retinal ganglion cells in culture. *Neuron* 1995;15:805–819.
43. Hefti F, ed. *Neurotrophic factors. Handbook of experimental pharmaceuticals,* 134th ed. Berlin, Heidelberg: Springer-Verlag, 1999.
44. Snider WD. Functions of the neurotrophins during nervous system development: what the knockouts are teaching us. *Cell* 1994;77:627–638.
45. Hanson MG Jr, Shen S, Wiemelt AP, et al. Cyclic AMP elevation is sufficient to promote the survival of spinal motor neurons *in vitro. J Neurosci* 1998;18: 7361–7371.
46. Hamburger V. The history of the discovery of the nerve growth factor. *J Neurobiol* 1993;24:893–897.
47. Barde YA. Neurotrophins: a family of proteins supporting the survival of neurons. *Prog Clin Biol Res* 1994; 390:45–56.
48. Acheson A, Conover JC, Fandl JP, et al. A BDNF autocrine loop in adult sensory neurons prevents cell death. *Nature* 1995;374:450–453
49. Bunge RP. Expanding roles for the Schwann cell: ensheathment, myelination, trophism and regeneration. *Curr Opin Neurobiol* 1993;3:805–809.
50. Son YJ, Thompson WJ. Schwann cell processes guide regeneration of peripheral axons. *Neuron* 1995;14:125–132.
51. Xu XM, Zhang SX, Li H, et al. Regrowth of axons into the distal spinal cord through a Schwann-cell–seeded mini-channel implanted into hemisected adult rat spinal cord. *Eur J Neurosci* 1999;11:1723–1740.
52. Sievers J, Bamberger C, Debus OM, et al. Regeneration in the optic nerve of adult rats: influences of cultured astrocytes and optic nerve grafts of different ontogenetic stages. *J Neurocytol* 1995;24:783–793.
53. Lindvall O, Kokaia Z, Bengzon J, et al. Neurotrophins and brain insults. *Trends Neurosci* 1994;17:490–496.
54. Isackson PJ. Trophic factor response to neuronal stimuli or injury. *Curr Opin Neurobiol* 1995;5:350–357.
55. Hoffer BJ, Hoffman A, Bowenkamp K, et al. Glial cell line–derived neurotrophic factor reverses toxin-induced injury to midbrain dopaminergic neurons *in vivo. Neurosci Lett* 1994;182:107–111.
56. Tomac A, et al. Protection and repair of the nigrostriatal dopaminergic system by GDNF *in vivo. Nature* 1995; 373:335–339.

Parkinson's Disease: Advances in Neurology, Vol. 91.
Edited by Ariel Gordin, Seppo Kaakkola, and Heikki Teräväinen
Lippincott Williams & Wilkins, Philadelphia © 2003

10

Estrogens and Aging

Marjo Tuppurainen and Seppo Saarikoski

Department of Obstetrics and Gynecology, Kuopio University Hospital, Kuopio; and Clinical Research Center, Bone and Cartilage Research Unit, University of Kuopio, Kuopio, Finland

Over the last hundred years, the average lifespan of women has increased dramatically (Table 10.1 and Fig. 10.1) (1), whereas the time of menopause, that is, the age at 1 year since last menstrual bleeding (2), has generally remained unchanged, being at the age of 51 years in most Western countries (3).

At menopause, the female endocrine picture changes dramatically. The ovary is the only endocrinological organ showing such a fast change during aging. Cyclical ovarian secretion of estradiol (17β-estradiol) disappears and estrogen deficiency appears as a result of physiological ovarian failure (4). The secretion of gonadotrophins, follicle-stimulating hormone, and luteinizing hormone increases massively because of the cessation of function of the estrogen feedback mechanism by inhibin in the hypothalamic-hypophyseal area (5). Before menopause, the ovaries produce more than 60% of the biologically active estrogen, estradiol, whereas the weaker estrogen, estrone, is derived from the metabolism of androstenedione by aromatization in peripheral tissues (6). After menopause, the estrone-to-estradiol ratio changes and adipose tissue becomes the main source of estrogen (6).

TABLE 10.1. *Estimated percentage of elderly (older than 65 yr)*

Yr	World	Europe	United States
1950	5.2	8.2	8.3
1975	5.6	11.4	10.5
2000	6.9	14.7	12.5
2025	10.4	21.0	18.8
2050	16.4	27.6	21.7

Source: United Nations Secretariat Department of Economic and Social Affairs Population Division. *World population prospects. The 1998 revision.* New York: United Nations, 1998. ESA/P/WP.150, with permission.

MENOPAUSAL SYMPTOMS

There is a wide distribution of organs containing receptors for estradiol, for example, skin, genitourinary organs, bone, and cardiovascular, gastrointestinal, and central nervous systems. Consequently, the clinical and metabolic scale of phenomena connected with aging and estrogen deficiency is multiple and varied (7). The most commonly encountered menopausal symptoms are hot flushes, which are experienced by 75% to 85% of Western women, but only 20% to 25% of women report symptoms as severe (8). These symptoms persist in 20% to 25% of women for more than 5 years (9). Estrogen deficiency leads to atrophy of the urogenital organs, seen, for example, in amenorrhea, shrinking of the myometrium, relaxation, and weakening of the pelvic floor, thinning of the vaginal and urethral epithelium, and urinary incontinence. Local genitourinary problems are seen in 70% to 85% of women after 4 to 5 years of ovarian failure if estrogen-replacement therapy (ERT)

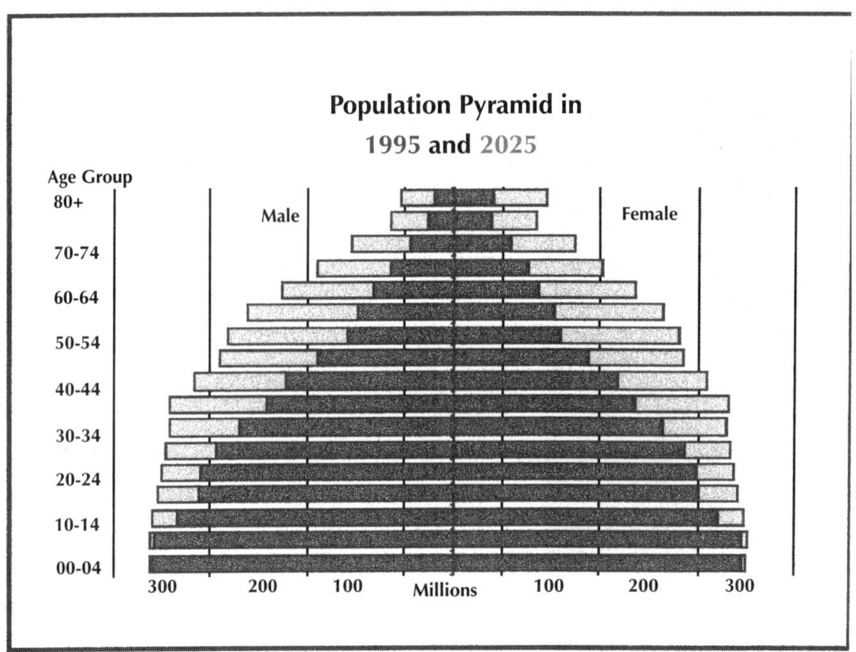

FIGURE 10.1. Prediction of world population. (From United Nations Secretariat Department of Economic and Social Affairs Population Division. *World population prospects. The 1998 revision.* New York: United Nations, 1998. ESA/P/WP.150, with permission.)

is not used (10). ERT is very effective against these symptoms.

Millions of postmenopausal women use hormone-replacement therapy (HRT), either unopposed or combined estrogen and progestin therapy. There is a wide variation in HRT use between different countries. The prevalence of HRT use has been reported to vary between 31% and 41% in Switzerland (11), 3% in Italy, and 25% in Germany (12). In the United States, the current use of HRT was 38% (13), as in the population-based Kuopio Osteoporosis Study, where the prevalence of current HRT use was 35% among 9,792 Finnish women aged 57.6 years (14).

Hormone-replacement Therapy and Cardiovascular Disease

The incidence of coronary heart disease (CHD) increases substantially after menopause, marking the end of the protective effect of endogenous estrogens against cardiovascular disease. CHD remains the leading cause of death in postmenopausal women around the world. Ovarian failure at menopause is associated with adverse effects on the walls of arterial vessels and the serum lipid profile. After menopause, total and low-density-lipoprotein (LDL) cholesterol levels increase, and high-density-lipoprotein cholesterol levels decrease. ERT reverses those changes (15,16). Estrogen also has a favorable action on the endothelial function such as the release of nitric oxide (17). Our studies show that the beneficial effect on serum lipids is also connected with the genotype apolipoprotein E4 (apoE4). Total cholesterol and LDL cholesterol levels responded more favorably to HRT in apoE4-negative women than in apoE4-positive women (18).

Results of randomized studies on ERT do not show such an unambiguous protective effect against CHD, although the beneficial metabolic changes brought about by ERT are well known (19). The Heart and Estrogen-Progestin Replacement Study (20) was a large randomized, controlled clinical trial designed to assess the effectiveness of HRT for secondary prevention of CHD among women with established CHD. In this study, the rate of subsequent CHD events was not lower for women using hormones. In addition, the Estrogen Replacement and Atherosclerosis (ERA) trial found no benefit from ERT or HRT in the progression of arteriosclerosis among postmenopausal women with angiographically documented coronary stenosis (21). The recent recommendation of the American Heart Association is that HRT should not be initiated for secondary prevention of CHD in postmenopausal women (22).

HRT may cause a transient increase in CHD risk among women with established heart disease, but not among healthy women. Several observational studies have looked at primary prevention—that is, the effect of HRT in women with no preexisting heart disease. In most meta-analyses, the reduction of the CHD events among HRT users is about 35% (23).

HRT and Stroke

Stroke remains the third leading cause of death after heart disease and cancer of women in most developed countries (24), leaving many survivors mentally and physically impaired. Stroke is the major cause of serious, long-term disability and the second leading cause of dementia after Alzheimer's disease (AD) (25). A recent thorough review (26) concludes that most studies suggest that HRT does not increase stroke risk. In addition, studies concerning fatal and nonfatal stroke reveal that estrogen may prevent the most lethal form of stroke or may improve stroke survival. Estrogen use has been associated with an 18% lower risk of mortality due to stroke (27).

HRT and Mortality

ERT is also associated with decreased mortality rates, and the risk of CHD in particular is clearly diminished. In a recent 12-year prospective study of 290,827 postmenopausal women (27), mortality from all causes was 18% lower among baseline estrogen users when compared with nonusers. The largest decrease in risk was against CHD (relative risk [RR], 0.66; 95% confidence interval [CI], 0.58–0.77) and other circulatory diseases (RR, 0.70; 95% CI, 0.74–0.89), particularly among the leanest women. The 34% lower risk of mortality due to CHD for baseline estrogen users found in that study (27) is similar to that observed in other previous studies (28–30). However, an important limitation of several observational studies of postmenopausal estrogens and mortality is that estrogen users typically have healthier lifestyles and a better cardiovascular profile than nonusers, which may explain, at least in part, the lower mortality rates for estrogen users (31,32).

HRT and Osteoporosis

Ovarian failure is closely related to the risk of osteoporosis. An accelerated phase of bone loss occurs during the 5-year period since menopause, being about 1% to 2% during the first years after menopause (33,34) and declining thereafter. Low bone density predicts bone fractures (35), particularly wrist, hip, and vertebral fractures. Early postmenopausal bone loss (36,37) and fractures (38) can be prevented with HRT. A recent meta-analysis concerning HRT and fractures found an overall 27% reduction in nonvertebral fractures, and for hip and wrist fractures, the effectiveness of HRT was greater, particularly for women younger than 60 years (39). In addition, HRT seems to have a beneficial effect on the balance maintenance system. In a study by Randell et al. (14), continuous use of HRT in early postmenopausal women (time since menopause is less than 5 years) was associated with a 30% decreased risk of nonslip-related falls.

ESTROGEN AND BRAIN

Estrogen receptors are found in several brain areas, for example, the hypothalamus and the preoptic area (40), and the hippocampi are rich of estrogen receptors (41).

The brain appears to be an important target organ for estrogen, leading to the assumption that estrogen might modify several cognitive and memory functions (42). The possible mechanisms of action are changes in cerebral blood flow; nerve growth factors; and many known effects on neurotransmitters including acetylcholine, monoamines, and γ-aminobutyric acid (43).

Advances in neuroscience have found correlations between estrogen and cognition (i.e., attention, learning, memory, language, constructive cognition, and judgment). The results of the effect of HRT on the cognitive function are still quite controversial. A recent thorough review and meta-analysis (44) concludes that women with clear menopausal symptoms showed improvements in verbal memory, vigilance, reasoning, and motor speed, but no change in other cognitive functions. In addition, ERT effectively improves sleep (45) but does not modify nocturnal breathing or periodic limb movement (46).

Estrogen is also related to several neurological diseases, particularly AD. The hippocampus, which has both α and β estrogen receptors (47), is particularly closely related with cognitive functions (48). AD primarily affects the hippocampus and destroys neurons and synaptic connections (49). Pathological characteristics of AD include neurofibrillary tangles and senile plaques (50).

The prevalence of AD among women is expected to double every 5 years after 65 years of age, reaching almost 50% at the age of 85 years (51). ERT has been suggested to be a protective factor against AD (52), but the mechanism underlying this phenomenon is unclear. One proposed explanation has been that the immune system modifies the effect of estrogen (53), as there have been suggestions that the immune system has a role in the development of AD (50). In addition, a recent meta-analysis (44) of observational studies suggested a 34% decreased risk of dementia among HRT users. However, some large studies (54,55) have suggested that ERT has no beneficial effects in secondary prevention or treatment of AD.

The role of estrogen in Parkinson's disease (PD) is highly disputed. However, Saunders-Pullman et al. (56) found a positive association between estrogen use and lower symptom severity in women with early PD not yet taking levodopa. These results indicate that estrogen therapy should not be avoided and may be beneficial in early PD, at least before the initiation of levodopa. A thorough review concerning PD and estrogen can be found in Chapter 11.

CONCLUSIONS

It is quite obvious that ERT is beneficial not only to treat climacteric symptoms, but also to the prevention of osteoporosis, fractures, and CHD in postmenopausal women. Minimizing climacteric symptoms improves the quality of life. Reduction of mortality and morbidity caused by CHD, osteoporosis, stroke, and AD may be achieved by the wide usage of estrogen in postmenopausal women. When considering the effects of estrogen in neurological diseases and conditions, we still have several open questions that remain to be answered.

Although scientific studies of the brain are in their infancy, numerous studies indicate that estrogen is essential to optimal brain function. The potential use of ERT to reduce the risk of AD and to ease the symptoms of PD may have a profound effect on women, their families, and society. Because of the controversy and the small sample sizes of prior studies, further investigations are needed. There is much work to be done to answer the many questions that remain regarding the effects of female hormones on women's health.

REFERENCES

1. United Nations Secretariat Department of Economic and Social Affairs Population Division. *World population prospects. The 1998 revision.* New York: United Nations, 1998. ESA/P/WP.150.
2. World Health Organization Scientific Group. *Research on the menopause in the 1990s.* Geneva, Switzerland: World Health Organization, 1996;866:1–107. Tech Report Series.

3. McKinlay SM, Brambilla BJ, Posner JG. The normal menopausal transition. *Maturitas* 1992;14:103–115.
4. Richardson SJ, Senikas V, Nelson JF. Follicular depletion during the menopausal transition: evidence for accelerated loss and ultimate exhaustion. *J Clin Endocrinol Metab* 1987;65:1231–1237.
5. Findlay JK, Xiao S, Shukovski L, et al. Novel peptides in ovarian physiology: inhibin, activin and follistatin. In: Adashi EY, Leung PCK, eds. *The Ovary*. New York: Raven Press, 1993:413–432.
6. Siiteri PK, MacDonald PC. Role of extraglandular estrogen in human endocrinology. In: Greep RO, Astwood E, eds. *Handbook of physiology: Endocrinology*, 2nd ed. Washington, DC: American Physiology Society, 1973:615–629.
7. Prior JC. Perimenopause: the complex endocrinology of the menopausal transition. *Endocr Rev* 1998;19:397–428.
8. Porter M, Penney GC, Russell D, et al. A population based survey of women's experience of the menopause. *Br J Obstet Gynaecol* 1996;103:1025–1028.
9. Huppert LC. Hormonal replacement therapy: benefits, risks, doses. *Med Clin North Am* 1987;71:23–39.
10. Cardozo L, Bachmann G, McClish D, et al. Meta-analysis of estrogen therapy in the management of urogenital atrophy in postmenopausal women: second report of the Hormones and Urogenital Therapy Committee. *Obstet Gynecol* 1998;92:722–727.
11. Schaad MA, Bonjour JP, Rizzoli R. Evaluation of hormone replacement therapy use by the sales figures. *Maturitas* 2000;34:185–191.
12. Oddens BJ, Boulet MJ, Lehert P, et al. Has the climacteric been medicalized? A study on the use of medication for climacteric complaints in four countries. *Maturitas* 1992;15:171–181.
13. Keating NL, Cleary RD, Rossi AS, et al. Use of hormone replacement therapy by postmenopausal women in the United States. *Ann Intern Med* 1999;130: 545–553.
14. Randell KM, Honkanen RJ, Komulainen MH, et al. Hormone replacement therapy and risk of falling in early postmenopausal women—a population-based study. *Clin Endocrinol* 2001;54:769–774.
15. Tuppurainen M, Heikkinen AM, Penttilä I, et al. Does vitamin D_3 have negative effects on serum levels of lipids? A follow-up study with a sequential combination of estradiol valerate and cyproterone acetate and/or vitamin D_3. *Maturitas* 1995; 22:55–61.
16. Godsland IF. Effects of postmenopausal hormone replacement therapy on lipid, lipoprotein, and apolipoprotein (a) concentrations: analysis of studies published from 1974–2000. *Fertil Steril* 2001;75:898–915.
17. Austin CE. Chronic and acute effects of oestrogens on vascular contractility. *J Hypertens* 2000;18:1365–1378.
18. Heikkinen AM, Niskanen L, Ryynänen M, et al. Is the response of serum lipids and lipoproteins to postmenopausal hormone replacement therapy modified by ApoE genotype? *Arterioscler Thromb Vasc Biol* 1999; 19:402–407.
19. Mendelsohn ME, Karas RH. The protective effects of estrogen on the cardiovascular system. *N Engl J Med* 1999;340:1801–1811.
20. Hulley S, Grady D, Bush T, et al. Randomized trial of estrogen plus progestin for secondary prevention of coronary heart disease in postmenopausal women. *JAMA* 1998;280:605–613.
21. Herrington DM, Reboussin DM, Brosnihan KB, et al. Effects of estrogen replacement on the progression of coronary-artery atherosclerosis. *N Engl J Med* 2000; 343:522–529.
22. Mosca L, Collins P, Herrington DM, et al. Hormone replacement therapy and cardiovascular disease: a statement for healthcare professionals from the American Heart Association. *Circulation* 2001;104:499–503.
23. Barrett-Connor E, Grady D. Hormone replacement therapy, heart disease, and other considerations. *Ann Rev Public Health* 1998;19:55–72.
24. World Health Organization. *The world health report*. Geneva: World Health Organization, 1998.
25. Skoog I, Nilsson L, Palmertz B, et al. A population-based study of dementia in 85-year olds. *N Engl J Med* 1993;328:153–158.
26. Paganini-Hill A. Hormone replacement therapy and stroke: risk, protection or no effect? *Maturitas* 2001;38: 243–261.
27. Rodriguez C, Calle EE, Patel AV, et al. Effect of body mass on the association between estrogen replacement therapy and mortality among elderly US women. *Am J Epidemiol* 2001;153:145–152.
28. Folsom AR, Mink PJ, Sellers TA, et al. Hormonal replacement therapy and morbidity and mortality in a prospective study of postmenopausal women. *Am J Public Health* 1995;85:1128–1132.
29. Schairer C, Lubin J, Troisi R, et al. Menopausal estrogen and estrogen-progestin replacement therapy and breast cancer risk. *JAMA* 2000;283:485–491.
30. Grodstein F, Stampfer MJ, Colditz GA, et al. Postmenopausal hormone therapy and mortality. *N Engl J Med* 1997;336:1769–1775.
31. Posthuma WF, Westendorp RG, Vandenbroucke JP. Cardioprotective effect of hormone replacement therapy in postmenopausal women: is the evidence biased? *Br Med J* 1994;308:1268–1269.
32. Matthews KA, Kuller LH, Wing RR, et al. Prior to use of estrogen replacement therapy, are users healthier than non-users? *Am J Epidemiol* 1996;143:971–978.
33. Kanis JA, Melton LJ, Christiansen C, et al. The diagnosis of osteoporosis. *J Bone Miner Res* 1994;9: 1137–1141.
34. Komulainen M, Tuppurainen MT, Kröger H, et al. Vitamin D and HRT: no benefit additional to that of HRT alone in prevention of bone loss in early postmenopausal women. A 2.5-year randomized placebo-controlled study. *Osteoporosis Int* 1997;7:126–132.
35. Kröger H, Tuppurainen M, Honkanen R, et al. Bone mineral density and risk factors for osteoporosis—a population-based study of 1600 perimenopausal women. *Calcif Tissue Int* 1994;55:1–7.
36. Lindsay R, Hart DM, Forrest C, et al. Prevention of spinal osteoporosis in oophorectomized women. *Lancet* 1980;2:1151–1154.
37. Komulainen M, Kröger H, Tuppurainen MT, et al. Prevention of femoral and lumbar bone loss with hormone replacement therapy and vitamin D_3 in early postmenopausal women: a population-based 5-year randomized trial. *J Clin Endocrinol Metab* 1999;84: 546–552.
38. Komulainen MH, Kröger H, Tuppurainen MT, et al. HRT and Vitamin D in prevention of non-vertebral fractures in postmenopausal women; a 5 year randomized trial. *Maturitas* 1998;31:45–54.

39. Torgerson D, Bell-Syer S. Hormone replacement therapy and prevention of non-vertebral fractures. A meta-analysis of randomized trials. *JAMA* 2001;285: 2891–2897.
40. Bixo M, Bäckström T, Winblad B, et al. Estradiol and testosterone in specific regions of the human female brain in different endocrine states. *J Steroid Biochem Mol Biol* 1995;55:297–303.
41. Reginster T, Shively C, Lewis C. Expression of estrogen receptor α and β transcripts in female monkey hippocampus and hypothalamus. *Brain Res* 1998;788: 320–322.
42. Shepherd JE. Effects of estrogen on cognition, mood, and degenerative brain diseases. *J Am Pharm Assoc (Washington)* 2001;41:221–228.
43. Di Paolo T. Modulation of brain dopamine transmission by sex steroids. *Rev Neurosci* 1994;5:27–41.
44. LeBlanc ES, Janowsky J, Chan BK, et al. Hormone replacement therapy and cognition: systematic review and meta-analysis. *JAMA* 2001;285:1489–1499.
45. Polo-Kantola P, Erkkola R, Irjala K, et al. Effect of short-term transdermal estrogen replacement therapy on sleep: a randomized, double-blind crossover trial in postmenopausal women. *Fertil Steril* 1999;71:873–880.
46. Polo-Kantola P, Rauhala E, Erkkola R, et al. Estrogen replacement therapy and nocturnal periodic limb movements: a randomized controlled trial. *Obstet Gynecol* 2001;97:548–554.
47. Pau CY, Pau KY, Spies HG. Putative estrogen receptor beta and alpha mRNA expression in male and female rhesus macaques. *Mol Cell Endocrinol* 1998;146: 59–68.
48. Pfaff DW. *Estrogen and brain function.* New York: Springer, 1980.
49. Silva I, Mor G, Naftolin F. Estrogen and the aging brain. *Maturitas* 2001;38:95–101.
50. Henderson VW. *Hormone therapy and the brain.* New York: Parthenon Publishing, 1999.
51. Evans DA. Estimated prevalence of Alzheimer's disease in the United States. *Milbank Q* 1990;68:267–289.
52. Waring SC, Rocca WA, Petersen RC, et al. Postmenopausal estrogen replacement therapy and risk of AD: a population-based study. *Neurology* 1999;52: 965–970.
53. Bechmann I, Mor G, Nilsen J, et al. FasL (CD95L, Apo1L) is expressed in the normal rat and human brain: evidence for the existence of an immunological brain barrier. *Glia* 1999;27:62–74.
54. Mulnard RA, Cotman CW, Kawas C, et al. for the Alzheimer's Disease Cooperative Study. Estrogen replacement therapy for treatment of mild to moderate Alzheimer disease. A randomized controlled trial. *JAMA* 2000;283:1007–1015.
55. Henderson VW, Paganini-Hill A, Miller BL, et al. Estrogen for Alzheimer's disease in women: randomized, double-blind, placebo-controlled trial. *Neurology* 2000; 54:295–301.
56. Saunders-Pullman R, Gordon-Elliott J, Parides M, et al. The effect of estrogen replacement on early Parkinson's disease. *Neurology* 1999;52:1417–1421.

Parkinson's Disease: Advances in Neurology, Vol. 91.
Edited by Ariel Gordin, Seppo Kaakkola, and Heikki Teräväinen
Lippincott Williams & Wilkins, Philadelphia © 2003

11

Estrogen and Parkinson's Disease

*Martin W. I. M. Horstink, *Elma Strijks, and †Dean E. Dluzen

**Department of Neurology, University Medical Centre, Nijmegen, The Netherlands; and †Department of Anatomy, Northeastern Ohio Universities, College of Medicine, Rootstown, Ohio*

Estrogens are steroid hormones derived from the precursor cholesterol. In the ovary, estrogens are produced, with the principal and most potent estrogen being 17β-estradiol (or simply, estradiol). In the testes, cholesterol is mainly converted to androgens, for example, testosterone, but small amounts of estradiol are also synthesized. Estrogens have effects on the nervous system that extend beyond the reproductive system, for example, the nigrostriatal dopaminergic system. Ovarian hormones are involved in cognition, dementia, and depression (1) (see Chapter 10). Although it is generally accepted that estrogens modulate the nigrostriatal system, the mechanisms of action are not fully understood, and results of experiments can be quite contradictory. Clinical evidence in patients with well-understood abnormalities in the dopaminergic system (i.e., Parkinson's disease [PD] and chorea) favors a dopaminergic action of estrogens. The discussion about the action of estrogens in PD is hampered by the fact that progesterone also modulates the nigrostriatal system. As far as animal experiments are concerned, we have focussed mainly on animal experiments in line with a dopaminergic action of estrogens. Estrogen receptors are found in brainstem dopaminergic neurons (2). However, many effects of estrogens on the nigrostriatal dopaminergic system are manifested in the absence of detectable classic estrogen receptors (3). A number of possible targets of estrogens have been found within the nigrostriatal dopaminergic system.

SYMPTOMATIC EFFECTS OF ESTROGENS

Pregnancy- and Contraceptive-induced Extrapyramidal Symptoms in Women

Contraceptives and pregnancy can induce chorea, a hyperdopaminergic phenomenon. It must be noted, however, that hormonal-induced chorea is only seldom seen in women, in spite of millions of pregnancies and users of contraceptives. Therefore, some kind of susceptibility to estrogens must be present in these women with chorea. Sydenham's chorea in childhood seems to confer a persistent hypersensitivity of dopaminergic activity (4). However, most reported patients with contraceptive-related chorea did not have Sydenham's chorea, so other causes of dopamine hypersensitivity to estrogens are probably involved (5–7). Some examples can include the following: moyamoya disease (8); antiphospholipid antibodies (9); lupus erythematosus (10,11); and Henoch–Schönlein purpura and congenital cyanotic heart disease (4). We do not know whether patients with chorea due to contraceptives are also predisposed to chorea gravidarum. The combination, however, is occasionally seen (12).

Influence of Menstrual Cycle and Exogenous Estrogens on Parkinson's Disease

Symptoms of PD can fluctuate with the menstrual cycle, which is thought by most authors to represent dopaminergic activity of estrogens. Estrogen levels show biphasic peaks, the first with ovulation and the second in the second half of the cycle. Before menstruation, the levels are at their nadir values. A premenstrual increase in parkinsonism is frequently seen (13,14), and patients with PD on levodopa therapy can experience worsening of parkinsonism after discontinuation of estrogens (15). We observed a young woman with PD demonstrating levodopa peak-dose and end-of-dose problems. Hyperkinesia increases at the preovulatory period, with a maximum in the ovulatory phase when estrogen levels are highest. Premenstrually, when estrogen levels are low, hyperkinesia clearly diminishes, whereas parkinsonism increases (Fig. 11.1). There are also reports that female patients with PD are more liable to have levodopa-induced dyskinesia than male patients (5,16). These observations suggest chorea with high levels and parkinsonism associated with low levels of estrogens—hence, a dopaminergic action of estrogens. However, data from two other reports question a dopaminergic effect of estrogens. Firstly, one report shows that parkinsonism increases in patients with PD treated with estrogen (17). Second, premenopausal women with PD demonstrated the expected biphasic estrogen peaks, but there was no significant correlation of severity of PD with serum levels of estrogens, although most women had a history of premenstrual worsening of PD (18).

There are four studies about the therapeutic effect of estrogen in PD. A retrospective analysis among 10,145 elderly female nursing home residents with PD, of which 195 received estrogen, found estrogen users to be more independent in activities of daily living, independent of age and cognitive impairment (19). In a placebo-controlled, randomized, double-blind trial, postmenopausal women with nonfluctuating PD and levodopa therapy took 2 mg of estradiol or placebo twice daily during 8 weeks. Although this dosage of estrogen is similar to the hormonal substitution therapy for postmenopausal complaints and postmenopausal osteoporosis, it should be noted that this dose produces lower serum levels than those observed in premenopausal women during the second half of their cycle. With this regimen, neither the Unified Parkin-

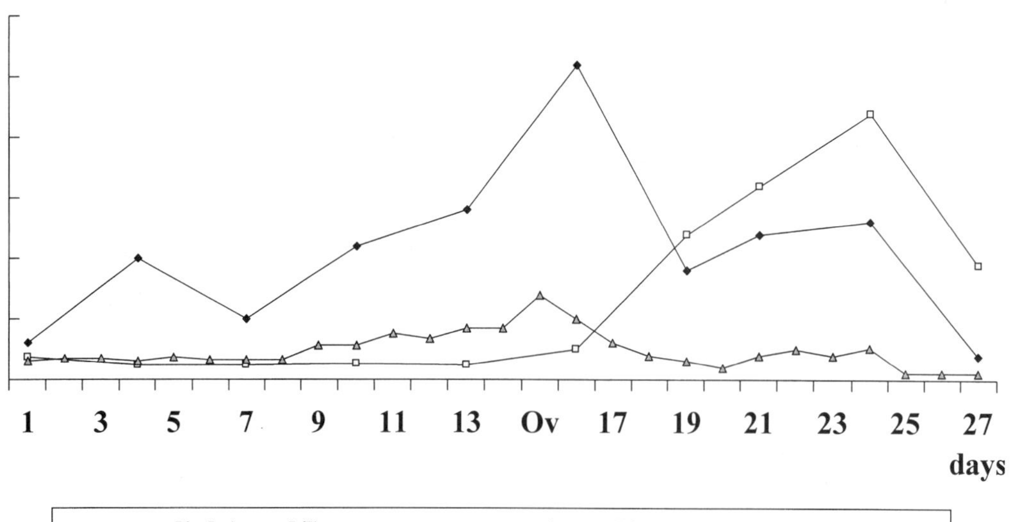

FIGURE 11.1. Female patient with Parkinson's disease and levodopa-induced hyperkinesia showing cycle-related changes in blood levels of estradiol and progesterone, as well as in the number of daily hours with levodopa-induced hyperkinesia. Hyperkinesia seems to fluctuate with levels of estrogen. (Ov, ovulation.)

son's Disease Rating Scale (UPDRS) motor examination part, nor subjective scores significantly improved with estrogen: UPDRS pretest scores, 10.57 ± 7.8; posttest scores, 13.14 ± 9.1 (mean ±SD) (20). And none of the patients with estrogen therapy reported any substantial improvement. Tsang et al. (21) administered estrogen or placebo during 8 weeks to a randomized group of patients with PD. Mean "on time" during waking hours significantly improved by 7% and mean "off time" by 4% in estrogen-treated patients. UPDRS part III scores (motor examination) improved by 3.5 ± 3.4 points. There was no improvement in UPDRS part II scores (activities of daily living), a timed tapping test, and the Hamilton Depression Scale. Blanchet et al. (22) examined women with fluctuating PD after 10 days of skin patches of estradiol or placebo. With this treatment, mean serum estradiol levels reached values as high as 24 times baseline. Estradiol significantly reduced the threshold dose necessary to provide antiparkinsonian efficacy with intravenously administered levodopa from 29 ± 4 mg to 21 ± 4 mg (p = .02).

The mean levodopa dose necessary to induce dyskinesias appeared to be somewhat lower (23 ± 5 mg) during estradiol treatment than with placebo (29 ± 5 mg), but the difference was not statistically significant (p = .17). Mean "on time" for placebo was 57% ± 2% of waking hours compared with 61% ± 4% with estradiol.

Dopaminergic Effects of Estrogen in Animal Experiments

Estrogens modulate dopamine activity in the nigrostriatal system (Fig. 11.2).

There are estrogen-dependent variations in basal extracellular concentration of striatal dopamine, in amphetamine-stimulated dopamine release, and in striatal dopamine-mediated behaviors (23). Most of these experiments are performed in ovariectomized female rats typically treated with the most potent estrogen, estradiol, or estradiol benzoate. Estrogens have the ability to increase dopamine concentrations by increasing tyrosine hydroxylase activity (24) and by decreasing dopamine breakdown. The possibility of estrogen-induced alterations in the function of

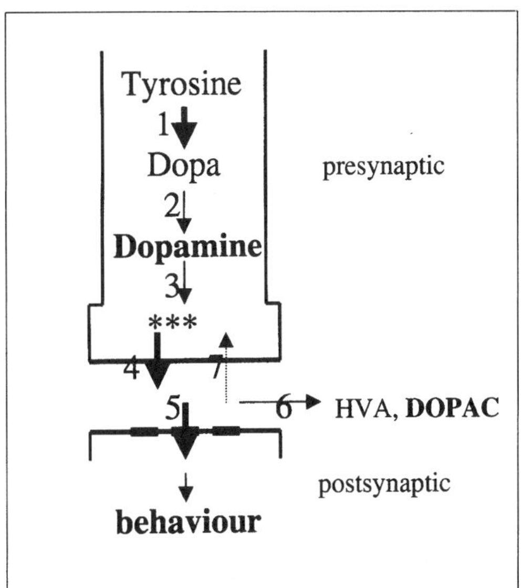

- 1 tyrosine hydroxylase
- 4 dopamine release
- 5 D2 receptors
- 6 MAO? COMT?
- 7 DAT
- behaviour (circling etc)

FIGURE 11.2. Left: Dopamine-related metabolism. Shown are (*enhanced names and arrows*) estrogen increases levels or activity and (*dotted arrow*) estrogen decreases activity. **Right:** Targets of estrogen. (HVA, homovanillic acid; DOPAC, 3,4-dihydroxyphenylacetic acid; DAT, dopamine transporter; *, presynaptic vesicles.)

monoamine oxidase (MAO) or catechol-*O*-methyltransferase (COMT) enzyme activity represents another potentially important modulatory action (25–27), but the limited data are not unequivocal and remain to be confirmed. Enhanced dopaminergic activity could also result from an increase in dopamine release, as shown by the fact that estrogens increase amphetamine-induced striatal dopamine release (28,29). Dopaminergic activity can also be enhanced by reducing the activity of dopamine reuptake by affecting the dopamine transporter (DAT). Ovariectomy in rats results in upregulation of DAT activity, an effect that is prevented by estradiol (30). Accordingly, the rate of dopamine uptake is significantly attenuated in steroid-treated animals (31). Estrogen has a similar effect on extracellular dopamine levels as the uptake blocker nomifensine, further suggesting that estradiol inhibits striatal dopamine uptake (32) and appears to exert this effect by decreasing the affinity of DAT for dopamine (33). Dopamine-mediated behavior can also be facilitated at the level of the dopamine receptor. Estrogens increase striatal dopamine D_2 receptor density and sensitivity, although the results are not fully uniform because both temporal and regional differences in D_2 findings are observed (34–37). Estrogens also modulate dopamine-mediated behavior. Female rats in estrus make more rotations than ovariectomized rats (23). Spontaneous locomotor activity decreases after ovariectomy, whereas estradiol reverses this effect (38), increases the number of rotations (35), and increases amphetamine-induced rotational behavior (37). Estrogen also potentiates the stereotypy induced by dopamine agonists in rats (39).

It must be noted, however, that the effects of estrogens (as mentioned) are not unequivocal. Many studies conclude that estrogens may have antidopaminergic effects (20,25, 40). For example, it has been reported that striatal D_2 receptors decrease after estrogen treatment (41), estrogen causes a downregulation of dopamine D_2 receptor messenger RNA in the striatum (38), and estrogen increases the density of DAT (42). In ovariectomized monkeys with midbrain lesions, which induce dopamine-sensitive dyskinesia, estrogen strongly reduces enhancement of dyskinesia by apomorphine (43). A similar antidopaminergic effect of estradiol on dyskinesia is seen in ovariectomized monkeys rendered parkinsonian by methylphenyltetrahydropyridine (MPTP). When the monkeys turn dyskinetic with levodopa, the dyskinesia reduces with estrogen (44).

A biphasic effect of estrogen could be one of the reasons that results may differ among studies. For example, administration of estrogen produces a significant reduction in the number of striatal dopaminergic receptors 10 hours after the last steroid injection, which is followed by an increase at 24 hours (45). Other factors that can account for the contradictory actions of estrogens are the age of the animals, confounding by progesterone, the dose, duration, and type of estrogen, the time interval between ovariectomy and administration of estrogen and the final measurement, and the method of measurements. Furthermore, the findings tested may originate from different loci within the nigrostriatal system or from different subpopulations of dopamine receptors.

ESTROGENS AND NEUROPROTECTION

Difference in Gender

In humans, there may exist some type of female resistance to parkinsonian neurodegeneration because many studies reveal a higher prevalence in men. Of 34 studies reviewed in which the gender of the patients was reported, 82% have a greater proportion of men (27). It must be noted, however, that studies relying on medical records are probably more biased than population-based surveys. Nevertheless, a number of formal epidemiological studies reveal a greater prevalence of PD in men (46–48). Swerdlow et al. (49) provide data from their patients and from seven other epidemiological studies, with a total of 1,835 patients and a male-to-female ratio of 1.5 : 1. However, a very large joint analysis comprising 18,506 subjects of seven community surveys in Europe yields no difference in prevalence between men (1.74%) and women (1.79%) (50). Furthermore, the segregation ratios of persons at risk in families with autosomal-dominant α-synuclein PD do not differ significantly (51–53). In these families, we counted 208 persons at risk: 120 men and 88 women. There were 88 patients with PD: 54 men and 34 women, yielding a segregation ratio for men of 45% and for women of 39% ($p = .23$; chi-square test). These segregation ratios suggest that men and women are equally at risk of acquiring α-synuclein PD. Finally, 101 patients with autosomal-recessive parkin gene parkinsonism also showed an equal number of male (N = 52) and female (N = 49) patients (54). So a male predominance in PD cannot be taken for certain.

In support of a gender difference in dopamine-modulating effect of estrogens is the impact of gender on the nigrostriatal system in experimental animals (55,56). Gender differences are also present in behavioral models, because amphetamine produces significantly fewer rotations in male versus female rats (57,58). Estrogens enhance amphetamine-stimulated release of dopamine in the striatum, but there is no effect in male rats (59). Methamphetamine and MPTP cause depletion in striatal dopamine levels, which are significantly greater in male than in female animals (27,60–62). Thus, in animals, there are sex differences in striatal dopamine and in the effect of estrogen on the striatal dopamine neurochemical and behavioral responses.

Clinical Evidence of Neuroprotection by Estrogens

Lyons et al. (16) reported that as PD progresses, gender differences emerge, with men exhibiting more severe parkinsonian motor features than women. Another study found that postmenopausal women with idiopathic PD, duration less than 5 years, not taking levodopa or agonists, who took estrogen at some point in the past had a lower UPDRS score (18.1 ± 10.8) than the group who had not taken estrogen (27.0 ± 15.1) (63). The earlier mentioned retrospective analysis among elderly female nursing home residents with PD, of which 195 received estrogen, found estrogen users to be more independent in activities of daily living (19). These studies could be interpreted as neuroprotection by estrogens, although a symptomatic effect cannot be ruled out. Furthermore, in a population-based community survey, postmenopausal estrogen use did not affect the risk of PD (64), and in another study (63), the age at onset was even lower by 5 years in women who had used estrogens. Both these latter facts do not support the hypothesis of estrogen neuroprotection in PD, so there is no firm unequivocal evidence of neuroprotection by estrogens in humans.

Neuroprotection in Animal Experiments

A more clear neuroprotective effect of estrogen on the nigrostriatal system is derived from animal experiments. As noted already, male animals show significantly greater reductions in striatal dopamine concentrations when treated with methamphetamine or MPTP than female animals. It is generally believed that MPTP acutely evokes dopamine release after uptake of its toxic metabolite 1-methyl-4-phenylpyridine (MPP^+) into terminals via the DAT and subsequently displaces dopamine from storage vesicles. Estrogens reduce the amount of dopamine depletion in the striatum after administration of methamphetamine, 6-hydroxydopamine, or MPTP (60–62,65–67). The combination of estrogen and the estrogen antagonist tamoxifen abolishes the striatal dopamine-sparing effect of estrogen on MPTP or methamphetamine toxicity (27,68). Estrogen inhibits dopamine uptake like that obtained with the uptake blocker nomifensine (32). These studies suggest that one means by which estrogen protects is by inhibiting DAT activity (27) and, hence, blocks the uptake of neurotoxins. Estrogen does not appear to be capable of restoring nigrostriatal dopaminergic neurons after methamphetamine-induced neurotoxicity (68). Unfortunately, there are no studies that examine a protective effect of estrogen on survival of dopaminergic neurons themselves, for example, with nigral cell counts. Callier et al. (69) used DAT levels as a measure of the integrity of nigral cells—an excellent method to diagnose PD in humans with CIT single-photon emission computed tomography (70)—and concluded that estrogen does not protect against MPTP-induced loss of dopamine terminals because DAT levels are extensively decreased in MPTP mice, in animals treated with either estrogen or placebo. However, if estrogen indeed inhibits DAT, as discussed already, the results probably indicate that MPTP destroys nigral cells, resulting in the loss of DAT and dopamine. But if estrogen is neuroprotective by reducing DAT activity, estrogen probably reduces DAT activity. Consequently, the cell and dopamine levels would be protected by estrogen because MPP^+ would not be taken up into nigral cells. The fact that striatal dopamine levels remained within the normal reference range in the estrogen-protected MPTP animals, whereas they are decreased in the nonprotected placebo group, is in favor of an estrogen-protection hypothesis. Whether neuroprotection via blocking of DAT-mediated uptake mechanisms into the nigral cells can be clinically related remains to be determined. Use of pesticides or herbicides and residency in rural areas are risk factors for PD (71). Moreover, it has been suggested that increased dopamine uptake through the DAT may contribute to PD resulting from intracellular dopamine metabolism, leading to oxidative stress and mitochondrial damage (72). In this regard, an estrogen-dependent inhibition of DAT function would diminish not only uptake of potential exogenous neurotoxins, but also excessive amounts of dopamine, which can produce nigrostriatal dopaminergic neurodegeneration. However, although such a mechanism represents an intriguing possibility, there are no firm arguments that the vast majority of PD is caused by exogenous or endogenous toxins. A major problem in discussing neuroprotection is that the exact cause of PD remains elusive. Recently, particular attention has focused on several conceptually distinct mechanisms such as genetics, oxidative stress, mitochondrial dysfunction, excitotoxicity, and apoptosis (73). Estrogens can act on a number of these conceptual domains. For example, estrogens could provide neuroprotection by reducing apoptosis (74) and oxidative stress (75).

CONCLUSIONS

Most studies with hormonal chorea or trials in PD suggest that estrogen exerts dopaminergic activity, although the measured effects are moderate. Remarkably, in clinical trials a dopaminergic effect is mainly shown in patients with fluctuating PD. Therefore, it is not unlikely that estrogen exerts a dopaminergic effect, mainly in patients with supersensitive dopamine receptors, which may be in accordance with the hypothesis of supersensitive dopamine receptors in hormonal chorea in women.

Neuroprotection-supporting arguments for estrogen on the nigrostriatal dopaminergic system, as derived from animal experiments, are much more easier to find than actual proof in patients with PD. However, the extension of these findings from animal models to clinical conditions remains open to discussion. The most convincing, but indirect, clinical support comes from studies concluding that PD is more prevalent in men than in women.

REFERENCES

1. Birge SJ. The role of ovarian hormones in cognition and dementia. *Neurology* 1997;48[Suppl 7]:S1–S41.
2. Heritage AS, Stumpf WQE, Sar M, et al. Brainstem catecholamine neurons are target sites for sex steroid hormones. *Science* 1980;207:1377–1380.
3. Di Paolo T. Modulation of brain dopamine transmission by sex steroids. *Rev Neurosci* 1994;5:27–42.
4. Nausieda PA, Koller WC, Weiner WJ, et al. Chorea induced by oral contraceptives. *Neurology* 1979;29: 1605–1609.
5. Nausieda PA, Bieliauskas LA, Bacon LD, et al. Chronic dopaminergic sensitivity after Sydenham's chorea. *Neurology* 1983;33:750–754.
6. Schipper HM. Neurology of sex steroids and oral contraceptives. *Neurol Clin* 1986;4:721–751.

7. Leys D, Destee A, Petit H, et al. Chorea associated with oral contraception. *J Neurol* 1987;235:46–48.
8. Pelletier J, Cabanot C, Levrier O, et al. Angiodysplasie de type Moya-Moya revelee par des mouvements anormaux involontaires choreiformes au cours d'une contraception orale. A propos de 2 cas. *Rev Neurol* 1997;153: 393–397.
9. Omdal R, Roalso S. Chorea gravidarum and chorea associated with oral contraceptives-diseases due to antiphospholipid antibodies? *Acta Neurol Scand* 1992;86: 219–220.
10. Mathur AK, Gatter RA. Chorea as the initial presentation of oral contraceptive induced systemic lupus erythematosus. *J Rheumatol* 1988;15:1042–1043.
11. Iskander MK, Khan M. Chorea as the initial presentation of oral contraceptive related systemic lupus erythematosus. *J Rheumatol* 1989;16:850–851.
12. Asherson RA, Gibson DG, Evans DW, et al. Diagnostic and therapeutic problems in two patients with antiphospholipid antibodies, heart valve lesions, and transient ischaemic attacks. *Ann Rheum Dis* 1988;47:947–953.
13. Quinn NP, Marsden CD. Menstrual-related fluctuations in Parkinson's disease. *Mov Disord* 1986;1:85–87.
14. Sandyk R. Estrogens and the pathophysiology of Parkinson's disease. *J Neurosci* 1989;45:119–122.
15. Shibayama H, Sato S, Sakata S, et al. Females are more liable to levodopa-induced dyskinesia in Parkinson's disease. *Parkinsonism Related Disord* 2001;7[Suppl]: S101.
16. Lyons KE, Hubble JP, Troster AI, et al. Gender differences in Parkinson's disease. *Clin Neuropharmacol* 1998;21:118–121.
17. Koller WC, Barr A, Biary N. Estrogen treatment of dyskinetic disorders. *Neurology* 1982;32:547–549.
18. Kompoliti K, Comella CL, Jaglin CA, et al. Menstrual-related changes in motoric function in women with Parkinson's disease. *Neurology* 2000;55:1572–1574.
19. Fernandez HH, Lapane KL. Estrogen use among nursing home residents with a diagnosis of Parkinson's disease. *Mov Disord* 2000;15:1119–1124.
20. Strijks E, Kremer JA, Horstink MW. Effects of female sex steroids on Parkinson's disease in postmenopausal women. *Clin Neuropharmacol* 1999;22:93–97.
21. Tsang KL, Ho SL, Lo SK. Estrogen improves motor disability in parkinsonian postmenopausal women with motor fluctuations. *Neurology* 2000;54:2292–2298.
22. Blanchet PJ, Fang J, Hyland K, et al. Short-term effects of high-dose 17 beta-estradiol in postmenopausal PD patients: a crossover study. *Neurology* 1999;53:91–95.
23. Becker JB. Gender differences in dopaminergic function in striatum and nucleus accumbens. *Pharmacol Biochem Behav* 1999;64:803–812.
24. Pasqualini C, Olivier V, Guibert B, et al. Acute stimulatory effect of estradiol on striatal dopamine synthesis. *J Neurochem* 1995;65:1651–1657.
25. Kompoliti K. Estrogen and movement disorders. *Clin Neuropharmacol* 1999;22:318–326.
26. Xie T, Ho SL, Ramsden D. Characterization and implications of estrogenic down-regulation of human catechol-*O*-methyltransferase gene transcription. *Mol Pharmacol* 1999;56:31–38.
27. Dluzen DE. Neuroprotective effects of estrogen upon the nigrostriatal dopaminergic system. *J Neurocytol* 2000;29:387–399.
28. Ohtani H, Nomoto M, Douchi T. Chronic estrogen treatment replaces striatal dopaminergic function in ovariectomized rats. *Brain Res* 2000;900:163–168.
29. Xiao L, Becker JB. Effects of estrogen agonists on amphetamine-stimulated striatal dopamine release. *Synapse* 1998;29:379–391.
30. Attali G, Weizman A, Gil-Ad I, et al. Opposite modulatory effects of ovarian hormones on rat brain dopamine and serotonin transporters. *Brain Res* 1997;756: 153–159.
31. Thompson TL. Attenuation of dopamine uptake *in vivo* following priming with estradiol benzoate. *Brain Res* 1999;10:164–167.
32. Disshon KA, Dluzen DE. Use of *in vitro* superfusion to assess the dynamics of striatal dopamine clearance: influence of estrogen. *Brain Res* 1999;842:399–407.
33. Disshon KA, Boja JW, Dluzen DE. Inhibition of striatal dopamine transporter activity by 17 beta-estradiol. *Eur J Pharmacol* 1998;345:207–211.
34. Levesque D, Di Paolo T. Modulation by estradiol and progesterone of the GTP effect on striatal D-2 dopamine receptors. *Biochem Pharmacol* 1993;45: 723–733.
35. Roy EJ, Buyer DR, Licari VA. Estradiol in the striatum: effects on behavior and dopamine receptors but no evidence for membrane steroid receptors. *Brain Res Bull* 1990;25:221–227.
36. Hruska RE, Ludmer LM, Pitman KT, et al. Effects of estrogen on striatal dopamine receptor function in male and female rats. *Pharmacol Biochem Behav* 1982;16: 285–291.
37. Rajakumar G, Chiu P, Chiu S, et al. 17 beta estradiol–induced increase in brain dopamine D-2 receptor: antagonism by MIF-1. *Peptides* 1987;8:997–1002.
38. Lammers CH, D'Souza U, Qin ZH, et al. Regulation of striatal dopamine receptors by estrogen. *Synapse* 1999; 34:222–227.
39. Chiodo LA, Caggiula AR, Saller CF. Estrogen potentiates the stereotypy induced by dopamine agonists in the rat. *Life Sci* 1981;28:827–835.
40. Van Harteveld C, Joyce JN. Effect of estrogen on the basal ganglia. *Neurosci Biobehav Rev* 1986;10:1–144.
41. Bazzett TJ, Becker JB. Sex differences in the rapid and acute effects of estrogen on striatal D_2 dopamine receptor binding. *Brain Res* 1994;637:163–172.
42. Morisette M, Di Paolo T. Effect of chronic estradiol and progesterone treatments of ovariectomized rats on brain dopamine uptake sites. *J Neurochem* 1993;60: 1876–1993.
43. Bedard P, Boucher R, Di Paolo T, et al. Interaction between estradiol, prolactin, and striatal dopaminergic mechanisms. *Adv Neurol* 1984;40:489–496.
44. Gomez-Mancilla B, Bedard PJ. Effect of estrogen and progesterone on L-DOPA induced dyskinesia in MPTP-treated monkeys. *Neurosci Lett* 1992;135:129–132.
45. Fernandez-Ruiz JJ, Amor JC, Ramos JA. Time-dependent effects of estradiol and progesterone on the number of striatal dopaminergic D_2-receptors. *Brain Res* 1989; 476:388–395.
46. Baldereschi M, Di Carlo A, Rocca WA, et al. Parkinson's disease and parkinsonism in a longitudinal study: two-fold higher incidence in men. ILSA Working Group. Italian Longitudinal Study on Aging. *Neurology* 2000;55:1358–1363.
47. Bower JH, Maraganore DM, McDonnell SK, et al. Influence of strict, intermediate, and broad diagnostic cri-

teria on the age- and sex-specific incidence of Parkinson's disease. *Mov Disord* 2000;15:819–825.
48. Kuopio AM, Marttila RJ, Helenius H, et al. Changing epidemiology of Parkinson's disease in southwestern Finland. *Neurology* 1999;52:302–308.
49. Swerdlow RH, Parker WD, Currie LJ, et al. Gender ratio differences between Parkinson's disease patients and their affected relatives. *Parkinsonism Related Disord* 2001;7:129–133.
50. de Rijk MC, Launer LJ, Berger K, et al. Prevalence of Parkinson's disease in Europe: a collaborative study of population-based cohorts. *Neurology* 2000;54[Suppl 5]: S21–S23.
51. Golbe LI, Di-Iorio G, Sanges G, et al. Clinical genetic analysis of Parkinson's disease in the Contursi kindred. *Ann Neurol* 1996;40:767–775.
52. Samii A, Markopoulou K, Wszolek ZK, et al. PET studies of parkinsonism associated with mutation in the alpha-synuclein gene. *Neurology* 1999;53:2097–2102.
53. Papadimitriou A, Veletza V, Hadjigeorgiou GM, et al. Mutated alpha-synuclein gene in two Greek kindreds with familial PD: incomplete penetrance? *Neurology* 1999;52:651–654.
54. Lucking CB, Durr A, Bonifati V, et al. A. Association between early-onset Parkinson's disease and mutations in the parkin gene. French Parkinson's Disease Genetics Study Group. *N Engl J Med* 2000;342:1560–1567.
55. Xiao L, Becker JB. Quantitative microdialysis determination of extracellular striatal dopamine concentration in male and female rats: effects of estrous cycle and gonadectomy. *Neurosci Lett* 1994;180:155–158.
56. McDermott JL, Liu B, Dluzen DE. Sex differences and effects of estrogen on dopamine and DOPAC release from the striatum of male and female CD^{-1} mice. *Exp Neurol* 1994;125:306–311.
57. Becker J-B, Robinson TE, Lorenz KA. Sex differences and estrous cycle variations in amphetamine-elicited rotational behavior. *Eur J Pharmacol* 1982;80:65–72.
58. Becker JB. Direct effect of 17 beta-estradiol on striatum: sex differences in dopamine release. *Synapse* 1990;5:157–164.
59. Castner SA, Xiao L, Becker JB. Sex differences in striatal dopamine: *in vivo* microdialysis and behavioral studies. *Brain Res* 1993;610:127–134.
60. Wagner GC, Tekirian TL, Cheo CT. Sexual differences in sensitivity to methamphetamine toxicity. *J Neural Transm Gen Sect* 1993;93:67–70.
61. Disshon KA, Dluzen DE. Estrogen reduces acute striatal dopamine responses *in vivo* to the neurotoxin MPP^+ in female, but not male rats. *Brain Res* 2000;868:95–104.
62. Miller DB, Ali SF, O'Callaghan JP, et al. The impact of gender and estrogen on striatal dopaminergic neurotoxicity. *Ann N Y Acad Sci* 1998;844:153–165.
63. Saunders-Pullman R, Gordon-Elliott J, Parides M, et al. The effect of estrogen replacement therapy on early Parkinson's disease. *Neurology* 1999;52:1417–1421.
64. Marder K, Tang MX, Alfaro B, et al. Postmenopausal estrogen use and Parkinson's disease with and without dementia. *Neurology* 1998;50:1141–1143.
65. Grandbois M, Morissette M, Callier S, et al. Ovarian steroids and raloxifene prevent MPTP-induced dopamine depletion in mice. *Neuroreport* 2000;11: 343–346.
66. Callier S, Morissette M, Grandbois M, et al. Neuroprotective properties of 17 beta-estradiol, progesterone, and raloxifene in MPTP C57Bl/6 mice. *Synapse* 2001; 41:131–138.
67. Dluzen D. Estrogen decreases corpus striatal neurotoxicity in response to 6-hydroxydopamine. *Brain Res* 1997;767:340–344.
68. Gao X, Dluzen DE. Tamoxifen abolishes estrogen's neuroprotective effect upon methamphetamine neurotoxicity of the nigrostriatal dopaminergic system. *Neuroscience* 2001;103:385–394.
69. Callier S, Morissette M, Grandbois M, et al. Stereospecific prevention by 17 beta-estradiol of MPTP-induced dopamine depletion in mice. *Synapse* 2000;37: 245–251.
70. Benamer TS, Patterson J, Grosset DG, et al. Accurate differentiation of parkinsonism and essential tremor using visual assessment of $[^{123}I]$-FP-CIT SPECT imaging: the $[^{123}I]$-FP-CIT study group. *Mov Disord* 2000;15: 503–510.
71. Veldman BA, Wijn AM, Knoers N, et al. Genetic and environmental risk factors in Parkinson's disease. *Clin Neurol Neurosurg* 1998;100:15–26.
72. Lee FJS, Liu F, Pristupa ZB, et al. Direct binding and functional coupling of α-synuclein to the dopamine transporters accelerate dopamine-induced apoptosis. *FASEB J* 2001;15:916–923.
73. Dunnett SB, Björklund A. Prospects for new restorative and neuroprotective treatments in Parkinson's disease. *Nature* 1999;399[Suppl]:A32–A39.
74. Sawada H, Ibi M, Kihara T, et al. Mechanisms of antiapoptotic effects of estrogens in nigral dopaminergic neurons. *FASEB J* 2000;14:1202–1214.
75. Sawada H, Ibi M, Kihara T, et al. Estradiol protects mesencephalic dopaminergic neurons from oxidative stress-induced neuronal death. *J Neurosci Res* 1998;54: 707–719.

Parkinson's Disease: Advances in Neurology, Vol. 91.
Edited by Ariel Gordin, Seppo Kaakkola,
and Heikki Teräväinen
Lippincott Williams & Wilkins, Philadelphia © 2003

12

Validating a Quality-of-Life Scale in Caregivers of Patients with Parkinson's Disease: Parkinson's Impact Scale (PIMS)

*Susan M. Calne, *Edwin Mak, †Jeanne Hall, †Marie-Jose Fortin, ‡Pamela King, ‡Germaine McInnes, ¶Linda Grantier, ¶Sherree Trecartin, and §Michael Schulzer

**Pacific Parkinson's Research Centre, University of British Columbia, Vancouver, Canada; †McGill Centre for Studies in Ageing, Montreal, Quebec, Canada; ‡Movement Disorders Clinic Glenrose Rehabiliation Hospital, Edmonton, Alberta, Canada; ¶Movement Disorders Clinic, Health Sciences Centre London, Ontario, Canada; §Victorian Order of Nurses, Saint John's, New Brunswick, Canada*

Quality of life (QoL) is difficult to define. In his book *Coping with Chronic Illness: Overcoming Powerlessness,* Miller (1) provides a working definition that we have chosen to use: QoL is a concept that "contains no consistent or universal meaning other than a general construct: to maximize satisfaction by living life to its fullest and functioning to the optimum of one's capability in all stages of life."

With appropriate symptomatic treatment, patients with Parkinson's disease (PD) may live a normal life span (2). After about 7 to 10 years, increasing disability and greater susceptibility to drug side effects leads these patients to require increasing amounts of physical and emotional support from a spouse, partner, or adult child. This need can last for 10 to 20 years in some cases, a longer period than for a patient with Alzheimer's disease (4.5 years) (3) and in many cases Huntington's disease (13.5 years) (4). Thus, a spouse, partner, or adult child may be providing some level of care over a very long period of time. Health-care providers do not always take into account the fact that a "caregiver" is rarely a trained nurse, usually fairly close in age to the patient, and may have his or her own health problems (5).

Although remaining at home is preferable, many patients with PD are eventually sufficiently disabled to need full-time nursing care in a facility. Sometimes this is not available, practical, or affordable, and the caregiver becomes a nurse working 24-hour shifts with little or no respite. The emotional and physical health of these caregivers is vital to the well-being and successful management of patients with PD. Health-care professionals caring for patients with PD need to consider the health of the primary caregiver when making treatment or lifestyle recommendations (5).

In the last 5 years, the QoL in PD has been measured using specifically designed scales (6–8). A major reason for measuring QoL is to assess the outcome of clinical trials and medical, surgical, and nursing treatment, because the importance of measuring the patient's subjective feelings, as well as the objective scores of disability, is now well recognized. Pharmaceutical companies routinely include the measurement of QoL in clinical trials to measure economic variables. Other reasons for measuring QoL are that level of disability and symptom relief are not the only factors affecting a patient's response to a chronic illness. Schrag et al. (9) have shown that other factors such as depression have a major influence on QoL in PD. Somatic symptoms of depression in the less severely affected patient with PD do not correlate with symptoms (10); it is when the illness is more advanced that a patient's mood disturbance more closely reflects the level of disability (11).

Over the last 5 years, the Parkinson's Impact Scale (PIMS) has been used in clinical trials and clinics (6). PIMS has been described elsewhere, but it includes 10 items inquiring into 10 areas of life: self-positive, self-negative, family, community, work, travel, leisure, safety, financial security, and sexuality. The rating scale fits onto one side of an 8- by 11-inch piece of paper, can be completed in less than 10 minutes, and takes fluctuations in symptoms ("on-off") into account. Guidelines for the definition of each item are provided. The scale includes two items not addressed by either Parkinson's Diseases Questionnaire-39 (PDQ-39) or Parkinson's Disease Quality of Life (PDQL) scales: financial security and sexuality, both of which are of the utmost importance in most people's lives. High item scores indicate a problem in a given area and can be used to determine the need for referral to the appropriate health-care department.

For psychometric purposes, item scores are assigned weights, so a global score can be derived with a simple calculator. The PIMS score correlates well with the Unified Parkinson's Disease Rating Scale (UPDRS) section II (activities of daily living) and section III (motor score), is sensitive, and is responsive to change over time (Schulzer et al., in press).

The impact of PD on caregivers has been examined, surveyed, and reported quite extensively, both qualitatively and by using various generic instruments, with similar results (12–16). In 1998, Glozman et al. (17) proposed a four-item scale for PD caregivers, but there is no evidence that it has been tested. The nurses who designed, tested, and published the PIMS (6) always felt that the instrument was flexible enough to be used in other settings and decided to test its reliability and validity in measuring the impact of PD on caregivers or partners of patients with PD.

METHODS

Subjects

The caregiver was defined as the primary person living at home full time with a patient with PD (partner or adult child). Caregivers had to be able to complete the scale without help, and they had to be fluent in either English or French. There were 110 female partners, 24 male partners, and 1 female adult child. Mean age of caregivers was 63.2 years (SD 10.8), mean duration of relationship was 35.6 years (SD 13.2), and mean duration of disease was 8.4 years (SD 5.6). The study was approved by the University Ethical Committees, and all subjects gave informed consent.

Recruitment

Five centers associated with the Parkinson Society Canada Clinical Assistance and Outreach Nursing Programs participated and recruited 97 English speaking and 38 French speaking subjects. Four centers were university-based movement disorder clinics staffed by neurologists with subspecialty training in movement disorders. The one outreach program nurse worked with the Victorian Order of Nurses, providing home visits to patients diagnosed with PD. Four of the centers had participated in the previous validity and reliability study (6).

Design

To assess the rating scale, the nurse in each of the five participating centers recruited between 10 and 38 subjects who spoke either English or French fluently and who were capable of giving informed consent. Subjects were recruited during a clinic visit with their partner with PD, or they responded to printed notices displayed in clinic waiting rooms. Subjects were informed that the study was to test the reliability and validity of the scale and it would not address specifically the impact of their partner's PD on their lives. Confidentiality was maintained by assigning blocks of identification numbers (IDs) to each center to use for their subjects, for the purposes of statistical analysis. Subjects provided their age, sex, years married (or together), and how long their patients had suffered from PD. Using either the English or the French language rating scale, subjects completed a baseline observation and were then asked to fill out the rating scale once a month on approximately the same date for 3 consecutive months. Subjects were asked to mail each scale as it was completed, and stamped addressed return envelopes were provided. We did not want subjects to refer to scores on earlier forms, to control for learning and memory bias. Subjects assigned a score to each question in column 1 (Table 1) if their partner's symptoms were stable over time (nonfluctuators). Subjects whose partners were experiencing random fluctuations (fluctuators) could assign scores to two other columns, 2a "best" ("on") and 2b "worst" ("off"). If a change in the patient's state from best to worst did not affect the caregiver's response to an item, then he or she assigned the same score to "best" and "worst."

Statistics

Total PIMS scores were analyzed for homogeneity across the five centres by means of analysis of variance. T-tests were used to compare total scores for respondents of age ≤ 65 vs. those of age > 65 and to compare total scores in females vs. males. An overall three-way analysis of variance was applied to analyze total scores simultaneously with respect to centre, age, gender, and their various interactions.

A. Individual item scores, each ranging from 0 to 4, were also analyzed across centers, ages, and genders by means of chi-square tests. Significant results were localized by means of standardized residual analyses. All the above analyses were carried out for caregivers who filled out column 1 (nonfluctuators) and for those who addressed columns 2a and 2b (fluctuators).
B. Test-retest reliability was evaluated by analyzing the total scores on the monthly (2–4) measurement occasions by means of repeated measures analyses of variance and by calculating the intraclass correlation coefficients of reliability (18). We also derived confidence intervals (CIs) for the reliability coefficients (19). Construct validity was established by examining the relationship between the total PIMS score and the corresponding length of time since diagnosis, by means of correlation analysis. The length of time since diagnosis represented an external, indirect measure of disease severity.
C. Factor analysis was performed to investigate the dimensions underlying the QoL instrument in caregivers of patients with PD. Both orthogonal (varimax) and oblique (Dquart) rotations were examined. The Cronbach α was calculated to assess the degree of internal consistency—that is, reliability in the responses to the various items in the questionnaire.
D. The sensitivity of the instrument to different levels of disease severity was analyzed by comparing the total PIMS scores for caregivers of nonfluctuators (column 1) to those of fluctuators at different stages of disease (column 2a and column 2b) by means of two-sample *t*-tests.
E. The responsiveness of the instrument to change in the caregivers' QoL, associated with change in the condition of the patients, as reflected in column 2a versus 2b, was analyzed by comparing the total scores in column 2a with those in column 2b by means of paired *t*-tests.
F. To support the results of the these analyses, all parametric tests were also reanalyzed by corresponding standard nonparametric methods.

RESULTS

The study was well received by the caregivers. One patient was hospitalized and died

TABLE 1. *Parkinson's Impact Scale (PIMS)*

- Please indicate by a number (0–4) what impact Parkinsonism has had on your life.
  0= no change, 1= slight, 2= moderate, 3= moderately severe, 4= severe.
- Use the definitions below to help you measure impact.

Self: (Positive)	*Refers to how positive you feel about yourself (self-worth, happiness, optimism)*
Self: (Negative)	*Refers how negative you feel about yourself (level of stress, anxiety or depression)*
Family Relationships:	*Refers to your spouse, partner, children and relatives that you consider part of your immediate family*
Community Relationships:	*Refers to your neighbours, friends, people you work with and those who provide you with services (store clerk, doctor, pastor, etc.)*
Work:	*Refers to your job andor the running of your home and your ability to support yourself and your family*
Travel:	*Refers to your ability to reach your destinations i.e.: work andor social*
Leisure:	*Refers to your ability to continue enjoyable activities (hobbies, sports, volunteering*
Safety:	*Refers to your ability to do what you want without injuring yourself or others (driving, being outdoors, in the kitchen, in the bathroom, etc.)*
Financial Security;	*Refers to your ability to support yourself and your family and pay your medical costs*
Sexuality:	*Refers to your ability to maintain a satisfactory sexual relationship*

- If your symptoms are stable complete column 1
- If your symptoms fluctuate complete columns 2a and 2b (best and worse)

	Column 1	Column 2a (Best)	Column 2b (Worst)
1. Self-positive			
2. Self-negative			
3. Family Relationships			
4. Community Relationships			
5. Work			
6. Travel			
7. Leisure			
8. Safety			
9. Financial Security			
10. Sexuality			

before her partner had completed the study, and one caregiver died during the study. One patient was in the hospital for 2 weeks during the time her partner was in the study. Center nurses collected the data for their center, reminding subjects if necessary and submitting completed data, as they became available. Two other subjects failed to complete the rating scales, in spite of having been reminded.

No significant differences were found in total scores among the five centers, the two age-groups, or the two genders. Item-by-center analysis did indicate an excess of higher scores in two centers (Ontario, Quebec) with respect to "travel" ($p = .02$). Item-by-age analysis showed a marginally significant excess of low scores for "travel" for the 65 or younger age-group ($p = .05$). Item-by-gender analysis indicated a significant excess in high

TABLE 2. *Correlation matrix for the ten items in the questionaire*

	SELF	FEEL	FAM	FRIEND	WORK	TRAVEL	LEIS	SAFE	FINAN
FEEL	0.68								
FAM	0.50	0.51							
FRIEND	0.36	0.48	0.68						
WORK	0.46	0.44	0.58	0.55					
TRAVEL	0.33	0.45	0.52	0.63	0.54				
LEIS	0.29	0.38	0.54	0.65	0.62	0.71			
SAFE	0.25	0.22	0.37	0.47	0.37	0.39	0.44		
FINAN	0.33	0.22	0.58	0.45	0.51	0.44	0.41	0.21	
SEX	0.26	0.35	0.45	0.37	0.40	0.51	0.50	0.26	0.33

scores among the men with respect to "safety" (p = .03), and a marginally significant excess in high scores in the men with respect to "work" (p = .05).

The test-retest intraclass correlation coefficient of reliability for caregivers of nonfluctuators was 0.80 (95% CI, 0.71–0.87). For caregivers of fluctuators, the intraclass correlation coefficient was 0.77 (95% CI, 0.64–0.87) in both their best and their worst states.

There was a highly significant correlation between the total PIMS score and the length of time since diagnosis ($r = 0.49$; $p < .0001$). Time since diagnosis was not significantly related to the age or the gender of the respondent.

Table 2 shows the correlation matrix for the 10 items in the questionnaire. Cronbach's alpha (α) was 89.1%. Factor analysis (varimax rotation) revealed four factors, which together accounted for 78.3% of the total variation in the data. Factor 1 represented "sex," "travel," and "leisure"; factor 2 accounted for "financial security," "family relationships," and "work"; factor 3 encompassed "self positive" and "self negative"; and factor 4 included "safety" and "community relationships." Table 3 shows the factor loadings on each of the four factors. Oblique rotations gave similar results.

To examine the sensitivity of the instrument to different levels of disease severity, a comparison of the mean total score for nonfluctuators with that of fluctuators in their best state showed marginally significant differences (effect size, 0.32; p = .05) (20). The mean total score for stable patients' caregivers was 10.17, and for those with fluctuators in their best state, the score was 12.66. The comparison of nonfluctuating patients to fluctuators in their worst state showed a very high sensitivity (effect size, 1.28; $p < .0001$), with a mean score for fluctuators in their worst state of 19.78.

Responsiveness in the caregivers' scores to change in the state of the patient was highly significant (standardized response mean, 1.60; $p < .0001$) (20).

Item-by-item comparison between the scores of the caregivers and those of patients with PD from our previous PIMS study (6) revealed that patients with PD had significantly higher scores on (i.e., were more concerned with) "self," "feelings," "work," "safety," and "financial security" (p = .03 to < .0001), whereas caregivers scored significantly higher than the patients with PD on "sexuality" (p = .003).

We have examined the effect of gender on the response to "sexuality" in both the care-

TABLE 3. *Factor loadings on each of the four factors*

	Factor 1	Factor 2	Factor 3	Factor 4
SEX	0.87			
TRAVEL	0.67			
LEIS	0.64			
FINAN		0.92		
FAM		0.63		
WORK		0.56		
SELF			0.88	
FEEL			0.87	
SAFE				0.90
FRIEND				0.56

givers and the PIMS patients (those for whom gender information was available). Briefly, in the caregivers, there was no significant difference between genders with respect to their concern with sexuality. There was a marginally significant difference between the genders in the PIMS patients, ($p = .058$), with the men showing greater concern with sexuality than the women. Comparing the female caregivers with the female PIMS patients with regard to the item *sexuality,* there was a highly significant gender-specific difference between the two subgroups ($p = .0096$), with the female caregivers being far more concerned with sexuality than the female patients.

DISCUSSION

Self-esteem, autonomy, and mood of patients with PD are affected by both their real and their perceived physical symptoms (6,21), although this may be more evident in patients who were younger at the onset of PD (9). Based on the authors' clinical experience there was no reason to think that this would be the case with caregivers. Both caregiver and patient fatigue and anxiety can exacerbate the patient's symptoms, which, in turn, affects the mood of both of them. Our results indicate that PIMS scores for the caregivers were homogeneous across the participating centers, across genders, and across ages, with no significant interactions among these factors. In particular, there was homogeneity between the English and the French versions of the scale. Caregivers' scores showed high test-retest reliability, and a high degree of internal consistency. Four factors accounted for most of the variation in the scores, namely, (a) "sex," "travel," and "leisure"; (b) "financial security," "family relationships," and "work"; (c) "self-positive" and "self negative"; and (d) "safety" and "community relationships."

Caregivers' PIMS scores showed a highly significant sensitivity to different levels of disease severity and a highly significant degree of responsiveness to change: A lapse in the patients' condition from a best to a worst state corresponded to a highly significant rise in the caregivers' PIMS score. These results underscore our initial premise when we developed the PIMS: that fluctuations in mobility must be taken into account when assessing QoL in PD. This study shows that disease severity has a significant effect on QoL, not only for the patients with PD but also for the caregiver, and confirms the observations of Carter et al. (12).

The caregivers rated the negative impact of PD most highly in three areas. These were, in order of priority, sexuality, travel, and leisure. Safety and community relationships were least important.

There was a preponderance of women partners in our study. In a cross-sectional French study Attias-Donfut (22) found that 86% of elderly men are cared for by women (43% spouses, 34% daughters, other women including daughters-in-law 9%). In contrast 59% of elderly women are cared for by other women (22). These figures are in agreement with a North American report that showed most elderly sick people are cared for by a female relative (72%). Seventy-three percent of men between the ages of 75 and 84 live with a caregiving spouse, compared with 30% of women. By age 85, 51% of men live with a spouse, compared with only 10% of women (23).

Most of our caregivers cited problems with sexuality as having the biggest impact on their lives. Sexual dissatisfaction among female partners of patients with PD has been described by both Basson (24) and Brown et al. (25). Nappi et al. (26) have recently provided a review on the topic. Brown et al. (25) relied on patient diaries, whereas Basson (24) interviewed 14 female partners at length, who all expressed sexual dissatisfaction as a result of hyposexuality (reduced arousal and low expectation of reaching orgasm). Twelve of the fourteen women identified two major determinants of low sexual desire, one of which was the fact that taking on the role of caregiver had significantly reduced their own sense of sexual need. Interestingly, in the study by Basson (24), some of the more affected patients with PD felt that it was difficult for them to see themselves as sexual beings when they were receiving so much "care" with activities of daily living. This might account for their lack of self-esteem, as shown in the original PIMS study. Our results show that sexual health and sexuality must be included in measurements of QoL. To date, PIMS is the only PD-specific instrument that can do this.

The high impact on the caregiver's ability to travel or pursue leisure activities outside the home is not surprising. If significantly disabled patients are still living at home with no outside support, the caregiver is required to be there most of the time. Attias-Donfut (22) found that when men were cared for by women, they received less help from local health units and support agencies. Male caregivers appear to find it easier to delegate and seek help (27), and women seem correspondingly unable to seek or accept help or are assumed to be able to cope (22). If care is being given a setting of mutual resentment, the caregiver may be unable to pursue independent activities without being made to feel guilty (28).

The lack of concern expressed by the caregivers over their safety may reflect the wording on the scale, which implies personal risk carrying out one's activities. In fact, however, physically fit caregivers are at risk for injury when assisting a disabled partner and should be included in physiotherapy assessments involving their partners (Carole Shaw, *personal communication, 1986*).

The low impact the caregivers attached to community relationships is not surprising because the activities included are those that must be carried out (shopping and banking) and will be the last activities to be given up. If caregivers have any respite, they may treasure time alone.

In summary, this is the first time a validated PD-specific instrument has been used to study the impact of PD on caregivers. Our findings emphasize that the impact on the caregiver is significant and yield further evidence for the high sensitivity of PIMS. We have now shown that PIMS is a reliable and valid psychometric instrument that can be used not only with patients with PD but also with caregivers in a clinical and research setting. PIMS is easy to use and is now available in three languages.

CONCLUSIONS

Caregivers rated, in order of importance, three major concerns: sexuality, travel, and leisure. There was less concern for safety and community relationships. The interesting differences shown by the patients' concern with safety and the caregivers' concerns with loss of sexuality deserve to be pursued in further independent studies. Notably PIMS can detect not only changes in the level of impact in patients who fluctuate between "on" and "off" but also the corresponding fluctuating levels of impact in their partners. In a clinical setting where one suspects caregiver burden, PIMS can be a useful quick way of identifying specific problems. In clinical or surgical trials, the impact of a patient's improvement or deterioration could be correlated with those of the primary caregiver.

ACKNOWLEDGMENTS

The authors thank Donald Calne for editorial assistance. This study was made possible by a grant from the British Columbia Parkinson Society in association with the Canadian office of Du Pont Pharma. Susan Calne acknowledges the support of the National Parkinson Foundation; Edwin Mak is supported by CIHR; Marie-Jose Fortin, Pamela King, Linda Grantier, and Sherree Trecartin acknowledge the support of Parkinson Society of Canada; Michael Schulzer is supported by the Parkinson Society British Columbia.

REFERENCES

1. Miller JE. *Coping with chronic illness: overcoming powerlessness.* Philadelphia: JB Lippincott Co, 1983.
2. Rajput AH, Uitti RJ, Rajput A, et al. Timely levodopa (LD) administration prolongs survival in Parkinson's disease. *Parkinsonism Relat Disord* 1997;3:159–165.
3. Monahan DJ, Hooker K. Caregiving and social support in two illness groups. *Social Work* 1997;42:278–287.
4. Hille ET, Siesling S, Vegter-van der Vlis M, et al. Two

centuries of mortality in ten large families with Huntington's disease: a rising impact of gene carriership. *Epidemiology* 1999;10:706–710.
5. Berry RA, Murphy JF. Well-being of caregivers of spouses with Parkinson's disease. *Clin Nurs Res* 1995; 4:373–386.
6. Calne S, Schulzer M, Mak E, et al. Validating a quality of life rating scale for Idiopathic Parkinsonism: Parkinson's Impact Scale (PIMS). *Parkinsonism Relat Disord* 1996;2:55–61.
7. de Boer AG, Wijker W, Speelman JD, et al. Quality of life in patients with Parkinson's disease: development of a questionnaire. *J Neurol Neurosurg Psychiatry* 1996; 61:70–74.
8. Peto V, Jenkinson C, Fitzpatrick R, et al. The development and validation of a short measure of functioning and well being for individuals with Parkinson's disease. *Qual Life Res* 1995;4:241–248.
9. Schrag A, Jahanshahi M, Quinn NP. What contributes to depression in Parkinson's disease? *Psychol Med* 2001;31:65–73.
10. Huber SJ, Freidenberg DL, Paulson GW, et al. The pattern of depressive symptoms varies with progression of Parkinson's disease. *J Neurol Neurosurg Psychiatry* 1990;53:275–278.
11. Gotham AM, Brown RG, Marsden CD. Depression in Parkinson's disease: a quantitative and qualitative analysis. *J Neurol Neurosurg Psychiatry* 1986;49:381–389.
12. Carter J, Stewart BJ, Archbold PG, et al. Living with a person who has Parkinson's disease: the spouse's perspective by stage of disease. *Mov Disord* 1998;13:20–28.
13. Habermann B. Spousal perspective of Parkinson's disease in middle life. *J Adv Nurs* 2000;31:1409–1415.
14. Lee KS, Merriman A, Owen A, et al. The medical, social, and functional profile of Parkinson's disease patients. *Singapore Med J* 1994;35:265–268.
15. Wallhagen MI, Brod M. Perceived control and well-being in Parkinson's disease. *West J Nurs Res* 1997;19: 11–25.
16. McRae C, Sherry P, Roper K. Stress and family functioning among caregivers of persons with Parkinson's disease. *Parkinsonism Related Disord* 2001;5:69–75.
17. Glozman JM, Bicheva KG, Fedorova NV. Scale of quality of life of caregivers (SQLC). *J Neurol* 1998;245 [Suppl 1]:S39–S41.
18. Fleiss JL. *The design and analysis of clinical experiments.* New York: Wiley & Sons, 1986.
19. Scheffé H. *The analysis of variance.* New York: Wiley & Sons, 1969.
20. Fayers PM, Machin D. Quality of life: assessment, analysis and interpretation. New York: John Wiley and Sons, 2000:338–341.
21. Poewe W, Luginger E. Depression in Parkinson's disease: impediments to recognition and treatment options. *Neurology* 1999;52[Suppl 3]:S2–S6.
22. Attias-Donfut C. The dynamics of elderly support: the transmission of solidarity patterns between generations. *Zeitschr Gerontol Geriatr* 2001;34:9–15.
23. Berlow E. *Room for improvement: lack of affordable, adaptable and accessible housing for mid-life and older women.* Older Women's League, 1993.
24. Basson R. Sexuality and Parkinson's disease. *Parkinsonism Relat Disord* 1996;2:177–187.
25. Brown RG, Jahanschi M, Quinn N, et al. Sexual function in patients with Parkinson's disease and their partners. *J Neurol Neurosurg Psychiatry* 1990;53:480–486.
26. Nappi R, Detaddei S, Veneroni F, et al. Sexual disorders in Parkinson's disease. *Funct Neurol* 2001;16:283–288.
27. Calne S. Nursing care of patients with idiopathic parkinsonism. *Nurs Times* 1994;90:38–39.
28. Calne S, Hurwitz T. *Adjustment, adaptation, and accommodation: psychosocial approaches to living with Parkinson's disease.* Miami: National Parkinson Foundation, 1997.

Parkinson's Disease: Advances in Neurology, Vol. 91.
Edited by Ariel Gordin, Seppo Kaakkola,
and Heikki Teräväinen
Lippincott Williams & Wilkins, Philadelphia

13

Genes and Oxidative Stress in Parkinsonism: cDNA Microarray Studies

*Silvia Mandel, *†Edna Grünblatt, †Peter Riederer, and *Moussa B. H. Youdim

**Eve Topf and U.S. National Parkinson's Foundation Centers of Excellence for Neurodegenerative Diseases, Bruce Rappaport Family Research Institute and Department of Pharmacology, Faculty of Medicine, Technion, Haifa, Israel; and †Bayrische Julius-Maximilians-University of Würzburg, Clinic and Polyclinic of Psychiatry and Psychotherapy, Department of Neurochemistry, Würzburg, Germany*

There have been numerous hypotheses concerning the etiology of Parkinson's disease (PD), including genetic aberrations, involvement of endogenous- and exogenous-derived neurotoxins, and oxidative stress (OS) due to the accumulation of reactive oxygen species (ROS). The current hypothesis concerning the pathogenesis of PD holds the belief that there is an ongoing selective OS and excessive iron accumulation that expresses itself with biochemical alterations compatible with this state (1–6) (see Chapter 8).

Much of our knowledge about substantia nigra (SN) dopaminergic neurodegeneration has come from studies with two neurotoxins that produce animal models for OS and a parkinsonism-like syndrome in rodents, primates, and other species. Both neurotoxins, namely 6-hydroxydopamine (6-OHDA) (7) and N-methyl-4-phenyl-1,2,3,6-tetrahydropyridine (MPTP) (8,9), cause the degeneration of nigrostriatal dopaminergic neurons with the subsequent loss of striatal dopamine (DA). These are considered relevant models of the disease and are thought to induce neurodegeneration via OS because iron chelators (e.g., desferrioxamine) (10–13); antioxidants (vitamin E) (14,15); the DA agonists apomorphine (16–18) and bromocriptine (19); glutathione analogs (20); and nitric oxide synthase (NOS) inhibitor (7NI, but not L-NAME) (21,22) have been described to prevent or attenuate their toxic effects.

The technique of the complementary DNA (cDNA) expression array is being extensively used to study global changes in gene expression in disease, model systems, and response to drug treatment (23–25). Recently, a first attempt to assess gene expression changes in nigrostriatal neurodegeneration employing gene microarray was reported by us (26,27).

In this chapter, we review the major gene changes in the nigrostriatum and DA cell bodies induced by a chronic MPTP regimen as assessed by the cDNA microarray, as well as the initial gene events that occur at a short time exposure to MPTP. This early gene expression will allow us to distinguish initial events from secondary effects arising from generalized cellular death.

GENE EXPRESSION IN CHRONIC MPTP INTOXICATION

Recently, we have reported a first attempt to assess gene expression changes in nigrostriatal neurodegeneration employing a gene microarray (26,27). In this study, MPTP-inducing parkinsonism neurotoxin given for 5 days caused elevation in the expression of genes related to OS, inflammation, glutamate excitotoxicity, and neurotrophic factor pathways, as well as in cell-cycle regulators and signal transduction molecules (Table 13.1). The initial gene expression changes obtained from cDNA hybridization studies were further verified by semiquantitative reverse transcriptase polymerase chain reaction (RT-PCR) and quantitative real-time RT-PCR techniques. MPTP upregulated the expression of growth factors including glial-cell–derived neurotrophic factor (GDNF) and epidermal growth factor (EGF); interleukin (IL-1R) type II, IL-1β, and IL-10; and lowered the expression of cytochrome P450 (CYP) 1A1 (involved in detoxification), tyrosine hydroxylase (TH) (the rate-limiting enzyme for DA metabolism), glutathione *S*-transferase, glutathione peroxidase precursor, nuclear factor-κB (NF-κB) p65 subunit and cyclin B2 (a G2/M-specific cell-cycle regulator) messenger RNAs (mRNAs).

The general increase in cytotoxic cytokines and cytokine receptors, together with the decrease in the inflammatory and iron-responsive transcription factor NF-κB p65 subunit mRNAs induced by MPTP, supports the involvement of inflammation in neurodegeneration (28-30). Activation and proliferation of microglia has been reported around and on top of dopaminergic neurons in idiopathic PD and in MPTP-treated animals (31,32). Increased chelatable iron in macrophages, microglia, and nigrostriatal dopaminergic neurons as seen in PD (31) may lead to OS and activation of NF-κB and gene regulation of IL-1β, IL-6, and tumor necrosis factor-α (TNF-α) (33,34). Indeed, a 70-fold increase in immunoreactive NF-κB in the nucleus of melanized dopaminergic neurons of patients with PD was previously reported (35).

Normal cellular metabolism produces oxidants, which are neutralized within cells by antioxidant enzymes and other antioxidants. An imbalance between oxidants and antioxidants has been postulated to lead to the degeneration of specific populations of neurons in neurodegenerative diseases. Indeed, mRNAs for both glutathione peroxidase precursor, involved in metabolizing hydrogen peroxide to water, and glutathione *S*-transferase have been decreased after 5 days of treatment with MPTP (26).

The increased expression of the neurotrophic factors GDNF and EGF may reflect a compensatory mechanism by stimulating the sprouting of the surviving neurons as suggested (36,37). This finding supports the validity of a gene-replacement therapeutic approach in animal models of PD using GDNF-encoding vectors (38).

TABLE 13.1. *Differential gene expression analysis in chronic 5-day MPTP-treated mice identified by Atlas mouse cDNA microarray*

Inflammation	**Oxidative stress**	**Neurotrophic**	**Iron related**
↑ IL-1β ↑ IL-1βR	↓ NADPH P450	↑ EGF ↑ NGF-α	↓ Transferrin receptor protein
↑ IL-6 ↑ IL-2R	↑ Glutathione peroxidase	↑ GDNF ↑ NGF-β	
↑ IL-7 ↑ IL-6R	↑ Glutathione transferase	↑ VEGF ↑ TGF-β	
↑ IL-10 ↑ IL-7R	↑ Glutathione reductase		
↓ iNOS ↑ IL-9R	↑ Oxidative stress-induced protein		
NF-κB p65 NF-κB p50			
Glutamate receptors	**Transporters & channels**	**Apoptosis & cell cycle**	**Hormone receptors**
↑ NMDA-R	↓ Glucose transporter 1	↓ Cyclin B2	↑ Prolactin R2
↑ AMPA-R	↓ Voltage-gated sodium channels	↓ cdk inhibitor protein 1	↑ LDL R
		↓ Cyclin B1	
		↓ cdk 4 & 6 inhibitors	
		↓ Caspase 11	
		↓ Caspase 7	

Source: Mandel S, Grünblatt E, Youdim M. cDNA microarray to study gene expression of dopaminergic neurodegeneration and neuroprotection in MPTP and 6-hydroxydopamine models: implications for idiopathic Parkinson's disease. *J Neurat Transm* 2000;60 Suppl]:117–124, with permission.

Effects of *R*- and *S*-Apomorphine on Gene Expression: *In Situ* Hybridization Analysis

We have previously reported that the D_1/D_2 agonist *R*-apomorphine and its non-DA receptor agonist *S*-isomer are potent radical scavengers and iron chelators and protect neurons from both 6-OHDA– and hydrogen peroxide–induced cell death (16). In addition, in mice, both *R*- and *S*-apomorphine significantly prevented the decline in DA and its metabolites 3,4-dihydroxyphenylacetic acid and homovanillic acid, as well as in the levels of reduced glutathione induced by MPTP (17,18). In our microarray and real-time PCR assays, the combined treatment of *R*-apomorphine and MPTP reversed the effect of MPTP alone on the expression of most genes analyzed.

R-apomorphine neuroprotection is attributed not only to DA receptor action but also to its radical-scavenging iron-chelating features (39–41). Apomorphine is a catechol-derived compound that is easily oxidizable and can therefore react with reactive oxygen species (ROS) (42). Similar to *R*-apomorphine, its enantiomer *S*-apomorphine, which is devoid of DA receptor agonism, prevented DA depletion and the elevated DA turnover and TH activity induced by MPTP, except that it was 10 times more effective than *R*-apomorphine (18). *In situ* hybridization analysis demonstrated that both *R*-apomorphine and *S*-apomorphine prevented the increase in TNF-α–induced protein, GDNF, and cyclin B2 mRNAs induced by MPTP in the SN. That both enantiomers of apomorphine prevented the effects of MPTP on the expression of these genes suggests that other pharmacological properties, besides DA receptor agonism, may also play a role in neuroprotection.

EARLY GENE EXPRESSION IN ACUTE MPTP INTOXICATION

The gene expression profile changes obtained after chronic administration of MPTP underline the importance of investigating the early cascade of molecular events leading finally to nigrostriatal DA neuronal cell death. Monitoring short-term gene alterations will provide a wider view and a more complex picture of the initial molecular events before dopaminergic neurodegeneration by MPTP. In a recent study, a time-dependent gene profile was investigated by means of quantitative real-time RT-PCR and *in situ* hybridization in the region of the nigrostriatum of mice acutely treated with a single dose (50 mg/kg) of MPTP for 3 hours, 6 hours, and 24 hours (43) (Fig. 13.1). At 3 hours of MPTP administration, the expression of GDNF, G2/M-specific cyclin B2, *N*-methyl D-aspartate (NMDA) receptor 2A, IL-1β, glutathione peroxidase, and glutathione reductase mRNAs was maximally induced, while that of TH was reduced. At 6 hours, there was an elevation in IL-10, IL-1R type II, OS-induced protein A170, parkin, NF-κB p65 and TH mRNAs, as well as a decrease in inducible NOS (iNOS) and NF-κB p105. At 24 hours, glutathione *S*-transferase and nicotinamide adenine dinucleotide phosphate CYP mRNAs levels were induced by MPTP.

A170 is a novel gene, whose expression was found to be induced by exposure of cells to OS (44). The OS-induced protein A170 mRNA was increased within 6 hours of a single MPTP dose. Its close structural similarity to the signal transduction substance 60- to 62-kd human lymphocyte protein suggests a possible role as a signal transduction mediator in MPTP-induced OS. This observation was further confirmed by *in situ* hybridization, which regionally localized the increased expression to the dopaminergic neurons of the SN (Fig. 13.2). Similar results were observed with GDNF after exposure to MPTP for 6 hours (Fig. 13.2) and with TNF-α–induced protein mRNAs (43).

These results revealed a dynamic and complex pattern of early gene expression in the nigrosriatum where inflammation and OS were evident, supporting the cDNA microarray studies obtained after chronic 5 days of treat-

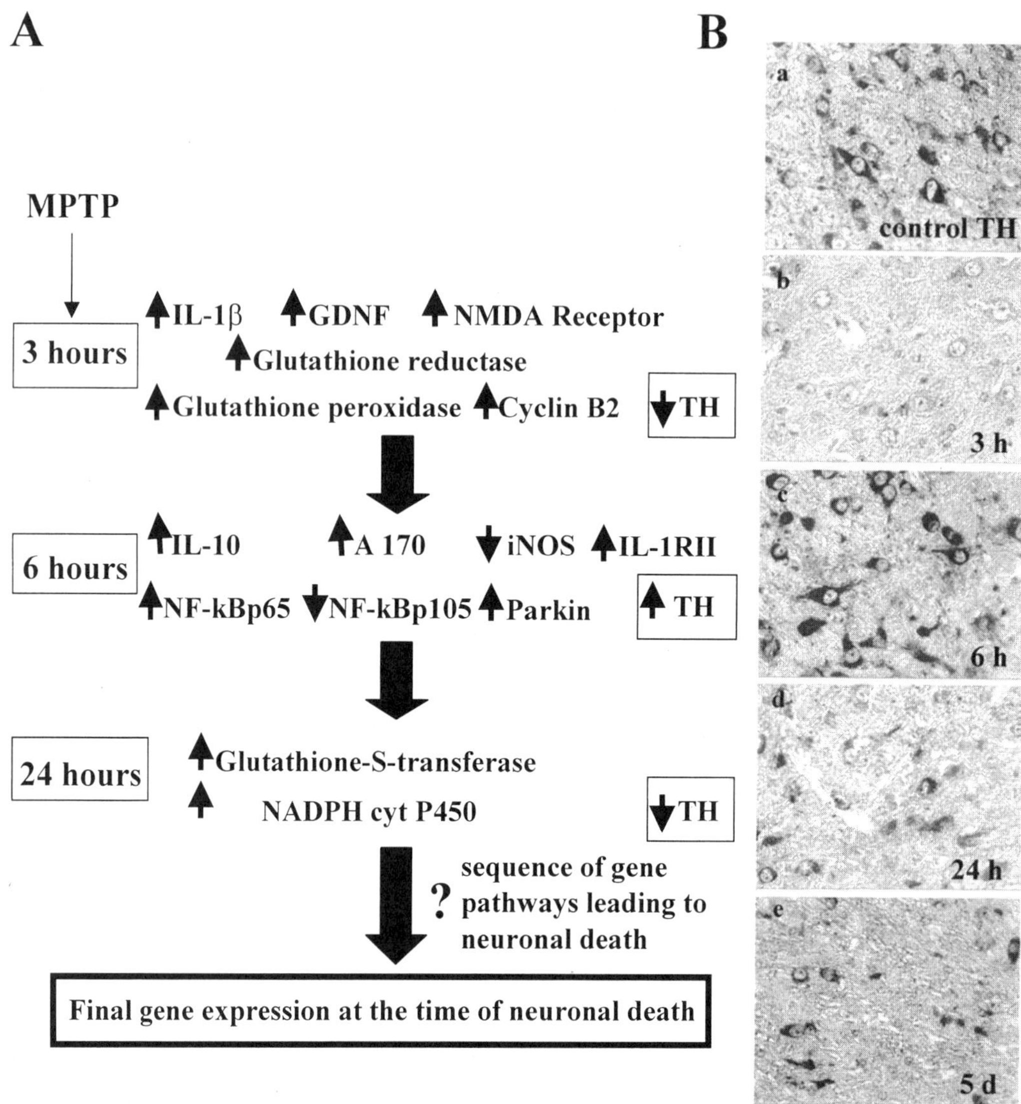

FIGURE. 13.1. Representative scheme of sequential early gene changes in the nigrostriatal pathway induced by acute MPTP treatment and their correlation with immunohistochemistry for tyrosine hydroxylase (TH). **A:** Mice were injected with a single dose of MPTP (50 mg/kg) for 3, 6, and 24 hours before testing. Measurement of differential gene expression was assessed by quantitative real-time polymerase cain reaction (PCR). The amount of each product was normalized to the housekeeping gene, β-actin. **B:** Parallel paraffin sections from MPTP-treated mice, at different time intervals, were reacted with mouse anti-TH antibody, followed by biotinylated second antibody, streptavidin peroxidase conjugate, and AEC substrate. TH-positive neurons were observed in the substantia nigra of control *(a)* and MPTP-treated mice for 3 hours *(b),* 6 hours *(c),* 24 hours *(d),* and 5 days *(e).* (From Mandel S, Grünblatt E, Maor G, et al. Early and late gene changes in MPTP mice model of Parkinson' disease employing cDNA micoarray. *Neurochem Res* 2002 (in press).

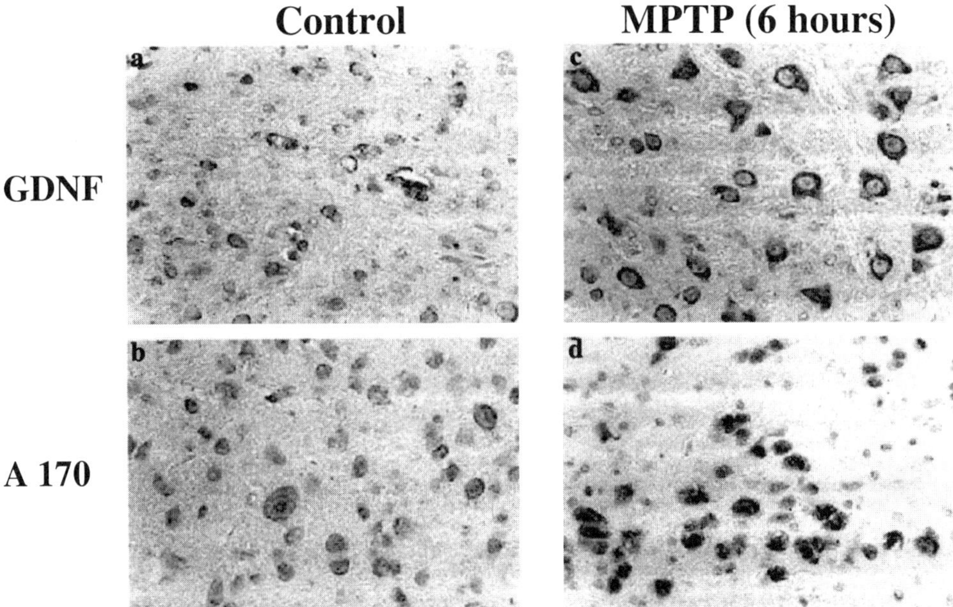

FIGURE 13.2. Representative photomicrographs illustrating glial-cell–derived neurotrophic factor (GDNF) and oxidative stress (OS) protein A170 *in situ* hybridization in the substantia nigra of saline-treated and acute 6-hour MPTP-intoxicated mice. After 6 hours of a single injection of MPTP (50 mg/kg), there was an increase in the expression of GDNF and OS–induced A170 messenger RNA levels inside the dopaminergic neurons in substantia nigra pars compacta. *In situ* hybridization was performed in paraffin-embedded brain tissue, as described in the "Methods" section. RNA sense probes were used as a negative control. (Scale bars = 50 μm.]

ment with MPTP and biochemical observations in idiopathic PD. In addition, the involvement of neurotrophic factors, the NMDA receptor, cell-cycle regulators, and antioxidant defenses has also been demonstrated.

SHORT-TERM REGULATION OF TH mRNA AND ITS PROTEIN

TH, the rate-limiting enzyme in the biosynthesis of catecholamines, is subjected to regulation at the level of transcription, alternative mRNA processing, regulation of RNA stability, translational control, and enzyme stability (45). TH mRNA and its protein levels were shown to be differentially affected by MPTP, as a result of the different exposure time intervals (43). The regulation of TH mRNA levels by MPTP correlated with changes in TH immunoreactivity in the SN. TH mRNA and its protein were substantially decreased in the SN as soon as 3 hours after a single MPTP injection, whereas an intense staining was observed after 6 hours of exposure to the toxin (Fig. 13.1A and B). Therefore, the increased or reduced TH protein levels may result from alterations in its mRNA. However, an additional effect of MPTP on TH enzyme stability and turnover cannot be ruled out. After chronic MPTP intoxication, the expression of TH protein was significantly lower than that in control mice because of dopaminergic cell-body loss (Fig. 13.1B). The abrupt drop in TH immunoreactivity 3 hours subsequent to MPTP administration may not be related to dopaminergic cell death; rather, it may be related to reduced protein synthesis or protein degradation because a prominent TH staining was observed 3 hours later.

IRON AND NEURODEGENERATION

One of the major pathology of PD and other progressive neurodegenerative diseases, is the accumulation of iron at those sites where the neurons degenerate (3,46). Numerous studies have shown that there is a progressive accumulation of iron and ferritin in patients with PD (1,31,47), specifically in the SN pars compacta (SNpc) and not the reticulum, even though the latter region has a higher iron content than the SNpc (31). Furthermore, iron has been observed in the rim of Lewy bodies where α-synuclein, ubiquitin, and TH are also present (31). Protein aggregation is now being considered as one important pathway for degeneration of neurons. α-Synuclein associated with the presynaptic membrane is not toxic; however, a number of recent studies (48–50) have shown that it forms toxic aggregates in the presence of iron and that this is considered to contribute to the formation of Lewy bodies via OS. The implication of the pivotal role for iron in dopaminergic neuron degeneration has been strengthened by the observations that both MPTP and 6-OHDA significantly increased iron in the SNpc of mice, rats, and monkeys treated with these neurotoxins (51–53) and iron chelators were neuroprotective in these models.

A major dilemma in the accumulation of iron within the SNpc and dopaminergic neurons (31,47) is that other metals have not been shown to accumulate in this area and that no explanation has been put forward as to how iron accumulates in the degenerating dopaminergic neurons. The pivotal importance of iron in neurodegeneration has taken a central place by the identification of two iron-regulatory element binding proteins 1 and 2 (IRP-1 and IRP-2) (54,55) and the divalent metal transporter 1, a metal transporter with a high affinity for iron (56). IRPs are cytosolic RNA binding proteins that respond to changes in the labile iron pool, to post-transcriptionally regulate the expression of the transferrin receptor (TfR) and ferritin, through binding to iron-responsive elements located in the untranslated region of their mRNA. When cells accumulate iron, IRPs lose their affinity for iron-responsive elements, allowing for ferritin synthesis and destabilization and degradation of TfR mRNA (57). The opposite occurs when cells are depleted of iron (low iron). In PD, both iron and ferritin are elevated while TfR is decreased.

Recent studies in knockout mice for IRP-2 have revealed accumulation of iron in the striatum with substantial bradykinesia and tremor (58). Furthermore, a number of genes have also been identified that alter iron and ferritin metabolism, which lead to neurodegenerative diseases (59,60). Our recent cDNA microarray observations have shown that MPTP increased the expression of numerous inflammatory and proapoptotic genes while antioxidant defense genes were downregulated (26,27). In addition, MPTP increased α-synuclein protein levels inside the dopaminergic neurons of the SNpc. It also decreased IRP-2 protein and the TfR mRNA (*unpublished data*), supporting previous studies on abnormal accumulation of iron in the SNpc in PD and in MPTP and 6-OHDA animal models (3,46,51,52). These events are completely reversed by pretreatment of mice with either *R*-apomorphine or (–)-epigallocatechin-3-gallate (EGCG) (*unpublished data*), both of which are known to possess iron-chelating properties and to completely prevent MPTP neurotoxicity, as does the iron chelator desferrioxamine in the 6-OHDA model (10).

The scenario of MPTP-induced neurotoxicity, which is linked to iron accumulation in the SN, resulting in OS and neurodegeneration, is depicted in Fig. 13.3. MPTP, like lipopolysaccharide (LPS) and interferon-γ (61), induces NOS, via activation of the inflammatory redox-sensitive transcription factor NF-κB, resulting in elevation of proinflammatory cytotoxic cytokine genes (IL-1β, IL-6) and cellular nitric oxide (NO) (62). MPTP causes nitration of TH (63) as one step in the degeneration of dopaminergic neurons. A similar nitration effect by NO is also observed for IRP-2 (64), resulting in degradation of IRP-2 with a consequential decrease in TfR mRNA levels and an increase in ferritin

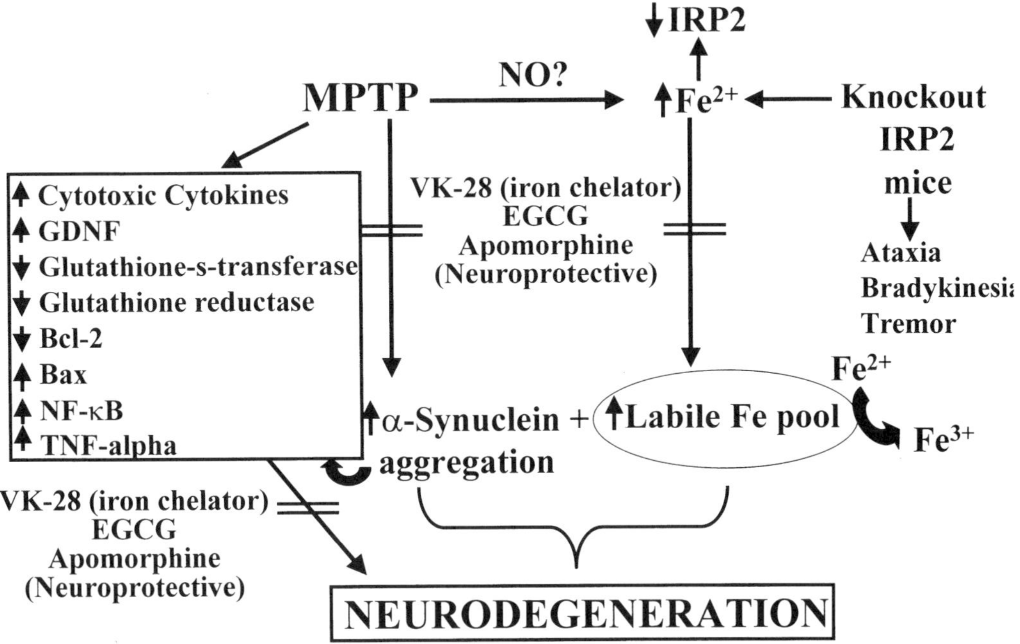

FIGURE 13.3. Schematic overview of the putative pathways participating in neurodegeneration, as induced by iron accumulation and oxidative stress (see text for explanation). (NO, nitric oxide; EGCG, (–)-epigallocatechin-3-gallate; IRP, iron-regulatory element binding protein; ROS, reactive oxygen species.)

synthesis. This modification in TH and IRP-2 leads to their degradation via the ubiquitin-proteosome pathway. These observations indicate that NO not only mediates modulation of TH activity but also plays a major role in controlling ferritin synthesis, which is increased in reactive microglia of the SNpc of parkinsonian brains, and consequently, iron metabolism in macrophages and neurons of the SNpc (65). The result is that free chelatable iron can then initiate OS and neurodegeneration. Both NOS inhibitors and iron chelators prevent MPTP neurotoxicity. Thus, iron chelation may be one other approach to neuroprotection. In considering the initiation of clinical trials of iron chelators in humans, the emphasis should be directed toward the development of novel centrally acting, nontoxic iron chelators. Unfortunately, most iron chelators including desferrioxamine do not cross the blood–brain barrier. However, apomorphine and EGCG have also been shown to possess iron-chelating properties, do penetrate the brain, and therefore should be considered for clinical use.

CONCLUSIONS

This chapter provides a wider, more complex picture of the initial molecular events before dopaminergic neurodegeneration by MPTP, further extending the gene expression profile obtained by a cDNA microarray in chronic MPTP-intoxicated mice. A dynamic and complex pattern of early gene expression in the nigrosriatum was revealed as a consequence of acute (3 to 24 hours) MPTP treatment, where involvement of genes related to OS and inflammatory processes was demonstrated. In addition, the implication of glutamate, NO, neurotrophic factors, cell-cycle regulators, and signal transduction molecules such as iNOS and NF-κB subunits, was also found. These results point to several factors as potential initiators of neuronal death, seen in chronic MPTP treatment, and firmly establish the roles of OS and inflammation, previously obtained by neurochemical and molecular studies.

This picture argues strongly that for therapy of neurodegenerative diseases, such as Parkinson's disease and Alzheimer's disease, the concept of single-drug intervention, as currently approached in most basic research and clinical trials, could no longer fulfill the requirements for the present millennium clinical therapeutics. Instead, strict drug protocols consisting of a cocktail of drugs with different pharmacological activities such as antioxidants, caspase inhibitors, antiinflammatory drugs, promoters of neurotrophic factor synthesis, and inhibitors of iNOS and glutamate excitotoxicity should be considered. We are presently comparing the MPTP-induced gene profile with that observed in 6-OHDA–treated rats and in human parkinsonian SN to elucidate how much homology they display.

REFERENCES

1. Riederer P, Sofic E, Rausch WD, et al. Transition metals, ferritin, glutathione, and ascorbic acid in parkinsonian brains. *J Neurochem* 1989;52:515–520.
2. Youdim MBH, Ben-Shachar D, Riederer P. The possible role of iron in the etiopathology of Parkinson's disease. *Mov Disord* 1993;8:1–12.
3. Gerlach M, Ben-Shachar D, Riederer P, et al. Altered brain metabolism of iron as a cause of neurodegenerative diseases? *J Neurochem* 1994;63:793–807.
4. Gotz ME, Kunig G, Riederer P, et al. Oxidative stress: free radical production in neural degeneration. *Pharmacol Ther* 1994;63:37–122.
5. Jenner P, Olanow CW. Oxidative stress and the pathogenesis of Parkinson's disease. *Neurology* 1996; 47[Suppl 3]:161–170.
6. Olanow CW, Youdim MBH. Iron and neurodegeneration: prospects for neuroprotection. In: Olanow CW, Jenner P, Youdim MBH, eds. *Neurodegeneration and neuroprotection in Parkinson's disease.* London: Academic Press, 1996:55–69.
7. Kostrzewa RM, Jacobowitz DM. Pharmacological action of 6-hydroxydopamine. *Pharmacol Rev* 1974;26: 199–288.
8. Davis GC, Williams AC, Markey SP, et al. Chronic parkinsonism secondary to intravenous injection of meperidine analogues. *Psychiatry Res* 1979;1:249–254.
9. Burns RS, Chiueh CC, Markey SP, et al. A primate model of parkinsonism: selective destruction of dopaminergic neurons in the pars compacta of the substantia nigra by *N*-methyl-4-phenyl-1,2,3,6-tetrahydropyridine. *Proc Natl Acad Sci USA* 1983;80:4546–4550.
10. Ben-Shachar D, Eshel G, Finberg JPM, et al. The iron chelator desferrioxamine (Desferal) retards 6-hydroxydopamine–induced degeneration of nigrostriatal neurons. *J Neurochem* 1991;56:1441–1444.
11. Lan J, Jiang DH. Excessive iron accumulation in the brain: a possible potential risk of neurodegeneration in Parkinson's disease. *J Neural Transm* 1997;104: 649–660.
12. Matarredona ER, Santiago M, Cano J, et al. Involvement of iron in MPP^+ toxicity in substantia nigra: protection by desferrioxamine. *Brain Res* 1997;773:76–81.
13. Santiago M, Matarredona ER, Granero L, et al. Neuroprotective effect of the iron chelator desferrioxamine against MPP^+ toxicity on striatal dopaminergic terminals. *J Neurochem* 1997;68:732–738.
14. Cadet JL, Katz M, Jackson-Lewis V, et al. Vitamin E attenuates the toxic effects of intrastriatal injection of 6-hydroxydopamine (6-OHDA) in rats: behavioral and biochemical evidence. *Brain Res* 1989;476:5–10.
15. Perumal AS, Gopal VB, Tordzro WK, et al. Vitamin E attenuates the toxic effects of 6-hydroxydopamine on free radical scavenging systems in rat brain. *Brain Res Bull* 1992;29:699–671.
16. Gassen M, Gross A, Youdim MBH. Apomorphine enantiomers protect pheochromocytoma (PC12) cells from oxidative stress induced by hydrogen peroxide and 6-hydroxydopamine. *Mov Disord* 1998;13:242–248.
17. Grünblatt E, Mandel S, Berkuzki T, et al. Apomorphine protects against MPTP-induced neurotoxicity in mice. *Mov Disord* 1999;14:612–618.
18. Grünblatt E, Mandel S, Maor G, et al. Effects of *R*-apomorphine and *S*-apomorphine on MPTP-induced striatal dopamine neuronal loss. *J Neurochem* 2001;77: 146–156.
19. Muralikrishnan D, Mohanakumar KP. Neuroprotection by bromocriptine against 1-methyl-4-phenyl-1,2,3,6-tetrahydropyridine-induced neurotoxicity in mice. *FASEB J* 1998;12:905–1012.
20. Di Monte D, Sandy MS, Smith MT. Increase efflux rather than oxidation is the mechanism of glutathione depletion by 1-methyl-4-phenyl-1,2,3,6-tetrahydropyridine (MPTP). *Biochem Biophys Res Commun* 1987; 148:153–160.
21. Schulz JB, Matthews RT, Beal MF. Role of nitric oxide in neurodegenerative diseases. *Curr Opin Neurol* 1995; 8:480–486.
22. Przedborski S, Jackson-Lewis V, Yokoyama R, et al. Role of neuronal nitric oxide in 1-methyl-4-phenyl-1,2,3,6-tetrahydropyridine (MPTP)–induced dopaminergic neurotoxicity. *Proc Natl Acad Sci USA* 1996;93: 4565–4571.
23. DeRisi J, Penland L, Brown PO, et al. Use of a cDNA microarray to analyze gene expression patterns in human cancer. *Nat Genet* 1996;14:457–460.
24. Lee CK, Klopp RG, Weindruch R, et al. Gene expression profile of aging and its retardation by caloric restriction. *Science* 1999;285:1390–1393.
25. Lockhart DJ, Winzeler EA. Genomics, gene expression and DNA arrays. *Nature* 2000;405:827–836.
26. Grünblatt E, Mandel S, Maor G, et al. Gene expression analysis in MPTP model of Parkinson's disease using cDNA microarray: effect of *R*-apomorphine. *J Neurochem* 2001;78:1–12.
27. Mandel S, Grünblatt E, Youdim M. cDNA microarray to study gene expression of dopaminergic neurodegenera-

tion and neuroprotection in MPTP and 6-hydroxydopamine models: implications for idiopathic Parkinson's disease. *J Neural Transm* 2000;60[Suppl]:117–124.
28. Mogi M, Harada M, Narabayashi H, et al. Interleukin (IL)-1 beta, IL-2, IL-4, IL-6 and transforming growth factor-alpha levels are elevated in ventricular cerebrospinal fluid in juvenile parkinsonism and Parkinson's disease. *Neurosci Lett* 1996;211:13–16.
29. Mogi M, Togari A, Ogawa M, et al. Effects of repeated systemic administration of 1-methyl-4-phenyl-1,2,3,6-tetrahydropyridine (MPTP) to mice on interleukin-1 beta and nerve growth factor in the striatum. *Neurosci Lett* 1998;250:25–28.
30. Bessler H, Djaldetti R, Salman H, et al. IL-1 beta, IL-2, IL-6 and TNF-alpha production by peripheral blood mononuclear cells from patients with Parkinson's disease. *Biomed Pharmacother* 1999;53:141–145.
31. Jellinger K, Paulus W, Grundke-Iqbal I, et al. Brain iron and ferritin in Parkinson's and Alzheimer's diseases. *J Neural Transm Parkinson Dis Dementia Sect* 1990;2:327–340.
32. Kohutnicka M, Lewandowska E, Kurkowska-Jastrzebska I, et al. Microglial and astrocytic involvement in a murine model of Parkinson's disease induced by 1-methyl-4-phenyl-1,2,3,6-tetrahydropyridine (MPTP). *Immunopharmacology* 1998;39:167–180.
33. Lin M, Rippe RA, Niemelä O, et al. Role of iron in NF-κB activation and cytokine gene expression by rat hepatic macrophages. *Am J Physiol* 1997;272:G1355–G1364.
34. Bowie A, O'Neill LA. Oxidative stress and nuclear factor-kappa B activation: a reassessment of the evidence in the light of recent discoveries. *Biochem Pharmacol* 2000;59:13–23.
35. Hunot S, Brugg B, Ricard D, et al. Nuclear translocation of NF-κB is increased in dopaminergic neurons of patients with Parkinson's disease. *Proc Natl Acad Sci USA* 1997;94:7531–7536.
36. Hadjiconstantinou M, Fitkin JG, Dalia A, et al. Epidermal growth factor enhances striatal dopaminergic parameters in the 1-methyl-4-phenyl-1,2,3,6-tetrahydropyridine–treated mouse. *J Neurochem* 1991;57:479–482.
37. Lin LF, Doherty DH, Lile JD, et al. GDNF: a glial cell line–derived neurotrophic factor for midbrain dopaminergic neurons. *Science* 1993;260:1130–1132.
38. Björklund A, Kirik D, Rosenblad C, et al. Towards a neuroprotective gene therapy for Parkinson's disease: use of adenovirus, AAV and lentivirus vectors for gene transfer of GDNF to the nigrostriatal system in the rat parkinson model. *Brain Res* 2000;886:82–98.
39. Ubeda A, Montesinos C, Playa M, et al. Iron-reducing and free-radical–scavenging properties of apomorphine and some related benzylisoquinolines. *Free Radical Biol Med* 1993;15:159–167.
40. Sam EE, Verbeke N. Free radical scavenging properties of apomorphine enantiomers and dopamine—possible implication in their mechanism of action in parkinsonism. *J Neural Transm Parkinson Dis Dementia Sect* 1995;10:115–127.
41. Gassen M, Glinka Y, Pinchasi B, et al. Apomorphine is highly potent free radical scavenger in rat mitochondrial fraction. *Eur J Pharmacol* 1996;308:219–225.
42. Gassen M, Youdim MBH. Free radical scavengers: chemical concepts and clinical relevance. *J Neural Transm* 1999;56:193–210.
43. Mandel S, Grünblatt E, Maor G, et al. Early and late gene changes in MPTP mice model of Parkinson's disease employing cDNA micoassay. *Neurochem Res* 2002 (in press).
44. Ishii T, Yanagawa T, Yuki K, et al. Low micromolar levels of hydrogen peroxide and proteasome inhibitors induce the 60-kDa A170 stress protein in murine peritoneal macrophages. *Biochem Biophys Res Com* 1997; 232:33–37.
45. Kumer SC, Vrana KE. Intricate regulation of tyrosine hydroxylase activity and gene expression. *J Neurochem* 1996;67:443–462.
46. Berg D, Gerlach M, Youdim MB, et al. Brain iron pathways and their relevance to Parkinson's disease. *J Neurochem* 2001;79:225–236.
47. Sofic E, Paulus W, Jellinger K, et al. Selective increase of iron in substantia nigra zona compacta of parkinsonian brains. *J Neurochem* 1991;56:978–982.
48. Ostrerova-Golts N, Petrucelli L, Hardy J, et al. The A53T alpha-synuclein mutation increases iron-dependent aggregation and toxicity. *J Neurosci* 2000;20:6048–6054.
49. Turnbull S, Tabner BJ, El-Agnaf OM, et al. Alpha-Synuclein implicated in Parkinson's disease catalyses the formation of hydrogen peroxide *in vitro. Free Radical Biol Med* 2001;30:1163–1170.
50. Ebadi M, Govitrapong P, Sharma S, et al. Ubiquinone (coenzyme Q10) and mitochondria in oxidative stress of Parkinson's disease. *Biol Signals Recept* 2001;10:224–253.
51. Monteiro HP, Winterbourn CC. 6-Hydroxydopamine releases iron from ferritin and promotes ferritin-dependent lipid peroxidation. *Biochem Pharmacol* 1989;38:4177–4182.
52. Mochizuki H, Imai H, Endo K, et al. Iron accumulation in the substantia nigra of 1-methyl-4-phenyl-1,2,3,6-tetrahydropyridine (MPTP)–induced hemiparkinsonian monkeys. *Neurosci Lett* 1994;168:251–253.
53. Temlett JA, Landsberg JP, Watt F, et al. Increased iron in the substantia nigra compacta of the MPTP-lesioned hemiparkinsonian African green monkey: evidence from proton microprobe element microanalysis. *J Neurochem* 1994;62:134–146.
54. Hentze MW, Kuhn LC. Molecular control of vertebrate iron metabolism: mRNA-based regulatory circuits operated by iron, nitric oxide, and oxidative stress. *Proc Natl Acad Sci USA* 1996;93:8175–8182.
55. Hanson ES, Leibold EA. Regulation of the iron regulatory proteins by reactive nitrogen and oxygen species. *Gene Expr* 1999;7:367–376.
56. Gunshin H, Mackenzie B, Berger UV, et al. Cloning and characterization of a mammalian proton-coupled metal-ion transporter. *Nature* 1997;388:482–488.
57. Schneider BD, Leibold EA. Regulation of mammalian iron homeostasis. *Curr Opin Clin Nutr Metab Care* 2000;3:267–273.
58. LaVaute T, Smith S, Cooperman S, et al. Targeted deletion of the gene encoding iron regulatory protein-2 causes misregulation of iron metabolism and neurodegenerative disease in mice. *Nat Genet* 2001;27:209–214.
59. Curtis AR, Fey C, Morris CM, et al. Mutation in the gene encoding ferritin light polypeptide causes dominant adult-onset basal ganglia disease. *Nat Genet* 2001; 28:350–354.
60. Zhou B, Westaway SK, Levinson B, et al. A novel pan-

tothenate kinase gene (*PANK2*) is defective in Hallervorden–Spatz syndrome. *Nat Genet* 2001;28:345–349.
61. Kim S, Ponka P. Effects of interferon-gamma and lipopolysaccharide on macrophage iron metabolism are mediated by nitric oxide–induced degradation of iron regulatory protein 2. *J Biol Chem* 2000;275:6220–6226.
62. Grunblatt E, Mandel S, Youdim MB. Neuroprotective strategies in Parkinson's disease using the models of 6-hydroxydopamine and MPTP. *Ann NY Acad Sci* 2000; 899:262–273.
63. Ara J, Przedborski S, Naini AB, et al. Inactivation of tyrosine hydroxylase by nitration following exposure to peroxynitrite and 1-methyl-4-phenyl-1,2,3,6-tetrahydropyridine (MPTP). *Proc Natl Acad Sci U S A* 1998;95: 7659–7663.
64. Kim S, Ponka P. Control of transferrin receptor expression via nitric oxide–mediated modulation of iron-regulatory protein 2. *J Biol Chem* 1999;274:33035–33042.
65. Jellinger KA. The pathology of Parkinson's disease. *Adv Neurol* 2001;86:55–72.

Parkinson's Disease: Advances in Neurology, Vol. 91.
Edited by Ariel Gordin, Seppo Kaakkola,
and Heikki Teräväinen
Lippincott Williams & Wilkins, Philadelphia © 2003

14

Is the Cause of Parkinson's Disease Environmental or Hereditary? Evidence from Twin Studies

Caroline M. Tanner

Clinical Research, Parkinson's Institute, Sunnyvale, California

The cause of Parkinson's disease (PD) has been controversial for more than a century. Rare forms caused by toxicants or genes have been described, but the cause of common sporadic PD remains unknown. Investigations in twins can be useful in the investigation of the causes of disease. First, twin studies provide information concerning the relative contribution of genetic and environmental factors to the cause of a disorder. In monozygotic twins, nuclear DNA is identical, although maternally derived mitochondrial DNA may differ. In dizygotic twins, about 50% of nuclear genetic material is identical. This proportion is the same in nontwin siblings. In diseases with primarily genetic causes, the rate of disease in monozygotic twins is much greater than that in dizygotic twins. If a disease has environmental causes, rates in monozygotic and dizygotic twins are not expected to differ. Second, twin pair case–control studies provide a powerful method for investigating the risk factors or protective factors for a disease. This chapter reviews twin studies in PD.

THE CAUSES OF PD

Purely genetic and purely environmental causes of parkinsonism have been described. Some of these are characterized by pure parkinsonism without signs of more extensive nervous system involvement. But most persons with PD have no history of familial disease or exposure to an environmental toxicant, followed by PD. The cause of most PD cases remains unknown, a source of much controversy and investigation.

Genetic Risk Factors

Mutations in three genes have been found to be associated with familial parkinsonism (1–4). Each has associated atypical features in some family members, and early age at onset is nearly universal. These mutations have not been found in sporadic disease (5,6). In other families, linkage has been associated with specific loci, but these, too, are unique to a few families, often with atypical features (7–9). In case–control studies, a history of another affected family member with PD was found in some persons with PD. The cause of such patterns is not known, and both nongenetic familial risk factors and "family bias" must be considered along with true genetic causes. All told, the forms of PD with a known or presumed genetic cause account for a small fraction of disease, likely 5% or less.

Environmental Risk Factors

The description of the cluster of parkinsonism produced by the neurotoxic pyridine, methylphenyltetrahydropyridine (MPTP), led to interest in an environmental cause of PD (10). MPTP-induced parkinsonism has clinical and pathological similarities to PD, suggesting that substances with similar mechanisms may cause PD. Compounds included in this category include inhibitors of mitochondrial complex I, such as rotenone. Paraquat, structurally similar to MPTP, has also been investigated. All of these chemicals cause nigral injury in animal models (11–13), and all are present in the environment. However, few cases of parkinsonism have been attributed to any of these agents, and most people with PD have no known exposure to chemicals established as causing parkinsonism.

Other Epidemiological Observations

Observations of patterns of PD in populations may yield clues to the cause of PD. Increasing age is the only definitive risk factor for PD. Male gender also appears to add to the risk of developing PD. Smoking cigarettes and drinking coffee are inversely associated with PD; that is, smokers and coffee drinkers are less likely to develop PD. The explanations for any of these patterns are unknown. Whether they reflect environmental or genetic risk factors remains a matter of debate. For example, the association of increasing age and PD risk may be due to a cumulative effect of either inborn metabolic characteristics or environmental exposures. Whether the underlying error is genetic or environmental remains controversial, but the debate is not a trivial one. The direction of research toward the cause of PD and its cure is very different if genes are thought to be the cause of PD than if environmental different if nongenetic factors are primary. A better understanding of the relative contribution of genetic and environmental factors to the cause of PD will, in turn, lead to a more focused, directed research effort. Studies of PD in twins provide an ideal opportunity to investigate the role of genes and environment in PD.

Challenges in Investigating PD

Any studies of PD are best understood in the context of the challenges posed by the clinical investigation of the disease. First, the clinical diagnosis of PD does not always predict typical pathological changes, even when the most stringent diagnostic criteria are used. Although the syndrome described by James Parkinson remains today as the cornerstone of clinical diagnostic criteria (bradykinesia, resting tremor, cogwheel rigidity, and postural reflex impairment) (14,15), these findings may also be found in other neurodegenerative syndromes including parkinsonism and drug-induced parkinsonism and familial parkinsonism. Whether these should be distinguished from PD in studies and whether this is possible even if desired are the difficult questions.

This difficulty in rendering a clinical diagnosis presents challenges in the conduct and interpretation of studies of PD in twins. First, among the difficulties is the lack of a diagnostic test. PD is determined most precisely at postmortem, when the characteristic pathology, coupled with a history of parkinsonism before death, provides definitive evidence. Few clinical studies can include postmortem confirmation of the clinical diagnosis. This introduces uncertainty into any investigation relying entirely or primarily on clinical findings. Moreover, PD is a relatively uncommon disorder, and cases of PD are not subject to universal reporting. Assembling a representative population of persons with PD is challenging. If cases are identified through clinics, those not seeking care are excluded, potentially introducing a bias. Investigations of the cause of PD are limited by the fact that PD is a late-life disorder. Thus, family history investigations are difficult because the presumed affected relatives are often dead, so diagnosis cannot be validated. Similarly, investigations of risk factors are difficult because recall of early life exposures is poor and because validation of these can be impossible.

EARLY WORK IN TWINS

Studies of twins or siblings are another approach used to investigate the determinants of PD (Table 14.1). In twin studies, the relative contribution of genetics and environment is determined by comparing concordance in

TABLE 14.1. *Concordance for Parkinson's disease from published twin studies, using the least stringent diagnostic criteria provided*

Study	Ascertainment method / Diagnosis method	Monozygotic pairs		Dizygotic pairs		Risk ratio (95% confidence interval)	Methodological concerns
		Concordant	Discordant	Concordant	Discordant		
Duvoisin et al., 1981 (20)	Clinical practice; advertisement Expert examination	4	44	1	18	1.58 (0.19–13.27)	Small sample size; ascertainment favors finding monozygotic twins and concordant pairs; examiners not blinded to zygosity; young age of twins studied; only monozygotic twins followed
Marsden, 1987 (22)	Advertisement	1	10	1	10	1.00 (0.07–14.05)	Small sample size; diagnosis uncertain; no follow-up
Marttila et al., 1988 (23)	Family doctor report Records linkage National health databases	0	18	1	13	0 (0–14.06)	Small sample size; diagnosis uncertain; no follow-up
Vieregge et al., 1992 (24)	Advertisement Expert examination	3	6	3	9	1.33 (0.35–5.13)	Small sample size; ascertainment favors finding monozygotic twins and concordant pairs; examiner not blinded to zygosity; no follow-up of pairs

monozygotic twins (who share all autosomal genes) and dizygotic twins (who share, on average, 50% of autosomal genes). If genetic factors are primary to the cause of PD, then concordance in monozygotic pairs will be high, whereas that in dizygotic pairs will be similar to disease rates in other siblings (sharing, on average, 50% of genes). Similar concordance rates in monozygotic and dizygotic twins suggest shared environment, particularly early life environment (as many twins separate after the teen years, particularly monozygotic twins).

Individual monozygotic twin pairs discordant (16,17) and concordant (18,19) have been described. But it was not until 1977 that a twin study method was used to investigate the relative contribution of genes and environment to PD. In 1977, Duvoisin et al. (20) initiated a collaborative study of PD in twins. They advertised for twins with PD in advocacy group newsletters, in adult twin registries, and through neurologists across the United States. They reviewed medical records and made attempts to examine all monozygotic pairs and an unselected subset of dizygotic pairs in whom one twin appeared to have PD. By 1983, they had examined 47 monozygotic pairs, 18 dizygotic pairs, and the survivors of 1 set of quadruplets (21). Of these, 43 monozygotic pairs were found to have PD in at least one brother, and 19 dizygotic pairs (including the quadruplets). Of these, one monozygotic pair was definitely concordant for typical PD (onset at ages 35 and 45). No dizygotic pairs were concordant for typical PD. If atypical parkinsonism were included, then 4 of 48 monozygotic and 1 of 19 dizygotic pairs were concordant. The authors concluded that concordance for parkinsonism is no more frequent in twins than would be expected from the age-specific incidence of the disease. Thus, they concluded that the main factors in the etiology of PD must be nongenetic.

Two other twin studies followed, with similar outcomes. Using an approach similar to that of Duvoisin et al. (11), Marsden (22) reported in a letter the results of a search for twins with PD through advertisement in the Parkinson's Disease Society's newsletter in the United Kingdom. Diagnosis was verified by contact with personal physicians. Of 22 pairs identified, 1 of 11 monozygotic and 1 of 11 dizygotic pairs were concordant for PD. The monozygotic pair had onset at ages 71 and 73, whereas the dizygotic pair had onset at ages 48 and 53. Marsden (22), too, concluded that inheritance seemed an unlikely cause of PD.

Marttila et al. (23) used a population-based approach, through records linkage, to identify twins with PD in Finland. They linked the Finnish Twin Cohort Registry with the Finnish Hospital Discharge Register and the Finnish Sickness Insurance Register and identified 42 PD cases in 41 twin pairs. The single concordant pair was a male dizygotic pair with onset at ages 55 and 56. Because this study identified twins from the entire Finnish population, the results were less likely to be biased due to the method of case identification. However, the most typical bias observed in twin studies is the greater response of monozygotic than dizygotic twins, which could theoretically result in an overestimate of monozygotic concordance. That was not observed in the preceding studies, despite that ascertainment was not population based.

Vieregge et al. (24) followed a similar recruitment method to those used by Duvoisin et al. (20) and Marsden (22), to identify twins with PD in Germany and Switzerland. Diagnosis was verified by personal examination. They identified 9 monozygotic and 12 dizygotic pairs, with PD in at least 1 twin. Of these, three monozygotic and three dizygotic pairs were concordant. The authors concluded that these findings did not establish a major genetic impact in the etiology of PD, although they argued that a genetic predisposition could not be ruled out.

Two groups further investigated the question of concordance in twins by using positron emission tomography (PET) imaging of striatal dopaminergic systems as a surrogate for affectedness. The hypothesis is that an abnormal dopaminergic system may be a marker of subsequent parkinsonism or may even be considered “preclinical parkinsonism.” The first study (25) identified 11 monozygotic and 7 dizygotic twin pairs from the United Kingdom and the Duvoisin et al. twin studies. All pairs were thought to be clinically discordant when recruited, although three of the “asymptomatic” twins in monozygotic pairs did have tremor when examined. Imaging studies found that 4 (40%) of 10 monozygotic and 2 (29%) of 7 dizygotic asymptomatic co-twins had reduced putamen ^{18}F-dopa uptake if the cutoff was greater than 2 SD below the normal mean. This greater concordance for abnormal putamen ^{18}F-dopa uptake in monozygotic than dizygotic twins was viewed as supportive of a genetic determinant to PD. Interestingly, however, if a slightly more stringent criterion for abnormal putamen ^{18}F-dopa uptake of 2.5 SD below the normal mean were used, only 1 (10%) of 10 monozygotic but 2 (29%) of 7 dizygotic pairs showed reduced uptake. If this criterion had been accepted, following the same reasoning, a different conclusion—that there is no evidence to support a genetic determinant to PD—would have been indicated.

A second study investigated some of the discordant twin pairs in the German and Swiss study (26). In this study, all of the clinically unaffected co-twins, irrespective of zygosity, were found to have abnormal ^{18}F-dopa uptake in at least one striatal measure (caudate, putamen, and rostrocaudal putaminal gradient). In addition, all clinically unaffected co-twins were found to have abnormalities on neuropsychological testing, particularly in verbal memory processing. If abnormalities of striatal ^{18}F-dopa uptake in clinically asymptomatic persons are in some way early signs of PD or susceptibility to PD, these results suggest that monozygotic and dizygotic twins are equally vulnerable. Such a pattern argues against a strong genetic determinant and in favor of shared environmental causes of the abnormality.

In summary, as of the early 1990s, no study had convincingly demonstrated greater monozygotic than dizygotic concordance for PD, and in all the preponderance of twin pairs studied were discordant for disease. Despite these seemingly definitive results, the advent of molecular genetics and more detailed investigation of one large multigenerational family prompted Duvoisin et al. (27) to reassess the U.S. twin study. They suggested that the prior studies and conclusions could not be viewed as conclusive. They based this assertion on several points. They argued that the numbers of twins studied were too small to disprove a substantial genetic contribution. Moreover, they argued that diagnostic criteria applied were too stringent. Using a much broader definition of “affected” (including dementia, cerebellar disorder, and other signs along with parkinsonism), they found 6 of 50 concordant monozygotic pairs and 1 of 19 concordant dizygotic pairs in a reanalysis of the 1988 report of Ward et al. (21). They concluded that the published twin studies neither excluded nor proved a genetic role in PD.

NAS/NRC WORLD WAR II VETERAN TWINS COHORT STUDY

We decided to address this controversy by performing a more rigorous study in twins. We investigated a large, unselected group of twins, the National Academy of Sciences/National Resource Council (NAS/NRC) World War II Veteran Twins Cohort (28). In the mid-1950s, the Medical Follow Up Agency of the Institute of Medicine of the NAS/NRC established a registry of approximately 32,000 white male twins, all of whom were born between 1917 and 1927 and were veterans of the U.S. Armed Services (29). Beginning in 1993, we conducted the first effort to directly contact all living members of the cohort, to identify twin pairs with PD in one or both twins. Twins with suspected PD, as identified by telephone screen, and their twin brothers were asked to undergo a standardized diagnostic evaluation performed by neurologists with expertise in PD. Final diagnoses were assigned by consensus of two movement disorders specialists unaware of zygosity or disease status in the twin brother, using diagnostic criteria based on the Core Assessment Program for Intracerebral Transplantations (30). Of 19,842 presumed living subjects in the NAS\NRC Registry, 14,436 were interviewed, 2,009 refused, and 3,397 were found to be dead or could not be located. Information for 2,716 of the dead or refusing subjects was available from proxy or other sources. A total of 193 twins were diagnosed with PD. Concordance-adjusted overall prevalence of PD was 8.7 per 1,000 (monozygotic, 8.7/1,000; dizygotic, 8.7/1,000). This prevalence estimate is similar to age-, race-, and gender-specific prevalence rates obtained using door-to-door studies (31), suggesting that any bias resulting from incomplete ascertainment is minimized.

If genetic factors are primary to the cause of PD, then concordance in monozygotic pairs (who are genetically identical) will be high, whereas that in dizygotic pairs will be similar to disease rates in other siblings (sharing, on average, 50% of genes). To assess the role of genetics in causing PD, we compared concordance for PD in monozygotic and dizygotic twins, as summarized briefly below (28). Pairwise concordance was defined as PD in both members of a pair. Concordance was calculated overall and by zygosity and age at diagnosis. Younger age at diagnosis was defined as PD diagnosed by age 50 or younger, reflecting the well-established near-exponential increase in incidence and prevalence of PD after age 50 (32). Results are shown in Table 14.2. Monozygotic and dizygotic concordance did not differ overall. For twins with onset after age 50, concordance rates were essentially identical in monozygotic and dizygotic twins. In the young-onset cases, however, monozygotic concordance was much increased. The overall similarity in concordance in monozygotic and dizygotic pairs is not consistent with a significant genetic cause of PD. In the less common young-onset parkinsonism, however, genetic factors are primary. This is consistent with the family studies already described, in which younger age at onset is a common clinical finding.

Although these results appear clear-cut, this twin study suffered from two important limitations: the lack of long-term follow-up and the inability to employ imaging studies as a method to ascertain preclinical disease. The underlying concern, of course, is that at least some of the clinically unaffected twins actually had preclinical disease, and that, had we been able to recognize those patients (with either longer term follow-up or imaging studies), it might have substantially altered our concordance data, and therefore the conclusions regarding the heritability of PD. We attempted to address these concerns in part through additional analyses of our findings. For example, differences in the duration of follow-up in monozygotic versus dizygotic pairs might lead to an underestimation of monozygotic concordance. However, we found similar duration of follow-up in monozygotic and dizygotic twins, about 9 years in each case. Estimation of incidence by zygosity similarly showed differences only in the twin pairs with onset before age 50 (Table 14.3). Finally, we used a broader definition of "affected" in the second twin, including twins with atypical parkinsonism, essential tremor

TABLE 14.2. *Pairwise concordance for Parkinson's disease*

	Concordant pairs		Discordant pairs		Pairwise concordance		Risk of concordance if MZ
	MZ	DZ	MZ	DZ	MZ	DZ	Relative risk (95% confidence interval)
Overall	11	10	60	80	15.5%	11.1%	1.39 (0.63–3.10)
First twin diagnosed <50 yr	4	2	0	10	100%	16.7%	6.00 (1.69–21.3)
First twin diagnosed >50 yr	7	8	58	68	10.8%	10.5%	1.02 (0.39–2.67)

DZ, dizygotic; MZ, monozygotic.

TABLE 14.3. *Incidence of Parkinson's disease in twin brothers of twins with the disease*

Incidence rates (1,000 subject-years)	Any zygosity	Monozygotic	Dizygotic	Relative risk (95% confidence interval)
All subjects	1.94	2.28	1.68	1.36 (0.58–3.20)
First twin diagnosis <50 yr	5.58	16.9	2.39	6.97 (1.28–37.8)
First twin diagnosis 51–65 yr	1.46	1.53	1.4	1.10 (0.22–5.44)
First twin diagnosis >65 yr	1.65	1.57	1.77	0.89 (0.24–3.29)

and dementia, alone or combined, as well as twins with PD. Again, we found no difference in concordance between monozygotic and dizygotic pairs.

FOLLOW-UP STUDIES

Recently, concern over these methodologic "loose ends" was highlighted by the work of Piccini et al. (33). In a study of 34 twins pairs, these investigators found that concordance for decreased putaminal ^{18}F-dopa uptake was higher in monozygotic than dizygotic twin pairs. Higher monozygotic concordance was most evident in the 19 pairs in whom longitudinal follow-up was possible, particularly when concordance was further defined to include an increased rate of loss of putaminal fluorodopa. However, only 56% of the original twins studied were included in this report. Whether similar results would have been found if all had been included remains unknown. Despite these reservations, this work was viewed by some as strong evidence in support of a genetic cause of PD. For example, Golbe (34), in an accompanying editorial, concluded that ". . . the role of genetics in PD . . . is central and indispensable."

More recently, a second follow-up of 23 twin pairs followed for 8 years had contradictory findings. Vieregge et al. (35) found similar clinical concordance for PD in monozygotic and dizygotic twins. Twins with prior decreased fluorodopa uptake on PET had not developed clinical PD. Because both studies are small in number and are subject to selection and other possible biases, a final interpretation of these different findings awaits confirmation in a larger unselected population. Also, importantly, the assumption that the radiographic finding (decreased striatal ^{18}F-dopa uptake as measured by PET) is a useful surrogate for either PD or susceptibility to PD is at present unknown. All of these questions will require further investigation.

POSTMORTEM STUDIES

Because the clinical diagnosis of PD is uncertain, even when experts render the diagnosis, postmortem confirmation of diagnosis remains the gold standard. In twins, such confirmation has been rare. Dickson et al. (36) recently report the postmortem findings in two members of the NAS/NRC twins cohort, both of whom were judged clinically concordant for PD during life. They found typical PD at postmortem examination, confirming this. Intriguingly, their conclusion based on this single concordant pair was that ". . . genetic factors are very important in the initiation of PD. . . ." It seems important to state that the observation of a single concordant pair or a single discordant pair does little to confirm or dispute the role of genetics in PD. In fact, concordance in a single pair can be the result of shared genes, shared environment, or some portion of both genetic and environmental factors. Observation of a pattern in a much larger population is needed for such an inference to be possible.

In counterpoint to the previously mentioned report, we recently presented a second postmortem report on one member of a monozygotic twin pair also judged to be clinically concordant for PD (37). In this case, however, postmortem findings were of typical multiple system atrophy, not of PD. Whether this will be the case for the brother still living is unknown, although it is of interest that neither twin had significant findings of dysautonomia during life. Just as the preceding pair cannot lead to the conclusion that genetic factors are important, this pair cannot lead to any.

INVESTIGATING RISK FACTORS IN TWINS

Studies in twins can be useful not only for the investigation of the relative contribution of genetics and environment to disease, but also for the identification of environmental risk factors for disease. In an investigation (38) of 31 monozygotic twin pairs identified from the study of Ward et al. (21), each twin was asked to respond to a series of questions about birth, childhood, and adult behaviors, such as birth order, medical history, head injury, and habits such as smoking cigarettes and drinking alcohol. When these were compared, the only statistically significant difference observed was that the twin with PD had smoked fewer cigarettes than had the twin without PD. In 13 discordant dizygotic pairs, there were no statistically significant differences.

We recently expanded on this observation in a larger sample of twins discordant for PD (39). We proposed that a study of smoking within twin pairs discordant for PD would allow the distinction between an inherent genetic predisposition to both PD and smoking from an independent action of cigarette smoke (and, possibly, nicotine) as a neuroprotective agent. We reasoned that because monozygotic twins are genetically identical, any difference found in monozygotic twins discordant for PD must be due to a biological action of cigarette smoke. We investigated lifelong cigarette smoking histories in 43 monozygotic and 50 dizygotic pairs discordant for PD. Correlation for smoking was high overall, particularly in monozygotic pairs. Despite this, the pack-years smoked by the twin without PD were greater than that in the twin with PD, most markedly in the monozygotic pairs. This relationship was also seen if pack-years were calculated until 10 or 20 years before PD onset, arguing against a disease-associated behavioral change. These data are compatible with a true biological protective effect of cigarette smoking, illustrating the unique insights to be gained from risk factor investigations in twins discordant for disease.

FUTURE DIRECTIONS

The question of whether longer duration of follow-up would change the pattern of concordance in the large NAS/NRC World War II Veteran Twins Cohort is now under investigation. Twin pairs discordant for PD are being reexamined to look for new clinical signs. In addition, striatal dopaminergic system function is being assessed using a ligand specific for the dopamine transporter (^{123}I-CIT) and single-photon emission computed tomography. Because this population is unselected, the bias inherent in studies identifying cases by advertisement, such as the imaging studies performed to date, is minimized. In particular, the tendency for those subjects with symptoms or frank disease to be more willing to volunteer for a study than those with no symptoms, resulting in an overestimation of concordance, will be minimized.

Another important direction will be the continued investigation of disease risk factors in twins. Because twins share genetic and environmental factors to a much higher degree than others, extending this work to include a risk factor investigation, will allow greater certainty that observed associations are of biological significance (40). First, genetic factors are almost perfectly controlled. For monozygotic twins, all genes encoded by nuclear DNA are identical, and the only possible genetic variance will derive from mitochondrial DNA. For dizygotic twins, on average 50% of genes will be shared, still a proportion much higher than would be expected in the genetically heterogeneous U.S. population. Second, many types of nongenetic exposures can be very similar within twin pairs (including behaviors such as cigarette smoking or coffee drinking). For these exposures, when measured as categories, it may be impossible to detect an effect no matter how large the sample size. This is illustrated in our study of cigarette smoking (described earlier) in which the category "ever smoking cigarettes" was not associated with PD (39). Yet, in this example, the actual dose of cigarette smoked (measured in pack-years) was greater in the twin without PD. This highlights an advantage of the case–control study within twin pairs, in which spurious associations of disease and exposures are minimized by the very similar experiences of the twin siblings. In effect, then, comparisons within twin pairs are the closest human approximation to the conditions required in well-designed laboratory studies using experimental animals, in which all animals in a given experiment are genetically identical, with identical environmental conditions, differing only by the single factor being tested in the experiment. By studying human twins, the uncertainty associated with traditional case–control comparisons, in which myriad potential confounding and biasing factors are possible, is greatly reduced.

CONCLUSIONS

The final challenge in investigating the cause of PD is to determine the interaction of genetic and environmental factors. In this area, too, studies of twins will be of importance, providing near-perfect (in monozygotic pairs) or very similar (in dizygotic pairs) genetic matching. Analogous to the advantage of the risk factor investigation posed earlier in this chapter, twin pairs provide a useful method for investigating gene–environment interactions. When specific genes are investigated in combination with well-quantified exposures in such a population, inference regarding the relationship between disease, exposure, and genotype will be clarified.

REFERENCES

1. Polymeropoulos M, Higgins J, Golbe L, et al. Mapping of a gene for PD to chromosome 4q21-q-23. *Science* 1996;274:1197–1199.
2. Kitada T, Asakawa S, Hattori N, et al. Mutations in the parkin gene case autosomal recessive juvenile parkinsonism. *Nature* 1998;392:605–608.
3. Hattori N, Matsumine H, Asakawa S, et al. Point mutations (Thr240Arg and Ala311Stop) in the parkin gene. *Biochem Biophy Res Comm* 1998;249:754–758.
4. Leroy E, Boyer R, Auburger G, et al. The ubiquitin pathway in PD. *Nature* 1998;395:451–452.
5. Chan P, Jiang X, Forno LS, et al. Absence of mutations in the coding region of the alpha-synuclein gene in pathologically proven PD. *Neurology* 1998;50:1136–1137.
6. Farrer M, Destee T, Becquet E, et al. Linkage exclusion in French families with probable Parkinson's disease. *Mov Disord* 2000;15:1075–1083.
7. Gasser T. Genetics of PD. *Clin Genet* 1998;54:259–265.
8. Farrer M, Gwinn-Hardy K, Hutton M, et al. The genetics of disorders with synuclein pathology and parkinsonism. *Hum Mol Genet* 1999;8:1901–1905.
9. Valente EM, Bentivoglio AR, Dixon PH, et al. Localization of a novel locus for autosomal recessive early-onset parkinsonism, *PARK6,* on human chromosome 1p35-p36. *Am J Hum Genet* 2001;68:895–900.
10. Langston JW, Ballard P, Tetrud JW, et al. Chronic parkinsonism in humans due to a product of meperidine-analog synthesis. *Science* 1983;219:979–980.
11. Langston JW. The etiology of PD with emphasis on the MPTP story. *Neurology* 1996;47[Suppl]:S153–S160.
12. Thiruchelvam M, Brockel BJ, Richfield EK, et al. Potentiated and preferential effects of combined paraquat and maneb on nigrostriatal dopamine systems: environmental risk factors for PD? *Brain Res* 2000;873:225–234.
13. Betarbet R, Sherer TB, MacKenzie G, et al. Chronic systemic pesticide exposure reproduces features of PD. *Nat Neurosci* 2000;3:1301–1306.
14. Parkinson J. *An essay on the shaking palsy.* London: Sherwood, Neeley, and Jones, 1817.
15. Gelb DJ, Oliver E, Gilman S. Diagnostic criteria for Parkinson's disease. *Arch Neurol* 1999;56:33–39.
16. Gudmundsson KR. A clinical survey of parkinsonism in Iceland. *Acta Neurol Scand* 1967;33:9–61.
17. Pembrey ME. Discordant identical twins, II: parkinsonism. *Practitioner* 1972;209:240–243.
18. Koller WC, O'Hara R, Nutt JG, et al. Monozygotic twins with PD. *Ann Neurol* 1986;19:402–405.
19. Jankovic J, Reches A. PD in monozygotic twins. *Ann Neurol* 1986;19:405–408.
20. Duvoisin RC, Eldridge R, Williams A, et al. Twin study of Parkinson's disease. *Neurology* 1981;31:77–80.
21. Ward CD, Duvoisin RC, Ince SE, et al. PD in 65 pairs of twins and in a set of quadruplets. *Neurology* 1983; 335:815–824.
22. Marsden CD. PD in twins. *J Neurol Neurosurg Psychiatry* 1987;50:105–106.
23. Marttila RJ, Kaprio J, Koskenvuo M, et al. PD in a nationwide twin cohort. *Neurology* 1988;38:1217–1219.
24. Vieregge P, Schiffke KA, Friedrich HJ, et al. PD in twins. *Neurology* 1992;42:1453–1461.
25. Burn DJ, Mark MH, Playford ED, et al. PD in twins studied with ^{18}F-dopa and positron emission tomography. *Neurology* 1992;42:1894–1900.
26. Holthoff VA, Vieregge P, Kessler J, et al. Discordant twins with PD: positron emission tomography and early signs of impaired cognitive circuits. *Ann Neurol* 1994; 36:176–182.
27. Johnson WG, Hodge SE, Duvoisin R. Twin studies and the genetics of PD—a reappraisal. *Mov Disord* 1990;5: 187–194.
28. Tanner CM, Ottman R, Goldman SM, et al. Parkinson's disease in twins: an etiologic study. *JAMA* 1999;281: 341–346.
29. Jablon S, Neel JV, Gershowitz H, et al. The NAS-NRC

twin panel: methods of construction of the panel, zygosity diagnosis, and proposed use. *Am J Hum Genet* 1967;19:133–161.
30. Langston JW, Widner H, Goetz CG, et al. Core Assessment Program for Intracerebral Transplantations (CAPIT). *Mov Disord* 1992;7:2–13.
31. Morgante L, Rocca WA, di Rosa AE, et al. Prevalence of PD and other types of parkinsonism: a door-to-door survey in three Sicilian municipalities. *Neurology* 1992; 42:1901–1907.
32. Tanner C, Goldman S. Epidemiology of PD. *Neurol Clin* 1996;14:317–335.
33. Piccini P, Brooks DJ. Etiology of PD: contributions from ^{18}F-DOPA positron emission tomography. *Adv Neurol* 1999;80:227–231.
34. Golbe LI. Alpha-synuclein and PD. *Mov Disord* 1999; 14:6–9.
35. Vieregge P, Hagenah J, Heberlein I, et al. PD in twins: a follow-up study. *Neurology* 1999;53:566–572.
36. Dickson D, Farrer M, Lincoln S, et al. Pathology of PD in monozygotic twins with a 20-year discordance interval. *Neurology* 2001;56:981–982.
37. Tanner CM. Progressive supranuclear palsy and multiple systems atrophy in twins. *Neurology* 2001;56[Suppl 3]:A221–A222.
38. Bharucha NE, Stokes L, Schoenberg BS, et al. A case–control study of twin pairs discordant for PD: a search for environmental risk factors. *Neurology* 1986; 36:284–288.
39. Tanner CM, Goldman SM, Aston DA, et al. Smoking and PD in twins. *Neurology* 2002;58:581–588.
40. Ottman R. Epidemiologic analysis of gene–environment interaction in twins. *Genet Epidemiol* 1994;11: 75–86.

Parkinson's Disease: Advances in Neurology, Vol. 91.
Edited by Ariel Gordin, Seppo Kaakkola,
and Heikki Teräväinen
Lippincott Williams & Wilkins, Philadelphia © 2003

15

Overview of the Genetics of Parkinsonism

Thomas Gasser

Department of Neurology, Klinikum Groβhadern, Ludwig-Maximilians-Universität, München, Germany

Parkinsonism is a clinically defined syndrome that is characterized by akinesia, rigidity, tremor, and postural instability. The most common cause of parkinsonism is Parkinson's disease (PD). PD is pathologically characterized by a rather selective degeneration of dopaminergic neurons of the substantia nigra, leading to a deficiency of dopamine in their striatal projection areas. Characteristic eosinophilic inclusions, the Lewy bodies, are found and have been considered essential for the pathological diagnosis of PD (1).

A recent major breakthrough was the mapping and cloning of a number of genes that cause monogenically inherited forms of parkinsonism with different associated pathologies and a variable, but overlapping, spectrum of clinical signs and symptoms. Although all of the mutations and loci identified so far appear to be responsible in only a small number of families, and their relevance for the vast majority of patients with PD is still unknown, there is considerable promise that the elucidation of the molecular pathways leading to monogenically inherited forms of parkinsonism will also allow insight into the common sporadic disorders and eventually allow the development of novel protective and therapeutic strategies.

MONOGENIC FORMS OF PD

A minority of patients with the typical clinical picture of PD have a positive family history compatible with a mendelian (autosomal-dominant or autosomal-recessive) inheritance. As a rule, age at onset in most of these cases is earlier, as compared with patients with sporadic disease, but no other specific clinical signs or symptoms distinguish familial from sporadic cases. Pathologically, there is degeneration of dopaminergic neurons of the substantia nigra. In some cases, as in parkin-associated parkinsonism, the pathological process appears to be highly selective, while in others, the degenerative process is more widespread (e.g., *PARK4*). In some families, there is more or less typical Lewy body pathology (*PARK1, PARK3*), while in others, there are atypical ubiquitin-positive inclusions (*PARK4*) or no Lewy bodies (*PARK2*). This observation indicates that different pathogenic processes are likely to lead to nigral cell death. Whether all those pathogenic processes are connected to a single cellular metabolic pathway and whether they have any relevance for the typical sporadic form of the disease remains to be determined. A summary of the genes and loci identified so far is given in Table 15.1.

AUTOSOMAL DOMINANTLY INHERITED PD

Five genetic loci have been identified by linkage studies to co-segregate with parkinsonism in families with dominant inheritance. To date, only one of these genes, α-synuclein, has been identified.

TABLE 15.1. *Genetically defined forms of Parkinson's disease and parkinsonism*

Locus	Inheritance	Onset	Pathology	Map position	Gene	Reference
PARK1	Dominant	40s	Nigral degeneration with Lewy bodies	4q21	α-Synuclein	(3)
PARK2	Recessive	20s	Nigral degeneration without Lewy bodies	6q25	Parkin	(29)
PARK3	Dominant	60s	Nigral degeneration with Lewy bodies, plaques and tangles in some	2p13	?	(14)
PARK4	Dominant	30s	Nigral degeneration with Lewy bodies, vacuoles in neurons of the hippocampus	4p16	?	(22)
PARK5	Dominant	~50	No pathology	4p14	Ubiquitin C-terminal hydrolase L1	(23)
PARK6	Recessive	~40	No pathology	1p35–37	?	(41)
PARK7	Recessive	~40	No pathology	1p38	?	(42)
PARK8	Dominant	~50	Nigral degeneraion, no distinctive inclusions	12	?	(1a)

Parkinson's Disease Caused by Mutations in the Gene for α-Synuclein (*PARK1*)

The first "PD gene" to be recognized was mapped to the long arm of chromosome 4 in a large family with dominant inheritance, relatively early age at onset (mean, 44 years), but otherwise typical PD with Lewy body pathology (2) and identified as the gene for α-synuclein. Only two point mutations have been recognized (3,4). The first mutation, which was found in the original Contursi family (Ala53Thr), has also been identified in several Greek kindreds (3,5,6). Haplotype analyses support the hypothesis that this is due to a founder effect (6). The second mutation was found in a small German pedigree (4).

The clinical picture in these families is compatible with idiopathic PD, although age at onset is somewhat lower (mean of about 45 years in the Contursi kindred) and progression appears to be more rapid than in sporadic cases (6,7). Pathology appears to be that of typical PD with Lewy body formation (8) but additional tau-pathology has been reported (8a).

The identification of α-synuclein as a "PD gene" led to the discovery that the encoded protein is one of the principle components of the Lewy body (9), which has always been considered to be the pathological hallmark of PD in both familial and sporadic cases. The currently favored hypothesis states that the amino acid changes in the α-synuclein protein associated with PD may favor a β-pleated sheet conformation, thereby leading to an increased tendency to form dimers and larger aggregates. The increased aggregability has been demonstrated *in vitro* (10–13). However, the precise relationship between the formation of aggregates and cell death is unknown and other mechanisms of pathogenesis may also be important. The normal function of α-synuclein is still largely unknown and may be irrelevant to the pathogenic process in PD because this is thought to result from a "gain" of a novel toxic function. A detailed discussion of the role α-synuclein in parkinsonian syndromes is presented in Chapter 17.

Parkinson's Disease Linked to Chromosome 2 (*PARK3*)

A second dominant locus has been described (*PARK3*), located on chromosome 2p13, in a subset of families with typical Lewy body pathology (14). Clinical features relatively closely resemble those of sporadic PD (15), including a similar mean age at onset (59 years in these families). Two of the families supporting linkage to this locus (families B and C) originated from a relatively small area in northern Germany and southern Denmark and share a common haplotype within the linked region, suggesting the existence of a founder effect. Based on haplotype analyses, the penetrance of the mutation was estimated to be 40%, suggesting that it might also play a role in apparently sporadic cases. So far, however, the founder haplotype has not been identified in other German patients with familial and sporadic PD (16,17), arguing against a recent and prevalent founder effect in Germany.

The gene has been mapped to a genetic distance of less than 3 cm (18). A large number of genes in this region, among them potential candidate genes such as the gene for transforming growth factor-α (19), or for sepiapterine reductase, dynactin, and semaphorin, have already been fully sequenced, but no mutation has been detected (18).

Follow-up examination over the years showed that in addition to parkinsonism, several members of chromosome 2–linked families showed signs of dementia, and neuropathology revealed, in addition to neuronal loss in the substantia nigra and typical brainstem Lewy bodies, the presence of neurofibrillary tangles and Alzheimer's plaques (20). Therefore, the underlying mutation may be associated with a range of phenotypes, which includes varying degrees of dementia and Alzheimer's disease pathology, as is also known for a subset of patients with idiopathic PD.

No other large families with linkage to 2p13 have been identified. However, recent resluts from a sib-pair study indicates a possible influence of this focus on age at onset in PD (20a).

Parkinsonism Dementia Linked to Chromosome 4p (PARK4)

A single family with parkinsonism with autosomal-dominant inheritance, originally described by Muenter et al. (21), has been linked to the short arm of chromosome 4 (22). Early onset (mean, 33.6 years) levodopa-responsive parkinsonism is the cardinal clinical feature in this family, but several atypical features have been described, including weight loss, dysautonomia, and dementia. Neuropathological changes include conspicuous vacuoles in the hippocampus and several other brain areas, in addition to nigral degeneration and Lewy body formation.

Despite the very striking phenotype (uniform onset in the mid-30s, rapid progression, and early death), there have been no other families described that conform to this clinical picture.

Parkinsonism Associated with a Mutation in the Gene for Ubiquitin Hydrolase L1 (*PARK5*)

A missense mutation in the gene for ubiquitin carboxy-terminal hydrolase L1 gene (*UCH-L1*), which is located on chromosome 4p (but outside the region supporting linkage in the Spellman-Muenter kindred, see above) has been identified in one affected family of German ancestry (23). This mutation was shown to reduce the enzymatic activity of ubiquitin hydrolase *in vitro.* The fact that this mutation again points to the importance of the proteasomal ubiquitination protein degradation pathway is intriguing (see discussion of parkin-related parkinsonism). To date, however, no other potentially pathogenic mutations of this gene have been identified (24, 25). In fact, another rare variant has been found in a family with PD, which did not segregate with the disease, raising doubts as to the pathogenic role (26).

AUTOSOMAL-RECESSIVE FORMS OF PARKINSONISM

One of the surprising recent developments was the recognition of the relatively high proportion of patients with early onset parkinsonism being caused by recessive mutations in a number of genes. So far, one of them, parkin (*PARK2*) has been cloned and extensively studied. Two others (*PARK6* and *PARK7*) have been mapped. The study of parkin-associated parkinsonism and parkin function has provided valuable insight into the molecular mechanisms of dopaminergic degeneration, particularly on the role of the cellular ubiquitination/protein degradation mechanisms in the disease process.

Autosomal-recessive Juvenile Parkinsonism (AR-JP) Caused by Mutations in the Gene for Parkin (*PARK2*)

Juvenile cases of parkinsonism with recessive inheritance were first recognized in Japan (27). Clinically, these patients suffer from levodopa-responsive parkinsonism and some show diurnal fluctuations, with symptoms becoming worse later in the day. Dystonia at the onset of the disease is quite common, and despite relatively slow progression, early and severe levodopa-induced motor fluctuations and dyskinesias may occur (27).

The genetic locus for AR-JP has been mapped to chromosome 6 (28), and mutations have been identified in a large gene in that region that was called parkin (29), a novel gene of, at that time, unknown function.

Parkin mutations turned out to be a common cause of parkinsonism with early onset, particularly in those with evidence of recessive inheritance. Nearly 50% of families from a population of sibling pairs collected by the European Consortium on Genetic Susceptibility in PD showed parkin mutations (30). A large number of mutations (deletions, insertions, point mutations, and even exon duplications and triplications) have been identified.

The European study population allowed the characterization of the clinical spectrum of parkin-associated parkinsonism. Mean age at onset in a European population was 32 years, progression of the disease was usually relatively slow, but levodopa-associated fluctuations and dyskinesias occurred frequently. Dystonia (usually in a lower extremity) at disease onset was found in about 40% of patients and brisk reflexes of the lower limbs were present in 44% (30). There was no discernible difference in the clinical phenotype between patients with missense mutations or truncating point mutations or deletions, suggesting that a complete loss of parkin function is associated with all of these mutations and with the full phenotype of early onset parkinsonism.

Although most patients became symptomatic in the third or fourth decade of life, the latest onset of the disease in the European series was at age 58 years, emphasizing that parkinsonism associated with parkin mutations is not necessarily "juvenile." More parkin-positive cases with late disease onset have been reported in the literature (31), but overall, parkin mutations are still very rare in sporadic late-onset PD. Although they seem to be responsible for most sporadic cases with onset before age 20 and are still rather common (25%) when onset is between 20 and 30, prevalence in older patients is almost certainly well below 5% (30).

The question of whether heterozygous mutations in the parkin gene can cause parkinsonism or are able to confer an increased susceptibility for typical late-onset PD is still unsettled. There is evidence from imaging studies (32) that heterozygotes may have mildly reduced uptake of fluorodopa in the basal ganglia. Furthermore, occasional families with heterozygous mutation carriers manifesting symptoms of PD have been described (31,33). In the absence of co-segregation, however, it is difficult to prove the causal relationship between genotype and phenotype. The observation of apparently heterozygous mutation carriers becoming symptomatic may also be explained by as yet undetected mutations in regulatory or intronic regions of the gene, which might affect splicing or transcription (30).

There is still relatively little information available on the neuropathology of molecularly confirmed cases of AR-JP. Severe and very selective degeneration of dopaminergic neurons and gliosis in the substantia nigra, but usually no Lewy bodies, have been described (34). The recent observation of typical ubiquitin-positive Lewy bodies in a patient with a parkin mutation (33) is difficult to reconcile with present concepts of the molecular pathogenesis of the disorder (see later discussion).

As mutations in parkin cause parkinsonism, in all likelihood, by a "loss-of-function" mechanism, the study of the normal function of parkin should provide insight into the molecular pathogenesis of the disorder. Several groups have now shown that parkin functions in the cellular ubiquitination/protein degradation pathway as a ubiquitin ligase (35,36). It is, therefore, conceivable that the loss of parkin function may lead to the accumulation of a non-ubiquitinated substrate, which is deleterious to the dopaminergic cell, but due to its non-ubiquitinated nature, does not accumulate in typical Lewy bodies (37). Several proteins have been shown to interact with parkin: an *O*-glycosylated form of α-synuclein (38), a protein associated with synaptic vesicles, CDCrel-1 (36), and a transmembrane protein, called the PAEL receptor (39) and synphilin, a protein interacting with alpha-synuclein, is intriguing. The possible interaction with α-synuclein and synphilin is intriguing, because it may provide the link between parkin-associated juvenile parkinsonism and typical late-onset PD (38,40). However, as both parkin and α-synuclein are widely expressed in the brain, this does not explain the striking selectivity of the degenerative process for dopaminergic neurons. The pael receptor, on the other hand, shows preferential expression in tyrosine hydroxylase–positive neurons (39). However, regional selectivity may well be caused by other factors—for example, the high burden of oxidative stress in dopaminergic neurons or by the lack of some, as yet undefined, compensatory mechanisms.

Recessive Early Onset Parkinsonism Linked to Chromosome 1 (*PARK6* and *PARK7*)

Very recently, two other recessive loci have been linked in families with early onset levodopa-responsive parkinsonism, both to chromosome 1: one in a large Sicilian family with four definitively affected members (the Marsala kindred). The phenotype was characterized by early onset (age range, 32 to 48 years) parkinsonism, with slow progression and sustained response to levodopa (41), which is similar to parkin-associated parkinsonism. Preliminary analyses suggest that this gene may also be responsible in more than a limited number of patients and families.

A second novel recessive locus, *PARK7*, has been mapped by van Duijn et al. (42), in a consanguineous Italian family. Again, the clinical picture is that of early onset, levodopa-responsive parkinsonism, but little else is known at this time.

GENETIC CONTRIBUTION TO SPORADIC PD

Although molecular genetic analysis has produced significant progress in families with parkinsonian phenotypes with mendelian inheritance, it must be remembered that in most cases, PD is a sporadic disorder. There is a subset of about 5% to 15% of families with more than one affected family member. Secondary cases are found more frequently among relatives of patients with PD than in an unaffected control population (43–45), but a clear mode of inheritance cannot be established. The type and the extent of a genetic contribution to nonmendelian PD is still controversial. A population-based case–control study indicates that the relative risk for first-degree family members of patients with PD is increased only on the order of 2 to 3 (46). A first segregation analysis was compatible with an inherited component to the age at onset of the disease, and not to the development of the disease itself (47); a second study of this kind (performed in Finland) confirmed a genetic factor in PD but was unable to distinguish between autosomal-dominant and autosomal-recessive inheritance (48).

A very large twin study indicates that genetic causes may be important, particularly in young-onset cases (onset before age 50 years) but appear negligible in those with onset at older than 50 years, a distinction that was also evident in one of the segregation studies (49).

Most attempts to identify the susceptibility genes, which are operative in these populations, have followed a candidate gene approach. Based on pathological, pathobiochemical, and epidemiological findings, hypotheses on the etiology of PD can be generated and genetic polymorphisms within, or closely linked to, genes that are thought to be involved in these pathways have been examined. Unfortunately, no consistent findings have emerged so far. A selection of genes studied are shown in Table 15.2. Despite a large number of initial positive results, findings have not been confirmed beyond doubt in any of these cases, indicating that studies with improved methodology (e.g., transmission disequilibrium testing [50] and the examination of haplotypes instead of single polymorphisms [51]) may be necessary.

A second approach to identify putative genetic risk factors for PD is the genome-wide analysis of a large population of small PD families (affected sibling pairs or affected pedigree members) with polymorphic DNA markers. The results of two of these studies have now become available (52,53). Several genomic regions with moderately positive lod scores (1.0 to 1.5) have been identified in these studies, but only a region on chromosome 9q appeared in both studies. However, one of the methodologic limitations of this type of study is that the identified regions are too large to be useful for the identification of specific candidate genes. Nevertheless, this approach will be valuable because it can be expanded to still larger patient populations and denser marker maps using single nucleotide polymorphisms, instead of the microsatellite markers commonly used today.

OTHER GENETIC DISORDERS PRESENTING WITH SIGNS AND SYMPTOMS OF PARKINSONISM

Recently, it has become apparent that a number of inherited neurodegenerative conditions that are neuropathologically and usually clinically clearly distinct from PD can present with signs and symptoms of parkinsonism and may sometimes, at least in initial stages of the disease, mimic idiopathic PD.

One of these disorders, the group of frontotemporal dementias with parkinsonism linked to chromosome 17 (FTDP-17), which are characterized by a pathological deposition of the microtubule-associated protein tau has received considerable attention (54). Mutations in the *tau* gene have been identified (55,56), located in exon-9, -10, -12, and -13,

TABLE 15.2. *Association studies in Parkinson's disease*

Candidate gene	Locus	Positive (or negative) association	No association
Dopaminergic transmission			
Dopamine D_2 receptor	11q22–23	(69)	(70)
Dopamine D_3 receptor	3q13.3		(70)
Dopamine D_4 receptor	11p15.5		(70)
Dopamine transporter	5p15.3	(71)	(69,72)
Tyrosine hydroxylase	11p15.5		(69)
Catechol-*O*-methyltransferase	22q12.1	(73)	(74)
Monoamine oxidase A	X		(75)
Monoamine oxidase B	Xp11.3	(76,77)	(78)
Heme oxygenase 1	22q12		(79)
Xenobiotic metabolism			
Debrisoquine-4-hydroxylase	22q13	(80–82)	(83,84)
Cytochrome P450 1A1	5q22–24		(85)
Paraoxonase 1	7q21.3	(86)	(87,88)
N-Acetyltransferase 2	8p23.1	(89,90)	(91)
Protein aggregation			
Apolipoprotein E	19q13.2	(92)	(93)
α-Synuclein	4q21.3–22	(92)	(94)
Ubiquitin carboxy-termal hydrolase L1	4p15	(95)	(96)

Note: Only a few studies are cited as representative examples.

or in adjacent intronic sequences, affecting the microtubule-binding repeat domain encoded by this part of the gene.

In most families, behavioral disturbances and dementia are the most prominent symptoms, with parkinsonism and other neurological disturbances such as supranuclear gaze palsy, pyramidal tract dysfunction, and urinary incontinence appearing to a variable degree during the later course of the disease. In other families, rapidly progressive levodopa-unresponsive parkinsonism with supranuclear gaze palsy is the leading symptom. Some mutations have been found to be associated with various clinical phenotypes, resembling Pick's disease, progressive supranuclear palsy (PSP), or corticobasal degeneration in different families and within single families (57).

A detailed discussion of inherited tau-related parkinsonian syndromes is presented in Chapter 16.

Other Tauopathies

PSP and corticobasal ganglionic degeneration (CBGD) are two other distinct entities with some overlapping clinical features, which are pathologically characterized by the deposition of abnormally phosphorylated tau protein. With very few notable exceptions, these disorders are sporadic, and no mutations in the coding region or in the splice sites of the *tau* gene have been identified in most patients.

Nevertheless, there appears to be a genetic susceptibility to the disease related to a particular haplotype of DNA markers surrounding the *tau* gene. Initially, Conrad et al. (58) observed that the "A0" allele of a dinucleotide repeat marker within the *tau* gene is highly associated, in homozygous form, with PSP. This allele was later found to be part of an extended haplotype (*H-1* haplotype) of more than 100 kb, which is usually inherited "en bloc" (59) and the strong association was confirmed. The same genetic background is found in patients with CBGD, supporting the close relationship between these two disorders (60).

Very recent evidence suggests that *tau* may also play a role in a subset of patients with clinically typical PD, indicating that the molecular pathways involved in neurodegeneration may be tightly interconnected (53,61).

Other Inherited Neurological Disorders Occasionally Presenting with Parkinsonism

The widespread use of molecular diagnosis in inherited neurological disorders has shown that the phenotypical spectrum of several disorders caused by expansions of CAG repeats may include late-onset levodopa-responsive parkinsonism or atypical parkinsonian syndromes. This has been shown for Huntington's disease (62,63) and for spinocerebellar ataxia type 2 (64) and type 3 (65,66).

Another inherited disorder occasionally presenting with parkinsonism is dopa-responsive dystonia (DRD). The phenotype is usually characterized by a childhood-onset dystonia, affecting the extremities first. Mild parkinsonism of adult onset has long been recognized as one clinical feature of the disease and may be the sole manifestation in some gene carriers (67). The positive family history of more typical childhood-onset DRD usually indicates the correct diagnosis. However, early onset parkinsonism not uncommonly presents with dystonia as a first symptom, making it difficult to distinguish from DRD in some cases. In fact, three of 22 cases with a phenotype of DRD proved to be due to mutations in the parkin gene (68).

CONCLUSIONS

The genetic findings in rare inherited forms of PD have contributed to our understanding of the clinical, neuropathological, and genetic heterogeneity of PD. The variability of clinical features, such as age at onset and occurrence of dementia or other associated features that has been found within single families, suggests that a single genetic cause (the pathogenic mutation in a given family) can lead to a spectrum of clinical manifestations. On the other hand, individuals with different genetic defects and different neuropathology may be clinically indistinguishable from each other and fulfill all presently accepted criteria of idiopathic PD. It is therefore apparent that a new genetic classification of PD, which is only partially congruent with the classic clinicopathological classification, is about to emerge.

There is convincing evidence that genetic factors play an important role in the etiology of at least a subset of patients with PD. Only a very small percentage of cases with dominant or recessive inheritance can probably be explained by mutations in the genes that have been identified so far (the genes for α-synuclein, ubiquitin carboxy-terminal hydrolase L1, and parkin) or by mutations in the as yet unidentified genes on chromosomes 1p, 2p, and 4p. The study of wild-type and mutated gene products will provide important insight into the molecular pathogenesis of nigral degeneration. However, it appears that intense efforts are still needed to unravel the full spectrum of etiological factors leading to the sporadic form of this common neurodegenerative disorder.

REFERENCES

1. Gibb WR, Lees AJ. The significance of the Lewy body in the diagnosis of idiopathic Parkinson's disease. *Neuropathol Appl Neurobiol* 1989;15:27–44.

1a. Funayama M, Hasegawa K, Kowa H, Saito M, Tsuji S, Obata F. A new locus for Parkinsons disease (PARK8) maps to chromosome 12p11.2-q13.1. *Ann Neurol* 2002; 51(3):296–301.

2. Polymeropoulos MH, Higgins JJ, Golbe LI, et al. Mapping of a gene for Parkinson's disease to chromosome 4q21-q23. *Science* 1996;274:1197–1199.

3. Polymeropoulos MH, Lavedan C, Leroy E, et al. Mutation in the α-synuclein gene identified in families with Parkinson's disease. *Science* 1997;276:2045–2047.

4. Krüger R, Kuhn W, Müller T, et al. Ala39Pro mutation in the gene encoding α-synuclein in Parkinson's disease. *Nat Genet* 1998;18:106–108.

5. Markopoulou K, Wszolek ZK, Pfeiffer RF. A Greek-American kindred with autosomal dominant, levodopa-responsive parkinsonism and anticipation. *Ann Neurol* 1995;38:373–378.

6. Papadimitriou A, Veletza V, Hadjigeorgiou GM, et al. Mutated alpha-synuclein gene in two Greek kindreds with familial PD: incomplete penetrance? *Neurology* 1999;52:651–654.

7. Golbe LI, Di Iorio G, Sanges G, et al. Clinical genetic analysis of Parkinson's disease in the Contursi kindred. *Ann Neurol* 1996;40:767–775.

8. Golbe LI, Di Iorio G, Bonavita V, et al. A large kindred with autosomal dominant Parkinson's disease. *Ann Neurol* 1990;27:276–282.

8a. Duda JE, Lee VM, Tojanowski JQ. Neuropathology of synuclein aggregates. *J Neurosci Res* 2000;61(2): 121–127.

9. Spillantini MG, Schmidt ML, Lee VM, et al. Alpha-synuclein in Lewy bodies. *Nature* 1997;388:839–840.

10. Goedert M, Spillantini MG, Davies SW. Filamentous nerve cell inclusions in neurodegenerative diseases. *Curr Opin Neurobiol* 1998;8:619–632.

11. Biere AL, Wood SJ, Wypych J, et al. Parkinson's disease associated alpha-synuclein is more fibrillogenic than beta- and gamma-synuclein and cannot cross-seed its homologs. *J Biol Chem* 2000;275:34574–34579.

12. Conway KA, Lee SJ, Rochet JC, et al. Acceleration of oligomerization, not fibrillization, is a shared property of both alpha-synuclein mutations linked to early-onset Parkinson's disease: implications for pathogenesis and therapy. *Proc Natl Acad Sci USA* 2000;97:571–576.

13. Conway KA, Harper JD, Lansbury PT. Accelerated *in vitro* fibril formation by a mutant alpha-synuclein linked to early-onset Parkinson disease. *Nat Med* 1998; 4:1318–1320.

14. Gasser T, Müller-Myhsok B, Wszolek ZK, et al. A susceptibility locus for Parkinson's disease maps to chromosome 2p13. *Nat Genet* 1998;18:262–265.

15. Wszolek ZK, Cordes M, Calne DB, et al. Hereditary Parkinson disease: report of 3 families with dominant autosomal inheritance. *Nervenarzt* 1993;64:331–335.

16. Gasser T, Bereznai B, Wieditz G, et al. Evaluation of a Danish/German founder haplotype at the *PARK3*-locus on chromosome 2p13. *Mov Disord* 1999;13[Suppl 2]: 103.

17. Klein C, Vieregge P, Hagenah J, et al. Search for the PARK3 founder haplotype in a large cohort of patients with Parkinson's disease from northern Germany. *Ann Hum Genet* 1999;63:285–291.

18. West AB, Zimprich A, Lockhart PJ, et al. Refinement of the *PARK3* locus on chromosome 2p13 and the analysis of 14 candidate genes. *Eur J Hum Genet* 2001;9: 659–666.

19. Zink M, Grimm L, Wszolek ZK, et al. Autosomal-dominant Parkinson's disease linked to 2p13 is not caused by mutations in transforming growth factor alpha (TGF alpha). *J Neural Transm* 2001;108:1029–1034.

20. Wszolek ZK, Gwinn-Hardy K, Wszolek EK, et al. Family C (German-American) with late onset parkinsonism: longitudinal observations including autopsy. *Neurology* 1999;52[Suppl 2]:A221.

20a. DeStefano AL, Lew MF, Golbe LI, Mark MH, Lazzarini AM, Guttman M, et al. PARK3 influences age at onset in Parkinson disease: a genome scan in the GenePD study. *Am J Hum Genet* 2002;70(5).

21. Muenter MD, Forno LS, Hornykiewicz O, et al. Hereditary form of parkinsonism–dementia. *Ann Neurol* 1998;43:768–781.

22. Farrer M, Gwinn-Hardy K, Muenter M, et al. A chromosome 4p haplotype segregating with Parkinson's disease and postural tremor. *Hum Mol Genet* 1999;8: 81–85.

23. Leroy E, Boyer R, Auburger G, et al. The ubiquitin pathway in Parkinson's disease. *Nature* 1998;395:451–452.

24. Harhangi BS, Farrer MJ, Lincoln S, et al. The Ile93Met mutation in the ubiquitin carboxy-terminal-hydrolase-L1 gene is not observed in European cases with familial Parkinson's disease. *Neurosci Lett* 1999;270:1–4.
25. Lincoln S, Vaughan J, Wood N, et al. Low frequency of pathogenic mutations in the ubiquitin carboxy-terminal hydrolase gene in familial Parkinson's disease. *Neuroreport* 1999;10:427–429.
26. Farrer M, Destee T, Becquet E, et al. Linkage exclusion in French families with probable Parkinson' s disease. *Mov Disord* 2000;15:1075–1083.
27. Ishikawa A, Tsuji S. Clinical analysis of 17 patients in 12 Japanese families with autosomal-recessive type juvenile parkinsonism. *Neurology* 1996;47:160–166.
28. Matsumine H, Saito M, Shimoda-Matsubayashi S, et al. Localization of a gene for an autosomal recessive form of juvenile parkinsonism to chromosome 6q25.2-27. *Am J Hum Genet* 1997;60:588–596.
29. Kitada T, Asakawa S, Hattori N, et al. Mutations in the parkin gene cause autosomal recessive juvenile parkinsonism. *Nature* 1998;392:605–608.
30. Lücking CB, Dürr A, Bonifati V, et al. Association between early-onset Parkinson's disease and mutations in the parkin gene. *N Engl J Med* 2000;342:1560–1567.
31. Klein C, Pramstaller PP, Kis B, et al. Parkin deletions in a family with adult-onset, tremor-dominant parkinsonism: expanding the phenotype. *Ann Neurol* 2000;48:65–71.
32. Hilker R, Klein C, Ghaemi M, et al. Positron emission tomographic analysis of the nigrostriatal dopaminergic system in familial parkinsonism associated with mutations in the parkin gene. *Ann Neurol* 2001;49:367–376.
33. Farrer M, Chan P, Chen R, et al. Lewy bodies and parkinsonism in families with parkin mutations. *Ann Neurol* 2001;50:293–300.
34. Takahashi H, Ohama E, Suzuki S, et al. Familial juvenile parkinsonism: clinical and pathologic study in a family. *Neurology* 1994;44:437–441.
35. Shimura H, Hattori N, Kubo S, et al. Familial Parkinson's disease gene product, parkin, is a ubiquitin-protein ligase. *Nat Genet* 2000;25:302–305.
36. Zhang Y, Gao J, Chung KK, et al. Parkin functions as an E2-dependent ubiquitin-protein ligase and promotes the degradation of the synaptic vesicle-associated protein, CDCrel-1. *Proc Natl Acad Sci USA* 2000;97: 13354–13359.
37. Kahle PJ, Leimer U, Haass C. Does failure of parkin-mediated ubiquitination cause juvenile parkinsonism? *Trends Biochem Sci* 2000;25:524–527.
38. Shimura H, Schlossmacher MG, Hattori N, et al. Ubiquitination of a new form of alpha-synuclein by parkin from human brain: implications for Parkinson's disease. *Science* 2001;293:263–269.
39. Imai Y, Soda M, Inoue H, et al. An unfolded putative transmembrane polypeptide, which can lead to endoplasmic reticulum stress, is a substrate of parkin. *Cell* 2001;105:891–902.
40. Chung KK, Zhang Y, Lim KL, et al. Parkin ubiquitinates the alpha-synuclein-interacting protein, synphilin-1: implications for Lewy-body formation in Parkinson's disease. *Nat Med* 2001;7:1144–1150.
41. Valente EM, Bentivoglio AR, Dixon PH, et al. Localization of a novel locus for autosomal recessive early-onset parkinsonism, park6, on human chromosome 1p35-p36. *Am J Hum Genet* 2001;68:895–900.
42. van Duijn CM, Dekker MC, Bonifati V, et al. *Park7,* a novel locus for autosomal recessive early-onset parkinsonism, on chromosome 1p36. *Am J Hum Genet* 2001; 69:629–634.
43. Bonifati V, Fabrizio E, Vanacore N, et al. Familial Parkinson's disease: a clinical genetic analysis. *Can J Neurol Sci* 1995;22:272–279.
44. Payami H, Larsen K, Bernard S, et al. Increased risk of Parkinson's disease in parents and siblings of patients. *Ann Neurol* 1994;36:659–661.
45. De Michele G, Filla A, Volpe G, et al. Environmental and genetic risk factors in Parkinson's disease: a case–control study in southern Italy. *Mov Disord* 1996;11:17–23.
46. Marder K, Tang MX, Mejia H, et al. Risk of Parkinson's disease among first-degree relatives: a community-based study. *Neurology* 1996;47:155–160.
47. Zareparsi S, Taylor TD, Harris EL, et al. Segregation analysis of Parkinson's disease. *Am J Med Genet* 1998; 80:410–417.
48. Moilanen JS, Myllylä VV, Autere JM, et al. Complex segregation analysis of Parkinson's disease in the Finnish population. *Hum Genet* 2001;108:184–189.
49. Tanner CM, Ottman R, Goldman SM, et al. Parkinson's disease in twins: an etiologic study. *JAMA* 1999;281: 341–346.
50. Spielman RS, Ewens WJ. A sibship test for linkage in the presence of association: the sib transmission/disequilibrium test. *Am J Hum Genet* 1998;62:450–458.
51. Seltman H, Roeder K, Devlin B. Transmission/disequilibrium test meets measured haplotype analysis: family-based association analysis guided by evolution of haplotypes. *Am J Hum Genet* 2001;68:1250–1263.
52. DeStefano AL, Golbe LI, Mark MH, et al. Genome-wide scan for Parkinson's disease: the GenePD Study. *Neurology* 2001;57:1124–1126.
53. Scott WK, Nance MA, Watts RL, et al. Complete genomic screen in Parkinson disease: evidence for multiple genes. *JAMA* 2001;286:2239–2244.
54. Spillantini MG, Goedert M. *Tau* gene mutations and *tau* pathology in frontotemporal dementia and parkinsonism linked to chromosome 17. *Adv Exp Med Biol* 2001; 487:21–37.
55. Hutton M, Lendon CL, Rizzu P, et al. Association of missense and 5'-splice-site mutations in *tau* with the inherited dementia FTDP-17. *Nature* 1998;393:702–705.
56. Hutton M. Missense and splice site mutations in *tau* associated with FTDP-17: multiple pathogenic mechanisms. *Neurology* 2001;56:S21–S25.
57. Reed LA, Wszolek ZK, Hutton M. Phenotypic correlations in FTDP-17. *Neurobiol Aging* 2001;22:89–107.
58. Conrad C, Andreadis A, Trojanowski JQ, et al. Genetic evidence for the involvement of *tau* in progressive supranuclear palsy. *Ann Neurol* 1997;41:277–281.
59. Baker M, Litvan I, Houlden H, et al. Association of an extended haplotype in the *tau* gene with progressive supranuclear palsy. *Hum Mol Genet* 1999;8:711–715.
60. Houlden H, Baker M, Morris HR, et al. Corticobasal degeneration and progressive supranuclear palsy share a common tau haplotype. *Neurology* 2001;56:1702–1706.
61. Martin ER, Scott WK, Nance MA, et al. Association of single-nucleotide polymorphisms of the *tau* gene with late-onset Parkinson's disease. *JAMA* 2001;286: 2245–2250.
62. Racette BA, Perlmutter JS. Levodopa responsive parkinsonism in an adult with Huntington's disease. *J Neurol Neurosurg Psychiatry* 1998;65:577–579.

63. Reuter I, Hu MT, Andrews TC, et al. Late onset levodopa responsive Huntington's disease with minimal chorea masquerading as Parkinson plus syndrome. *J Neurol Neurosurg Psychiatry* 2000;68:238–241.
64. Gwinn-Hardy K, Chen JY, Liu HC, et al. Spinocerebellar ataxia type 2 with parkinsonism in ethnic Chinese. *Neurology* 2000;55:800–805.
65. Tuite PJ, Rogaeva EA, St George Hyslop PH, et al. Dopa-responsive parkinsonism phenotype of Machado–Joseph disease: confirmation of 14q CAG expansion. *Ann Neurol* 1995;38:684–687.
66. Gwinn-Hardy K, Singleton A, O'Suilleabhain P, et al. Spinocerebellar ataxia type 3 phenotypically resembling Parkinson's disease in a black family. *Arch Neurol* 2001;58:296–299.
67. Nygaard TG, Trugman JM, de Yebenes JG, et al. Dopa-responsive dystonia: the spectrum of clinical manifestations in a large North American family. *Neurology* 1990;40:66–69.
68. Tassin J, Durr A, Bonnet AM, et al. Levodopa-responsive dystonia: GTP cyclohydrolase I or parkin mutations? *Brain* 2000;123:1112–1121.
69. Plante Bordeneuve V, Taussig D, Thomas F, et al. Evaluation of four candidate genes encoding proteins of the dopamine pathway in familial and sporadic Parkinson's disease: evidence for association of a DRD2 allele. *Neurology* 1997;48:1589–1593.
70. Nanko S, Ueki A, Hattori M, et al. No allelic association between Parkinson's disease and dopamine D_2, D_3, and D_4 receptor gene polymorphisms. *Am J Med Genet* 1994;54:361–364.
71. Le Couteur DG, Leighton PW, McCann SJ, et al. Association of a polymorphism in the dopamine-transporter gene with Parkinson's disease. *Mov Disord* 1997;12: 760–763.
72. Leighton PW, Le Couteur DG, Pang CC, et al. The dopamine transporter gene and Parkinson's disease in a Chinese population. *Neurology* 1997;49:1577–1579.
73. Yoritaka A, Hattori N, Yoshino H, et al. Catechol-*O*-methyltransferase genotype and susceptibility to Parkinson's disease in Japan. *J Neural Transm* 1997; 104:1313–1317.
74. Xie T, Ho SL, Li LS, et al. G/A1947 polymorphism in catechol-*O*-methyltransferase (COMT) gene in Parkinson's disease. *Mov Disord* 1997;12:426–427.
75. Hotamisligil GS, Girmen AS, Fink JS, et al. Hereditary variations in monoamine oxidase as a risk factor for Parkinson's disease. *Mov Disord* 1994;9:305–310.
76. Costa P, Checkoway H, Levy D, et al. Association of a polymorphism in intron 13 of the monoamine oxidase B gene with Parkinson disease. *Am J Med Genet* 1997;74: 154–156.
77. Kurth JH, Kurth MC, Poduslo SE, et al. Association of a monoamine oxidase B allele with Parkinson's disease. *Ann Neurol* 1993;33:368–372.
78. Ho SL, Kapadi AL, Ramsden DB, et al. An allelic association study of monoamine oxidase B in Parkinson's disease. *Ann Neurol* 1995;37:403–405.
79. Kimpara T, Takeda A, Watanabe K, et al. Microsatellite polymorphism in the human heme oxygenase-1 gene promoter and its application in association studies with Alzheimer and Parkinson disease. *Hum Genet* 1997; 100:145–147.
80. Wilhelmsen KC, Wszolek ZK. Is there a genetic susceptibility to idiopathic parkinsonism? *Parkinson Related Disord* 1995;1:73–84.
81. Armstrong M, Daly AK, Cholerton S, et al. Mutant debrisoquine hydroxylation genes in Parkinson's disease. *Lancet* 1992;339:1017–1018.
82. Smith CA, Gough AC, Leigh PN, et al. Debrisoquine hydroxylase gene polymorphism and susceptibility to Parkinson's disease. *Lancet* 1992;339:1375–1377.
83. Diederich N, Hilger C, Goetz CG, et al. Genetic variability of the CYP2D6 gene is not a risk factor for sporadic Parkinson's disease. *Ann Neurol* 1996;40:463–465.
84. Gasser T, Müller-Myhsok B, Supala A, et al. The CYP2D6B-allele is not over-represented in a population of German patients with idiopathic Parkinson's disease. *J Neurol Neurosurg Psychiatry* 1996;61:518–520.
85. Takakubo F, Yamamoto M, Ogawa N, et al. Genetic association between cytochrome P450IA1 gene and susceptibility to Parkinson's disease. *J Neural Transm Gen Sect* 1996;103:843–849.
86. Akhmedova SN, Yakimovsky AK, Schwartz EI. Paraoxonase 1 Met-Leu 54 polymorphism is associated with Parkinson's disease. *J Neurol Sci* 2001;184:179–182.
87. Wang J, Liu Z. No association between paraoxonase 1 (*PON1*) gene polymorphisms and susceptibility to Parkinson's disease in a Chinese population. *Mov Disord* 2000;15:1265–1267.
88. Taylor MC, Le Couteur DG, Mellick GD, et al. Paraoxonase polymorphisms, pesticide exposure and Parkinson's disease in a Caucasian population. *J Neural Transm* 2000;107:979–983.
89. Agundez JA, Jimenez-Jimenez FJ, Luengo A, et al. Slow allotypic variants of the *NAT2* gene and susceptibility to early-onset Parkinson's disease. *Neurology* 1998;51:1587–1592.
90. Bandmann O, Vaughan JR, Holmans P, et al. Association of slow acetylator genotype for *N*-acetyltransferase 2 with familial Parkinson's disease. *Lancet* 1998;350: 1136–1139.
91. Harhangi BS, Oostra BA, Heutink P, et al. *N*-acetyltransferase-2 polymorphism in Parkinson's disease: the Rotterdam study. *J Neurol Neurosurg Psychiatry* 1999; 67:518–520.
92. Kruger R, Vieira-Saecker AM, Kuhn W, et al. Increased susceptibility to sporadic Parkinson's disease by a certain combined alpha-synuclein/apolipoprotein E genotype. *Ann Neurol* 1999;45:611–617.
93. Whitehead AS, Bertrandy S, Finnan F, et al. Frequency of the apolipoprotein E epsilon 4 allele in a case–control study of early onset Parkinson's disease. *J Neurol Neurosurg Psychiatry* 1996;61:347–351.
94. Parsian A, Racette B, Zhang ZH, et al. Mutation, sequence analysis, and association studies of alpha-synuclein in Parkinson's disease. *Neurology* 1998;51: 1757–1759.
95. Maraganore DM, Farrer MJ, Hardy JA, et al. Case–control study of the ubiquitin carboxy-terminal hydrolase L1 gene in Parkinson's disease. *Neurology* 1999;53: 1858–1860.
96. Mellick GD, Silburn PA. The ubiquitin carboxy-terminal hydrolase-L1 gene S18Y polymorphism does not confer protection against idiopathic Parkinson's disease. *Neurosci Lett* 2000;293:127–130.

Parkinson's Disease: Advances in Neurology, Vol. 91.
Edited by Ariel Gordin, Seppo Kaakkola, and Heikki Teräväinen
Lippincott Williams & Wilkins, Philadelphia © 2003

16

Hereditary Tauopathies and Parkinsonism

*Zbigniew K. Wszolek, *Yoshio Tsuboi, †Mathew Farrer, *Ryan J. Uitti, and †Mike L. Hutton

**Department of Neurology and the †Neuroscience Research Laboratory, Mayo Clinic, Jacksonville, Florida*

HEREDITARY TAUOPATHIES

Tau is an intracellular protein that promotes assembly and stabilization of microtubules (1). Microtubules are cellular structures responsible for axonal transport. Tau protein consists of six major isoforms resulting from splicing of exon-2, -3, or -10 of the *tau* gene located on the long arm of chromosome 17. In the physiological state of the adult brain, the ratio of 3-repeat (3R) to 4-repeat (4R) tau remains equal to 1 (2).

Hyperphosphorylation of tau leads to less solubility and formation of pathological filaments and inclusions (3). Disorders with pathological neuronal and glial tau accumulation are known as tauopathies (4). Tauopathies include movement disorders such as progressive supranuclear palsy (PSP), corticobasal ganglionic degeneration (CBGD), and neurodegeneration with brain iron accumulation (NBIA-1); dementive disorders such as Alzheimer's disease, Pick's disease, and dementia pugilistica; and "overlap" syndromes with both movement disorders and dementia components such as parkinsonism–dementia complex of Guam, subacute sclerosing panencephalitis, Niemann–Pick disease type C, and others (5). From the perspective of genetic aspects, the major familial tauopathy is a frontotemporal dementia and parkinsonism linked to chromosome 17 (FTDP-17). The mutations on the *tau* gene in FTDP-17 disorders can lead to accumulation of either 3R or 4R *tau* isoforms. On the other hand, only 4R *tau* isoforms accumulate in PSP and CBGD. Mainly 3R *tau* isoforms accumulate in Pick's disease. In Alzheimer's disease, the ratio of 3R to 4R tau remains equal to 1 (5–7).

HISTORY OF FTDP-17

The term "FTDP-17" was introduced during an international consensus conference held in Ann Arbor, Michigan, in 1996. Then, only 13 kindreds were definitely or probably linked to the *wld* locus on chromosome 17 (8). On the basis of available clinical information from these 13 kindreds, the clinical features of FTDP-17 were elucidated. They were grouped into three major categories: behavioral, cognitive, and motor disturbances. The *behavioral disturbances* included impaired social conduct, hyperorality, hyperphagia, obsessive stereotyped behavior, and psychosis. The *cognitive disturbances* included disturbed executive functions, whereas visuospatial, orientation, and common memory functions were relatively preserved until late in the illness. The most frequently observed *motor disturbances* consisted of parkinsonism characterized by rigidity, bradykinesia, postural instability, and poor response to dopaminergic therapy. This occurred either early or late in the illness. The other *motor disturbances* included dystonia, spasticity, supranuclear gaze palsy, and even weakness due to amyotrophy.

PROGRESS IN THE STUDY OF FTDP-17 SINCE 1996

Since the consensus conference the major progress has been in the area of molecular genetics. Missense and deletion mutations have been identified in the *tau* gene on chromosome 17 (9–11). To date, 26 different mutations have been reported located on exon-1, -9, -10, -12, and -13 and intron after exon-10 in the *tau* gene (Table 16.1). These mutations were described in 62 separately ascertained families.

Progress has been made in understanding clinical aspects of FTDP-17. Previously unpublished clinical and pathological information has become available on some of the original 13 families. The identification of new families demonstrates that FTDP-17 occurs in a worldwide distribution.

Fifteen families were identified in the United States; 12 in Japan; 8 in Great Britain; 7 each in France and the Netherlands; 5 in Canada; 2 each in Australia, Italy, and Germany; and 1 each in Spain and Sweden. It is impossible to estimate the prevalence and incidence indices of FTDP-17. It is still an extremely rare condition. From published reports, the estimated total number of affected patients from all 62 known families is 470, including deceased individuals. The most prevalent mutation is exon-10 P301L missense mutation. It has been identified in 21 separately ascertained kindreds with 148 affected individuals. The second most frequent mutation is exon-10 5′ splice site plus 16 intronic mutation described in eight separately ascertained families, including 78 affected individuals. The exon-10 N279K missense mutation is the third most prevalent mutation, present in five separately ascertained kindreds with 52 affected family members.

PHENOTYPICAL AND GENOTYPICAL CORRELATIONS

The average age at symptomatic disease onset of FTDP-17 is 49 years (range, 25 to 76 years; data from 50 families). The average duration of the disease is 8.5 years (range, from 2 to 26 years; data from 33 families) (12).

The phenotypical presentation of FTDP-17 kindreds is extremely variable (Table 16.2). It varies not only with different mutations but also among kindreds with the same mutation. In addition, affected individuals from the same family may present with different clinical phenotypes. The personality and behavioral changes are probably the most frequent clinical features because they are seen in almost all described kindreds. In contrast, the occurrence of dementia and parkinsonism is more variable. Depending on the clinical presentation, the FTDP-17 families can be divided into two major groups:

1. Families with dementia-predominant phenotype
2. Families with parkinsonism-predominant phenotype

In general, non–exon-10 missense mutations lead to a dementia-predominant phenotype. Motor symptoms such as parkinsonism, eye movement abnormalities, dystonia, and upper and lower motor neuron dysfunction are rarely seen in patients with these mutations. On the other hand, many if not most of

TABLE 16.1. *Known mutations in frontotemporal dementia and parkinsonism linked to chromosome 17 (FTDP-17)*

Site	Mutation			
		Non–exon 10 mutations		
Exon 1	R5W	R5H		
Exon 9	K257T	I260V	G272V	
Exon 12	V337M	E342V	K369I	
Exon 13	G389R	R406W		
		Exon 10 and splice-site mutations		
Exonic	N279K	Δ280K	L284L	delN296
	N296N	N296H	P301L	P301S
5′ Splice site	S305N (−2)	S305S (−1)	+3	+11
	+12	+13	+14	+16

TABLE 16.2. *Clinical features that can indicate specific mutations in the* tau *gene*

	Mutations not in exon 10					
	Exon 1	Exon 9	Exon 12	Exon 13	Mutations in exon 10	Exon 10 5′ splice-site mutations
Age at onset, yr						
≤30					P301S	
31–40				G389R	delN296	−2
41–50		G272V	E342V		N279K P301L	+3 +11 +14 +16
≥51	R5H		V337M	R406W	L284L S305S del280K	+12 +13
Duration, yr						
≤5	R5H			G389R	del280 delN296	−2
6–10		G272V	E342V		N279K L284L P301L P301S	−1 +11 +12
11–15			V337M			+3 +14 +16
>15				R406W		
First sign						
Parkinsonism					N279K P301L delN296	−1 +3 +11
Dementia	R5H			R406W	L284L delN296	+3 +12
Personality change		G272V	V337M E342V		P301L	−2 −1 +12 +14 +16
Parkinsonism						
Early prominent					N279K delN296	−1 +11
Late prominent					P301S	+3 +12 +14 +16
Rare minimal		G272V			P301L	−2
Dementia						
Early prominent				R406W		−1 +12
Late prominent		G272V	V337M		del280K L284L P301L P301S	−2 +3 +11 +13
Rare minimal					N279K	
Personality change						
Early prominent		G272V	V337M	R406W	del280K L284L P301L P301S	−2 −1 +12 +14 +16
Eye movement abnormalities					N279K P301S delN296	−1 +3
Epilepsy					P301S	
Myoclonus			V337M		P301S	+11
Pyramidal signs					N279K	−1 +3 +12
Amyotrophy					P301L	+14

affected individuals harboring the exon-10 missense and intronic mutations develop parkinsonism-predominant phenotype quite frequently in the early stages of their illness. However, some of these families, particularly those with P301L mutation, demonstrate considerable phenotypical variation.

It is plausible to speculate that these phenotypical variations are due to different basic molecular mechanisms occurring in these families. Available autopsy data in families with non–exon-10 missense mutations usually demonstrate widespread cortical neuronal pathological features with the presence of straight filaments composed of six *tau* isoforms. On the other hand, autopsy data from families with exon-10 missense and 5′ splice-site intronic mutations reveal cortical and subcortical neuronal and glial pathological features with the presence of filamentous formations containing 4R *tau* isoforms. However, there are some families without available pathological data. Consequently, these types of correlations need further verification.

CLINICAL PRESENTATION OF SELECTED MUTATIONS AND KINDREDS

The exon-10 P301L missense mutation is the most prevalent FTDP-17 mutation. It has been identified in 22 separately ascertained kindreds with worldwide distribution (9,13–21). It is thought that the founder effect may be involved in some of the Dutch and French Canadian families (M. L. Hutton, *personal communication, 2001*). The usual presenting symptoms include personality and behavioral changes, particularly disinhibition and language difficulties, but in some cases, parkinsonism is present from the onset of the illness (Seattle family D). However, parkinsonian signs usually develop late in the disease. On autopsy, neuronal loss in the substantia nigra is almost always evident, even in cases with minimal or nonparkinsonian symptoms (13–21).

The exon-10 P301S missense mutation affects three kindreds: Italian, German, and Japanese (22–24). The phenotype of the German kindred is dominated by the occurrence of a severe seizure disorder unresponsive to conventional anticonvulsive therapy. Some of the affected individuals from this kindred even died of status epilepticus. Thus, the clinical presentation of this mutation extends our knowledge of the FTDP-17 phenotype. Interestingly, seizures are not observed in the Italian and Japanese kindreds. On the other hand, myoclonus was seen in German and Italian families, but not in Japanese kindreds. Rapidly progressive dementia and parkinsonism were present in all three families.

The exon-10 5′ splice-site plus 14 intronic mutation has been described in a family with

FIGURE 16.1. Pallido-ponto-nigral degeneration (*PPND*) family pedigree. The PPND family has been investigated since September 23, 1987. The pedigree was revised and updated February 8, 2001 for men (*squares*) and women (*circles*), with affected family members (*fully darkened squares or circles*) also shown. A diagonal line through a square or a circle indicates a deceased person. A dot in the center of the square or a circle represents only historical data available, with limited information on date and place of birth and death. "B" indicates date of birth. A number inside the enlarged symbols indicates age at death. An arrow indicates index case. Four branches of the PPND family designated as A, B, C, and D are outlined in four different shades. A founder of each branch is a child of a woman (II-3) who was born in 1854 and died at age 32 years. Thus, about 130 years separate the presently living descendants of these four branches' founders. The family members from different branches settled in different geographical locations; individuals from branch A mostly settled in Iowa and Arizona, from branch B in Montana and Washington, from branch C in Iowa, and from branch D in Missouri. The PPND family pedigree is still incomplete. The individual III-1, according to family notes, was drafted into the military service and never returned home. There are no records available on individuals of IV-1, 2, and 3 and their descendants. There are also no records on descendants of V-10 and 12. There is then a possibility that the PPND family is much larger than depicted in this pedigree, that there are other affected individuals in the United States who are alive, and that there are more individuals at risk of developing this illness.

dementia–disinhibition–parkinsonism–amyotrophy complex. This is the first kindred linked to chromosome 17 (25,26) and is still the only one that harbors this specific mutation. The family exhibits signs of personality changes, frontotemporal dementia, parkinsonism, and amyotrophy. There is a long (up to about 20 years) prodromal phase characterized by behavioral aberrations such as excessive religiosity, inappropriate sexual advances, overeating, and shoplifting. It is also the only kindred or mutation associated with amyotrophy.

The exon-10 N279K missense mutation was originally described in the pallido-ponto-nigral degeneration (PPND) family (27–29). This kindred is the largest among all FTDP-17 families (Fig. 16.1). The affected individu-

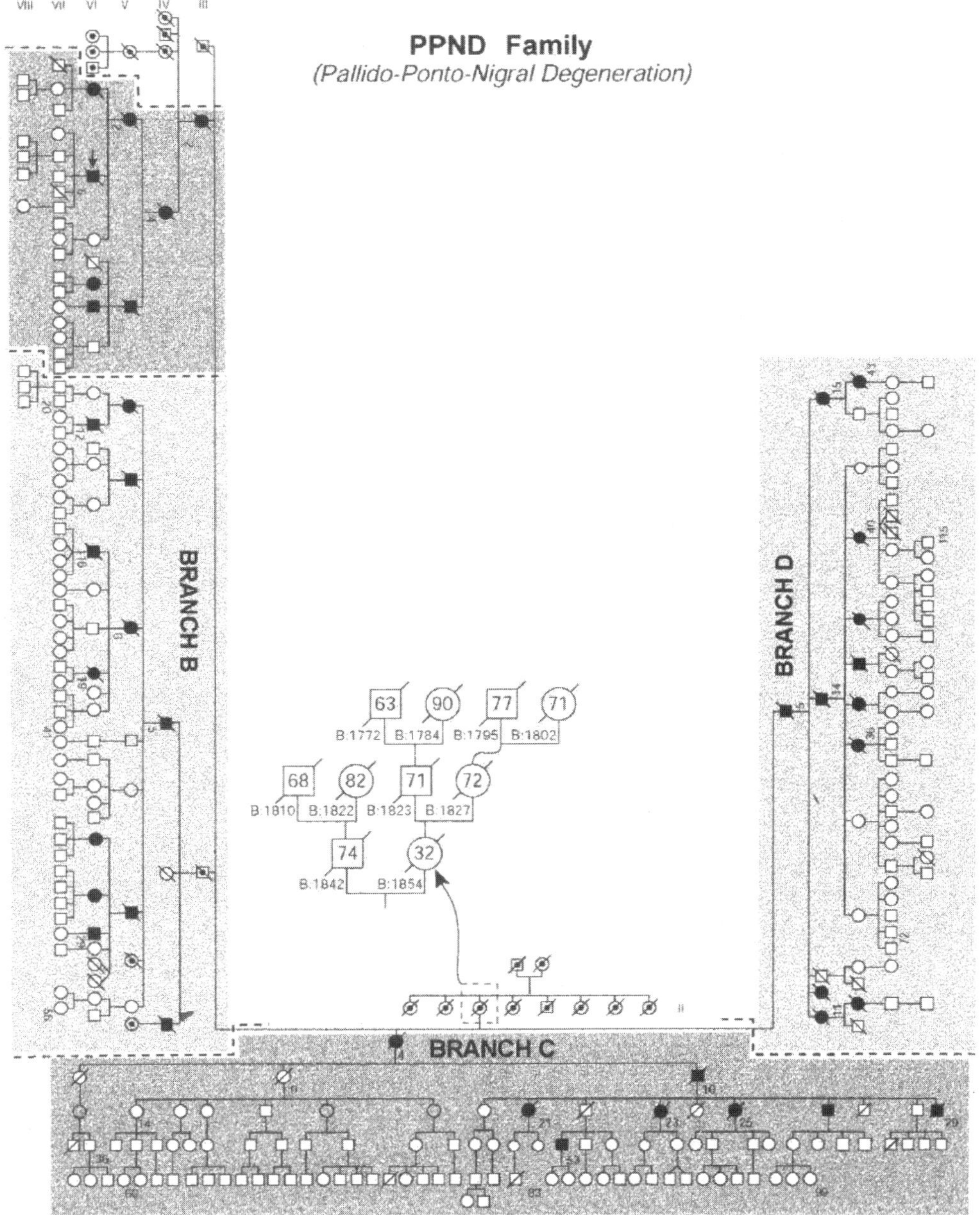

als usually present with parkinsonian features, including bradykinesia, rigidity, and postural instability. However, about one third of affected individuals present with either personality changes or dementia alone or in combination with parkinsonism. The clinical features also include dystonia unrelated to medications, eye movement abnormalities (Fig. 16.2), pyramidal tract dysfunction, frontal lobe release signs, perseverative vocalizations, and bladder incontinence. Response to levodopa therapy is seen only in the initial stage of the disease.

This family has four branches established by the children of the first known affected individual who was born in 1854 and who died at age 32 years (Fig. 16.1). Thus, more than 130 years separate these four branches of the family. The geographical residence and the professions also vary among the individuals from these branches. It is then plausible to hypothesize that some environmental factors influence the significant differences in phenotypical presentation observed among the four branches of this family. Another explanation of these differences may be related to the presence of unknown susceptibility or modifying genes.

Recently, the same mutation was found in three additional families: one from France and two from Japan (30–32). Haplotyping analysis revealed that the PPND French and Japanese families are not related to each other, but both Japanese families share a common founder (33). Yet, another Japanese family has been discovered by Drs. Kobayashi and Mizuno (*personal communication, 2001*).

Retrospective review of available medical records on affected individuals from the PPND family demonstrates differences in

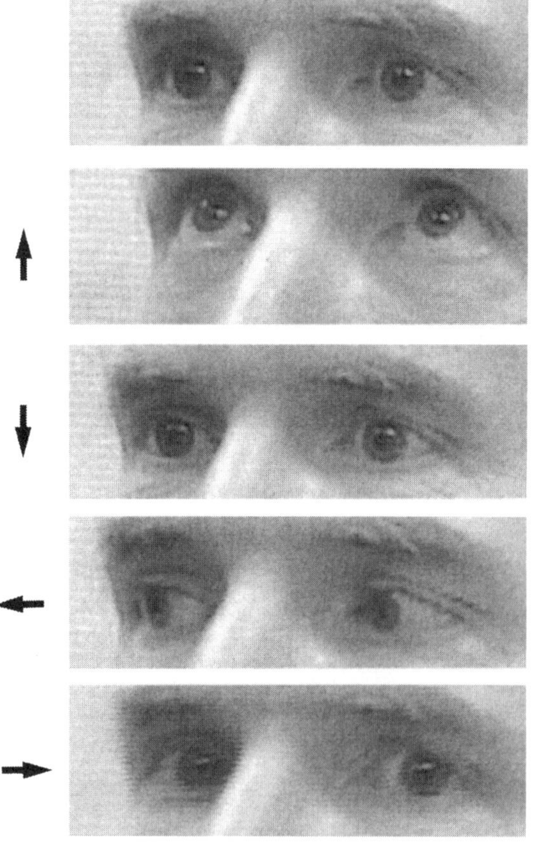

FIGURE 16.2. Affected individual from the (PPND) family. Individual VI-9 (Fig. 16.1). Last time examined by Z. K. W. at age 43 years in March 2000 and followed since 1988. The first five examinations were performed at the time when he was healthy but considered to be an at-risk individual (his father died of PPND). His first symptoms developed at age 41 years. His first symptom was tremor in his left lower limb (rare initial presentation). These photographs were taken during his last examination and demonstrate vertical gaze palsy and impairment of downgaze. The vertical gaze palsy is one of the most characteristic clinical features in sporadic progressive supranuclear palsy (PSP) cases. Sporadic PSP, corticobasal ganglionic degeneration, and PPND (N279K mutation) are all four repeat tauopathies.

clinical presentation among the four family branches (Table 16.3). The average age at onset for branch A is 40 years and that for branch C is 47 years. Interestingly, all seven affected individuals from branch C presented with parkinsonism, but only four of them responded to dopaminergic therapy and only for an average of 9 months. Four of seven affected individuals from branch A also initially presented with parkinsonism, but the response to dopaminergic therapy was longer in two of three treated individuals, lasting 12 months. Affected individuals from branches A and B usually presented with a mixture of signs more characteristic of CBGD-like phenotype. By contrast, most affected individuals from branches C and D usually presented with a PSP-like phenotype. This analysis is limited because no systematic longitudinal studies were performed on all individuals. The data were collected from sources, including the medical records of primary physicians, neurologists, and other specialists, as well as from personal examinations by one of us (Z. K. W.). Molecular genetic studies demonstrated the presence of the *H-1* allele in all 21 tested affected individuals from the PPND family. The N279K mutation has occurred on an *H-1* genotype background. Apolipoprotein E allele genotyping demonstrated no common pattern.

USEFUL CLINICAL CRITERIA FOR DIAGNOSING FTDP-17

As outlined already, FTDP-17 remains a rare neurological condition. Nevertheless, it should be considered in the differential diagnosis in the presence of the following:

- Age at neurological symptom onset between the third and fifth decades
- Rapid disease progression
- Personality and behavioral abnormalities
- Frontotemporal dementia
- Parkinsonism-plus disorders (bradykinesia, rigidity, postural instability, paucity of resting tremor, and poor or no response to dopaminergic therapy), frequently with early falls and supranuclear gaze palsy; somewhat similar to sporadic PSP presentation; less commonly apraxia, dystonia, and lateralization; somewhat similar to sporadic CBGD

TABLE 16.3. *Clinical and molecular genetic studies of four branches of pallido-ponto-nigral degeneration family (N = 33)*

Variable	A	B	C	D
N	7	10	7	9
Range and mean age at onset (yr)	36–45 40	32–46 41	41–56 47	41–58 45
Range and mean disease duration (yr)	5–10 7	6–19 10	2–16 8	6–13 9
Initial sign(s) (%)	P (58) PC (14) PC+D (14) D (14)	P (10) PC (20) PC+D (10) D (40) P+D (20)	P (100)	P (45) PC (11) P+D (11) P+PC (33)
"+" Response to dopaminergic treatment and its duration (n = 19), % and mo	2/3 (67) 12	2/5 (40) 9	4/6 (67) 9	1/5 (20) 12
H1/H2 haplotype (n = 21)	H1/H1 = 4/4	H1/H1 = 5/6 H1/H2 = 1/6	H1/H1 = 4/5 H1/H2 = 1/5	H1/H1 = 6/6
ApoE allele (n = 21)	3.3 = 4/4	2.4 = 1/6 3.3 = 3/6 3.4 = 2/6	2.3 = 2/5 3.4 = 3/5	3.3 = 4/6 3.4 = 2/6
Predominant phenotype	CBGD	CBGD	PSP	PSP

CBGD, corticobasal ganglionic degeneration; D, dementia; P, parkinsonism; PC, personality changes; PSP, progressive supranuclear palsy.

- Occasionally, progressive speech difficulties from the onset of the illness
- At times, poorly controlled with standard anticonvulsant therapy; seizure disorder superimposed on dementia and parkinsonism
- Positive family history
- Variability in clinical presentation among family members from the same kindred and among different families, even with the same mutation

DIRECTIONS FOR FUTURE CLINICAL RESEARCH ON FTDP-17

Despite significant progress in understanding FTDP-17, there are still many clinical areas that require further exploration. Future research is needed to assess autonomic nervous system involvement, sleep abnormalities, and pupillary and eye movement dysfunction. Affected individuals from the PPND family frequently report insomnia. Sleep studies are needed to delineate this dysfunction and to determine if a rapid eye movement behavior disorder is associated with FTDP-17. Personality and cognitive deficits await more detailed neuropsychological examinations. Structural and functional imaging have been performed in only some FTDP-17 kindreds. Positron emission tomography examinations using newer radiotracers will help demonstrate the nature of neuronal dysfunction of vulnerable cell populations.

Presymptomatic genetic testing has been performed on several at-risk individuals in the PPND family. However, most of them have chosen not to proceed with such testing because of the lack of effective symptomatic or curative therapy (34). This lack of interest in presymptomatic testing is similar to that encountered among the at-risk individuals for Huntington's disease. It remains to be seen how at-risk individuals from other kindreds will react to the possibility of such testing. There are no known therapies for FTDP-17. It is hoped that the development of transgenic mice will provide an opportunity to test therapeutic agents soon (35). We believe that there is also a need for a Second International Conference on FTDP-17. Such a forum can provide the opportunity to discuss the clinical, molecular genetic, and pathological progress on this disorder and delineate further research directions.

HEREDITARY PARKINSONISM, DEPRESSION, WEIGHT LOSS, CENTRAL HYPOVENTILATION—PERRY'S SYNDROME

The first family that presented with parkinsonism, depression, weight loss, and central hypoventilation was described by Perry et al. (36,37) in 1975. Later, four additional families with an identical phenotype were described in Canada, the United States, the United Kingdom, and France (38–41). Recently, two other families with this syndrome have been discovered: one in Japan and one in Turkey (42) (Dr. Elibol, *personal communication, 2001*) (Table 16.4). The disease progression is relentless, leading to death in 4 to 8 years. Affected individuals die either suddenly or of respiratory failure (38,39). The most consistent clinical features of this syndrome include parkinsonism and hypoventilation. Pathological findings reveal the presence of severe neuronal loss and gliosis mainly in the substantia nigra, with or without scarce Lewy bodies (36–42). This syndrome has been inherited in an autosomal-dominant fashion. The phenotype of this kindred differs from that other familial autosomal-dominant or autosomal-recessive parkinsonian syndromes linked to known mutations and loci.

We are trying to establish collaborations with researchers who described families with this syndrome to form a consortium and proceed with linkage analysis. We hope that the research on these families can be resurrected and blood samples collected. All known families are too small to accomplish successful linkage analysis studies. However, if considered as a group, there is potential to find linkage and even to proceed with a mutation search. We invite all researchers following families with this syndrome to collaborate with us on this project.

TABLE 16.4. *A review of previously reported families with parkinsonism, depression, weight loss, and central hypoventilation and a newly discovered Japanese family*

Report	Mean age at onset (range, yr)	Mean disease duration (range, yr)	Initial signs	Clinical feature				Response to levodopa	Other	Pathological feature
				P	D	WL	HV			
Perry et al. (36,37)	48 (42–52)	5 (4–6)	D, WL	+	+	+	+	–	Suicide in one	Cell loss in SN; few LBs
Purdy et al. (38)	46	2.5 (2–3)	D, WL	+	+	+	+	–	Sudden death in one	Cell loss in SN, mild cell loss in caudate nucleus, globus pallidus, pons, and medulla; few LBs
Roy et al. (39)	51 (45–57)	3 (3–4)	P, D	+	+	+	+	+	Sudden death in three	Cell loss in SN, mild cell loss in locus ceruleus; no LB
Lechevalier et al. (40)	52 (45–57)	7 (6–8)	P, D	+	+	+	+	+	Died of respiratory failure in two	Cell loss in SN and dorsal medullary nuclei; no LB
Bhatia et al. (41)	39 (35–43)	3.5 (3–4)	P	+	+	–	–	+	Sudden death in one	Cell loss in SN and locus ceruleus, two LBs in SN, one LB in bnM
Japanese family (42)	41 (38–43)	6	P, D	+	+	+	+	+	Suicide in one	Cell loss in SN and locus ceruleus; no LB

bnM, basal nucleus of Meynert; D, depression; HV, hypoventilation; LB, Lewy body; P, parkinsonism; SN, substantia nigra; WL, weight loss.

TABLE 16.5. *Familial parkinsonism with known mutations or loci*

Chromosome/ gene	Inheritance pattern	Range of age at disease onset (mean) (yr)	Phenotype	Response to levodopa
1p35–36	AR	32–48 (41)	PD	Good
1p36	AR	27–40 (33)	PD	Good
2p13	AD	36–89 (58)	PD	Good
4p14–15/*UCH-L1*	AD	49–51 (50)	PD	Good
4p15	AD	24–48 (30's)	PD with dementia	Good
4q21/*α-synuclein*	AD	20–85 (46)	PD with dementia	Good
6q25.2–27/*parkin*	AR	6–58 (26)	PD	Good
17q21–22/*tau*	AD	32–58 (41)	FTDP-17	Poor

AD, autosomal dominant; AR, autosomal recessive; FTDP-17, frontotemporal dementia and parkinsonism linked to chromosome 17; PD, Parkinson's disease; UCH-L1, ubiquitin carboxy-terminal hydrase L1.
Data from references 43–49.

HEREDITARY PARKINSONISM

Familial aspects of Parkinson's disease have become an exciting and active field of movement disorders due to continuous progress in molecular genetic techniques. The present state of this research is outlined in Table 16.5. The known parkinsonian loci and mutations have been identified on chromosomes 1p, 2p, 4p, 4q, 6q, and 17q (43–49). There is no doubt that more mutations responsible for familial parkinsonism will be identified. The role of susceptibility genes in Pick's disease and parkinsonian-plus syndromes also awaits further exploration.

Correspondence: Zbigniew K. Wszolek, M.D., Department of Neurology, Mayo Clinic, 4500 San Pablo Road, Jacksonville, FL 32224, USA.

REFERENCES

1. Goedert M. Neurofibrillary pathology of Alzheimer's disease and other tauopathies. *Prog Brain Res* 1998; 117:287–306.
2. Hong M, Zhukareva V, Vogelsberg-Ragaglia V, et al. Mutation-specific functional impairments in distinct *tau* isoforms of hereditary FTDP-17. *Science* 1998;282: 1914–1917.
3. Mailliot C, Sergeant N, Bussiere T, et al. Phosphorylation of specific sets of *tau* isoforms reflects different neurofibrillary degeneration processes. *FEBS Lett* 1998;433:201–204.
4. Spillantini MG, Goedert M, Crowther RA, et al. Familial multiple system tauopathy with presenile dementia: a disease with abundant neuronal and glial tau filaments. *Proc Natl Acad Sci USA* 1997;94:4113–4118.
5. Arvanitakis Z, Wszolek ZK. Recent advances in the understanding of tau protein and movement disorders. *Curr Opin Neurol* 2001;14:491–497.
6. Dickson DW. Neurodegenerative diseases with cytoskeletal pathology: a biochemical classification. *Ann Neurol* 1997;42:541–544.
7. Spillantini MG, Goedert M. Tau protein pathology in neurodegenerative diseases. *Trends Neurosci* 1998;21: 428–433.
8. Foster NL, Wilhelmsen K, Sima AA, et al. Frontotemporal dementia and parkinsonism linked to chromosome 17: a consensus conference. *Ann Neurol* 1997;41: 706–715.
9. Hutton M, Lendon CL, Rizzu P, et al. Association of missense and 5′-splice-site mutations in tau with the inherited dementia FTDP-17. *Nature* 1998;393:702–705.
10. Poorkaj P, Bird TD, Wijsman E, et al. Tau is a candidate gene for chromosome 17 frontotemporal dementia. *Ann Neurol* 1998;43:815–825.
11. Spillantini MG, Murrell JR, Goedert M, et al. Mutation in the tau gene in familial multiple system tauopathy with presenile dementia. *Proc Natl Acad Sci USA* 1998; 95:7737–7741.
12. Reed LA, Wszolek ZK, Hutton M. Phenotypic correlations in FTDP-17. *Neurobiol Aging* 2001;22:89–107.
13. Bird TD, Nochlin D, Poorkaj P, et al. A clinical pathological comparison of three families with frontotemporal dementia and identical mutations in the tau gene (P301L). *Brain* 1999;122:741–756.
14. Nasreddine ZS, Loginov M, Clark LN, et al. From genotype to phenotype: a clinical, pathological, and biochemical investigation of frontotemporal dementia and parkinsonism (FTDP-17) caused by the P301L tau mutation. *Ann Neurol* 1999;45:704–715.
15. Heutink P, Stevens M, Rizzu P, et al. Hereditary frontotemporal dementia is linked to chromosome 17q21-q22: a genetic and clinicopathological study of three Dutch families. *Ann Neurol* 1997;41:150–159.
16. Spillantini MG, Crowther RA, Kamphorst W, et al. Tau pathology in two Dutch families with mutations in the microtubule-binding region of tau. *Am J Pathol* 1998; 153:1359–1363.
17. Mirra SS, Murrell JR, Gearing M, et al. Tau pathology in a family with dementia and a P301L mutation in tau. *J Neuropathol Exp Neurol* 1999;58:335–345.
18. Dumanchin C, Camuzat A, Campion D, et al. Segrega-

tion of a missense mutation in the microtubule-associated protein *tau* gene with familial frontotemporal dementia and parkinsonism. *Hum Mol Genet* 1998;7: 1825–1829.

19. Rizzu P, Van Swieten JC, Joosse M, et al. High prevalence of mutations in the microtubule-associated protein tau in a population study of frontotemporal dementia in the Netherlands. *Am J Hum Genet* 1999;64: 414–421.
20. Houlden H, Baker M, Adamson J, et al. Frequency of tau mutations in three series of non-Alzheimer's degenerative dementia. *Ann Neurol* 1999;46:243–248.
21. Kodama K, Okada S, Iseki E, et al. Familial frontotemporal dementia with a P301L tau mutation in Japan. *J Neurol Sci* 2000;176:57–64.
22. Bugiani O, Murrell JR, Giaccone G, et al. Frontotemporal dementia and corticobasal degeneration in a family with a P301S mutation in tau. *J Neuropathol Exp Neurol* 1999;58:667–677.
23. Sperfeld AD, Collatz MB, Baier H, et al. FTDP-17: an early-onset phenotype with parkinsonism and epileptic seizures caused by a novel mutation. *Ann Neurol* 1999; 46:708–715.
24. Yasuda M, Yokoyama K, Nakayasu T, et al. A Japanese patient with frontotemporal dementia and parkinsonism by a tau P301S mutation. *Neurology* 2000;55: 1224–1227.
25. Lynch T, Sano M, Marder KS, et al. Clinical characteristics of a family with chromosome 17–linked disinhibition–dementia–parkinsonism–amyotrophy complex. *Neurology* 1994;44:1878–1884.
26. Wilhelmsen KC, Lynch T, Pavlou E, et al. Localization of disinhibition–dementia–parkinsonism–amyotrophy complex to 17q21-22. *Am J Hum Genet* 1994;55: 1159–1165.
27. Clark LN, Poorkaj P, Wszolek Z, et al. Pathogenic implications of mutations in the tau gene in pallido-ponto-nigral degeneration and related neurodegenerative disorders linked to chromosome 17. *Proc Natl Acad Sci USA* 1998;95:13103–13107.
28. Reed LA, Schmidt ML, Wszolek ZK, et al. The neuropathology of a chromosome 17–linked autosomal dominant parkinsonism and dementia ("pallido-ponto-nigral degeneration"). *J Neuropathol Exp Neurol* 1998; 57:588–601.
29. Wszolek ZK, Pfeiffer RF, Bhatt MH, et al. Rapidly progressive autosomal dominant parkinsonism and dementia with pallido-ponto-nigral degeneration. *Ann Neurol* 1992;32:312–320.
30. Delisle MB, Murrell JR, Richardson R, et al. A mutation at codon 279 (N279K) in exon 10 of the *tau* gene causes a tauopathy with dementia and supranuclear palsy. *Acta Neuropathol (Berlin)* 1999;98:62–77.
31. Yasuda M, Kawamata T, Komure O, et al. A mutation in the microtubule-associated protein tau in pallido-nigroluysian degeneration. *Neurology* 1999;53:864–868.
32. Arima K, Kowalska A, Hasegawa M, et al. Two brothers with frontotemporal dementia and parkinsonism with an N279K mutation of the *tau* gene. *Neurology* 2000; 54:1787–1795.
33. Tsuboi Y, Baker M, Hutton M, et al. Families with N279K mutation on the tau gene: clinical, molecular genetic, and pathological studies. *Neurology* 2001; 56[Suppl 3]:A126.
34. McRae CA, Diem G, Yamazaki TG, et al. Interest in genetic testing in pallido-ponto-nigral degeneration (PPND): a family with frontotemporal dementia with parkinsonism linked to chromosome 17. *Eur J Neurol* 2001;8:179–183.
35. Lewis J, McGowan E, Rockwood J, et al. Neurofibrillary tangles, amyotrophy and progressive motor disturbance in mice expressing mutant (P301L) tau protein. *Nat Genet* 2000;25:402–405.
36. Perry TL, Bratty PJ, Hansen S, et al. Hereditary mental depression and parkinsonism with taurine deficiency. *Arch Neurol* 1975;32:108–113.
37. Perry TL, Wright JM, Berry K, et al. Dominantly inherited apathy, central hypoventilation, and Parkinson's syndrome: clinical, biochemical, and neuropathologic studies of 2 new cases. *Neurology* 1990; 40:1882–1887.
38. Purdy A, Hahn A, Barnett HJ, et al. Familial fatal parkinsonism with alveolar hypoventilation and mental depression. *Ann Neurol* 1979;6:523–531.
39. Roy EP III, Riggs JE, Martin JD, et al. Familial parkinsonism, apathy, weight loss, and central hypoventilation: successful long-term management. *Neurology* 1988;38:637–639.
40. Lechevalier B, Schupp C, Fallet-Bianco C, et al. Familial parkinsonian syndrome with athymhormia and hypoventilation. *Rev Neurol* 1992;148:39–46.
41. Bhatia KP, Daniel SE, Marsden CD. Familial parkinsonism with depression: a clinicopathological study. *Ann Neurol* 1993;34:842–847.
42. Tsuboi Y, Wszolek ZK, Kusuhara T, et al. Japanese family with parkinsonism, depression, weight loss, and central hypoventilation *Neurology* 2002;58:1025–1030.
43. Valente EM, Bentivoglio AR, Dixon PH, et al. Localization of a novel locus for autosomal recessive early-onset parkinsonism, *PARK6,* on human chromosome 1p35-p36. *Am J Hum Genet* 2001;68:895–900.
44. Gasser T, Muller-Myhsok B, Wszolek ZK, et al. A susceptibility locus for Parkinson's disease maps to chromosome 2p13. *Nat Genet* 1998;18:262–265.
45. Leroy E, Boyer R, Auburger G, et al. The ubiquitin pathway in Parkinson's disease. *Nature* 1998;395:451–452.
46. Farrer M, Gwinn-Hardy K, Muenter M, et al. A chromosome 4p haplotype segregating with Parkinson's disease and postural tremor. *Hum Mol Genet* 1999;8: 81–85.
47. Polymeropoulos MH, Lavedan C, Leroy E, et al. Mutation in the alpha-synuclein gene identified in families with Parkinson's disease. *Science* 1997;276: 2045–2047.
48. Matsumine H, Saito M, Shimoda-Matsubayashi S, et al. Localization of a gene for an autosomal recessive form of juvenile parkinsonism to chromosome 6q25.2-27. *Am J Hum Genet* 1997;60:588–596.
49. van Duijn CM, Dekker MC, Bonifati V, et al. Park7, a novel locus for autosomal recessive early-onset parkinsonism, on chromosome 1p36. *Am J Hum Genet* 2001; 69:629–634.

Parkinson's Disease: Advances in Neurology, Vol. 91.
Edited by Ariel Gordin, Seppo Kaakkola,
and Heikki Teräväinen
Lippincott Williams & Wilkins, Philadelphia © 2003

17

α-Synuclein and Parkinson's Disease

Lawrence I. Golbe

Department of Neurology, University of Medicine and Dentistry of New Jersey, Robert Wood Johnson Medical School, New Brunswick, New Jersey

An important piece of the puzzle of Parkinson's disease (PD) has been moving into place since 1997. A detailed understanding of the mechanism of the toxic action of α-synuclein, once attained, may fully delineate the cause of PD. It may represent the final step necessary to identify multiple potential new targets for prophylactic treatment of PD.

NORMAL α-SYNUCLEIN

Function

α-Synuclein is a relatively abundant protein of neuronal cytoplasm. It localizes with synaptic vesicles. Its primary normal function, far from fully understood, appears to be stabilization of dopamine vesicles during and after transport from cell bodies to synaptic terminals, at which point it may somehow regulate the synaptic store of vesicles and inhibit excessive synaptic release (1–4). α-Synuclein knockout mice do not develop neuronal loss or overt parkinsonism but do exhibit subtle changes in dopaminergic function (1).

In addition to its function at dopaminergic synapses, α-synuclein has chaperone properties and stress protein properties, helping to keep other proteins from aggregating under conditions of cellular stress (5,6). For example, α-synuclein protects glutathione *S*-transferase and aldolase from heat-induced precipitation (5). It also regulates secretory vesicles in platelets (7) and binds and transports fatty acids (8).

Structure

α-Synuclein is a small protein, with only 140 amino acids. Under normal conditions, it exhibits no particular secondary structure (9). Its amino end bears four imperfect repeats of an 11–amino acid sequence that includes the 6–amino acid consensus sequence KTKEGV (10). Five to eight amino acids separate successive repeats. This large segment of α-synuclein allows binding of the protein to lipid membranes. There is a very hydrophobic middle region, and at the carboxy end, there is a negatively charged highly acidic area that mediates interactions with other proteins (9,11,12). On binding to lipid membranes, α-synuclein and other natively unfolded proteins assume a more rigid, α-helical structure at the amino end (12). α-Synuclein is posttranslationally modified via phosphorylation by G-protein–coupled receptor kinases. This impairs the ability of α-synuclein to interact with phospholipids (13). It is also glycosylated to a form that interacts with parkin, as described below. Defects in posttranslational modification of α-synuclein are good candidates for pathogenetic factors in PD.

Interactions

The carboxy terminal of α-synuclein mediates interactions with other proteins. The normal physiological interactions of α-synuclein are only starting to be unraveled and remain little more than a series of fragmentary observations. However, a full understanding of the normal function of α-synuclein may be of secondary importance to the question of PD. The role of α-synuclein in PD pathogenesis appears to be a toxic gain of function, rather than hypofunction.

A yeast two-hybrid screening technique revealed a novel protein, dubbed synphilin-1, which may help anchor α-synuclein to yet other proteins involved in vesicle physiology (14). However, mutations in synphilin-1 appear not to contribute to the cause of PD (15).

Another yeast two-hybrid screen revealed an interaction with a component of the proteasome system, Tat binding protein 1 (16). α-Synuclein inhibits phospholipase D_2, which may help regulate endocytosis at the cell membrane. This supports other observations suggesting that α-synuclein is involved in vesicular transport.

Involvement in the microtubule-associated protein (MAP) kinase pathway by α-synuclein is suggested by the co-localization of that protein with Elk-1, which is known to bind to one MAP kinase (17). α-Synuclein also binds with high avidity to MAP1B, which is found with α-synuclein in Lewy bodies (18).

Tau, another MAP, occurs at the periphery of some Lewy bodies and binds to α-synuclein (19). An interaction of α-synuclein with tau is further supported by the recent finding of an allelic association of PD with the same *tau* allele that occurs in the primary tauopathies progressive supranuclear palsy and corticobasal degeneration (20).

The human dopamine transporter (DAT) complexes with α-synuclein to facilitate clustering of DAT in the presynaptic membrane of dopaminergic neurons. This promotes entry of dopamine with its attendant toxicity (21).

Degradation

Under normal conditions, a large fraction of α-synuclein molecules emerge from the translational process misfolded. The pathway by which excessive, defective, or damaged α-synuclein is degraded may play an important role in the pathogenesis of PD. This appears to occur via the ubiquitin-proteasomal pathway (22,23). In fact, experimental inhibition of proteasomal function reproduces the formation of both α-synuclein–rich aggregates and apoptotic cell death (23,24).

Parkin plays an important role in preparing ubiquitin for its role in this process. A recent investigation of the α-synuclein–parkin interactions unexpectedly found that only a form of α-synuclein that interacts with parkin is one that is glycosylated at some of its hydroxyl groups (25). Genetically determined defects in parkin, as occur in about half of all cases of autosomal-recessive juvenile parkinsonism, permit accumulation of *O*-glycosylated α-synuclein in neurons. The relevance of this phenomenon to sporadic PD remains unclear, but we must consider the possibility that all PD may arise from disordered interaction between parkin and α-synuclein (26). This possibility was strengthened by the recent anecdotal description of typical Lewy bodies in the brain of a patient with PD and compound heterozygous parkin mutations (27).

The mutant α-synuclein associated with autosomal-dominant familial PD is degraded more slowly than the wild type (22). α-Synuclein that has formed insoluble aggregates not only fails to be degraded by the proteasome but also actually appears to clog the proteasome, preventing it from degrading soluble α-synuclein (28).

ABNORMAL α-SYNUCLEIN

Relationship with Alzheimer's Disease

The first clue of a relationship of α-synuclein to neurodegenerative disorders was the 1993 observation that a fragment of that protein comprising the amino acids 61 to 95 is a component of amyloid plaques in Alzheimer's disease (29). One of the several aliases of α-synuclein is therefore non–amyloid-component precursor (NACP). At least one more recent publication, however, has failed to find α-synuclein in amyloid plaques (30). In 1995, the *NACP* gene sequence was found to be homologous to that of the rat synuclein gene and mapped to human chromosome 4q (31,32).

Relationship with PD

The first demonstration of a relationship of α-synuclein to PD itself came in 1996 with the linkage analysis of a large Italian American family, the Contursi kindred (33,34). This family was unusually well suited for linkage analysis because the high penetrance of the trait and the large sibship sizes permitted ascertainment of the necessary number of affected living individuals. The critical region at chromosome 4q21-22 included approximately 100 known genes (35). The leading candidates among these included, by virtue of its known relation to Alzheimer's plaques, α-synuclein. Sequencing of the candidates revealed a G209A substitution in the gene for α-synuclein (36). It is a missense mutation, producing a threonine for alanine substitution at amino acid 53, dubbed PARK1. Groups worldwide then screened series of patients with PD for PARK1 (37–40), finding it only in a few families of Greek origin (36,41–46).

Haplotype analysis shows that the affected Greek patients share with the affected members of the Contursi kindred a haplotype spanning 4q21-22 (M. Polymeropoulos, *personal communication,* 1998), demonstrating a probable founder effect. In fact, Greece and southern Italy, the origin of the Contursi kindred, have been in close contact over the centuries. The Contursi kindred would have been interpreted as six separate families if not for the genealogical effort that found a common ancestor in the early eighteenth century (34). Similar genealogical work is not possible in Greece, where those records have been destroyed by political conflict.

Several groups have sequenced the coding regions of the α-synuclein gene in series of patients with familial and sporadic PD. The lone positive result was found (47) in a German family with a mutation close to that of the Italian and Greek families, with a G for C substitution at nucleotide 88. This substitutes proline for the alanine at amino acid 30. (This mutation is also called PARK1.) Both mutations substitute a more hydrophobic for the relatively hydrophilic alanine in a segment of the protein between consensus repeats in the N-terminal region. The A30P patients suffered onset of PD in their 50s, slightly later than the mean age in the A53T families. Correspondingly, most of the abnormal *in vitro* properties of A30P α-synuclein are slightly less marked than those of A53T α-synuclein (48).

There has been one report that the co-occurrence of an allele of a polymorphism in the promoter region of α-synuclein and the 4 allele of apolipoprotein E is 12-fold more frequent in patients with PD than in control subjects (49). This was refuted by a subsequent larger, negative study of similar design (50), but an association of this promoter region polymorphism with PD was confirmed by a recent report that a haplotype that includes that allele is more frequent in patients with PD than in control subjects (51). Unfortunately, an attempt to measure α-synuclein in the cerebrospinal fluid as a convenient biomarker for PD was unsuccessful (52).

Properties of Mutant α-Synuclein

Both of the known PD-associated α-synuclein mutants, A53G and A30T, increase the molecule's vulnerability to oxidative stress induced by hydrogen peroxide, 1-methyl-4-phenylpyridine (MPP^+) (53,54) and a variety of other insults (55). The mode of cell death in cultured neuronal cells transfected with mutant or wild-type α-synuclein is apoptotic (55).

Perhaps the most important abnormal property of the two known *PARK1* mutants is their increased aggregability (56,57). Experimental C-terminal truncation of α-synuclein via loss of the last 20 amino acids also enhances aggregation (53,58) and most α-synuclein in Lewy bodies, in fact, is so truncated (59). Although the site of the two *PARK1* mutations is in the hydrophilic N-terminal portion of the α-synuclein molecule among the consensus repeats, the portion of the molecule necessary and sufficient to its self-aggregation is a

12–amino acid stretch from residue 71 to 82 in the middle of the hydrophobic portion (60).

Abnormal Aggregation

Lewy bodies, the pathological hallmark of PD, have been known for many years to stain strongly for ubiquitin and to include more than 20 other protein and lipid components. After the relationship of α-synuclein to rare forms of hereditary PD was discovered, the "backbone" of the Lewy body was found to be α-synuclein, even in patients with no α-synuclein mutation (59,61–63).

Normal α-synuclein self-aggregates readily. At lower concentrations, it tends to form oligomers, but at higher concentrations, it forms larger aggregates (2). A53G and A30T mutant α-synuclein self-aggregate more avidly than wild-type α-synuclein (64). This process appears to be caused not by reduced solubility, but by more rapid nucleation rates of the mutants relative to the wild type (65). The resulting aggregates assume a β-pleated sheet formation, like amyloid in the plaques of Alzheimer's disease (48,57,66,67).

Proaggregate Factors

α-Synuclein aggregates more readily under conditions of oxidative stress (6,68). This property appears to be central to the pathogenesis of PD, where dopamine metabolism creates a normal baseline condition of unusual free radical presence. Retrospective epidemiological data suggest that patients with PD have experienced more exposure than controls to herbicides and/or pesticides, which exert oxidative stress.

A most intriguing observation is that α-synuclein itself produces hydrogen peroxide when exposed to Fe^{2+} ion (69). This raises the possibility that under some conditions, α-synuclein can catalyze the production of oxidative species that cause it to aggregate.

Increased concentration of calcium or iron also promotes oligomeric aggregation of α-synuclein (70,71). This process may constitute a step in one of the vicious cycles involved in the pathogenesis of neuronal loss in PD proposed in this chapter.

Another potent cause of α-synuclein proaggregate formation is either *PARK1* mutation (72). The observation that oligomers of mutant α-synuclein form more readily and persist longer than oligomers of wild-type α-synuclein supports the important hypothesis that oligomers are neurotoxic.

Toxins and α-Synuclein

The best animal model of PD, at least until the advent of α-synuclein transgenic models discussed later in this chapter, is the methylphenyltetrahydropyridine (MPTP) model (73). However, a shortcoming of this model has been the probable absence of Lewy bodies. But pathological examination of nigral neurons of baboons in the early stages of MPTP intoxication reveals the beginnings of α-synuclein aggregates in degenerating cell bodies, away from the normal synaptic location of α-synuclein (74). Such aggregates have also been observed in nigral neurons of rats exposed to rotenone, like MPP^+ (the toxic metabolite of MPTP), a mitochondrial complex I toxin (75). α-Synuclein *in vitro* forms fibrils more quickly in the presence of rotenone, dieldrin, or paraquat (76). These important findings show that exogenous toxins alone, without a concomitant genetic defect, can produce nigral pathology associated with α-synuclein aggregation. The implication is that impairment of α-synuclein biochemistry is integral to parkinsonism caused by mitochondrial toxins. Further work will attempt to clarify whether mature α-synuclein aggregates are necessary to toxic parkinsonism or merely a byproduct of the pro–α-synuclein-aggregation effect of oxidative stress.

Part of that answer is provided by the observation that α-synuclein is specifically nitrated both in MPTP parkinsonism (77) and in human PD brain (78). This provides additional support for the hypothesis that the abnormal behavior of α-synuclein in PD is related to oxidative stress.

Mechanism of Toxicity of α-Synuclein Oligomers

Aggregated α-synuclein is now known to be selectively toxic to dopaminergic neurons (79). Recent work has shown that the "protoaggregates" or "oligomers" of α-synuclein, not the mature aggregates, are the toxic species (80). The oligomers attack lipid membranes, particularly those of dopamine vesicles, causing transient permeabilization and leakage of toxic dopamine into the cytoplasm (81). The oligomers may also compromise the mitochondrial membrane (82), degrading the transmembrane potential and inducing apoptotic signals (83,84). The cell membrane itself may also be vulnerable to attack by α-synuclein oligomers, permitting entry of calcium that induces apoptosis (85).

α-SYNUCLEIN TRANSGENIC ANIMAL MODELS OF PD

Drosophila Model

Before the discovery of a relationship between α-synuclein and PD, the available animal models of PD did not reproduce the development of Lewy bodies. But Feany and Bender in 2000 (86) reported strains of *Drosophila,* which normally has no α-synuclein, expressing normal human α-synuclein and each of the two known PD-associated mutant α-synucleins. These flies exhibited progressive loss of motor ability starting in midlife and α-synuclein–positive aggregates in degenerating dopaminergic neurons. The motor effect was more pronounced in the flies expressing *PARK1* mutant than wild type α-synuclein. The aggregates resembled Lewy bodies in their fibrillary structure. These changes were specific for dopaminergic neurons, but as in human PD, not all dopaminergic neurons were involved. Unanswered questions relevant to the utility of this model are whether the motor deficit responds to pharmacological dopaminergic stimulation and, indeed, whether that deficit is the result of the observed dopaminergic neuronal loss, rather than the result of some functional loss without an anatomical correlate (87).

Mouse Models

Mouse models have not mimicked human PD nearly as well as the *Drosophila* model. One mouse overexpressing normal α-synuclein (88) showed granular, rather than fibrillar, inclusions. Some of these were located in the nuclei, which is not the case for Lewy bodies of PD. Most important, dopaminergic neuronal loss was absent, although there was variable loss of dopamine terminals, and there was only minimal motor impairment. This model used a platelet-derived growth factor (PDGF) promotor.

Mouse models using a Thy-1 promotor (89–91) and expressing either wild-type or *PARK1* mutant α-synuclein show exclusively cytoplasmic Lewy body–like α-synuclein–positive aggregates and progressive motor loss. However, nigral neuronal loss was absent, as with the PDGF promotor model, and there was major motor neuron pathology, a feature not seen in PD.

A mouse model using a tyrosine hydroxylase (TH) promoter gave even more discouraging results, with no behavioral change or neuronal pathology, except for accumulation of α-synuclein in dopaminergic cells without Lewy body formation (92). Another A30P α-synuclein mouse under control of a TH promoter, moreover, was no more sensitive to MPTP than wild-type controls, contrary to expectations based on *in vitro* cell preparations (93).

SUMMARY AND CONCLUSIONS: HYPOTHETICAL ETIOLOGY AND PATHOGENESIS OF PD

The top row in Figure 17.1 shows the five known etiologies of PD: parkin (*PARK2*) mutations, *PARK1* mutations, genetic detoxification defects, excessive toxin exposure, and mitochondrial mutations. The relative importance of these five etiologies, either in any in-

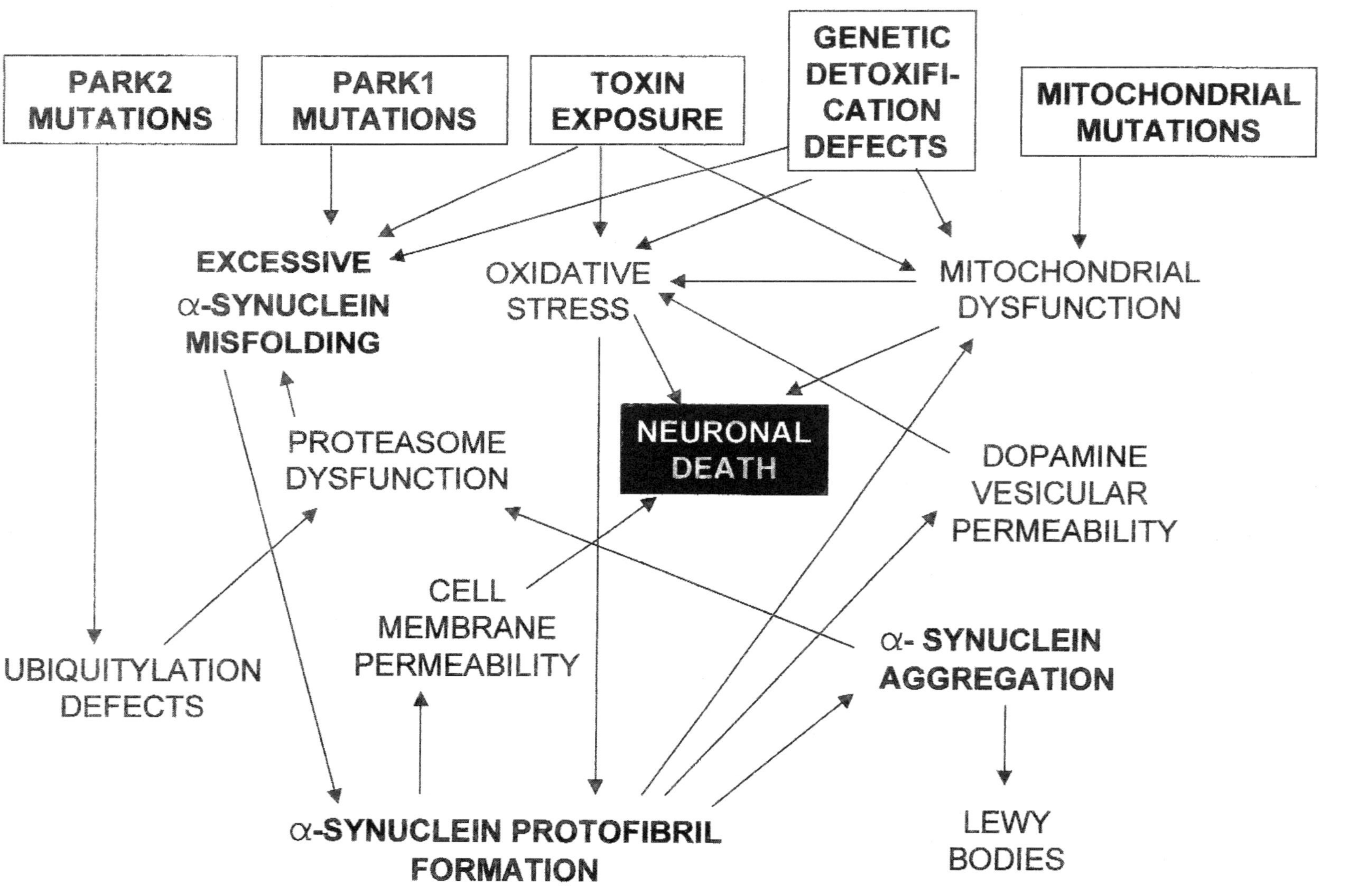

FIGURE 17.1. Hypothetical pathogenesis of Parkinson's disease.

dividual patient or in the total PD population, is unknown. In very few cases, only one of these is operative.

There is no theoretical reason why other etiological factors could not exist.

In this hypothetical scheme, the proximate causes of neuronal death are oxidative stress and mitochondrial dysfunction leading to apoptotic neuronal death. The diagram shows the paths from the five etiologies to this ultimate outcome. Most of these paths involve a vicious cycle, which may explain why the clinical course in PD begins gradually and accelerates with time.

PARK2 mutations impair ubiquitylation. This impairs proteasomal function, which permits accumulation of those α-synuclein molecules that under normal conditions by chance emerge misfolded from the process of translation. *PARK1* mutations themselves produce misfolded α-synuclein. Regardless of its genesis, the misfolded α-synuclein aggregates into protofibrils, which permeabilize dopamine vesicles, releasing dopamine, which produces oxidative stress. The α-synuclein protoaggregates may also permeabilize mitochondria, reducing their transmembrane potential, inducing an apoptotic cascade, and producing oxidative stress. They may also permeabilize the cell membrane, permitting entry of calcium, which also serves as an apoptotic signal.

The α-synuclein protofibrils and/or their mature aggregates appear to clog the proteasome.

This impairs disposal of misfolded α-synuclein, thereby permitting accumulation of more protofibrils.

Excessive exposure to toxins, particularly certain pesticides that are not fully characterized, or a hereditary deficiency of detoxification mechanisms in the setting of lesser exposure can promote α-synuclein misfolding and aggregation. This would presumably feed into the mechanism described earlier. Toxin exposure, genetically deficient detoxification, and mitochondrial genetic defects can also damage mitochondrial function, producing a cellular energy deficit and aggravating the oxidative stress.

The mature α-synuclein aggregates form Lewy bodies, which may have the salutary effect of removing the aggregates from access to proteasomes, where they would exert a toxic effect, described earlier. The sequestration of mature α-synuclein aggregates into Lewy bodies would also shift the equilibrium away from the injurious protoaggregates in the direction of mature aggregates, which appear not to be able to permeabilize lipid membranes. There is no evidence that Lewy bodies themselves are deleterious.

ACKNOWLEDGMENTS

Supported by a Center of Excellence Grant from the American Parkinson's Disease Association. I thank Roger C. Duvoisin, inspiration and guidance always.

REFERENCES

1. Abeliovich A, Schmitz Y, Farinas I, et al. Mice lacking α-synuclein display functional deficits in the nigrostriatal dopamine system. *Neuron* 2001;25:239–252.
2. Narayanan V, Scarlata S. Membrane binding and self-association of α-synuclein. *Biochemistry* 2001;40: 9927–9934.
3. Jensen PH, Nielsen MH, Jakes R, et al. Binding of a α-synuclein to rat brain vesicles is abolished by familial Parkinson's disease mutation. *J Biol Chem* 2001;273: 26292–26294.
4. Murphy DD, Rueter SM, Trojanowski JQ, et al. Synucleins are developmentally expressed, and α-synuclein regulates the size of the presynaptic vesicular pool in primary hippocampal neurons. *J Neurosci* 2001;20: 3214–3220.
5. Kim TD, Paik SR, Yang CH, et al. Structural changes in α-synuclein affect its chaperone-like activity *in vitro. Protein Sci* 2000;9:2489–2496.
6. Souza JM, Giasson BI, Lee VM-Y, et al. Chaperone-like activity of synucleins. *FEBS Lett* 2001;474:116–119.
7. Hashimoto M, Yoshimoto M, Sisk A, et al. NACP, a synaptic protein involved in Alzheimer's disease, is differentially regulated during megakaryocyte differentiation. *Biochem Biophys Res Comm* 2001;237:611–616.
8. Sharon R, Goldberg MS, Bar-Josef I, et al. α-Synuclein occurs in lipid-rich high molecular weight complexes, binds fatty acids and shows homology to the fatty acid–binding proteins. *Proc Natl Acad Sci USA* 2001; 98:9110–9115.
9. Weinreb PH, Zhen W, Poon AW, et al. NACP, a protein implicated in Alzheimer's disease and learning, is natively unfolded. *Biochemistry* 2001;35:13709–13715.
10. Maroteaux L, Campanelli JT, Scheller RH. Synuclein: a neuron-specific protein localized to the nucleus and presynaptic nerve terminal. *J Neurosci* 1988;8: 2804–2815.

11. Clayton DF, George JM. The synucleins—a family of proteins involved in synaptic function, plasticity, neurodegeneration and disease. *Trends Neurosci* 2001;21: 249–254.
12. Eliezer D, Kutluay E, Bussell R, et al. Conformational properties of α-synuclein in its free and lipid-associated states. *J Mol Biol* 2001;307:1061–1073.
13. Pronin AN, Morris AJ, Surguchov A, et al. Synucleins are a novel class of substrates for G protein–coupled receptor kinases. *J Biol Chem* 2001;275:26515–26522.
14. Engelender S, Kaminsky Z, Guo X, et al. Synphilin-1 associates with α-synuclein and promotes the formation of cytosolic inclusions. *Nature Genet* 2001;22:110–114.
15. Bandopadhyay R, de Silva R, Khan N, et al. No pathogenic mutations in the synphilin-1 gene in Parkinson's disease. *Neurosci Lett* 2001;307:125–127.
16. Ghee M, Fournier A, Mallet J. Rat α-synuclein interacts with Tat binding protein 1, a component of the 26S proteasomal complex. *J Neurochem* 2001;75:2221–2224.
17. Iwata A, Miura S, Kanazawa I, et al. α-Synuclein forms a complex with transcription factor Elk-1. *J Neurochem* 2001;77:239–252.
18. Jensen PH, Islam K, Kenney J, et al. Microtubule-associated protein 1B is a component of cortical Lewy bodies and binds α-synuclein filaments. *J Biol Chem* 2001; 275:21500–21507.
19. Jensen PH, Hager H, Nielsen MS, et al. α-Synuclein binds to tau and stimulates the protein kinase A–catalyzed tau phosphorylation of serine residues 262 and 356. *J Biol Chem* 2001;274:25481–25489.
20. Golbe LI, Lazzarini AM, Spychala JR, et al. The tau A0 allele in Parkinson's disease. *Mov Disord* 2001;16: 442–447.
21. Lee FJS, Liu F, Pristupa ZB, et al. Direct binding and functional coupling of α-synuclein to the dopamine transporters accelerate dopamine-induced apoptosis. *FASEB J* 2001;15:916–926.
22. Bennett MC, Bishop JF, Leng Y, et al. Degradation of α-synuclein by proteasome. *J Biol Chem* 2001;274: 33855–33858.
23. Rideout HJ, Larsen KE, Sulzer D, et al. Proteasomal inhibition leads to formation of ubiquitin/α-synuclein–immunireactive inclusions in PC12 cells. *J Neurochem* 2001;78:899–908.
24. McLean PJ, Kawamata H, Hyman BT. α-Synuclein–enhanced green fluorescent protein fusion proteins form proteasome sensitive inclusions in primary neurons. *Neuroscience* 2001;104:901–912.
25. Shimura H, Schlossmacher MG, Hattori N, et al. Ubiquitination of a new form of α-synuclein by parkin from human brain: implications for Parkinson's disease. *Science* 2001;293:263–269.
26. Haass C, Kahle PJ. Parkin and its substrates. *Science* 2001;293:224–225.
27. Farrer M, Chan P, Chen R, et al. Lewy bodies and parkinsonism in families with parkin mutations. *Ann Neurol* 2001;50:293–300.
28. Bence NF, Sampat RM, Kopito RR. Impairment of the ubiquitin-proteasome system by protein aggregation. *Science* 2001;292:1552–1555.
29. Ueka K, Fukushima H, Masliah E, et al. Molecular cloning of cDNA encoding an unrecognized component of amyloid in Alzheimer's disease. *Proc Natl Acad Sci U S A* 1993;90:11282–11286.
30. Bayer TA, Jakala P, Hartmann T, et al. α-Synuclein accumulates in Lewy bodies in Parkinson's disease and dementia with Lewy bodies but not in Alzheimer's disease—amyloid plaque cores. *Neurosci Lett* 2001;266: 213–216.
31. Campion D, Martin C, Heilig R, et al. The NACP/synuclein gene: chromosomal assignment and screening for alterations in Alzheimer's disease. *Genomics* 2001;26: 254–257.
32. Chen X, Rohan de Silva HA, Pettenati MJ, et al. The human NACP/α-synuclein gene: chromosome assignment to 4q21.3-q22 and *Taq*I RFLP analysis. *Genomics* 2001; 26:425–427.
33. Golbe LI, Di Iorio G, Bonavita V, et al. A large kindred with autosomal dominant Parkinson's disease. *Ann Neurol* 1990; 27:276–282.
34. Golbe LI, Di Iorio G, Sanges G, et al. Clinical genetic analysis of Parkinson's disease in the Contursi kindred. *Ann Neurol* 1996;40:767–775.
35. Polymeropoulos MH, Higgins JJ, Golbe LI, et al. Mapping of a gene for Parkinson's disease to chromosome 4q21-q23. *Science* 2001;274:1197–1199.
36. Polymeropoulos MH, Lavedan C, Leroy E, et al. Mutation in the α-synuclein gene identified in families with Parkinson's disease. *Science* 2001;276:2045–2047.
37. Chan P, Jiang X, Forno LS, et al. Absence of mutations in the coding region of the α-synuclein gene in pathologically proven Parkinson's disease. *Neurology* 2001; 50:1136–1137.
38. Scott WK, Stajich JM, Yamaoka LH, et al. Genetic complexity and Parkinson's disease. *Science* 2001;277: 388–389.
39. Muñoz E, Oliva R, Obach V, et al. Identification of Spanish familial Parkinson's disease and screening for the Ala53Thr mutation of the α-synuclein gene in early onset patients. *Neurosci Lett* 2001;235:57–60.
40. Izumi Y, Morino H, Oda M, et al. Genetic studies in Parkinson's disease with an α-synuclein/NACP gene polymorphism in Japan. *Neurosci Lett* 2001;300: 125–127.
41. Markopoulou K, Wszolek ZK, Pfeiffer RF, et al. Reduced expression of the G209A α-synuclein allele in familial parkinsonism. *Ann Neurol* 2001;46:374–381.
42. Papadimitriou A, Veletza V, Hadjigeorgiou GM, et al. Mutated α-synuclein gene in two Greek kindreds with familial PD: incomplete penetrance? *Neurology* 2001; 52:651–654.
43. Athenassiadou A, Voutsinas, Psiouri L, et al. Genetic analysis of families with Parkinson disease that carry the Ala53Thr mutation in the gene encoding α-synuclein. *Am J Hum Genet* 2001;65:555–558.
44. Veletza S, Bostatzopoulos S, Hantzigeorgiou G, et al. Alpha-synuclein mutation associated with familial Parkinson's disease in two new Greek kindreds. *J Neurol* 2001;246[Suppl 1]:43.
45. Spira PJ, Sharpe DM, Halliday G, et al. Clinical and pathological features of a parkinsonian syndrome in a family with an ala53thr α-synuclein mutation. *Ann Neurol* 2001;49:313–319.
46. Papapetropoulos S, Paschalis C, Athanassiadou A, et al. Clinical phenotype in patients with α-synuclein Parkinson's disease living in Greece in comparison with patients with sporadic Parkinson's disease. *J Neurol Neurosurg Psychiatry* 2001;70:662–665.

47. Krüger R, Kuhn W, Müller T, et al. Ala30Pro mutation in the gene encoding α-synuclein in Parkinson's disease. *Nat Genet* 2001;18:106–108.
48. Narhi L, Wood SJ, Steavenson S, et al. Both familial Parkinson's disease mutations accelerate α-synuclein aggregation. *J Biol Chem* 2001;274:9843–9846.
49. Krüger R, Kuhn W, Müller T, et al. Increased susceptibility to sporadic Parkinson's disease by a certain combined α-synuclein/apolipoprotein E genotype. *Ann Neurol* 2001;45:611–617.
50. Khan N, Grahan E, Dixon P, et al. Parkinson's disease is not associated with the combined α-synuclein/apolipoprotein E susceptibility genotype. *Ann Neurol* 2001;49:665–668.
51. Farrer M, Maraganore DM, Lockhart P, et al. α-Synuclein gene haplotypes are associated with Parkinson's disease. *Hum Mol Genet* 2001;10:1847–1851.
52. Jakowec MW, Petzinger GM, Sastry S, et al. The native form of α-synuclein is not found in the cerebrospinal fluid of patients with Parkinson's disease or normal controls. *Neurosci Lett* 2001;253:13–16.
53. Kanda S, Bishop JF, Eglitis MA, et al. Enhanced vulnerability to oxidative stress by α-synuclein mutations and C-terminal truncation. *Neuroscience* 2001;97: 279–284.
54. Ko LW, et al. Sensitization of neuronal cells to oxidative stress with mutated human α-synuclein. *J Neurochem* 2001;75:2546–2554.
55. Lee M, Hyun DH, Halliwell B, et al. Effect of the overexpression of wild-type or mutant α-synuclein on cell susceptibility to insult. *J Neurochem* 2001;76: 998–1009.
56. Conway KA, Harper JD, Lansbury PT. Accelerated *in vitro* fibril formation by a mutant α-synuclein linked to early-onset Parkinson's disease. *Nat Med* 2001;4: 1318–1320.
57. El-Agnaf OMA, Jakes R, Curran MD, et al. Effects of the mutations Ala30 to Pro and Ala53 to Thr on the physical and morphological properties of α-synuclein protein implicated in Parkinson's disease. *FEBS Lett* 2001;440:67–70.
58. Crowther RA, Jakes R, Spillantini MG, et al. Synthetic filaments assembled from C-terminally truncated α-synuclein. *FEBS Lett* 2001;436:309–312.
59. Baba M, Nakajo S, Tu P-H, et al. Aggregation of α-synuclein in Lewy bodies of sporadic Parkinson's disease and dementia with Lewy bodies. *Am J Pathol* 2001;152:879–884.
60. Giasson, Murray IVJ, Trojanowski JQ, et al. A hydrophobic stretch of 12 amino acid residues in the middle of α-synuclein is essential for filament assembly. *J Biol Chem* 2001;276:2380–2386.
61. Spillantini MG, Schmidt ML, Lee VM-Y, et al. α-Synuclein in Lewy bodies. *Nature* 2001;388:840–841.
62. Spillantini MG, Crowther RA, Jakes R, et al. α-Synuclein in filamentous inclusions of Lewy bodies from Parkinson's disease and dementia with Lewy bodies. *Proc Natl Acad Sci U S A* 2001;95:6469–6473.
63. Irizarry MC, Growdon W, Gomez-Isla T, et al. Nigral and cortical Lewy bodies and dystrophic nigral neurites in Parkinson's disease and cortical Lewy body disease contain α-synuclein immunoreactivity. *J Neuropathol Exp Neurol* 2001;57:334–337.
64. Giasson BI, Uryu K, Trojanowski JQ, et al. Mutant and wild type human α-synucleins assemble into elongated filaments with distinct morphologies *in vitro. J Biol Chem* 2001;274:7619–7622.
65. Wood SJ, Wypych J, Steavenson S, et al. α-Synuclein fibrillogenesis is nucleation-dependent: implications for the pathogenesis of Parkinson's disease. *J Biol Chem* 2001;274:19509–19512.
66. Conway KA, Harper JD, Lansbury PT. Fibrils formed *in vitro* from α-synuclein and two mutant forms linked to Parkinson's disease are typical amyloid. *Biochemistry* 2001;39:2552–2562.
67. Serpell LC, Berriman J, Jakes R, et al. Fiber diffraction of synthetic α-synuclein filaments shows amyloid-like cross-beta conformation. *Proc Natl Acad Sci USA* 2001; 97:4897–4902.
68. Hashimoto M, Hsu LJ, Xia Y, et al. Oxidative stress induces amyloid-like aggregate formation of NACP/α-synuclein *in vitro. Neuroreport* 2001;10:717–721.
69. Turnbull S, Tabner BJ, El-Agnaf OMA, et al. α-Synuclein implicated in Parkinson's disease catalyses the formation of hydrogen peroxide *in vitro. Free Rad Biol Med* 2001;30:1163–1170.
70. Ostrerova-Golts N, Petrucelli L, Hardy J, et al. The A53T α-synuclein mutation increases iron-dependent aggregation and toxicity. *J Neurosci* 2001;20: 6048–6054.
71. Nielsen MS, Vorum H, Lindersson E, et al. Ca^{2+} binding to α-synuclein regulates ligand binding and oligomerization. *J Biol Chem* 2001;276:22680–22684.
72. Rochet JC, Conway KA, Lansbury PT. Inhibition of fibrillization and accumulation of prefibrillar oligomers in mixtures of human and mouse α-synuclein. *Biochemistry* 2001;39:10619–10626.
73. Heikkila RE, Manzino L, Cabbat FS, et al. Effects of 1-methyl-4-phenyl-1,2,3,6-tetrahydropyridine (MPTP) and several of its analogues on the dopaminergic nigrostriatal pathway in mice. *Neurosci Lett* 1985;58: 133–137.
74. Kowall NW, Hantraye P, Brouillet E, et al. MPTP induces α-synuclein aggregation in the substantia nigra of baboons. *NeuroReport* 2001;11:211–213.
75. Betarbet R, Sherer TB, MacKenzie G, et al. Chronic systemic pesticide exposure reproduces features of Parkinson's disease. *Nat Neurosci* 2001;3:1301–1306.
76. Uversky VN, Li J, Fink AL. Pesticides directly accelerate the rate of α-synuclein fibril formation: a possible factor in Parkinson's disease. *FEBS Lett* 2001;500: 105–108.
77. Przedborski S, Chen QP, Vila M, et al. Oxidative post-translational modifications of α-synuclein in the MPTP mouse model of Parkinson's disease. *J Neurochem* 2001;76:637–640.
78. Duda JE, Giasson BI, Chen Q, et al. Widespread nitration of pathological inclusions in neurodegenerative synucleinopathies. *Am J Pathol* 2001;157:1439–1445.
79. Forloni G, Bertani I, Calella AM, et al. α-Synuclein and Parkinson's disease: selective neurodegenerative effect of α-synuclein fragment on dopaminergic neurons *in vitro* and *in vivo. Ann Neurol* 2001;47:632–640.
80. Volles MJ, Lee S-J, Rochet J-C, et al. Vesicle permeabilization by protofibrillar α-synuclein: implications for the pathogenesis and treatment of Parkinson's disease. *Biochemistry* 2001;40:7812–7819.
81. Tabrizi SJ, Orth M, Wildinson JM, et al. Expression of

mutant α-synuclein causes increased susceptibility to dopamine toxicity. *Hum Mol Genet* 2001;9:2683–2689.
82. Hsu LJ, Sagarra Y, Arroyo A, et al. α-Synuclein promotes mitochondrial deficit and oxidative stress. *Am J Pathol* 2001;157:401–410.
83. Saha AR, Ninkina NN, Hanger DP, et al. Induction of neuronal death by α-synuclein. *Eur J Neurosci* 2001;12: 3073–3077.
84. Tanaka Y, Engelender S, Igarashi S, et al. Inducible expression of mutant α-synuclein decreases proteasome activity and increases sensitivity to mitochondria-dependent apoptosis. *Hum Mol Genet* 2001;10:919–926.
85. Gomez-Tortosa E, Sanders JL, Newell K, et al. Cortical neurons expressing calcium binding proteins are spared in dementia with Lewy bodies. *Acta Neuropathol* 2001; 101:36–42.
86. Feany MB, Bender WW. A *Drosophila* model of Parkinson's disease. *Nature* 2001;404:394–398.
87. Beal MF. Experimental models of Parkinson's disease. *Nat Rev Neurosci* 2001;2:325–332.
88. Masliah E, Rockenstein E, Veinbergs I, et al. Dopaminergic loss and inclusion body formation in α-synuclein mice: implications for neurodegenerative disorders. *Science* 2001;287:1265–1269.
89. van der Putten H, Wiederhold K-H, Probst A, et al. Neuropathology in mice expressing human α-synuclein. *J Neurosci* 2001;20:6021–6029.
90. Kahle PJ, Neumann M, Ozmen L, et al. Subcellular localization of wild-type and Parkinson's disease–associated mutant α-synuclein in human and transgenic mouse brain. *J Neurosci* 2001;20:6365–6373.
91. Sommer B, Barbieri S, Hofele K, et al. Mouse models of α-synucleinopathy and Lewy pathology. *Exp Gerontol* 2001;35:1389–1403.
92. Matsuoka Y, Vila M, Lincoln S, et al. Lack of nigral pathology in transgenic mice expressing human α-synuclein driven by the tyrosine hydroxylase promoter. *Neurobiol Dis* 2001;8:535–539.
93. Rathke-Hartlieb S, Kahle PJ, Neumann M, et al. Sensitivity to MPTP is not increased in Parkinson's disease–associated mutant α-synuclein transgenic mice. *J Neurochem* 2001;77:1181–1184.

Parkinson's Disease: Advances in Neurology, Vol. 91.
Edited by Ariel Gordin, Seppo Kaakkola,
and Heikki Teräväinen
Lippincott Williams & Wilkins, Philadelphia © 2003

18

Functional Brain Imaging in Parkinson's Disease

Maren Carbon, Christine Edwards, and David Eidelberg

Center for Neurosciences, North Shore–Long Island Jewish Research Institute and Movement Disorders Center, North Shore University Hospital, Manhasset, New York

This chapter focuses on recent work with positron emission tomography (PET), emphasizing the changes in regional brain function and network activity that occur during antiparkinsonian therapy. Although dopamine metabolism PET techniques illustrate the primary pathology in Parkinson's disease (PD) (as summarized in Chapter 6), cerebral blood flow and glucose metabolism analyses are useful for understanding the effects of dopamine loss on the activity of spatially remote but functionally interconnected brain areas. In particular, the identification and quantification of brain networks add a link between clinical impairment and brain dysfunction. In this chapter, we show that the successful treatment of PD is associated with improved regional brain function and suppression of pathological network activity.

THE PARKINSON'S DISEASE–RELATED PATTERN

We have used ^{18}F-fluorodeoxyglucose (^{18}F-FDG) PET in PD and developed a new statistical modeling approach to identify a disease-related regional metabolic brain network covariance. In PD, this network, termed PD-related pattern (PDRP), is characterized by covarying pallidal, thalamic, and pontine hypermetabolism associated with relative decreases in the lateral premotor cortex (PMC), the supplementary motor area (SMA), the dorsolateral prefrontal cortex (DLPFC), and the parietooccipital association regions (1–3) (Fig. 18.1). Previous studies on resting glucose metabolism in PD have already described metabolic changes in the lentiform nucleus (4). However, our network modeling approach broadened the scope of functional pathology to include areas known to be particularly involved in the planning and performance of voluntary movement in healthy subjects (5–7). These specific areas are impaired in brain activation studies of patients with PD performing freely chosen joystick and finger-extension movements (8,9).

The statistical modeling approach that we have developed for network identification is a form of principal component analysis, known as the scaled subprofile model (10–12). This analysis not only demonstrates the functional connectivity of various brain regions but also supplements the anatomical information by quantifying the expression of the covariance pattern in individual subjects.

Applying this technique, the PDRP network precisely discriminates patients with PD and controls in various subsequent populations (3). The PDRP network is detectable early in the course of the illness (13), and its expression in individual patients consistently correlates with motor disability and advancing disease duration (14–16). PDRP expression has been found to relate to the akinetic rigid symptoms of PD, rather than tremor. Indeed, PDRP activity was found to be similarly elevated in patients with PD both with and

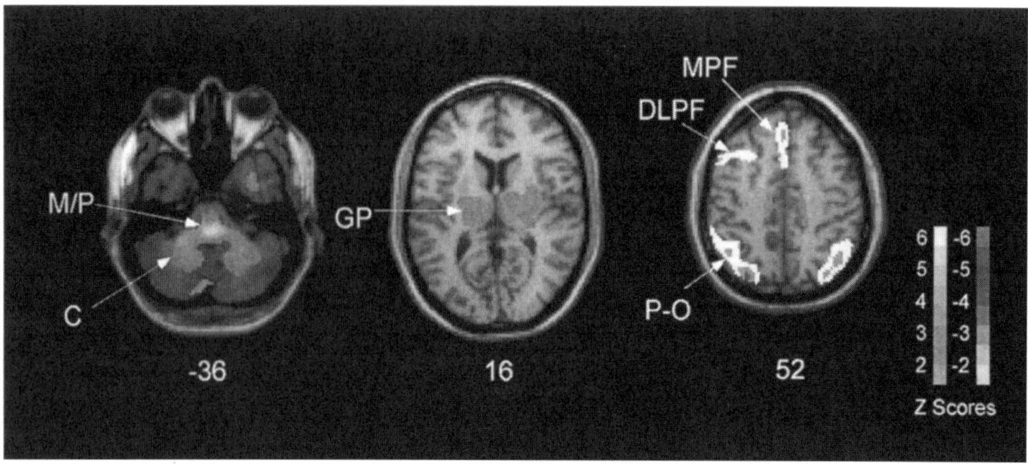

FIGURE 18.1. Three axial slices taken from whole-brain voxel-based network analysis. The metabolic data represent the regions that contribute significantly to the PD-related covariance pattern. The numbers under each slice are in millimeters relative to the anteroposterior commissure line. Voxels with region weights greater than $Z = 1.5$ are color-coded red-yellow, and region weights less than $Z = -1.5$ are color-coded blue-purple. (M/P, midbrain/pons; C, cerebellum; GP, globus pallidus; DLPF, dorsolateral prefrontal cortex; MPF, medial prefrontal cortex; PO, parietooccipital cortex.) (From Moeller JR, Nakamura T, Mentis MJ, et al. Reproducibility of regional metabolic covariance patterns: comparison of four populations. *J Nucl Med* 1999;40:1264–1269, with permission.)

without tremor. Those with significant tremor expressed an additional independent network, involving metabolic activity of the thalamus bilaterally and the pons (17). PDRP expression can also reliably distinguish atypical parkinsonian syndromes (13,15,18). This suggests that this network does not simply reflect a particular symptom constellation, but that it is the metabolic consequence of presynaptic nigrostriatal dopamine loss. We confirmed this notion by demonstrating that the expression of the PDRP correlates not only with the clinical disease severity, but also with striatal dopamine deficiency as determined by ^{18}F-fluorodopa PET (1). More recently, we have demonstrated the reproducibility of the PDRP in multiple PD populations scanned on different tomographs (3,19), as well as in single-photon emission computed tomography perfusion data (15).

In summary, the PDRP represents a dynamic network of regional metabolic changes in PD, identified through an entirely data-driven statistical approach. It is noteworthy that the topography of this pattern corresponds with the anatomy of cortical-striatal-pallidal-thalamic-cortical motor pathways (CSPTC), identified using invasive methods in experimental animal models (20,21). The PDRP quantifies the abnormal functional activity of the motor CSPTC in living patients.

Internal globus pallidus (GPi) output is one crucial pathophysiological link between basal ganglia function and motor cortex function. Increased pallidal inhibitory outflow has been suggested to be the pathophysiological correlate of akinesia in PD (22). Because glucose metabolism reflects synaptic activity, we tested the hypothesis that intraoperatively recorded spontaneous single-unit GPi firing rates would correlate with preoperative cerebral glucose metabolism (23). Interestingly, GPi firing rates highly correlated with ventral thalamic glucose metabolism, but not with metabolic changes in the motor cortex. Moreover, using regional covariance analysis, we identified a significant brain network that correlated with spontaneous GPi firing rates.

The topography of this pattern resembled the PDRP, being characterized by pallidothalamic and brainstem metabolic activity. Thus, the PDRP is likely to have a physiological and a statistical basis as an imaging descriptor of parkinsonism.

INTERVENTIONAL MODULATION OF BRAIN GLUCOSE METABOLISM IN PD

Having established the PDRP as a functional marker of parkinsonism, we investigated the effects of antiparkinsonian interventions on the activity of this network. Although various surgical interventions for PD have become widespread in clinical practice, the pathophysiological effects of surgery are not clearly understood (22). Over the past several years, we have studied the effects of several stereotaxic interventions on resting glucose metabolism. In particular, we examined the hypothesis that effective antiparkinsonian therapy is associated with modulation of PDRP network activity. We considered the notion that interventions targeting specific CSPTC nodes lead to significant reductions in PDRP expression, and that the degree of network modulation correlates with clinical improvement. Furthermore, we localized the regional changes in cerebral metabolism that occurred after each investigation and determined whether these changes correlated with clinical response. (The results are summarized in Table 18.1 and Figure 18.2.) To quantify network expression in different cohorts and treatment conditions, we developed an automated computational method to compute pattern expression in individual subjects (13, 16,24). This algorithm is blind to operative status (pre, post; on, off) and to therapeutic intervention (drug, lesioning, deep brain stimulation [DBS]).

In a cohort of subjects undergoing unilateral pallidotomy, the preoperative abnormal elevation in glucose metabolism in the lentiform nucleus and thalamus declined after surgery, concomitant with an increase in SMA metabolism (25). This pattern of operative change closely resembled the PDRP topography, reflecting a correction in brain function that was highly correlated with clinical outcome after surgery. Interestingly, clinical improvement in both limbs correlated with the degree of network suppression that was achieved after pallidal lesioning.

In a subsequent FDG PET study of GPi DBS, we assessed seven patients off medication, comparing brain glucose metabolism on and off stimulation (26). As in pallidotomy,

TABLE 18.1. *Changes in glucose metabolism with antiparkinsonian therapy*

Intervention	Percent change in motor score	Correlation of change in PDRP induced by intervention with change in motor score	Regional changes by intervention
Ventral pallidotomy	30.9%	$r = 0.84$ $p = .01$	↑ PMC ↑ primary motor cortex ↑ dorsolateral prefrontal cortex
Globus pallidus internalis deep brain stimulation	36.0%	$r = 0.66$ $p < .03$	↑ PMC cerebellum
Subthalamotomy	41.4%	$r = 0.79$ $p < .0001$	↓ Globus pallidus internalis ↓ ventral thalamus ↓ midbrain substantia nigra ↓ pons ↑ cerebellum
Levodopa infusion	30.6%	$r = 0.78$ $p < .04$	↓ primary motor cortex ↓ ventral thalamus ↓ putamen ↓ cerebellum

PDRP, Parkinson's disease–related pattern; PMC, premotor cortex.

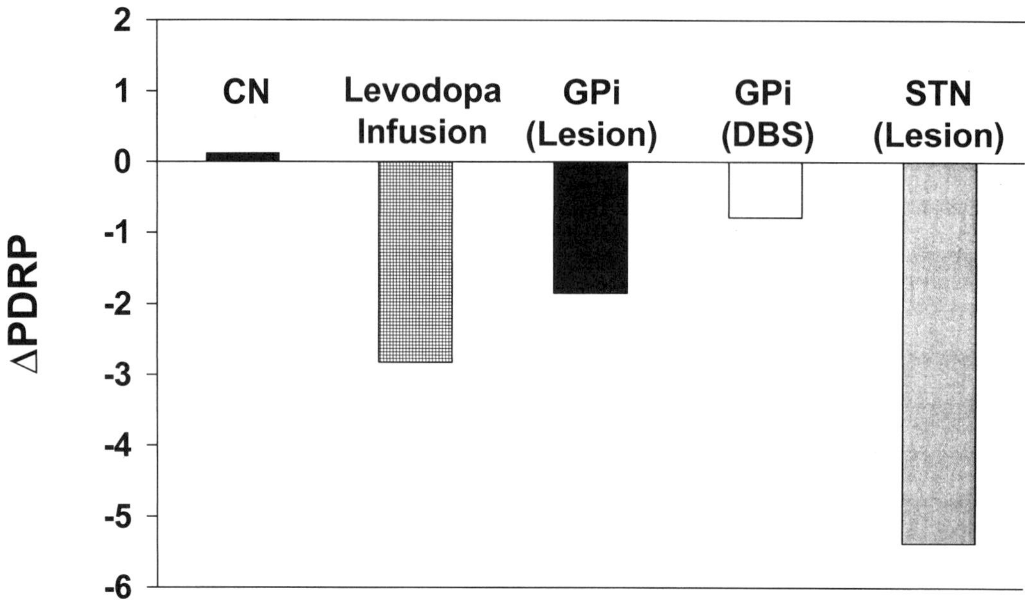

FIGURE 18.2. Bar graph illustrating relative changes in the expression of the Parkinson's disease–related pattern *(Δ PDRP)* (see text) during antiparkinsonian therapy with levodopa infusion (37), and unilateral ventral pallidotomy (25), pallidal deep brain stimulation (DBS) (26), and subthalamotomy (19). In the case of hemispheric lesioning (the internal segment of the globus pallidus [GPi] and the subthalamic nucleus [STN]), *Δ PDRP* reflects subject score differences before and 3 to 6 months after surgery. In the case of GPi DBS, this measure reflects changes in network expression off and on 12 hours of pallidal stimulation. In the case of levodopa infusion, this measure reflects changes occurring after acute steady-state intravenous administration of the drug. For surgical interventions, *Δ PDRP* reflects changes in network activity in the operated-on hemispheres. With levodopa infusion, the PDRP changes were averaged across hemispheres. The control data *(CN)* represent *Δ PDRP* values for the unoperated-on contralateral hemispheres in the unmedicated state.

GPi stimulation consistently reduced PDRP expression; the degree of network suppression correlated significantly with the improvement in Unified Parkinson's Disease Rating Scale (UPDRS) motor ratings during stimulation. Furthermore, regional analysis showed a stimulation-induced metabolic increase in the resting metabolism in the PMC ipsilateral to stimulation and in the cerebellum bilaterally. The metabolic increase in the PMC correlated significantly with the clinical change. As in pallidotomy, the primary metabolic change mediating the motor improvement is located in premotor cortical areas that are anatomically related to the globus pallidus (27).

Modulation of the PDRP was demonstrated also in a subsequent study of seven patients undergoing unilateral subthalamotomy (19). FDG PET and network analysis revealed a highly significant reduction in the expression of the PDRP in all operated-on hemispheres, correlating with a significant reduction in UPDRS motor scores. At the same time, no changes in the non–operated-on hemispheres were observed. The maximum reduction in surgical glucose metabolism was located in the midbrain, spanning the magnetic resonance imaging–confirmed lesion site, as well as in the substantia nigra pars reticulata (SNpr). Additional metabolic decreases were present in the ipsilateral GPi and the ventral thalamus, and in the pons, in the area of the pedunculopontine nucleus (PPN). These areas receive major inhibitory output from the GPi and SNpr in animal models of parkinsonism (28). Functionally, the PPN is thought to regulate gait initiation, other stereotyped movements, and postural control (29). In keeping with our observations in pallidal stimulation, we further noticed metabolic increases in the ipsilateral cerebellar hemisphere and dentate nucleus.

In addition to surgical interventions, we assessed metabolic changes associated with dopaminergic pharmacotherapy. As suggested by the correlation of the PDRP network with striatal dopamine deficiency and in keeping with our general hypothesis, acute intravenous levodopa infusion in PD led to a significant reduction in network activity, paralleling clinical motor improvement (30). Regional analysis revealed localized metabolic decreases with levodopa infusion in the putamen, the primary site of levodopa action. Significant metabolic reductions were also present downstream in the thalamus and cerebellum.

In summary, these studies show that successful antiparkinsonian therapy, regardless of the mechanism of intervention, is mediated by PDRP suppression. The degree of network modulation correlates consistently with clinical outcome. Thus, the PDRP network may be valuable as a reliable *in vivo* marker of symptomatic therapy of PD and for the investigation of new therapeutic agents.

INTERVENTIONAL MODULATION OF MOTOR ACTIVATION IN PD

Using new three-dimensional PET techniques (31), we measured motor-activation responses during interventions with $H_2{}^{15}O$ PET. These studies were performed in the same PET sessions as the resting state assessments of glucose use cited earlier. In this series of experiments, we tested the hypothesis that interventional suppression of the PDRP activity facilitated brain activation during motor execution. We furthermore determined whether specific aspects of abnormal movement in PD such as timing and spatial errors were selectively improved by therapy, and whether these changes were associated with localized alterations in the neural activity within the CSPTC loops and related pathways.

In these studies, subjects performed a paced sequence of predictable reaching movements on a digitizing tablet with the dominant right hand. Movements were directed to targets on a computer display (32). Individual subjects performed this timed reaching task with identical individual experimental constraints (movement extent and rate) in both treatment conditions (26,30).

GPi DBS induced a significant enhancement of motor-activation responses in the SMA and in the sensorimotor cortex and caudal SMA contralateral to the moving hand (26). During stimulation, a reduction in initiation time consistent with improved akinesia was achieved. This improvement was correlated with an increase in regional cerebral blood flow (rCBF) in the left sensorimotor cortex, the right cerebellum, and the left ventrolateral thalamus. It has been suggested that the excessive inhibitory pallidal outflow to the thalamus, a crucial feature in the pathophysiology of akinesia (33), results in altered thalamic glucose metabolism (23). Our current results may illustrate that a DBS-induced reduction of this inhibitory pallidal output serves as a basis for enhanced physiological activation, associated with facilitated rCBF in the thalamus.

Concomitantly, GPi DBS reduced the mean and variability of spatial errors. This improvement was correlated with an rCBF increase in left sensorimotor cortex and both cerebellar hemispheres, the latter associated with online corrections in spatial error in normal subjects (34). Despite that movement-onset time and spatial accuracy were partly mediated by the same regions, they were statistically unrelated in our PD cohort. Although the pallidum does not directly project to cerebellar areas, it is possible that the stimulation-induced changes in the cerebellar hemispheres are mediated via pallidal projections to the PPN (23,35).

These findings contrast with our investigations of brain activation subsequent to intravenous levodopa administration titrated to achieve a comparable clinical benefit (36). Because levodopa infusion reduces PDRP expression in resting glucose metabolism, we hypothesized that this would also facilitate brain activation during movement (30). Using the motor-execution task described earlier and with H_2O PET, we found that levodopa infusion increased activation responses in the posterior putamen and in the ventral thalamus and pons.

In contrast to GPi DBS, levodopa infusion *increased* spatial errors. Interestingly, as in the DBS experiments, these changes correlated with treatment-mediated alterations in cerebellar cortical activity.

Additionally, levodopa produced a significant improvement of movement time, a physiological descriptor of parkinsonian bradykinesia. This improvement was correlated with increased activation-induced rCBF in the putamen contralateral to the moving hand. These observations support the notion of a reversal of abnormal function in CSPTC loops with antiparkinsonian treatment. A specific effect of levodopa appears to be a reversal of abnormal elevation of putaminal glucose metabolism at rest (37), which, in turn, facilitates putaminal activation during movement.

Summarizing our observations of altered brain activation by antiparkinsonian treatment, we confirmed our hypothesis that suppression of the PDRP in the resting state is associated with a facilitation of regional activation at specific nodes of the motor CSPTC loop and related circuits. Despite this commonality of metabolic network modulation, specific therapies appear to enhance motor activation in different regional network elements depending on the primary site of intervention.

CONCLUSIONS

Metabolic neuroimaging with PET has advanced from describing the resting metabolic landscape of PD to providing a quantitative assessment of therapeutic interventions. In the future, this approach may prove useful in testing new drugs and surgical treatment strategies. This methodology may also be applicable to the study of more complex motor functions such as learning, as well as in delineating the basis for cognitive and affective manifestations of parkinsonism.

ACKNOWLEDGMENTS

This work was supported by National Institutes of Health ROI NS 35069 and K24 NS 02101, and by grants from the Parkinson Disease Foundation and the American Parkinson Disease Association. The authors acknowledge the valuable contributions of their colleagues in the Neuroscience Center and the Cyclotron/PET Facility of the North Shore–Long Island Jewish Research Institute.

REFERENCES

1. Eidelberg D, Moeller JR, Dhawan V, et al. The metabolic anatomy of Parkinson's disease: complementary [^{18}F]fluorodeoxyglucose and [^{18}F]fluorodopa positron emission tomographic studies. *Mov Disord* 1990;5(3): 203–213.
2. Eidelberg D, Moeller JR, Dhawan V, et al. The metabolic topography of parkinsonism. *J Cereb Blood Flow Metab* 1994;14:783–801.
3. Moeller JR, Nakamura T, Mentis MJ, et al. Reproducibility of regional metabolic covariance patterns: comparison of four populations. *J Nucl Med* 1999; 40(8):1264–1269.
4. Wolfson LI, Leenders KL, Brown LL, et al. Alterations of regional cerebral blood flow and oxygen metabolism in Parkinson's disease. *Neurology* 1985;35(10): 1399–1405.
5. Deecke L. Electrophysiological correlates of movement initiation. *Rev Neurol (Paris)* 1990;146:612–619.
6. deJong BM, Willemsen AT, Paans AM. Brain activation related to the change between bimanual motor programs. *Neuroimage* 1999;9:290–297.
7. Freund HJ. Premotor area and preparation of movement. *Rev Neurol (Paris)* 1990;146:543–547.
8. Jahanshahi M, Jenkins IH, Brown RG, et al. Self-initiated versus externally triggered movements, I: an investigation using measurement of regional cerebral blood flow with PET and movement-related potentials in normal and Parkinson's disease subjects. *Brain* 1995;118: 913–933.
9. Playford ED, Jenkins IH, Passingham RE, et al. Impaired mesial frontal and putamen activation in Parkinson's disease: a positron emission tomography study. *Ann Neurol* 1992;32:151–161.
10. Alexander GE, Moeller JR. Application of the scaled subprofile model to functional imaging in neuropsychiatric disorders: a principal component approach to modeling brain function in disease. *Hum Brain Mapping* 1994;2:1–16.

11. Eidelberg D, Edwards C, Mentis M, et al. Movement disorders: Parkinson's disease. In: Mazziotta JC, Toga AW, Frackowiak RSJ, eds. *Brain mapping: the disorders.* San Diego: Academic Press, 2000:241–261.
12. Moeller JR, Strother SC. A regional covariance approach to the analysis of functional patterns in positron emission tomographic data. *J Cereb Blood Flow Metab* 1991;11:A121–135.
13. Eidelberg D, Moeller JR, Ishikawa T, et al. Early differential diagnosis of Parkinson's disease with ^{18}F-fluorodeoxyglucose and positron emission tomography. *Neurology* 1995;45:1995–2004.
14. Eidelberg D, Moeller JR, Ishikawa T, et al. Assessment of disease severity in parkinsonism with fluorine-18-fluorodeoxyglucose and PET. *J Nucl Med* 1995;36: 378–383.
15. Feigin A, Pillai V, Fukuda M, et al. ECD/SPECT in the differential diagnosis of parkinsonism. *Mov Disord* 2002 *(in press).*
16. Moeller JR, Eidelberg D. Divergent expression of regional metabolic topographies in Parkinson's disease and normal ageing. *Brain* 1997;120:2197–2206.
17. Antonini A, Moeller JR, Nakamura T, et al. The metabolic anatomy of tremor in Parkinson's disease. *Neurology* 1998;51:803–810.
18. Eidelberg D, Takikawa S, Moeller JR, et al. Striatal hypometabolism distinguishes striatonigral degeneration from Parkinson's disease. *Ann Neurol* 1993;33: 518–527.
19. Su P, Ma Y, Fukuda M, et al. Metabolic changes following subthalamotomy for advanced Parkinson's disease. *Ann Neurol* 2001;50:514–520.
20. Alexander GE, Crutcher MD, DeLong MR. Basal ganglia-thalamocortical circuits: parallel substrates for motor, oculomotor, "prefrontal" and "limbic" functions. *Prog Brain Res* 1990;85:119–146.
21. Wichmann T, DeLong MR. Functional and pathophysiological models of the basal ganglia. *Curr Opin Neurobiol* 1996;6:751–758.
22. Marsden C, Obeso J. The functions of the basal ganglia and the paradox of stereotaxic surgery in Parkinson's disease. *Brain* 1994;117:877–897.
23. Eidelberg D, Moeller JR, Kazumata K, et al. Metabolic correlates of pallidal neuronal activity in Parkinson's disease. *Brain* 1997;120:1315–1324.
24. Moeller JR, Ishikawa T, Dhawan V, et al. The metabolic topography of normal aging. *J Cereb Blood Flow Metab* 1996;16:385–398.
25. Eidelberg D, Moeller JR, Ishikawa T, et al. Regional metabolic correlates of surgical outcome following unilateral pallidotomy for Parkinson's disease. *Ann Neurol* 1996;39:450–459.
26. Fukuda M, Mentis MJ, Ma Y, et al. Networks mediating the clinical effects of pallidal brain stimulation for Parkinson's disease: a PET study of resting-state glucose metabolism. *Brain* 2001;124:1601–1609.
27. Middleton FA, Strick PL. Basal ganglia and cerebellar loops: motor and cognitive circuits. *Brain Res Rev* 2000;31:236–250.
28. Mitchell IJ, Clarke CE, Boyce S, et al. Neural mechanisms underlying parkinsonian symptoms based upon regional uptake of 2-deoxyglucose in monkeys exposed to 1-methyl-4-phenyl-1,2,3,6-tetrahydropyridine. *Neuroscience* 1989;32:213–226.
29. Pahapill PA, Lozano AM. The pedunculopontine nucleus and Parkinson's disease. *Brain* 2000;123:1767–1783.
30. Feigin A, Ghilardi MF, Fukuda M, et al. Effects of levodopa infusion on motor activation responses in Parkinson's disease. *Neurology* 2002 *(in press).*
31. Dhawan V, Kazumata K, Robeson W, et al. Quantitative brain PET: comparison of 2D and 3D acquisition on the GE Advance Scanner. *Clin Positron Imaging* 1998;1: 135–144.
32. Ghilardi M, Ghez C, Moeller J, et al. Patterns of regional brain activation associated with different aspects of motor learning. *Brain Res* 2000;871:127–145.
33. DeLong MR. Primate models of movement disorders of basal ganglia origin. *Trends Neurosci* 1990;13: 281–285.
34. Jueptner M, Weiller C. A review of differences between basal ganglia and cerebellar control of movements as revealed by functional imaging studies. *Brain* 1998;121: 1437–1449.
35. Parent A, Hazrati LN. Functional anatomy of the basal ganglia, I: The cortico-basal ganglia-thalamo-cortical loop. *Brain Res Rev* 1995;20:91–127.
36. Ghilardi MF, Ghez CP, Feigin A, et al. Motor sequence learning in Parkinson's disease: differential effects of levodopa and DBS. *Neurology* 2001;56:A147.
37. Feigin A, Fukuda M, Dhawan V, et al. Metabolic correlates of levodopa response in Parkinson's disease. *Neurology* 2001;57:2083–2088.

Parkinson's Disease: Advances in Neurology, Vol. 91.
Edited by Ariel Gordin, Seppo Kaakkola,
and Heikki Teräväinen
Lippincott Williams & Wilkins, Philadelphia © 2003

19

Single-Photon Emission Tomography and Dopamine Transporter Imaging in Parkinson's Disease

Kenneth Marek, Danna Jennings, and John Seibyl

Department of Neurology, The Institute for Neurogenerative Disorders, New Haven, Connecticut

Imaging in Parkinson's disease (PD) has emerged as a bridge to help translate our understanding of the pathophysiology of PD into meaningful clinical tools and new therapies.

In vivo functional imaging uses specific chemical ligands as tags or markers to neurochemically dissect the dopaminergic deficit in PD and related disorders. The strengths and limitations of *in vivo* functional imaging studies depend on the imaging technology used to measure brain neurochemistry and the ligand or biochemical marker used to tag a specific brain neurochemical system. Positron emission tomography (PET) and single-photon emission computed tomography (SPECT) have been the primary techniques used to study the dopaminergic system in PD and related disorders (1,2). Both SPECT and PET are sensitive methods of measuring *in vivo* neurochemistry. Although generally PET cameras have better resolution than SPECT cameras, SPECT studies may be technologically and clinically more feasible, particularly for large clinical studies and in clinical practice. The choice of imaging modality is ultimately determined by the specific study questions and study design. Specific markers for the dopaminergic system have been widely used to evaluate patients with PD including ^{18}F-fluorodopa (3–8), ^{11}C-vesicular monoamine transporter type 2 (VMAT2) (9–11) and dopamine transporter (DAT) ligands (12–16). DAT is a protein that is located on the dopamine presynaptic nerve terminal. Therefore, these ligands directly measure dopamine terminal integrity and degeneration. DAT SPECT imaging has been increasingly used both in clinical studies and in the clinical practice of PD. This chapter focuses on the recent studies using DAT ligands and SPECT as a potential tool to aid in PD diagnosis, to assess PD progression, and to identity at-risk individuals for PD.

IMAGING THE DOPAMINE TRANSPORTER

The value of DAT radioligands in PD and related disorders derives from postmortem studies showing loss of dopaminergic neurons and concomitant DAT target sites located on presynaptic terminals. Ongoing degeneration results in a progressive reduction in the radiolabeled marker uptake in those regions containing DAT striatum. Hence, DAT ligands used as imaging agents have the advantage of a high density of target sites in a region of brain relevant to the pathophysiological process (Fig. 19.1).

DAT imaging agents are cocaine analogues with nanomolar affinity at the DAT (17–22). These ligands are chemically modified to al-

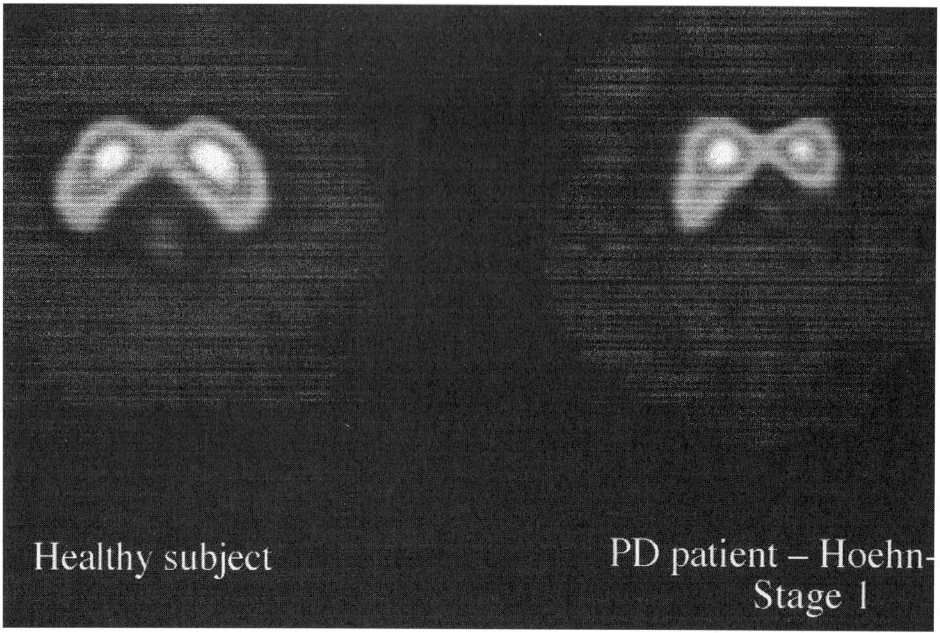

FIGURE 19.1. Single-photon emission computed tomography (SPECT) ^{123}I-β-CIT images from a patient with mild Parkinson's disease (PD) and from an age-matched healthy subject. Note the asymmetrical reduction in ^{123}I-β-CIT uptake is more marked in the putamen than in the caudate in the patient. Regions of interest were drawn based on co-registered magnetic resonance imaging. Levels of SPECT activity are color-encoded from low (*black*) to high (*yellow/white*).

ter the rapid metabolism of cocaine at the ester linkage to provide more *in vivo* stability of the parent compound. Nonetheless, the kinetic properties of DAT radiotracers are quite different with regard to plasma protein binding, permeability across the blood–brain barrier, binding affinity, selectivity for the DAT, and elimination. These differences are highly meaningful to the applications of the DAT ligand for imaging (23). For example, although a given DAT tracer may distinguish PD from healthy controls based on the qualitative appearance of striatal uptake, the ability to distinguish the longitudinal changes in severity of PD may be more difficult for tracers with relatively poorer signal-to-noise properties (lower specific to nonspecific brain uptake) (Table 19.1). The quantitative properties of the radiotracer must be well understood to assess disease progression. Specifically, does the imaging signal provide a measure that is related to B_{max}, the density of DAT, and/or the integrity of dopaminergic neurons? This question requires detailed validation of the radiopharmaceutical and imaging technology, including a careful characterization of the reproducibility of the outcome measure, the potential effect of symptomatic treatments on

TABLE 19.1. *Comparative differences between some SPECT DAT radioligands*

SPECT tracer	^{123}I-β-CIT	^{123}I-FP-CIT	^{99m}Tc-TRODAT	^{123}I-Altropane
Time to peak uptake	Protracted 8–18 hr	Rapid 2–3 hr	Rapid 2–3 hr	Rapid 0.5–1 hr
Washout phase	Prolonged	Prolonged	Intermediate	Rapid
DAT binding affinity	1.4 nM Ki	3.5 nM Ki	9.7 nM Ki	6.62 nM IC_{50}
DAT:SERT selectivity	1.7:1	2.8:1	26:1	28:1
SPECT target: background-to-tissue ratio	High	High	Low	Low

DAT, dopamine transporter; SERT, serotonin transporter; SPECT, single-photon emission computed tomography.

the imaging outcome measure, and others, as well as the consideration of regulation of DAT density in the face of the disease process (24–29).

For some tracers, absolute quantitation of the DAT signal may require invasive methods involving full kinetic modeling, whereas other DAT tracers have a pharmacokinetic profile, which simplifies the methods for signal quantification. For example, the unusual binding kinetics of ^{123}I-β-CIT, with a protracted period of stable specific radiotracer uptake in the brain and extremely slow elimination from the DAT sites in striatum permit reproducible quantitative determination of DAT density using a simple tissue ratio method (30,31). For DAT tracers with faster washout from specific binding sites, this simple ratio technique will overestimate the density of binding sites in healthy striatum relative to PD (32), although these tracers may permit better visual discrimination of diseased from control cases.

Several radioligands have been developed that bind to the DAT and may provide a measure of dopamine terminal integrity. None of these tracers is commercially available in North America, although one tropane derivative of cocaine (fluoropropyl-CIT [FP-CIT], DATSCAN) is available as a ^{123}I-labeled tracer in Europe. Of the DAT SPECT tracers in development, ^{123}I-β-CIT, ^{123}I-FP-CIT, ^{123}I-altropane, and ^{99m}Tc-TRODAT have been the most widely evaluated DAT agents (14,33,34) for SPECT imaging and ^{18}F-CFT (WIN 35,428) for PET (19,35,36).

DOPAMINE TRANSPORTER IMAGING FOR DIAGNOSING PARKINSON'S DISEASE AND RELATED DISORDERS

The initial human imaging studies of DAT SPECT distribution in brain focused on the ability of the imaging technique to distinguish PD from controls and the correlation of the imaging signal with clinical assessment of disease severity. This represents the application of DAT SPECT imaging both as a trait marker (is the disease present?) and a state marker (how severe is the disease?). DAT SPECT imaging in patients with very early PD has helped the understanding of premorbid interval, the length of time between initiation of the pathophysiological process and the first appearance of clinical symptoms. In most patients with PD, the early course of the disorder is characterized by unilateral onset of motor symptoms with subsequent bilateralization of symptoms, although right-to-left asymmetry of motor impairment persists throughout the clinical course. Imaging studies of DAT consistently demonstrate bilateral alterations in the tracer uptake in the striatum of patients with unilateral symptoms (37–39). In these patients, imaging of DATs shows about a 50% reduction in the putamen contralateral to the symptomatic side and a 25% reduction in the putamen ipsilateral to the symptom side relative to age-matched healthy subjects (Fig. 19.1). Based on these studies and estimates that most patients with hemi-PD develop bilateral symptoms in 3 to 6 years, it is possible to develop a preliminary estimate of (a) the amount of signal loss in the striatum at the time symptoms become manifest and (b) a backward extrapolation of the data to an estimate of the time required for symptoms to first appear—that is, the premorbid interval. Using untested assumptions including a linear progression of signal loss, DAT imaging studies suggest a premorbid period of approximately 5 to 7 years (40).

In several large, multicenter studies assessing DAT SPECT imaging to determine clinical diagnosis, patients with PD were distinguished from age-matched healthy controls with more than 95% sensitivity and 92% to 94% specificity (Table 19.2). This is similar to the discriminative ability of ^{18}F-fluorodopa PET, another presynaptic marker and measure of dopamine metabolism. Striatal uptake for DAT tracers also correlates with clinical rating scales of PD severity like the Unified Parkinson's Disease Rating Scale (UPDRS), suggesting DAT imaging may provide a marker both for the presence of disease and for the severity of the pathological process (41–43). Furthermore, consistent with postmortem evaluation of the regional pattern of dopaminergic loss in PD, DAT imaging indicates greater signal loss

TABLE 19.2. *Summary of some larger studies evaluating DAT radioligands in diagnostic assessment of Parkinson's disease compared with healthy controls*

Study	Tracer	Subjects	Findings	Comments
Parkinson Study Group (45)	^{123}I-β-CIT	60 PDism, 14 ET, 22 HS	PDism vs/HS & ET, sensitivity = 0.98, specificity = 0.83	Muliticenter, core lab visual read, quantitative read 0.96 sensitivity, 0.94 specificity
The ^{123}I-FP-CIT Study Group (61)	^{123}I-FP-CIT	128 PDism, 27 ET, 35 HS	PDism, sensitivity = 0.95, specificity = 0.93	Multicenter, core lab visual read
Huang et al. (62)	^{99m}Tc TRODAT-1	34 PD, 17 HS	Good discrimination between PD and HS	Some groups overlap of striatal uptake ratios
Mozley et al. (42)	^{99m}Tc TRODAT-1	42 PD, 61 HS	Good discrimination between PD and HS	Some groups overlap of striatal uptake ratios
Schwarz et al. (63)	^{123}I-IPT	28 PD, 9 HS	Excellent discrimination between PD and HS	Only one PD subject overlapped with control

DAT, dopamine transporter; ET, essential tremor; HS, healthy subjects; PDism, Parkinsonism (idiopathic Parkinson's disease, progressive supranuclear palsy, multiple system atrophy, corticobasilar degeneration).

in the caudate relative to the putamen, and within the putamen greater impairment in posterior and lateral regions.

Distinguishing between PD and related parkinsonisms (parkinsonian-plus syndromes) such as progressive supranuclear palsy, striatonigral degeneration is important due to differences in prognosis and treatment response among these disorders. Pathologically, many parkinsonism patients are also characterized by nigrostriatal dopamine neuron loss, hence changes in uptake are noted on DAT imaging. Similar to idiopathic PD, the pathology in these related disorders manifests as reduction of *in vivo* DAT striatal uptake. The severity of DAT loss alone does not distinguish between PD and other causes of parkinsonism. However, the pattern of loss in parkinsonism is less region specific than in idiopathic PD with the putamen and caudate more equally effected (44–48). Striatal uptake in these disorders is also more symmetrical than in idiopathic PD. DAT SPECT can discriminate between PD and other causes of parkinsonism with a sensitivity of about 75% to 80%. The more extensive pathology associated with Parkinson's syndrome may be reflected in abnormalities in postsynaptic dopamine receptor imaging. Postsynaptic D_2/D_3 receptor densities are normal or slightly elevated in idiopathic PD. Hence, a strategy of imaging presynaptic and postsynaptic dopaminergic sites or metabolic imaging may serve to distinguish PD from other related parkinsonisms (44,49).

DOPAMINE TRANSPORTER IMAGING FOR EVALUATING DISEASE PROGRESSION AND DISEASE-MODIFYING TREATMENTS

Studies of the rate of neurodegenerative change and factors that affect the progression of motor symptoms are largely indirect and based on postmortem evaluations of the brains of individuals who die after varying disease duration (50,51). Better information about disease progression in individuals with PD is becoming increasingly important as neuroprotective or neurorestorative strategies for PD are developed and tested. Rational targeting of these agents to appropriate patients and evaluation of their efficacy requires clear understanding of those factors that influence the variability of disease onset and progression. Such information can inform diagnosis and the timing of initiation of drug treatment. For example, if the neurodegenerative process in PD extends over a period of many decades before the initial motor manifestations in some patients, the value of a neuroprotective strategy could be diminished compared with its value in individuals with a more acute disease process.

Phenomenological observations about the clinical course in PD may serve as a guide to understanding the pathophysiology and direct the focus of research questions using imaging. Patients with PD usually present with subtle motor symptoms that progress over many years. Longitudinal evaluation of PD progression of motor impairment indicates both a high degree of variability between patients in their rates of disease progression and variability within an individual over the course of illness. These clinical studies of PD suggest patients early in the course of their disease progress faster than those in later stages of illness (52). It is not clear what factors affect the variability in clinical motor symptoms.

DAT SPECT imaging permits the serial within-patient assessment of the progression of the dopaminergic defects over the illness course. These studies have been performed with both DAT and ^{18}F-fluorodopa, demonstrating in early patients a progressive loss from baseline of approximately 6% to 10% per year of both ^{18}F-fluorodopa and DAT uptake in patients with early PD (26,27,29) (Fig. 19.2). The rate of dopamine signal loss in these studies is about 10-fold to 15-fold greater than that in healthy subjects, which demonstrates a clearly measurable DAT signal loss of approximately 6% per decade based on large cross-sectional studies (30). Although conclusions about progression of the disease based on markers such as DAT are limited by small sample sizes, it is again also possible to use these data to determine premorbid intervals similar to that described earlier using imaging data in patients with hemi-PD. Consistent with the cross-sectional data and information obtained in imaging studies of patients with hemi-PD described earlier, serial DAT SPECT imaging study data similarly suggest

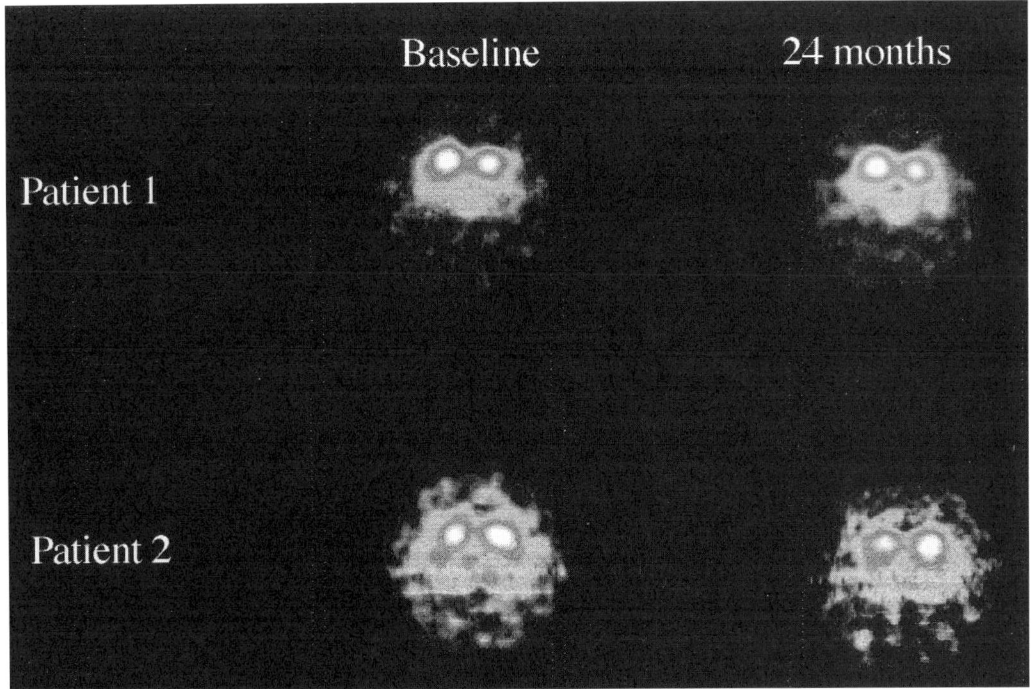

FIGURE 19.2. Sequential single-photon emission computed tomography (SPECT) ^{123}I-β-CIT images of in subjects with Parkinson's disease demonstrating the progression of dopaminergic degeneration during the scanning interval. Levels of SPECT activity are color-encoded from low (*black*) to high (*yellow/white*).

that neurodegeneration in PD is an ongoing process originating about 5 to 10 years before development of symptoms of PD.

In longitudinal studies that have used both imaging and clinical measures of symptom severity in progressing patients with PD, there has been limited correlation between motor measures of progression and changes in the imaging signal (26,53). This is an apparent paradox, because cross-sectional studies of patients with PD show excellent correlation of motor measures and imaging outcomes. However, these same cross-sectional studies show in very early hemi-PD patients no correlation between changes in the striatum occurring on the side ipsilateral to symptoms and motor scores. Hence, it is likely that the sensitivity of the imaging measure is much higher and/or measures a more elementary level of pathophysiological change in patients. On the other hand, the expression of motor symptoms may involve the interplay of compensatory neurochemical systems downstream from the primary pathophysiological event. In a longitudinal study of patients with PD imaged serially over 4 years with ^{123}I-β-CIT SPECT, the correlation between changes in the loss of signal over time and UPDRS motor score became statistically significant only as study duration increased (54). Finally, another crucial factor for the lack of motor and imaging correlation cited in studies evaluating both ^{18}F-fluorodopa PET and DAT SPECT imaging in progressing patients with PD is the inability to achieve complete washout of medications in patients.

What are some factors that could influence the progression dopaminergic loss over time? A number of different models have been proposed for the processes that initiate and serve to maintain the ongoing process of neuronal loss in PD. One compelling model suggests that a possible mechanism for ongoing neuronal degeneration in PD involves transport and compartmentalization of neurotoxic compounds, including dopamine, into presynaptic terminals by the DAT and their sequestration into synaptic vesicles by the vesicular transporter VMAT2 (55). Work with the toxins producing experimental parkinsonism—6-hydroxydopamine and the active metabolite (1-methyl-4-phenylpyridine) of methylphenyltetrahydropyridine—suggests a crucial role of the level of DAT and VMAT2 expression in modulating the toxic effects of these agents on dopaminergic neurons (56). These toxins can produce free radicals and reactive species that may alter important cell proteins when they are concentrated in the cytosol of cells (57). DAT could thus pump selective toxins into cells while the vesicular transporter (VMAT2) sequesters the toxins into vesicles, thereby reducing cytosolic concentrations.

Recent DAT SPECT imaging studies in progressing patients with PD have been consistent with this hypothesis. In particular, studies of PD progression using ^{123}I-β-CIT SPECT have identified groups of individuals who are fast progressors and slow progressors. Interestingly, retrospective analyses indicate that the individuals whose rate of DAT binding loss was the most rapid had the highest average initial levels of DAT binding (26). This result is consistent with the idea that neurons with greater functional DAT expression might demonstrate faster rates of neuronal degeneration, although other explanations are plausible. Another possible explanation is that differences in rates of progression in patients with PD may be due to functionally significant polymorphisms at key regulatory sites for dopamine neuronal toxicity, the DAT and VMAT2. It is possible that a relative slowing in the rate of progression of dopaminergic damage over time could be subserved by selection of the initially most-robustly expressing neurons. If DAT densities in remaining neurons were lower than those in initially damaged cells, for example, then slower toxin transport into these remaining dopaminergic neurons could slow the progression of their death. Neurons could also downregulate DAT expression to prolong their survival and, thus, slow the rate of progression of clinical symptoms. These hypotheses are speculative but lend themselves to direct testing using imaging markers of DAT and VMAT2 in patients with PD.

Most importantly, longitudinal imaging studies with DAT ligands and other markers have markedly affected the design of therapeutic studies of neurodegenerative disorders (58). As therapies are developed and tested, which may be neuroprotective or neurorestorative treatments (i.e., therapeutic approaches that attempt to modulate the ongoing pathophysiological disease process), imaging provides an essential objective endpoint for changes in neurodegeneration. Although imaging endpoints must be complemented by enduring clinical functional changes, imaging has become useful to demonstrate changes in the rate of neurodegeneration. Several ongoing trials for protective and restorative drugs have used or will use imaging as one of several endpoints for degeneration in studies of PD (59,60). It may be possible to incorporate information from the DAT SPECT images to stratify those patients who might be the best candidates for a neuroprotective and/or restorative trials.

CONCLUSIONS

DAT SPECT imaging has emerged as an important tool for the assessment of PD and related disorders. The range of clinical research questions from accurate and early diagnoses of an at-risk population, monitoring the disease progression with an aim to improve understanding of the factors implicated in the initiation and promulgation of neuronal loss and to aid in the evaluation of disease-modifying treatments for the disorder, represents the mature application of neuroreceptor imaging technologies to important clinical questions and serves as a model for the use of these methods in other neurodegenerative disorders.

As simpler tools to screen large populations are developed to identify preclinical at-risk individuals for neurodegenerative disorders, DAT SPECT imaging can be widely used to establish and monitor the onset and progression of neurodegeneration. Finally, as treatments become available that target both the mechanisms that initiate and subsequently promote the course of disease progression, having precise information about a patient's neurochemical status and potential at-risk status will lead to improvements in clinical management.

REFERENCES

1. Phelps M. Positron emission tomography (PET). In: Mazziota J, Gilman S, eds. *Clinical brain imaging: principles and applications.* Philadelphia: FA Davis Co, 1992:71–107.
2. Lassen N, Holm S. Single photon emission computerized tomography (SPECT). In: Mazziota J, Gilman S, eds. *Clinical brain imaging: principles and Applications.* Philadelphia: FA Davis Co, 1992:108–134.
3. Leenders K, Antonini A. PET ^{18}F-Fluorodopa (FD) uptake and disease progression in Parkinson's disease. *Neurology* 1995;45:A220.
4. Eidelberg D, Moeller JR, Ishikawa T, et al. Early differential diagnosis of Parkinson's disease with ^{18}F-fluorodeoxyglucose and positron emission tomography. *Neurology* 1995;45:1995–2005.
5. Snow BJ, Tooyama J, McGreer EG, et al. Human positron emission tomographic [^{18}F]fluorodopa studies correlate with dopamine cell counts and levels. *Ann Neurol* 1993;34:324–330.
6. Piccini P, Brooks DJ. Etiology of Parkinson's disease: contributions from ^{18}F-DOPA positron emission tomography. *Adv Neurol* 1999;80:227–231.
7. Brooks DJ. Advances in imaging Parkinson's disease. *Curr Opin Neurol* 1997;10:327–331.
8. Sawle GV, Playford ED, Burn DJ, et al. Separating Parkinson's disease from normality. Discriminant function analysis of fluorodopa F-18 positron emission tomography data. *Arch Neurol* 1994;51:237–243.
9. Frey KA, Koeppe RA, Kilbourn MR. Imaging the vesicular monoamine transporter. *Adv Neurol* 2001;86: 237–247.
10. Frey KA, Wieland DM, Kilbourn MR. Imaging of monoaminergic and cholinergic vesicular transporters in the brain. *Adv Pharmacol* 1998;42:269–272.
11. Frey KA, Koeppe RA, Kilbourn MR, et al. Presynaptic monoaminergic vesicles in Parkinson's disease and normal aging. *Ann Neurol* 1996;40:873–884.
12. Brücke T, Asenbaum S, Pirker W, et al. Measurement of the dopaminergic degeneration in Parkinson's disease with [^{123} I]β-CIT and SPECT. *J Neural Transm* 1997;22 [Suppl 50]:9–24.
13. Booij T, Tissingh G, Boer G. [^{123}I]FP-SPECT shows a pronounced decline of striatal dopamine transporter labeling in early and advanced Parkinson's disease. *J Neurol Neurosurg Psychiatry* 1997;62:133–140.
14. Fischman AJ, Bonab AA, Babich JW, et al. Rapid detection of Parkinson's disease by SPECT with altropane: a selective ligand for dopamine transporters. *Synapse* 1998;29:128–141.
15. Innis RB, Seibyl JB, Scanley BE, et al. Single photon emission computed tomographic imaging demonstrates loss of striatal dopamine transporters in Parkinson's disease. *Proc Natl Acad Sci USA* 1993;90:11965–11969.

16. Tatsch K, Schwarz J, Mozley PD, et al. Relationship between clinical features of Parkinson's disease and presynaptic dopamine transporter binding assessed with [123I]IPT and single-photon emission tomography. *Eur J Nucl Med* 1997;24:415–421.
17. Boja JW, Patel A, Carroll FJ, et al. [125I]-RTI-55: a potent ligand for dopamine transporters. *Eur J Pharmacol* 1991;194:133–134.
18. Brouard A, Pelaprat D, Boja JW, et al. Potent cocaine analogs inhibit [3H]dopamine uptake in rat mesencephalic cells in primary cultures: pharmacological selectivity of embryonic cocaine sites. *Brain Res Dev* 1993;75:13–17.
19. Coulter CL, Happe HK, Bergmann DA, et al. Localization and quantification of the dopamine transporter: comparison of [3H]WIN 35,428 and [125I]RTI-55. *Brain Res* 1995;690:217–224.
20. Fujita M, Shimada S, Fukuchi K, et al. Distribution of cocaine recognition sites in rat brain: *in vitro* and *ex vivo* autoradiography with [125I]RTI-55. *J Chem Neuroanat* 1994;7:13–23.
21. Staley JK, Basile M, Flynn DD, et al. Visualizing dopamine and serotonin transporters in the human brain with the potent cocaine analogue [125I]RTI-55: *in vitro* binding and autoradiographic characterization. *J Neurochem* 1994;62:549–556.
22. Volkow ND, Gatley SJ, Fowler JS, et al. Long-lasting inhibition of *in vivo* cocaine binding to dopamine transporters by 3 beta-(4-iodophenyl)tropane-2-carboxylic acid methyl ester: RTI-55 or beta CIT. *Synapse* 1995; 19:206–211.
23. Abi-Dargham A, Gandelman MS, DeErausquin GA, et al. SPECT imaging of dopamine transporters in human brain with iodine-123-fluoroalkyl analogs of beta-CIT. *J Nucl Med* 1996;37:1129–1133.
24. Ahlskog JE, Uitti RJ, O'Connor MK, et al. The effect of dopamine agonist therapy on dopamine transporter imaging in Parkinson's disease. *Mov Disord* 1999;14: 940–946.
25. Innis RB, Marek KL, Sheff K, et al. Effect of treatment with L-dopa/carbidopa or L-selegiline on striatal dopamine transporter SPECT imaging with [123I]beta-CIT. *Mov Disord* 1999;14:436–442.
26. Marek K, Innis R, van Dyck G, et al. [123I]beta-CIT SPECT imaging assessment of the rate of Parkinson's disease progression. *Neurology* 2001;57:2089–2094.
27. Pirker W, Djamshidian S, Asenbaum S, et al. The progression of dopaminergic degeneration in Parkinson's disease and atypical parkinsonism: a longitudinal β-CIT SPECT study. *Neurology* 2001;56[Suppl 3]:A268.
28. Seibyl JP, Marek K, Sheff K, et al. Test/retest reproducibility of [123I]β-CIT SPECT brain measurement of dopamine transporters in Parkinson's disease patients. *J Nucl Med* 1997;38:1453–1461.
29. Staffen W, Mair A, Unterrainer J, et al. Measuring the progression of idiopathic Parkinson's disease with [123I] beta-CIT SPECT. *J Neural Transm* 2000;107:543–552.
30. van Dyck CH, Seibyl JP, Malison RT. Age-related decline in dopamine transporters: analysis of striatal subregions, nonlinear effects, and hemispheric asymmetries. *Am J Geriatr Psychiatry* 2002;10:36–43.
31. Laruelle M, Wallace E, Seibyl JP, et al. Graphical, kinetic, and equilibrium analyses of *in vivo* [123I] beta-CIT binding to dopamine transporters in healthy human subjects. *J Cereb Blood Flow Metab* 1994;14:982–994.
32. Seibyl JP, Marek K, Sheff K, et al. Iodine-123-beta-CIT and iodine-123-FPCIT SPECT measurement of dopamine transporters in healthy subjects and Parkinson's patients. *J Nucl Med* 1998;39:1500–1508.
33. Seibyl JP. Single-photon emission computed tomography of the dopamine transporter in parkinsonism. *J Neuroimaging* 1999;9:223–228.
34. Kung MP, Stevenson DA, Plossl K, et al. [99mTc]TRODAT-1: a novel technetium-99m complex as a dopamine transporter imaging agent. *Eur J Nucl Med* 1997;24: 372–380.
35. Frost JJ, Rosier AJ, Reich SG, et al. Positron emission tomography imaging of the dopamine transporter with 11C-WIN 35,428 reveals marked decline in mild Parkinson's disease. *Ann Neurol* 1993;34:423–431.
36. Rinne JO, Laihinen A, Nagren K, et al. PET examination of the monoamine transporter with [11C]beta-CIT and [11C]beta-CFT in early Parkinson's disease. *Synapse* 1995;21:97–103.
37. Marek KL, Seibyl JP, Zoghbi SS, et al. [I-123]CIT SPECT imaging demonstrates bilateral loss of dopamine transporters in hemi-Parkinson's disease. *Neurology* 1996;46:231–237.
38. Guttman M, Burkholder J, Kish SJ, et al. [11C]RTI-32 PET studies of the dopamine transporter in early dopa-naive Parkinson's disease. *Neurology* 1997;48: 1578–1583.
39. Booij J, Andringa G, Rijks LJ, et al. [123I]FP-CIT binds to the dopamine transporter as assessed by biodistribution studies in rats and SPECT studies in MPTP-lesioned monkeys. *Synapse* 1997;27:183–190.
40. Marek K. Dopaminergic dysfunction in parkinsonism: new lessons from imaging. *Neuroscientist* 1999;5: 333–339.
41. Benamer HT, Patterson J, Wyper DJ, et al. Correlation of Parkinson's disease severity and duration with 123I-FP-CIT SPECT striatal uptake. *Mov Disord* 2000;15: 692–698.
42. Mozley PD, Scheider JS, Acton PD, et al. Binding of [99mTc]TRODAT-1 to dopamine transporters in patients with Parkinson's disease and in healthy volunteers. *J Nucl Med* 2000;41:584–589.
43. Seibyl JP, Marek KL, Quinlan D, et al. Decreased single-photon emission computed tomographic [123I]beta-CIT striatal uptake correlates with symptom severity in Parkinson's disease. *Ann Neurol* 1995;38:589–598.
44. Varrone A, Marek KL, Jennings D, et al. [(123)I]beta-CIT SPECT imaging demonstrates reduced density of striatal dopamine transporters in Parkinson's disease and multiple system atrophy. *Mov Disord* 2001;16: 1023–1032.
45. Parkinson Study Group. A multicenter assessment of dopamine transporter imaging with DOPAscan/SPECT in parkinsonism. *Neurology* 2000;55:1540–1547.
46. Ilgin N, Zubieta J, Reich SG, et al. PET imaging of the dopamine transporter in progressive supranuclear palsy and Parkinson's disease. *Neurology* 1999;52: 1221–1226.
47. Messa C, Volonte MA, Fazio F, et al. Differential distribution of striatal [123I]beta-CIT in Parkinson's disease and progressive supranuclear palsy, evaluated with single-photon emission tomography. *Eur J Nucl Med* 1998; 25:1270–1276.
48. Pirker W, Asenbaum S, Bencsits G, et al. [123I]beta-CIT SPECT in multiple system atrophy, progressive

supranuclear palsy, and corticobasal degeneration. *Mov Disord* 2000;15:1158–1167.
49. Ichise M, Kim YJ, Ballinger JR, et al. SPECT imaging of the pre- and postsynaptic dopaminergic alterations in L-dopa–untreated PD. *Neurology* 1999;52:1206–1214.
50. McGeer PL, Itagaki S, Akiyama H, et al. Rate of cell death in parkinsonism indicates active neuropathological process. *Ann Neurol* 1988;24:574–576.
51. Fearnley J, Lees A. Ageing and Parkinson's disease: substantia nigra regional selectivity. *Brain* 1991;114: 2283–2301.
52. Lee CS, Schulzer M, Mak EK, et al. Clinical observations on the rate of progression of idiopathic parkinsonism. *Brain* 1994;117:501–507.
54. Brooks DJ. Morphological and functional imaging studies on the diagnosis and progression of Parkinson's disease. *J Neurol* 2000;247[Suppl 2]:11–18.
54. Jennings D, Innis RB, Seibyl JP, Marek K. [^{123}I]β-CIT and SPECT assessment of progression in early and late Parkinson's disease. *Neurology* 2000;56[Suppl 3]:A74.
55. Uhl G. Hypothesis: the role of dopaminergic transporters in selective vulnerability of cells in Parkinson's disease. *Ann Neurol* 1998;43:555–560.
56. Takahashi N, Miner LL, Sora I, et al. VMAT2 knockout mice: heterozygotes display reduced amphetamine-conditioned reward, enhanced amphetamine locomotion, and enhanced MPTP toxicity. *Proc Natl Acad Sci U S A* 1997;94:9938–9943.
57. Wang YM, Gainetdinov RR, Fumagalli F, et al. Knockout of the vesicular monoamine transporter 2 gene results in neonatal death and supersensitivity to cocaine and amphetamine. *Neuron* 1997;19:1285–1296.
58. Shoulson I. Experimental therapeutic of neurodegenerative disorders: unmet needs. *Science* 1998;282: 1072–1074.
59. Parkinson Study Group. Dopamine transporter brain imaging to assess the effects of pramipexole vs. levodopa on Parkinson's disease progression. *JAMA* 2002; 287:1653–1661.
60. Brooks D, Rakshi JS, Pavese N, et al. Relative rates of progression of early Parkinson's disease patients started on either a dopamine agonist (ropinirole) or levodopa: 2-year and 5-year follow-up ^{18}F-dopa PET findings. *Neurology* 2000;54[Suppl 3]:A113.
61. Benamer TS, Patterson J, Grosset DG, et al. Accurate differentiation of parkinsonism and essential tremor using visual assessment of [^{123}I]-FP-CIT SPECT imaging: the [^{123}I]-FP-CIT study group. *Mov Disord* 2000;15: 503–510.
62. Huang WS, Lin SZ, Lin JG, et al. Evaluation of early-stage Parkinson's disease with ^{99m}Tc-TRODAT-1 imaging. *J Nucl Med* 2001;42:1303–1308.
63. Schwarz J, Tatsch K, Linke R, et al. Measuring the decline of dopamine transporter binding in patients with Parkinson's disease using ^{123}I-IPT and SPECT. *Neurology* 1997;48[Suppl]:A208.

Parkinson's Disease: Advances in Neurology, Vol. 91.
Edited by Ariel Gordin, Seppo Kaakkola,
and Heikki Teräväinen
Lippincott Williams & Wilkins, Philadelphia © 2003

20

Mechanisms of Motor Complications in Treatment of Parkinson's Disease

Ajit Kumar, Zhigao Huang, and Raúl de la Fuente-Fernández

Pacific Parkinson's Research Centre, Vancouver Hospital and Health Centre, University of British Columbia, Vancouver, British Columbia, Canada

Long-term dopaminomimetic therapy is often complicated by the emergence of variations of motor response in a substantial proportion of patients with Parkinson's disease (PD). These motor complications are often related to levodopa treatment, although they may also be encountered with the use of synthetic dopamine (DA) agonists. Clinically, motor complications of treatment take the form of fluctuations of bradykinesia, rigidity, and tremor, often in combination with dyskinesias. Up to 50% of patients with PD experience motor fluctuations after 5 years of treatment (1). Dyskinesias occur in a similar proportion of patients with PD. The classification of motor complications associated with treatment in PD is listed in Tables 20.1 and 20.2.

Two factors appear to be important in the genesis of levodopa-related motor complications:

1. Progressive nigrostriatal degeneration reflecting progression of PD
2. Long-term use of levodopa

It has been observed that motor complications related to treatment positively correlate with both duration of PD and duration of levodopa therapy (2,3). Although the exact mechanisms of these complications are far from clear, research over the past few years has given some indicators. Different research groups have demonstrated, with differing emphasis, changes at various levels including the presynaptic dopaminergic nerve terminals, the postsynaptic medium spiny striatal neurons, and further downstream. In addition, the peripheral pharmacokinetics of levodopa was once postulated to play a major part. However, results from recent research suggest that central mechanisms are more important than peripheral pharmacokinetics in the pathogenesis of motor complications related to levodopa treatment. Even among the central

TABLE 20.1. *Motor Fluctuations Associated with Dopaminomimetic Treatment in Parkinson's Disease*

- **"Wearing off"** (predictable end-of-dose and morning akinesia)
- **"On-off"** (sudden unpredictable changes in motor response)
- "**Inhibitory** response" (worsening at the beginning or end of dose)

TABLE 20.2. *Levodopa-Related Dyskinesias*

- **Related to the "off" state**
  "Off" dystonia (including early morning dystonia)
- **Related to the "on" state**
  Peak-dose choreoathetosis
  Peak-dose dystonia
  Biphasic choreoathetosis/dystonia
  Myoclonus Asterixis

mechanisms, the relative importance of each is unsettled. It is likely that multiple mechanisms that influence each other operate in concert. An overview of these changes based on evidence from current research is described in the following paragraphs.

PHARMACOKINETICS OF LEVODOPA

Peripheral pharmacokinetics of levodopa is influenced at the level of the gut where it is absorbed, as well as at the level of the blood–brain barrier (BBB) where it is transported into the brain. Levodopa is absorbed in the proximal small intestine. High protein intake and slowing of gastric emptying by meals or anticholinergics retard levodopa absorption. Large neutral amino acids compete with levodopa for absorption in the gut, as well as for transportation across the BBB. Reports conflict on the clinical significance of levodopa metabolites, 3-*O*-methyldopa (3-OMD) in particular, in competing with levodopa for transportation across the BBB (4). Although peripheral pharmacokinetic factors may influence fluctuations and dyskinesias, several studies have demonstrated the relative insignificance of peripheral pharmacokinetic mechanisms in the pathogenesis of motor complications (5,6). For this reason, we focus on alterations that occur at the cellular and molecular levels in presynaptic dopaminergic nerve terminals and postsynaptic medium spiny neurons in the striatum.

PRESYNAPTIC CHANGES

Degeneration of presynaptic nigrostriatal dopaminergic nerve terminals plays a role in the genesis of levodopa-related motor complications. In the subclinical stage of PD, despite progressive degeneration of dopaminergic nerve terminals, levels in the synaptic cleft are maintained fairly constant (7). This is accomplished by compensatory mechanisms. There is increased synthesis of DA, augmentation of discharge frequency of dopaminergic neurons, action of DA at adjacent denervated synapses, and perhaps activation of previously silent synapses (8). Experimental studies in cynomolgus monkeys reveal an increase in the DA metabolites/DA ratio after methylphenyltetrahydropyridine (MPTP) treatment (9–11). This increase in the value of the ratio of DA metabolites to DA would suggest increased synthesis that residual nigrostriatal neurons undertake to maintain dopaminergic homeostasis (12). An increase in DA release per pulse has been observed in *in vitro* experiments (13). However, based on the model of partially denervated striatum in the rat, some others argue that increased DA release per pulse is unlikely to be an effective compensatory mechanism (14). Fluorodopa positron emission tomography (PET) studies measure *in vivo* the functional integrity of the nigrostriatal DA system in PD. Fluorodopa uptake reflects decarboxylation activity and vesicular storage. (±)-α-^{11}C-dihydrotetrabenazine (DTBZ) is a radio-labeled ligand that binds to the vesicular monoamine transporter type 2. In patients with PD, fluorodopa uptake has been found to be upregulated compared with DTBZ binding (15). This observation is likely to derive from upregulation of aromatic L-amino acid decarboxylase activity. Whether tyrosine hydroxylase, the rate-limiting enzyme in the synthesis of DA, is also upregulated in PD remains unknown. The net result of these changes is increased capacity of the remaining dopaminergic neurons to decarboxylate exogenous levodopa. This should help buffer oscillations of DA levels in the synaptic cleft with levodopa usage, particularly in the early stage of PD (3).

With further progression of PD, the capacity to store DA synthesized from exogenous levodopa is diminished and fluctuations in motor function manifest. It is generally thought that the progressive loss of nigrostriatal terminals is responsible for levodopa-related end-of-dose motor fluctuations in PD (16). Fluorodopa uptake, which correlates with DA cells in the substantia nigra (17), is reduced by 28% in the putamen of fluctuators compared with stable responders (18). A positive correlation between striatal dopaminergic nerve terminal deficiency and the ability of exogenous levodopa to increase synaptic DA level binding has been observed using PET scanning (19). This suggests that DA turnover increases with disease progression. We proposed increased DA turnover results in swings in synaptic DA level, and this is an important mechanism in the pathogenesis of motor complications in PD. We confirmed this prediction using the ^{11}C-raclopride displacement model (20). The estimated increase in synaptic DA level 1 hour after levodopa administration was three times greater in fluctuators than in stable patients with PD. Four hours after levodopa administration, only stable responders maintained elevated synaptic DA levels (20). Interestingly, these changes in synaptic DA levels not only preceded the recurrence of clinically apparent motor fluctuations but also were independent of differences in severity of nigrostriatal damage (i.e., both groups had similar motor scores at the time the PET scans were done). One factor that has repeatedly been found to correlate with motor fluctuations is the age of the patient. The younger the age at onset of PD, the greater the incidence of motor fluctuations (21).

In advanced PD, changes in cerebrospinal fluid levels of DA and its metabolites correlate with motor function (22). This also suggests a decreased buffering capacity in the pathogenesis of motor fluctuations. Levodopa is also decarboxylated to DA in serotonergic neurons and other dopa decarboxylase–containing cells (23). DA leaks out of the cell compartment as soon as it is synthesized and reaches postsynaptic receptors by volume transmission. This could be another contributing mechanism for motor fluctuations.

Some argue that the increased DA efflux observed in partially denervated animals is due to a decrease in the rate at which DA is removed from extracellular fluid by remaining terminals, rather than due to increased DA release (13,24). The plasma membrane dopamine transporter (DAT) is the most important mechanism for clearing DA from the synapse and is a major determinant of the amount of DA available for receptor stimulation. Direct measurements of DA concentration in the striatal extracellular space in both intact and 6-hydroxydopamine (6-OHDA) rats after levodopa treatment have shown that elevation of extracellular DA induced by exogenous levodopa is not altered by a selective DA reuptake inhibitor in lesioned animals (25,26). DAT messenger RNA per dopaminergic neuron decreases in PD. This suggests downregulation of DAT (27). A similar study has demonstrated that D-*threo*-^{11}C-methylphenidate (MP) binding (which is a marker for DAT) is reduced to a greater extent than DTBZ binding in PD (15). This also supports the view that DAT may be downregulated in PD. In addition, chronic levodopa treatment is associated with a decrease in MP binding to striatal DAT sites (28). This indicates that DAT is sensitive to pharmacological manipulation.

POSTSYNAPTIC CHANGES

Evidence from a large body of research emphasizes the role of changes that occur distal to the nigrostriatal endings in the pathogenesis of motor complications. Alterations have been described in several interrelated neurochemical systems, and at the molecular level, in the striatal medium spiny neurons. Degeneration of presynaptic DA nerve terminals eventually leads to marked variations of DA levels in the synaptic cleft after administration of levodopa. This pulsatile exposure of the postsynaptic medium spiny neuron to DA has been proposed to set off a cascade of changes at the receptor level and further downstream.

DOPAMINE RECEPTORS

Changes in DA receptors, particularly the D_2 receptor, have long been considered responsible for fluctuations and dyskinesias; however, whether this is actually so remains unclear. Zeng et al. (29) found that D_1 and D_2

receptor densities in the normal monkey striatum were not altered after chronic levodopa treatment, irrespective of the occurrence of dyskinesia. One hypothesis is that dyskinesia may result from overstimulation of D_1 receptors. In support of this view, dyskinetic movements in hemiparkinsonian rats sensitized by chronic pulsatile levodopa administration have been successfully blocked by oligonucleotide antisense to D_1 receptor (30). However, results from studies on D_1 receptor binding are not consistent with this hypothesis. Nigrostriatal lesions generally induce no changes in this receptor subtype in patients with PD (31–33) or MPTP-lesioned primates (34,35).

Another hypothesis focuses on the role of D_2 receptors. Experimental work and postmortem studies on human and parkinsonian brains have demonstrated D_2 upregulation (9,36,37). However, treatment with long-acting D_2 agonists, such as bromocriptine, ropinirole, or pergolide, induces little or no dyskinesia in levodopa-naive patients with PD or MPTP-lesioned primates (38–40). Finally, PET studies have failed to show *in vivo* differences in D_1 or D_2 binding between dyskinetic and nondyskinetic patients (41).

It has also been proposed that changes in second-messenger systems coupled to DA receptors could contribute to motor complications in PD. Upregulation of alpha subunits of G_s, G_{olf}, and G_i, shown in the striatum of 6-OHDA rats, may be an indicator of this (42,43).

OTHER RECEPTORS

Glutamate Receptors

Medium spiny neurons in the striatum receive glutamatergic afferents from the cortex and express glutamatergic receptors including the *N*-methyl D-aspartate (NMDA), α-amino-3-hydroxy-5-methyl-4-isoxazole (AMPA), and metabotropic subtypes. NMDA receptors are known to be critical for neuronal development, synaptic transmission, learning, and memory (44,45). NMDA receptors have a dual character: They are both ligand gated and voltage dependent (46). NMDA receptors are heteroisomeric complexes comprising of NMDAR1 and various NMDAR2 subunits. NMDAR1, NMDAR2A, and NMDAR2B subunits are detected in the striatum in humans (47,48). NMDAR1 is concerned with the formation of functional NMDA channels, whereas NMDAR2 subunits regulate the biochemical properties of the receptors (49). NMDA receptors are modulated by protein phosphorylation. Tyrosine phosphorylation regulates channel properties such as opening and conductance, whereas serine/threonine phosphorylation regulates anchoring to cell membranes (50,51). Studies in 6-OHDA parkinsonian rats have shown an increase in the phosphorylation of NMDAR subunits. Such increases in phosphorylation become more marked when the 6-OHDA rats develop altered motor responses to levodopa treatment (51).

Tyrosine phosphorylation affects the NMDAR2B subunit, whereas serine/threonine phosphorylation affects the NMDAR2A subunit. It has been suggested that this phosphorylation involves second-messenger systems linking them to adjacent DA receptors (7). DA receptors presumably activate striatal kinases such as cyclic adenosine monophosphate (cAMP), protein kinase A (PKA), calcium/calmodulin-dependent protein kinase II (CaMK II), and tyrosine kinases (50,51). Evidence supporting this includes reduction of phosphorylation, both serine/threonine and tyrosine, as well as improvement in motor responses, after intrastriatal injections of striatal kinase inhibitors such as KN-93, which inhibits CaMK II (50), or genestein, which inhibits tyrosine kinase (7). The net result of increased phosphorylation of NMDA receptor subunits is heightened sensitization of these receptors. How this translates into altered motor responses is unclear. Presumably, alterations of glutamatergic cortical input to the striatal medium spiny neurons modify the efferent activity of these striatal cells (7). Changes in the subthalamic-pallidal glutamatergic pathways have also been postulated to play a role in the genesis of motor complications related to treatment of PD (52–54).

Further evidence of NMDA receptor involvement stems from studies showing improvement in levodopa-related dyskinesias after the administration of NMDA antagonists, both in animals and in humans. In animal models, NMDA antagonists extend the duration of motor response to chronic levodopa treatment (55) and reduce dyskinesias (56,57). Similarly, NMDA receptor antagonists, such as dextromethorphan (58), amantadine (59,60), and memantine (61), significantly attenuate motor fluctuations and dyskinesias in PD.

AMPA glutamate receptors have also been suggested to contribute to parkinsonian symptoms and levodopa-associated motor response alterations in PD. The AMPA antagonist NBQX has been shown to improve motor responses to levodopa in parkinsonian rats (62).

Opioid Transmission

Changes in opioid transmission in the basal ganglia have been observed with long-term dopaminomimetic therapy (63,64). Dynorphin and enkephalin are co-transmitters of γ-amino butyric acid (GABA) in the direct and indirect pathways of the basal ganglia circuitry, respectively (65,66). The direct pathway of the basal ganglia arises from GABA-containing striatal medium spiny neurons and projects to the internal segment of the globus pallidus (GPi) and substantia nigra pars reticulata (SNpr) (67). These direct GABAergic striatal output neurons coexpress excitatory D_1 receptors, substance P, and dynorphin. The indirect pathway arises from striatal GABA-containing medium spiny neurons and projects to the external segment of the globus pallidus and hence to the GPi via the subthalamic nucleus (67). These indirect GABAergic striatal output neurons coexpress inhibitory D_2 receptors and enkephalin.

In levodopa-treated MPTP-lesioned primates, and in postmortem studies of levodopa-treated patients with PD, striatal preproenkephalin-A mRNA levels are elevated, whereas levels of preprotachykinin mRNA are within the normal range (63,64,68,69). Increased opioid transmission has also been observed by PET in patients with PD with dyskinesias (70). The reason for induction of increased opioid transmission is unclear but may involve interactions between the dopaminergic and opioid systems (71,72). How increased opioid transmission may result in motor complications is also far from clear. Alteration of GABA transmission by increased levels of dynorphin and enkephalin in the direct and indirect pathways, respectively, could be a key factor (73).

Blockade of opioid transmission using either a nonselective opioid receptor antagonist (naltrexone), a μ-opioid receptor antagonist (cyprodime), or a δ-opioid receptor antagonist (naltrindole) reduces dyskinesias in MPTP-lesioned marmosets without affecting the antiparkinsonian effects of levodopa (74).

Adenosine Receptors

A_1 and A_{2a} are the subtypes of adenosine receptors in the human basal ganglia. A_1 receptor stimulation inhibits cAMP formation. In contrast, A_{2a} receptor stimulation increases cAMP formation. A_1 receptors are more abundant in the direct pathway (75), whereas A_{2a} receptors predominate in the indirect pathway (76). A_1-D_1 and A_{2a}-D_2 antagonistic interactions occur at the membrane level (77,78). There is some evidence that these interactions may contribute to worsening parkinsonian symptoms in animal models (79). Treatment of MPTP-lesioned monkeys with A_{2a} antagonists not only improves parkinsonian symptoms but also reduces dyskinesias (80,81).

Role of Immediate Early Genes

Inductions of delta-FosB (DFB) (and its isoforms), which is a Fos-related antigen, and JunD have been shown in the striatum of 6-OHDA rats (82). Such changes can be increased by pulsatile dopaminomimetic treatment (83).

DFB and JunD form a dimer, the AP1 complex. Another isoform of DFB combines with a smaller, fast, migrating form of JunD to form another dimer, the pAP1 complex. These dimers act as primers, presumably binding to as yet unidentified genes that regulate synthesis of NMDA receptors, DA receptors, enkephalin, and dynorphin (83). Thus, excessive induction of Immediate Early Genes (IEG) by pulsatile dopaminomimetic therapy may be an early step that sets off a series of changes contributing to the development of motor complications.

FLUCTUATIONS AND DYSKINESIAS

Fluctuations in motor response can be classified as "wearing off," which occur at the end of the interval between doses, and "on-off," which refers to random fluctuations in motor response that are unrelated to the time of levodopa doses (84). A common pathophysiological mechanism may underlie both, although they are clinically distinct (85). Among dyskinesias, peak-dose dyskinesia is most common (86).

In patients who develop fluctuations, whether of the "wearing-off" type or the "on-off type," pharmacodynamic changes occur in the antiparkinsonian effect in relation to levodopa administration. These include shortening of the latency of response, steepening of the dose–response slope, and decreased duration of action (87–89). Presynaptic changes in the DA nerve terminals, particularly decreased buffering capacity and increased DA turnover, can account for part of the "wearing-off" effect. However, a multitude of postsynaptic changes in relation to DA denervation and chronic dopaminergic therapy can also contribute to the pathogenesis of this motor complication. Both presynaptic and postsynaptic factors are also likely to be involved in the pathogenesis of the "on-off" phenomenon.

Two types of clinical responses to levodopa are recognized. The short-duration response, which is an improvement in motor function that lasts for minutes to hours, and the long-duration response that builds up over days to weeks of continuous levodopa therapy (90). Whereas the short-duration response tends to parallel the rise and fall of plasma levodopa levels, there are indicators that the long-duration response may be mediated by postsynaptic changes (91). Although fluctuations mainly reflect changes in the short-duration response, the seemingly smooth clinical response to levodopa in early PD is probably related to the long-duration response (91).

The steepening of the dose–response curve in fluctuations tends to narrow the dose of levodopa that produces the antiparkinsonian effect, eventually leading to a situation in which the response is suddenly observed only at a particular dose, resembling an "all-or-none" phenomenon. In this situation, even slight variations of the pharmacokinetics of levodopa, and thus striatal DA, can result in a highly variable antiparkinsonian response (85). This is particularly so when the dose of levodopa is at or just more than threshold levels. This mechanism may contribute to the "on-off" effect.

Another phenomenon encountered in patients with PD is a transient worsening of motor function below the baseline at the beginning or at the end of a dose of levodopa. This is the "inhibitory response" (92,93). DA receptors with a different affinity for DA as compared with those (postsynaptic) that mediate improvement in motor function have been postulated to be involved because the stimulation of these presynaptic receptors could suppress endogenous DA release (94). There is PET evidence supporting this notion (95). It remains uncertain whether alterations in presynaptic DA receptors play a significant role in the pathogenesis of motor complications.

CONCLUSIONS

At the presynaptic level, changes in DA turnover, in DAT, or in presynaptic DA receptor regulation may play a role. At the postsynaptic level, we have already mentioned that some authors favor alterations in the indirect pathway as a major contributing factor. Others, however, favor the direct pathway. Still others stress the importance of NMDA receptor sensitization or changes in other neurochemical systems (opioid or adenosine). We have too many explanations and insufficient evidence to choose between them.

ACKNOWLEDGMENTS

The authors express their gratitude to Donald B. Calne, DM, FRSC, for his inspirational guidance in writing this chapter, and Susan Calne, RN, for skillful editing. Raúl de la Fuente-Fernández is supported by the Pacific Parkinson's Research Institute (Vancouver, BC, Canada).

REFERENCES

1. Sweet RD, McDowell FH. The "on-off" response to chronic L-DOPA treatment of parkinsonism. *Adv Neurol* 1974;5:331–338.
2. Lesser RP, Fahn S, Snider SR, et al. Analysis of the clinical problems in parkinsonism and the complications of long-term levodopa therapy. *Neurology* 1979;29: 1253–1260.
3. Saint-Hilaire MH, Feldman RG. The "on-off" phenomenon in Parkinson's disease. In: Joseph AB, Young RR, eds. *Movement disorders in neurology and neuropsychiatry.* Boston: Blackwell Scientific Publications, 1999: 180–184.
4. Nutt JG, Woodward WR, Gancher ST, et al. 3-*O*-methyldopa and the response to levodopa in Parkinson's disease. *Ann Neurol* 1987;21:584–588.
5. Fabbrini G, Juncos J, Mouradian MM, et al. Levodopa pharmacokinetic mechanisms and motor fluctuations in Parkinson's disease. *Ann Neurol* 1987;21:370–376.
6. Gancher ST, Nutt JG, Woodward WR. Peripheral pharmacokinetics of levodopa in untreated, stable, and fluctuating parkinsonian patients. *Neurology* 1987;37: 940–944.
7. Chase TN, Konitsiotis S, Oh JD. Striatal molecular mechanisms and motor dysfunction in Parkinson's disease. *Adv Neurol* 2001;86:355–360.
8. Bezard E, Gross CE. Compensatory mechanisms in experimental and human parkinsonism: towards a dynamic approach. *Prog Neurobiol* 1998;55:93–116.
9. Bezard E, Dovero S, Prunier C, et al. Relationship between the appearance of symptoms and the level of nigrostriatal degeneration in a progressive 1-methyl-4-phenyl-1,2,3,6-tetrahydropyridine–lesioned macaque model of Parkinson's disease. *J Neurosci* 2001;21: 6853–6861.
10. Di Paolo T, Bedard P, Daigle M, et al. Long-term effects of MPTP on central and peripheral catecholamine and indoleamine concentrations in monkeys. *Brain Res* 1986;379:286–293.
11. Elsworth JD, Taylor JR, Sladek JR Jr, et al. Striatal dopaminergic correlates of stable parkinsonism and degree of recovery in old-world primates one year after MPTP treatment. *Neuroscience* 2000;95:399–408.
12. Zigmond MJ, Abercrombie ED, Berger TW, et al. Compensations after lesions of central dopaminergic neurons: some clinical and basic implications. *Trends Neurosci* 1990;13:290–296.
13. Stachowiak MK, Keller RW Jr, Stricker EM, et al. Increased dopamine efflux from striatal slices during development and after nigrostriatal bundle damage. *J Neurosci* 1987;7:1648–1654.
14. Garris PA, Christensen JR, Rebec GV, et al. Real-time measurement of electrically evoked extracellular dopamine in the striatum of freely moving rats. *J Neurochem* 1997;68:152–161.
15. Lee CS, Samii A, Sossi V, et al. *In vivo* positron emission tomographic evidence for compensatory changes in presynaptic dopaminergic nerve terminals in Parkinson's disease. *Ann Neurol* 2000;47:493–503.
16. Fabbrini G, Mouradian MM, Juncos JL, et al. Motor fluctuations in Parkinson's disease: central pathophysiological mechanisms. Part I. *Ann Neurol* 1988; 24: 366–371.
17. Snow BJ, Tooyama I, McGeer EG, et al. Human positron emission tomographic (^{18}F)fluorodopa studies correlate with dopamine cell counts and levels. *Ann Neurol* 1993;34:324–330.
18. de la Fuente-Fernández R, Pal PK, Vingerhoets FJG, et al. Evidence for impaired presynaptic dopamine function in parkinsonian patients with motor fluctuations. *J Neural Transm* 2000;107:49–57.
19. Tedroff J, Pedersen M, Aquilonius SM, et al. Levodopa-induced changes in synaptic dopamine in patients with Parkinson's disease as measured by [^{11}C] raclopride displacement and PET. *Neurology* 1996;46:1430–1436.
20. de la Fuente-Fernández R, Lu JQ, Stossi V, et al. Biochemical variations in the synaptic level of dopamine precede motor fluctuations in Parkinson's disease: PET evidence of increased dopamine turnover. *Ann Neurol* 2001;49:298–303.
21. Quinn N, Critchley P, Marsden CD. Young onset Parkinson's disease. *Mov Disord* 1987;2:73–91.
22. Cedarbaum JM, Olanow CW. Dopamine sulfate in ventricular cerebrospinal fluid and motor function in Parkinson's disease. *Neurology* 1991;41:1567–1570.
23. Melamed E, Hefti F, Wurtman RJ. Nonaminergic striatal neurons convert exogenous L-dopa to dopamine in parkinsonism. *Ann Neurol* 1980;8:558–563.
24. Snyder GL, Keller RW Jr, Zigmond MJ. Dopamine efflux from striatal slices after intracerebral 6-hydroxydopamine: evidence for compensatory hyperactivity of residual terminals. *J Pharmacol Exp Ther* 1990;253: 867–876.
25. Abercrombie ED, Bonatz AE, Zigmond MJ. Effects of L-dopa on extracellular dopamine in striatum of normal and 6-hydroxydopamine–treated rats. *Brain Res* 1990; 525:36–44.
26. Miller DW, Abercrombie ED. Role of high-affinity dopamine uptake and impulse activity in the appearance of extracellular dopamine in striatum after administration of exogenous L-DOPA: studies in intact and 6-hydroxydopamine–treated rats. *J Neurochem* 1999;72: 1516–1522.
27. Uhl GR, Walther D, Mash D, et al. Dopamine transporter messenger RNA in Parkinson's disease and control substantia nigra neurons. *Ann Neurol* 1994;35: 494–498.
28. Guttman M, Stewart D, Hussey D, et al. Influence of L-

dopa and pramipexole on striatal dopamine transporter in early PD. *Neurology* 2001;56:1559–1564.

29. Zeng BY, Pearce RK, MacKenzie GM, et al. Chronic high dose L-dopa treatment does not alter the levels of dopamine D-1, D-2 or D-3 receptor in the striatum of normal monkeys: an autoradiographic study. *J Neural Transm* 2001;108:925–941.
30. Van Kampen JM, Stoessl AJ. Effects of oligonucleotide antisense to dopamine D_{1a} receptor messenger RNA in a rodent model of levodopa-induced dyskinesia. *Neuroscience* 2000;98:61–67.
31. Pierot L, Desnos C, Blin J, et al. D_1 and D_2-type dopamine receptors in patients with Parkinson's disease and progressive supranuclear palsy. *J Neurol Sci* 1988; 86:291–306.
32. Raisman R, Cash R, Ruberg M, et al. Binding of [^{3}H] SCH 23390 to D-1 receptors in the putamen of control and parkinsonian subjects. *Eur J Pharmacol* 1985;113: 467–468.
33. Rinne JO, Rinne JK, Laakso K, et al. Dopamine D-1 receptors in the parkinsonian brain. *Brain Res* 1985;359: 306–310.
34. Calon F, Goulet M, Blanchet PJ, et al. Levodopa or D_2 agonist induced dyskinesia in MPTP monkeys: correlation with changes in dopamine and GABA receptors in the striatopallidal complex. *Brain Res* 1995;680:43–52.
35. Gagnon C, Bedard PJ, Di Paolo T. Effect of chronic treatment of MPTP monkeys with dopamine D-1 and/or D-2 receptor agonists. *Eur J Pharmacol* 1990;178: 115–120.
36. Jaber M, Robinson SW, Missale C, et al. Dopamine receptors and brain function. *Neuropharmacology* 1996; 35:1503–1519.
37. Seeman P, Bzowej NH, Guan HC, et al. Human brain D_1 and D_2 dopamine receptors in schizophrenia, Alzheimer's, Parkinson's, and Huntington's diseases. *Neuropsychopharmacology* 1987;1:5–15.
38. Lees AJ, Stern GM. Sustained bromocriptine therapy in previously untreated patients with Parkinson's disease. *J Neurol Neurosurg Psychiatry* 1981;44:1020–1023.
39. Pearce RK, Banerji T, Jenner P, et al. *De novo* administration of ropinirole and bromocriptine induces less dyskinesia than L-dopa in the MPTP-treated marmoset. *Mov Disord* 1998;13:234–241.
40. Rascol O. Ropinirole, clinical profile. In: Olanow CW, Obeso JA, eds. *Beyond the decade of the brain.* Kent: Wells Medical Ltd, 1997:163–176.
41. Turjanski N, Lees AJ, Brooks DJ. *In vivo* studies on striatal dopamine D_1 and D_2 site binding in L-dopa–treated Parkinson's disease patients with and without dyskinesias. *Neurology* 1997;49:717–723.
42. Butkerait P, Wang HY, Friedman E. Increases in guanine nucleotide binding to striatal G proteins is associated with dopamine receptor supersensitivity. *J Pharmacol Exp Ther* 1994;271:422–428.
43. Marcotte ER, Sullivan RM, Mishra RK. Striatal G-proteins: effects of unilateral 6-hydroxydopamine lesions. *Neurosci Lett* 1994;169:195–198.
44. Moriyoshi K, Masu M, Ishii T, et al. Molecular cloning and characterization of the rat NMDA receptor. *Nature* 1991;354:31–37.
45. Schwarzschild MA, Cole RL, Meyers MA, et al. Contrasting calcium dependencies of SAPK and ERK activations by glutamate in cultured striatal neurons. *J Neurochem* 1999;72:2248–2255.
46. Smith CUM. Ligand-gated ion channels. In: *Elements of molecular neurobiology,* 2nd ed. Chichester: John Wiley and Sons, 1996:186–214.
47. Kosinski CM, Standaert DG, Counihan TJ, et al. Expression of *N*-methyl-D-aspartate receptor subunit mRNAs in the human brain: striatum and globus pallidus. *J Comp Neurol* 1998;390:63–74.
48. Wollmuth LP, Kuner T, Seeburg PH, et al. Differential contribution of the NR1- and NR2A-subunits to the selectivity filter of recombinant NMDA receptor channels. *J Physiol* 1996;491:779–797.
49. Wollmuth LP, Kuner T, Sakmann B. Adjacent asparagines in the NR2-subunit of the NMDA receptor channel control the voltage-dependent block by extracellular Mg^{2+}. *J Physiol* 1998;506:13–32.
50. Oh JD, Del Dotto P, Chase TN. Protein kinase A inhibitor attenuates levodopa-induced motor response alterations in the hemi-parkinsonian rat. *Neurosci Lett* 1997;228:5–8.
51. Oh JD, Russell DS, Vaughan CL, et al. Enhanced tyrosine phosphorylation of striatal NMDA receptor subunits: effect of dopaminergic denervation and L-DOPA administration. *Brain Res* 1998;813:150–159.
52. Mitchell IJ, Carroll CB. Reversal of parkinsonian symptoms in primates by antagonism of excitatory amino acid transmission: potential mechanisms of action. *Neurosci Biobehav Rev* 1997;21:469–475.
53. Schmidt WJ, Kretschmer BD. Behavioural pharmacology of glutamate receptors in the basal ganglia. *Neurosci Biobehav Rev* 1997;21:381–392.
54. Starr MS, Starr BS, Kaur S. Stimulation of basal and L-DOPA–induced motor activity by glutamate antagonists in animal models of Parkinson's disease. *Neurosci Biobehav Rev* 1997;21:437–446.
55. Engber TM, Papa SM, Boldry RC, et al. NMDA receptor blockade reverses motor response alterations induced by levodopa. *Neuroreport* 1994;5:2586–2588.
56. Blanchet PJ, Konitsiotis S, Chase TN. Amantadine reduces levodopa-induced dyskinesias in parkinsonian monkeys. *Mov Disord* 1998;13:798–802.
57. Papa SM, Chase TN. Levodopa-induced dyskinesias improved by a glutamate antagonist in parkinsonian monkeys. *Ann Neurol* 1996;39:574–578.
58. Verhagen ML, Blanchet PJ, van den Munckhof P, et al. A trial of dextromethorphan in parkinsonian patients with motor response complications. *Mov Disord* 1998; 13:414–417.
59. Del Dotto P, Pavese N, Gambaccini G, et al. Intravenous amantadine improves levodopa-induced dyskinesias: an acute double-blind placebo-controlled study. *Mov Disord* 2001;16:515–520.
60. Luginger E, Wenning GK, Bosch S, et al. Beneficial effects of amantadine on L-dopa–induced dyskinesias in Parkinson's disease. *Mov Disord* 2000;15:873–878.
61. Merello M, Nouzeilles MI, Cammarota A, et al. Effect of memantine (NMDA antagonist) on Parkinson's disease: a double-blind crossover randomized study. *Clin Neuropharmacol* 1999;22:273–276.
62. Marin C, Jimenez A, Bonastre M, et al. Non-NMDA receptor–mediated mechanisms are involved in levodopa-induced motor response alterations in parkinsonian rats. *Synapse* 2000;36:267–274.
63. Herrero MT, Augood SJ, Hirsch EC, et al. Effects of L-DOPA on preproenkephalin and preprotachykinin gene expression in the MPTP-treated monkey striatum. *Neuroscience* 1995;68:1189–1198.
64. Morissette M, Goulet M, Soghomonian JJ, et al. Pre-

proenkephalin mRNA expression in the caudate-putamen of MPTP monkeys after chronic treatment with the D_2 agonist U91356A in continuous or intermittent mode of administration: comparison with L-DOPA therapy. *Brain Res Mol Brain Res* 1997;49:55–62.
65. Del Fiacco M, Paxinos G, Cuello AC. Neostriatal enkephalin-immunoreactive neurones project to the globus pallidus. *Brain Res* 1982;231:1–17.
66. Gerfen CR, Young WS. Distribution of striatonigral and striatopallidal peptidergic neurons in both patch and matrix compartments: an *in situ* hybridization histochemistry and fluorescent retrograde tracing study. *Brain Res* 1988;460:161–167.
67. Wichmann T, DeLong MR. Models of basal ganglia function and pathophysiology of movement disorders. *Neurosurg Clin North Am* 1998;9:223–236.
68. Jolkkonen J, Jenner P, Marsden CD. L-DOPA reverses altered gene expression of substance P but not enkephalin in the caudate-putamen of common marmosets treated with MPTP. *Brain Res Mol Brain Res* 1995;32:297–307.
69. Nisbet AP, Foster OJ, Kingsbury A, et al. Preproenkephalin and preprotachykinin messenger RNA expression in normal human basal ganglia and in Parkinson's disease. *Neuroscience* 1995;66:361–376.
70. Piccini P, Weeks RA, Brooks DJ. Alterations in opioid receptor binding in Parkinson's disease patients with levodopa-induced dyskinesias. *Ann Neurol* 1997;42: 720–726.
71. Schad CA, Justice JB Jr, Holtzman SG. Differential effects of delta- and mu-opioid receptor antagonists on the amphetamine-induced increase in extracellular dopamine in striatum and nucleus accumbens. *J Neurochem* 1996;67:2292–2299.
72. Yoshida Y, Koide S, Hirose N, et al. Fentanyl increases dopamine release in rat nucleus accumbens: involvement of mesolimbic mu- and delta-2-opioid receptors. *Neuroscience* 1999;92:1357–1365.
73. Maneuf YP, Mitchell IJ, Crossman AR, et al. On the role of enkephalin cotransmission in the GABAergic striatal efferents to the globus pallidus. *Exp Neurol* 1994;125: 65–71.
74. Henry B, Fox SH, Crossman AR, et al. Mu- and delta-opioid receptor antagonists reduce levodopa-induced dyskinesia in the MPTP-lesioned primate model of Parkinson's disease. *Exp Neurol* 2001;171:139–146.
75. Ferre S, O'Connor WT, Svenningsson P, et al. Dopamine D_1 receptor–mediated facilitation of GABAergic neurotransmission in the rat strioentopenduncular pathway and its modulation by adenosine A_1 receptor–mediated mechanisms. *Eur J Neurosci* 1996; 8:1545–1553.
76. Schiffmann SN, Jacobs O, Vanderhaeghen JJ. Striatal restricted adenosine A_2 receptor (RDC8) is expressed by enkephalin but not by substance P neurons: an *in situ* hybridization histochemistry study. *J Neurochem* 1991; 57:1062–1067.
77. Ferre S, Fredholm BB, Morelli M, et al. Adenosine-dopamine receptor–receptor interactions as an integrative mechanism in the basal ganglia. *Trends Neurosci* 1997;20:482–487.
78. Fuxe K, Ferre S, Zoli M, et al. Integrated events in central dopamine transmission as analyzed at multiple levels. Evidence for intramembrane adenosine A_{2a}/dopamine D_2 and adenosine A_1/dopamine D_1 receptor interactions in the basal ganglia. *Brain Res Brain Res Rev* 1998;26:258–273.
79. Fuxe K, Strömberg I, Popoli P, et al. Adenosine receptors and Parkinson's disease. Relevance of antagonistic adenosine and dopamine receptor interactions in the striatum. *Adv Neurol* 2001;86:345–353.
80. Grondin R, Bedard PJ, Hadj TA, et al. Antiparkinsonian effect of a new selective adenosine A_{2a} receptor antagonist in MPTP-treated monkeys. *Neurology* 1999;52: 1673–1677.
81. Kanda T, Tashiro T, Kuwana Y, et al. Adenosine A_{2a} receptors modify motor function in MPTP-treated common marmosets. *Neuroreport* 1998;9:2857–2860.
82. Vallone D, Pellecchia MT, Morelli M, et al. Behavioural sensitization in 6-hydroxydopamine–lesioned rats is related to compositional changes of the AP-1 transcription factor: evidence for induction of FosB- and JunD-related proteins. *Brain Res Mol Brain Res* 1997;52: 307–317.
83. Calon F, Grondin R, Morissette M, et al. Molecular basis of levodopa-induced dyskinesias. *Ann Neurol* 2000; 47:S70–S78.
84. Quinn NP. Classification of fluctuations in patients with Parkinson's disease. *Neurology* 1998;51[Suppl]: S25–S29.
85. Chase TN, Oh JD. Striatal mechanisms and pathogenesis of parkinsonian signs and motor complications. *Ann Neurol* 2000;47[Suppl]:S122–S129.
86. Fahn S. The spectrum of levodopa-induced dyskinesias. *Ann Neurol* 2000;47:S2–S9.
87. Contin M, Riva R, Martinelli P, et al. Longitudinal monitoring of the levodopa concentration–effect relationship in Parkinson's disease. *Neurology* 1994;44: 1287–1292.
88. Nutt JG, Woodward WR, Carter JH, et al. Effect of long-term therapy on the pharmacodynamics of levodopa. Relation to on-off phenomenon. *Arch Neurol* 1992;49:1123–1130.
89. Sohn YH, Metman LV, Bravi D, et al. Levodopa peak response time reflects severity of dopamine neuron loss in Parkinson's disease. *Neurology* 1994;44:755–757.
90. Nutt JG, Holford NH. The response to levodopa in Parkinson's disease: imposing pharmacological law and order. *Ann Neurol* 1996;39:561–573.
91. Nutt JG. Fluctuations in response to treatment for Parkinson's disease. *Adv Neurol* 2001;86:361–366.
92. Merello M, Lees AJ. Beginning-of-dose motor deterioration following the acute administration of levodopa and apomorphine in Parkinson's disease. *J Neurol Neurosurg Psychiatry* 1992;55:1024–1026.
93. Nutt JG, Gancher ST, Woodward WR. Does an inhibitory action of levodopa contribute to motor fluctuations? *Neurology* 1988;38:1553–1557.
94. Paalzow GHM, Paalzow LK. L-DOPA: how it may exacerbate parkinsonian symptoms. *Trends Pharmacol Sci* 1986;7:15–19.
95. de la Fuente-Fernández R, Lim AS, Sossi V, et al. Apomorphine-induced changes in synaptic dopamine levels: positron emission tomography evidence for presynaptic inhibition. *J Cereb Blood Flow Metab* 2001;21: 1151–1159.

Parkinson's Disease: Advances in Neurology, Vol. 91.
Edited by Ariel Gordin, Seppo Kaakkola,
and Heikki Teräväinen
Lippincott Williams & Wilkins, Philadelphia © 2003

21

The Management of Patients with Early Parkinson's Disease

*Olivier Rascol, *C. Brefel-Courbon, †P. Payoux, and ‡J. Ferreira

**Department of Clinical Pharmacology and Pharmacovigilance, Clinical Investigations Centre, INSERM; †Department of Nuclear Medicine, Toulouse University Hospital, Toulouse, France; and ‡Department of Neurology, Egas Moniz Research Centre, Lisbon University Hospital, Lisbon, Portugal*

The management of patients with early Parkinson's disease (PD) involves different steps. The first one is to establish the diagnosis of "idiopathic" PD. Then the patient and his or her family should be adequately informed and get the appropriate answers to their questions about PD: causes, symptoms, progression, prognosis, genetic transmission, treatments, ongoing research, and future perspectives. It is also important at this stage to evaluate the individual and specific needs and expectations of each patient because these can be markedly different according to age, profession, culture, hobbies, mood, cognition, and comorbidity. Based on this ground, the next step is to choose the most adequate therapeutic option and to start follow-up.

This chapter does not cover all these aspects but focuses on how to choose the first antiparkinsonian medication in a drug-naive patient with early PD. Recently, several algorithms have been published in an effort to simplify and standardize the numerous possible pharmacological options presently available (1). The objective of this review is not to produce or reproduce another algorithm but to discuss and illustrate some of the factors contributing to the final therapeutic decision.

NEUROPROTECTIVE MEDICATIONS

Over time, motor symptoms of PD progressively worsen. The need for symptomatic medications increases, the quality of their effects deteriorates, and nonmotor symptoms develop. A major therapeutic goal is therefore to limit this process. Secondary prevention, once PD has been diagnosed, aims at slowing down, stopping, or even reversing neuronal death. According to various known biochemical pathways that may play a role in cell death, several drugs are potential candidates for neuroprotection (2).

If a neuroprotective agent proved safe and clinically efficacious, this drug would probably be systematically prescribed in nearly all patients, as soon as PD is diagnosed and ideally before the symptoms occur. Until now, unfortunately, none of the medications that have been tested proved to influence clinically relevant endpoints regarding "neuroprotection" in randomized clinical trials (RCTs). Therefore, there is presently no clinical evidence to recommend any neuroprotective agent to treat PD. Any intervention remains, at best, investigational. Because several agents are currently under study at PD centers, clinicians should consider referring interested patients immediately after diagnosis and before prescribing symptomatic treatments to participate in phase II or phase III trials.

SYMPTOMATIC TREATMENT OF EARLY PD

Symptomatic medications are only initiated if the patient and his or her physician agree that functional disability requires drug intervention. Then comes the choice among the different potential options. Anticholinergics were discovered one century ago (3) and remained the only choice until levodopa usefulness was established in the late 1960s (4). In these times, there were not many alternative options, and the decision was rather easy. Within the last three decades, other medications were approved for the treatment of PD: monoamine oxidase B (MAO-B) inhibitors (selegiline); catechol-*O*-methyltransferase (COMT) inhibitors (entacapone only because tolcapone cannot be used in patients with early PD due to hepatic toxicity) dopamine (DA) agonists (bromocriptine, lisuride, pergolide, piribedil, cabergoline, pramipexole, and ropinirole); and amantadine. With now a dozen of different drugs available (not even considering combination strategies), it is more difficult to decide which one should be started first. Does this matter? Does this have the same impact on immediate and long-term outcomes?

Ideally, any treatment should be simple, efficacious, safe, and cost-effective. Choosing a given drug to achieve this objective is driven by a complex combination of different factors. Doctors sometimes base their choice on pathophysiological concepts. They should rather be influenced by the level of clinical evidence, mainly relying on the results of clinical trials. The opinion leaders' influence, personal scientific background, individual empirical experience, marketing pressure, and socioeconomic and cultural environments also have their own impact. We shall give some examples.

THE IMPACT OF PATHOPHYSIOLOGICAL CONCEPTS ON CLINICAL PRACTICE IN THE MANAGEMENT OF EARLY PD

The discovery in the late 1960s of DA depletion in the striatum of patients with PD provided a strong pathophysiological rationale to use levodopa (and other DA agents) in the treatment of PD. Since then, this strategy proved quite successful, and levodopa still remains the "gold standard" for the treatment of PD.

Some years ago, however, the question of a putative negative impact of levodopa therapy on PD progression was put forward because DA metabolism produces free radicals. Based on *in vitro* data and according to the pathophysiological concept that oxidative stress causes neurodegeneration, many physicians became reluctant to prescribe levodopa early. They rather delayed its use as much as possible, to "protect" the remaining neurons from this potential toxicity. Until now, the question of levodopa "toxicity" remained controversial, in spite of several public debates among international experts, usually referring to preclinical data in the context of conflicting marketing stakes (5). Recently, a group of opinion leaders published a "consensus statement" that concluded that there was no clinical demonstration that levodopa was toxic *in vivo* in PD (6). In spite of this reassurance, everyone has not been convinced yet, and several people, including patients with PD, remain concerned. One can hope that adequate RCTs, such as the Earlier vs. Later L-Dopa study (7), will provide sufficient objective clinical evidence to close the discussion.

More recently, a newer pathophysiological theory became quite popular to discuss how patients with early PD should be treated. This is known as continuous DA stimulation (CDS) (8). This concept is largely used by various drug companies to base their marketing strategy on. Briefly, preclinical data obtained in 6-hydroxydopamine–treated rats and methylphenyltetrahydropyridine-intoxicated monkeys show that a parkinsonian brain cannot adequately buffer the peaks of DA concentrations elicited by the intermittent administration of short-acting drugs such as oral levodopa. This nonphysiological pulsatile DA stimulation may induce a cascade of abnormal responses in the basal ganglia: dysregulation of striatal DA and non-DA receptors, abnormal intracellular signaling of striatal neurones, abnormal output of the basal ganglial motor loop, and abnormal motor behaviors such as the "on-off" phenomenon and dyskinesias. Based on this concept, doctors are now encouraged to deliver as early as possible the most continuous DA stimulation, to prevent the occurrence of long-term motor complications. From a pharmacokinetic perspective, there are many drugs that can be proposed to achieve CDS: levodopa controlled-release (CR) formulations because they reduce peak plasma concentrations (C_{max}) and prolong (apparent) elimination half-life, entacapone because it prolongs levodopa elimination half-life without increasing its C_{max}, and most available DA agonists because they have a longer elimination half-life than standard levodopa. Accordingly, one can speculate that all these drugs should be used early in the management of PD. The hypothesis is attractive, but theories should be challenged and we need to prove such concepts on clinical grounds. In the context of CDS, one should not forget, for example, that the early use of CR levodopa failed to prevent motor complications in two large RCTs (9,10). Moreover, although we lack head-to-head comparisons, another challenging observation is that cabergoline, with its long elimination half-life (about 70 hours), does not seem to reduce the risk of long-term motor complications much more than lisuride, with its short half-life (3 hours) (11,12). In this context, in the absence of any clinical evidence in patients with early PD and based solely on animal data, pathophysiological concepts, and marketing claims, can we agree that an expensive drug such as entacapone should be systematically combined as soon as levodopa is initiated to treat *de novo* nonfluctuating patients? It is crucial to incorporate the level of clinical evidence in our decision strategy (13).

THE MOVEMENT DISORDERS SOCIETY EVIDENCE-BASED ASSESSMENT OF ANTIPARKINSONIAN INTERVENTIONS

The Movement Disorders Society (MDS) recently established and funded an initiative to review the different available antiparkinsonian therapeutic interventions according to the robustness of the corresponding published clinical evidence. This endeavor was aimed at organizing and making accessible this information to improve physicians' knowledge of the available evidence. This should help us incorporate this background into our own decision strategy. The approach followed was to develop an evidence-based review in which therapeutic interventions were classified accordingly with a specified set of criteria regarding efficacy, clinical usefulness, and safety (Table 21.1). Such classification was agreed upon by consensus among a panel of MDS experts. The scientific basis for that classification was defined as all identified original articles (MEDLINE and Cochrane Library, English peer-reviewed literature) that reported on RCTs that enrolled a minimum of 20 patients with established diagnosis of PD, used objective scales for measuring target symptoms, and had a minimum of 4 weeks of treatment follow-up. This scientific basis is most appropriate to establish efficacy, but much less so for safety, because RCTs are not designed to identify rare adverse reactions. Therefore, other sources, beside RCTs, were used for safety (post–marketing surveillance and regulatory publications). The usefulness of these therapeutic interventions was put into perspective according to type of clinical problems. Several of these clinical problems are crucial to consider when managing patients with early PD, namely efficacy of treatment as monotherapy and prevention of motor

TABLE 21.1. *Standard definitions of the terms used to qualify efficacy, clinical usefulness, and safety of therapeutic interventions*

Efficacy	
Efficacious	Evidence shows that the intervention has a positive effect on studied outcomes (at least one good-quality randomized controlled trial).
Efficacy likely	Evidence suggests but is not sufficient to show that the intervention has a positive effect on studied outcomes.
Efficacy unlikely	Evidence suggests that the intervention does not have a positive effect on studied outcomes.
Nonefficacious	Evidence shows that the intervention does not have a positive effect on studied outcomes.
Insufficient evidence	There are no data available, or available data do not provide enough evidence either for or against the use of the intervention in treatment of Parkinson's disease.
Clinical usefulness	
Clinically useful	For a given situation, evidence available is sufficient to conclude that the intervention provides clinical benefit.
Possibly useful	For a given situation, evidence available suggests but is insufficient to conclude that the intervention provides clinical benefit.
Investigational	Available evidence is insufficient to support the use of the intervention in clinical practice, but further study is warranted.
Not useful	For a given situation, available evidence is sufficient to say that the intervention provides no clinical benefit.
Safety	
Acceptable risk without specialized monitoring.	
Acceptable risk with specialized monitoring.	
Unacceptable risk.	
Insufficient evidence to make conclusions on the safety of the intervention.	

complication. The entire MDS evidence-based research document will be published as a supplement of the *Journal of Movement Disorders.* We shall briefly summarize its conclusions referring to early PD.

Drug Efficacy as Monotherapies

The MDS evidence-based research concluded that of the available antiparkinsonian medications used as monotherapy in early PD, there was enough clinical evidence to conclude that *efficacious* drugs were levodopa (standard and CR formulations); four agonists (dihydroergocryptine, pergolide, pramipexole, and ropinirole); and selegiline (Table 21.2). Standard levodopa has never been tested against placebo, but the effect size of levodopa treatment, once the appropriate dose is achieved, is so remarkably large that it could be established beyond reasonable doubt without the need of RCTs on the basis of open

TABLE 21.2. *Symptomatic interventions for the treatment of parkinsonism (motor features) as monotherapies in patients with early Parkinson's disease*

	Efficacious	Likely efficacious	Insufficient evidence
Medications	Standard levodopa Controlled-release levodopa	Bromocriptine Lisuride	Apomorphine Cabergoline Piribedil
	Dihydroergocriptine Pergolide Pramipexole Ropinirole Seligiline	Anticholinergics Amantadine	 Entacapone[a] Tolcapone[a]
Surgery			All interventions
Rehabilitation			All interventions

[a]Based on their mechanism of action, catechol-*O*-methyltransferase inhibitors are not considered as efficacious when used as monotherapy in Parkinson's disease, but no published clinical trial was identified.

control experiments. Moreover, subsequently, levodopa proved more efficacious than several DA agonists in RCTs such as bromocriptine (14), ropinirole (15), and pramipexole (16). CR levodopa was compared with standard levodopa in several studies with equivalent improvement in parkinsonism at short-term and long-term evaluation (17). Several agonists improved parkinsonism better than placebo: pergolide (18), dihydroergocryptine (19), pramipexole (20), and ropinirole (21). Likewise, selegiline (22) has also been compared with placebo treatment in RCTs and improved parkinsonism. Others drugs such as bromocriptine, lisuride, cabergoline, amantadine, and anticholinergics were considered *likely efficacious* as monotherapy in PD, because they were tested in RCTs of lower quality or in studies without placebo control, but consistently showed improvement in treatment compared with baseline evaluation. Data on other monotherapy treatments were insufficient to include because of lack of adequate evidence to draw conclusions or conflicting results on their efficacy.

There are nearly no published RCTs comparing a given drug as monotherapy with another one, with the exception of one study comparing ropinirole with bromocriptine (23). This study showed a slight but significantly greater improvement with ropinirole in patients not receiving selegiline. The clinical relevancy of such a small difference remains to be established. Conversely, in most RCTs comparing levodopa with others medications, levodopa proved more efficacious. This is why in most long-term follow-up studies, agonists are generally initiated as monotherapy and are supplemented later with small doses of open-labeled levodopa if and when patients need a complement to keep control over parkinsonism. No comparative data are available between agonists and amantadine, selegiline, anticholinergics, or entacapone.

Prevention of Motor Complications

Another important clinical issue when initiating the treatment of a patient with PD is to estimate the impact of this initial treatment on long-term outcome, particularly regarding late motor complications (fluctuations and dyskinesias). This has been considered with a growing interest in the last few years because such motor complications are frequent, difficult to treat, disabling, and may be at least partly irreversible.

In spite of the CDS hypothesis, predicting that the early use of CR levodopa formulations should reduce the risk of long-term motor complication, the MDS evidence-based research concluded that the early use of CR levodopa is *not efficacious* in preventing the long-term occurrence of motor complications, based on two large standard levodopa controlled RCTs (9,10). In the advent of the CDS hypothesis, some physicians are also sometimes prescribing levodopa, divided into six or more daily doses from the initiation of treatment. There is no clinical evidence to support this practice.

The only medications considered by the MDS evidence-based research as *efficacious* therapies in reducing the risk of motor complication when used early in the treatment of PD were three DA agonists: cabergoline (11), ropinirole (24), and pramipexole (16) (Table 21.3). In these RCTs, levodopa was usually used an adjunct early or late to the agonist to keep control over parkinsonism when the antiparkinsonian effect of the agonist monotherapy was waning (see previous section, "Drug Efficacy as Monotherapies"). Bromocriptine was considered *likely efficacious* based on lower quality levodopa controlled trials (25,26). The fact that four different agonists proved *efficacious* or *likely efficacious* suggests that this property might be a "class effect." However, in the absence of adequate published RCTs or because of conflicting results, it was concluded that there are *insufficient data to conclude* on this effect of other agonists like lisuride, pergolide, and piribedil. There also were *insufficient data to conclude* on the use of any other compounds, including MAO-B and COMT inhibitors. This is particularly true for entacapone, and it is worth noting that in spite of CDS prediction, there is

TABLE 21.3. *Preventive interventions for motor complications in levodopa-naive patients with Parkinson's disease*

	Efficacious	Likely efficacious	Nonefficacious	Insufficient data
Medications	Cabergoline Pramipexole	Bromocriptine	Standard levodopa	Apomorphine
				Dihydroergocriptine
	Ropinirole		Controlled-release levodopa	Lisuride Pergolide Piribedil Selegiline Entacapone Tolcapone Amantadine Anticholinergics
Surgery				All interventions
Rehabilitation				All interventions

yet no clinical evidence that the early combination of entacapone and levodopa does or does not improve long-term outcome of patients, particularly regarding dyskinesia.

SAFETY

It is beyond the scope of this chapter to review in detail all known side effects of antiparkinsonian medications. As already pointed out, the scientific data to base conclusions on for safety cannot be restricted to RCTs, particularly because such trials are never powered to identified rare and/or idiosyncratic adverse reactions that are nevertheless clinically meaningful. Therefore, for the safety part of a risk/benefit assessment, other sources must be reviewed including post–marketing surveillance, pharmacovigilance, and regulatory publications, such as those issued by the Committee of Proprietary Medicinal Product in Europe and the Food and Drug Administration in the United States.

It is common knowledge that all dopaminergic medications including levodopa and DA agonists share a similar safety profile, reflecting excessive DA stimulation. The most frequent adverse effects are nausea, vomiting, hypotension, confusion, and hallucinations. There are not many head-to-head objective comparisons between the different dopaminergic agents. All agonists have very similar safety profiles (except for pulmonary and retroperitoneal fibrosis, which may be less frequent with non-ergot compounds). All agonists are empirically reported to induce more nausea, hypotension, and hallucinations than levodopa. This is not well documented in double-blind RCTs, except for hallucinations (16,24). Common adverse effects of amantadine include confusion, hallucination, edema, and livido reticularis. With antimuscarinic agents, the most frequent adverse reactions are urinary retention, constipation, dry mouth, increase in intraocular pressure, and confusion.

Such safety profiles are obviously crucial to consider when initiating a treatment. For example, cognitively impaired or elderly patients are unlikely to tolerate DA agonists or anticholinergics and might be better managed with standard levodopa. This is common knowledge, and we shall rather concentrate in this review (mainly for length concerns) on two specific side effects that caused recent controversies: mortality on selegiline and "sleep attacks" on DA agonists.

A few years ago, concerns about selegiline safety were raised because of an increased mortality rate in the levodopa plus selegiline arm of a large levodopa controlled RCT conducted in patients with early PD (27). Subsequent metaanalysis and smaller RCTs failed to reproduce or support this finding (28). In the absence of clear confirmatory reports, there are still insufficient data to conclude, although most prescribers now consider this risk unlikely in spite of some small studies reporting an increased cardiovascular risk due to orthostatic hypotension and autonomic nerve system dysfunction on selegiline (29).

"Sleep attacks" have also been a major concern in the past years. The alert was generated when Frucht et al. (30) reported on eight patients with PD who complained of having motor vehicle accidents due to falling asleep at the wheel on pramipexole or ropinirole. Such observations led to regulatory driving restrictions. Inappropriate daytime somnolence and "sleep attacks" have been subsequently reported with nearly all dopaminergic antiparkinsonian medications, including most DA agonists, including apomorphine (31), bromocriptine (32), pergolide (33), lisuride (32), pergolide (32), cabergoline (34), as well as levodopa monotherapy (35) and entacapone (36). There is an obvious need for pharmacological epidemiological studies (including age-matched healthy volunteers) to establish which drugs are the main risk factors for such sleep episodes and whether any drug is at greater risk than the others. In a recent cross-sectional survey conducted in nearly several hundreds of patients with PD and aged-matched healthy volunteers, we observed that age and duration of levodopa therapy were the two main risk factors (J. Ferreira et al., *unpublished data*). Among the patients who were receiving a DA agonist in this survey, the percentage of those reporting "sleep attacks" was similar to that of those receiving bromocriptine, ropinirole, lisuride, and piribedil. However, a recent metaanalysis reported that the risk of somnolence in patients taking pramipexole and ropinirole was greater than that of patients taking levodopa (37).

COST-DRIVEN DECISIONS

Drug costs may not be seen as a major concern when making a therapeutic decision, particularly for doctors and patients living in countries with a good social security system. It is, however, a major problem from a public health perspective, and it is sometimes the most crucial factor in countries with less effective social insurance. The daily costs of different antiparkinsonian medications can vary from 1 to 10 Fr. The most recently marketed drugs are usually the most expensive ones, but not necessarily the most efficacious or the safest ones. Table 21.4 shows an estimation of the daily cost of different antiparkinsonian medications in France. It is obvious that the three cheapest drugs are also the three oldest ones: Anticholinergics, amantadine, and levodopa cost less than 3 Fr a day. Then there is a group of more expensive (and less "old") drugs, namely selegiline, piribedil, lisuride, and bromocriptine costing from 5 to 20 Fr per day. Finally, the most expensive treatments (more than 20 Fr per day) are the most recently launched ones, including entacapone, ropinirole, and pergolide. (Pergolide was only marketed in France in 2001.)

TABLE 21.4. *Daily costs (France)*

Trihexyphenidyl (Artane 10 mg/d)	1.56 Fr
Amantadine (Mantadix 300 mg/d)	2.20 Fr
L-dopa (Modopar 300 mg/d)	2.97 Fr
Selegiline (Leurquin 10 mg/d)	6.00 Fr
Piribedil (Trivastal 200 mg/d)	9.73 Fr
Lisuride (Dopergine 1.5 mg/d)	12.09 Fr
Bromocriptine (Bromokin 30 mg/d)	13.99 Fr
Entacapone (Comtan 600 mg/d)	19.29 Fr
Ropinirole (Requip 15 mg/d)	35.73 Fr
Pergolide (Celance 3 mg/d)	43.24 Fr

Other direct, as well as indirect and intangible, costs should be considered, and because Table 21.4 is simplistic, it cannot summarize all economic aspects related to the management of early PD. However, it is interesting to look at such simple data, particularly keeping in mind that many of these drugs are not so different regarding efficacy and safety.

CONCLUSIONS

In conclusion, clearly any practitioner will base his or her therapeutic decision to initiate treatment in a given patient with PD on a combination of several considerations. The weight of these different factors varies markedly from one patient to another; from one physician to another; and from one country to another, according to age, needs, efficacy, safety, empirical and technical experience, and personal, cultural, and socioeconomic conditions. In regions with a low economic level and a poor social security system, for example, theoretical hypotheses such as "CDS" and long-term concerns about motor complications might not be seen realistically as crucial factors when initiating therapy. The cheapest and most efficacious treatments are those that allow the treatment of the largest number of patients and will be the most appropriate pragmatic choices. In richer countries, there is more space for long-term concerns, attractive but speculative theories, and marketing pressure that obviously has a stronger impact. We believe that an evidence-based approach should be promoted and favored as much as possible to help make the most adequate decisions. This is often a difficult task because it is not so easy to have access to the appropriate data, to analyze them, and to make clear conclusions. This is why working groups such as the Cochrane and the MDS evidence-based research have been initiated.

REFERENCES

1. Olanow CW, Watts RL, Koller WC. An algorithm (decision tree) for the management of Parkinson's disease: treatment guidelines. *Neurology* 2001;56[Suppl]: S1–S88.
2. Mizuno Y, Mori H, Kondo T. Potential of neuroprotective therapy in Parkinson's disease. *CNS Drugs* 1994; 1:45–56.
3. Lang AE, Blair RDG. Anticholinergic drugs and amantadine in the treatment of Parkinson's disease. In: Calne DB, ed. *Handbook of experimental pharmacology: drugs for the treatment of Parkinson's diseases,* vol 88. Berlin, Heidelberg: Springer-Verlag, 1989.
4. Cotzias GC, Papavasiliou PS, Gellene R. Modification of parkinsonism—chronic treatment with levodopa. *N Engl J Med* 1969;280:337–345.
5. Murer MG, Raisman-Vozari, Gershanik O. Levodopa in Parkinson's disease. Neurotoxicity issue laid to rest? *Drug Safety* 1999;21:339–352.
6. Agid Y, Ahlskog E, Albanese A, et al. Levodopa in the treatment of Parkinson's disease: a consensus meeting. *Mov Disord* 1999;14:911–913.
7. Fahn S. Parkinson disease, the effect of levodopa, and the ELLDOPA trial. Earlier vs. Later L-Dopa. *Arch Neurol* 1999;56:529–535.
8. Olanow CW, Schapira AHV, Rascol O. Continuous dopamine-receptor stimulation in early Parkinson's disease. *Trends Neurosci* 2000;23[Suppl]:S117–S126.
9. Dupont E, Anderson A, Boas J, et al. Sustained-release Madopar HBS compared with standard Madopar in the long-term treatment of *de novo* parkinsonian patients. *Acta Neurol Scand* 1996;93:14–20.
10. Block G, Liss C, Scott R, et al. Comparison of immediate-release and controlled release carbidopa/levodopa in Parkinson's disease. A multicenter 5-year study. *Eur Neurol* 1997;37:23–27
11. Rinne UK, Bracco F, Chouza C, et al. Early treatment of Parkinson's disease with cabergoline delays the onset of motor complications. *Drugs* 1998;55[Suppl 1]: S23–S30.
12. Rinne UK. Lisuride, a dopamine agonist in the treatment of early Parkinson's disease. *Neurology* 1989; 39:336–339.
13. Sackett DL, Richardson WS, Rosenberg W, et al. *Evidence-based medicine: how to practice and teach EBM.* New York: Churchill Livingstone, 1997.
14. Parkinson's Disease Research Group in the United Kingdom. Comparisons of therapeutic effects of levodopa, levodopa and selegiline, and bromocriptine in patients with early, mild Parkinson's disease: three year interim report. *Br Med J* 1993;307:469–472.
15. Rascol O, Brooks DJ, Brunt ER, et al, for the 056 Study Group. Ropinirole in the treatment of early Parkinson's disease: a 6-month interim report of a 5-year levodopa-controlled study. *Mov Disord* 1998;13:39–45.
16. Parkinson Study Group. Pramipexole versus levodopa as initial treatment for Parkinson's disease: a randomized controlled trial. *JAMA* 2000;284:1931–1938.
17. Koller WC, Hutton JT, Tolosa E, et al, and the Carbidopa/Levodopa Study Group. Immediate-release and controlled-release carbidopa/levodopa in PD: a 5-year randomized multicenter study. *Neurology* 1999;53: 1012–1019.
18. Barone P, Bravi D, Bermejo-Pareja F, et al. Pergolide monotherapy in the treatment of early Parkinson's disease: a randomized, controlled study. *Neurology* 1999; 53:573–579.
19. Bergamasco B, Frattola L, Muratorio A, et al. Alpha-dihydroergocryptine in the treatment of *de novo* parkinsonian patients: results of a multicentre, randomised, double-blind, placebo-controlled study. *Acta Neurol Scand* 2000;101:372–380.
20. Shannon KM, Bennett JP, Friedman JH, for the Pramipexole Study Group. Efficacy of pramipexole, a novel dopamine agonist, as monotherapy in mild to moderate Parkinson's disease. *Neurology* 1997;49: 724–728.
21. Adler CH, Sethi KD, Hauser RA, et al. Ropinirole for the treatment of early Parkinson's disease. *Neurology* 1997;49:393–399.
22. Parkinson Study Group. Impact of deprenyl and tocopherol treatment of Parkinson's disease in DATATOP subjects not requiring levodopa. *Ann Neurol* 1996;39: 29–36.
23. Korczyn AD, Brooks DJ, Brunt ER, et al, on behalf of the 053 Study Group. Ropinirole versus bromocriptine in the treatment of early Parkinson's disease: 6-month interim report of a 3-year study. *Mov Disord* 1998;13: 46–51.
24. Rascol O, Brooks DJ, Korczyn AD, et al, for the 056 Study Group. A five-year study of the incidence of dyskinesia in patients with early Parkinson's disease who were treated with ropinirole or levodopa. *N Engl J Med* 2000;342:1484–1491.
25. Montastruc JL, Rascol O, Senard JM, et al. A ran-

domised controlled study comparing bromocriptine to which levodopa was later added, with levodopa alone in previously untreated patients with Parkinson's disease: a five year follow-up. *J Neurol Neurosurg Psychiatry* 1994;57:1034–1038.
26. Przuntek H, Welzel D, Gerlach M, et al. Early institution of bromocriptine in Parkinson's disease inhibits the emergence of levodopa-associated motor side effects. Long-term results of the PRADO study. *J Neural Transm* 1996;103:699–715.
27. Lees AJ. Parkinson's Disease Research Group of the United Kingdom. Comparison of therapeutic effects and mortality data of levodopa and levodopa combined with selegiline in patients with early, mild Parkinson's disease. *Br Med J* 1995;311:1602–1607.
28. Olanow CW, Myllylä VV, Sotaniemi KA, et al. Effect of selegiline on mortality in patients with Parkinson's disease: a meta-analysis. *Neurology* 1998;51:825–830.
29. Churchyard A, Mathias CJ, Lees AJ. Selegiline-induced postural hypotension in Parkinson's disease: a longitudinal study on the effects of drug withdrawal. *Mov Disord* 1999;14:246–251.
30. Frucht S, Rogers JD, Greene PE, et al. Falling asleep at the wheel: motor vehicle mishaps in persons taking pramipexole and ropinirole. *Neurology* 1999;52: 1908–1910.
31. Homann CN, Wenzel K, Suppan K, et al. Sleep attacks after acute administration of apomorphine. *Mov Disord* 2000;15[Suppl]:P585
32. Ferreira JJ, Galitzky M, Montastruc JL, et al. Sleep attacks and Parkinson's disease treatment. *Lancet* 2000; 355:1333–1334.
33. Scharpira AHV. Sleep attacks (sleep episodes) with pergolide. *Lancet* 2000;355:1332.
34. Ebersbach G, Norden J, Tracik F. Sleep attacks in Parkinson's disease: polysomnographic recordings. *Mov Disord* 2000;15[Suppl 3]:S89.
35. Ferreira JJ, Thalamas C, Montastruc JL, et al. Levodopa monotherapy can induce "sleep attacks" in Parkinson's disease patients. *J Neurol* 2001;248:426–427.
36. Tracik F, Ebersbach G. Sudden daytime sleep onset in Parkinson's disease: polysomnographic recordings. *Mov Disord* 2001;16:500–506.
37. Etiman M, Samii A, Takkouche B, et al. Increased risk of somnolence with the new dopamine agonists in patients with Parkinson's disease: a meta-analysis of randomised controlled trials. *Drug Safety* 2001;24: 863–868.

Parkinson's Disease: Advances in Neurology, Vol. 91.
Edited by Ariel Gordin, Seppo Kaakkola,
and Heikki Teräväinen
Lippincott Williams & Wilkins, Philadelphia © 2003

22

Treatment of Advanced Parkinson's Disease: An Evidence-based Analysis

Christopher G. Goetz

*Department of Neurological Sciences and Department of Pharmacology,
Rush University/Rush-Presbyterian-St. Luke's Medical Center, Chicago, Illinois*

From a clinical perspective, patients with Parkinson's disease (PD) can be divided into three prototypical categories with mild, moderate, or severe impairment. In mild cases, research and clinical treatment efforts focus on concepts of neuroprotection and "levodopa sparing" (see Chapter 21). As the disease progresses and patients develop moderate disability, the usual treatment is levodopa (1). The hallmark of moderate PD is a stable response to medication without motor complications. The third category of patients are those with advanced disease, defined here as those with progressive motor impairment in spite of levodopa therapy and with an unstable medication response, leading to motor complications that include fluctuations and dyskinesias. In addition to progressive parkinsonism and motor complications, many of these patients also experience nonmotor complications including dysautonomia, depression, and hallucinations (2). This summary analyzes treatments applicable to patients with advanced PD already on levodopa. The two components of advanced PD, progressive parkinsonism and motor complications, are considered separately and then integrated. The methodology used is an evidence-based analysis, and the cited literature emphasizes results from randomized controlled trials, otherwise known as level I (3). Unless otherwise specified, only studies with at least 20 enrolled subjects that used standardized assessment measures and involved at least 4 weeks of therapy are considered (Table 22.1). This methodology allows different therapies to be evaluated with similar criteria. It places priority on the importance of randomization and controlled observations. Whereas nonrandomized controlled trials (level II) and open-label studies or case histories (level III) can offer other types of clinical information, the reliance on data from randomized controlled trials is particularly valuable to assessments of treatment efficacy. A comprehensive evidence-based medical review of treatment strategies for all phases of PD has been prepared by the Movement Disorders Society and is the core document on which this summary is based (4). Although the format of that work is different from that of this discussion and the final draft is still in preparation, the author has used the project's materials to provide herein his own conclusions. The following definitions are used: *efficacious* means that the body of evidence, including at least

TABLE 22.1. *Criteria used for evaluation of studies on efficacy of treatments*

- Randomized, controlled clinical trials
- Inclusion of only patients with advanced Parkinson's disease on levodopa/carbidopa or levodopa/benserazide
- At least 20 subjects
- At least 4 weeks of treatment
- Use of standardized tools for measuring the target behavior being assessed

one level I study with the criteria of Table 22.1 and with a control group receiving standard medical therapy for PD, permits a conclusion that the intervention is useful in managing the target behavior under consideration; *likely efficacious* means that the body of evidence consistently suggests efficacy but is not substantial enough to establish the treatment as efficacious; *insufficient* means that the body of data is inadequate or conflicting, so no conclusions can be offered. *Not likely efficacious* means that the body of evidence suggests that a given treatment is not effective in managing the target behavior under consideration. *Not efficacious* means that the body of evidence permits the conclusion that the intervention is not useful in managing the target behavior under consideration.

TREATMENT OF PRIMARY MOTOR SIGNS OF ADVANCED PARKINSON'S DISEASE

Several adjunctive treatments to levodopa are *efficacious* in managing the motor signs of progressive parkinsonism in patients with advanced PD taking levodopa (Table 22.2). These treatments include four dopamine (DA) agonists (bromocriptine, pergolide, cabergoline, and pramipexole) and entacapone. Standard levodopa was never tested against placebo in controlled trials. Because of its longstanding acceptance as a standard of efficacy in PD and its current use as part of the operative definition of advanced PD, standard levodopa is not specifically reviewed in this summary. Nonetheless, just as superiority to placebo is evidence of efficacy, equivalency to standard levodopa is considered strong support of effective treatment of PD. Based on such comparative trials, the long-acting levodopa formulation is also considered *efficacious* in advanced PD. Treatments that are likely *efficacious* include apomorphine, pallidotomy, and deep brain stimulation (DBS) of the pallidum or subthalamic nucleus (STN). Data on several other treatments listed in Table 22.2 are *insufficient* to draw conclusions.

Medications

Agonists

Bromocriptine

Several level I studies meeting the criteria in Table 22.1 have examined the efficacy of bromocriptine on parkinsonism in patients with advanced PD who are already being treated with levodopa. Four were placebo controlled, and six were active comparator trials using another DA agonist: cabergoline in one, pergolide in three, lisuride in one, and pramipexole in one. One study compared dif-

TABLE 22.2. *Efficacy data on agonists as treatment of primary motor aspects of advanced Parkinson's disease in levodopa-treated subjects*

	Efficacious	Likely efficacious	Insufficient data
Medications	Bromocriptine Pergolide Cabergoline Pramipexole Slow-release levodopa[a] Entacapone	Apomorphine	Lisuride Ropinirole Anticholinergics Amantadine Selegiline Tolcapone
Surgical treatments		Pallidotomy Pallidal DBS Subthalamic DBS	Thalamotomy Thalamic DBS Subthalamotomy Fetal transplantation

Note: DBS, deep brain stimulation.

[a]Conclusion based on equivalency between study drug and standard levodopa. Because of its longstanding acceptance as a standard of efficacy in Parkinson's disease and its current use is part of the operative definition of advanced Parkinson's disease, standard levodopa is not specifically reviewed in this summary.

fering regimens of bromocriptine titration and one study compared bromocriptine/levodopa therapy with tolcapone/levodopa. Whereas the focus of several of these studies was on motor fluctuations or dyskinesias, the design permitted clear assessment of changes in the primary signs of parkinsonism as well.

In the four placebo-controlled trials, bromocriptine doses ranged up to 100 mg per day, but the mean dose was approximately 20 mg per day (5–8). Parkinsonian scales varied but significantly improved in all four studies compared with placebo. In one, the levodopa dose was significantly reduced (5). In the study by Guttman (8), an additional arm included pramipexole treatment in association with levodopa. When added to levodopa, both drugs were superior to placebo. Motor impairment scores were slightly better in the subjects taking pramipexole, but no statistically significant differences between bromocriptine and pramipexole occurred. Adverse effects with bromocriptine included orthostatic dizziness, insomnia, nausea, and hallucinations. In a double-blind randomized comparison of a seven-step versus a three-step titration schedule of bromocriptine to 15 mg per day, both treatments significantly improved parkinsonian signs and had similar side effects (9). As a group, the studies comparing bromocriptine with other agonists support the placebo-controlled data, showing that when bromocriptine is added to levodopa, parkinsonism significantly improves compared with baseline function (10–14). The primary assessment tool in these studies was the Unified Parkinson's Disease Rating Scale (UPDRS). Bromocriptine was equivalent to the other agonists in some studies, although two found pergolide to be superior in abating parkinsonism (12,13). A final study compared bromocriptine with tolcapone and found equivalent UPDRS motor scores with the two treatments, both being superior to baseline function on levodopa alone (15). For side effects, bromocriptine, compared to tolcapone, induced more hallucinations (10% vs. 1%) and orthostatic hypotension (23% vs. 6%), but fewer muscle cramps (7% vs. 21%) and dystonia (1% vs. 14%). Dyskinesias were frequent with both drugs (bromocriptine, 38%; tolcapone, 51%). As a group, these many trials adequately establish that bromocriptine is *efficacious* as an adjunctive therapy to levodopa in patients with advanced PD.

Pergolide

Four studies (12,13,15,16) document pergolide efficacy in patients with advanced PD on levodopa therapy. In the only large level I randomized placebo-controlled study, Olanow et al. (16) documented that the total parkinsonism score significantly improved on pergolide compared with placebo. Further, the sample that improved at least 25% over their baseline scores was 56% on pergolide versus only 25% on placebo. Assessments of activities of daily living (ADL) also significantly improved on pergolide compared with placebo. Adverse reactions were more frequent with pergolide and, as with bromocriptine, included increased dyskinesias, nausea, hallucinations, dizziness, and sleep disruption. The other three studies compared pergolide with bromocriptine (11–13). They document significant improvement over baseline parkinsonism scores with pergolide treatment, and two studies showed superiority of pergolide over bromocriptine at the doses studied (see above) (12,13). This body of evidence adequately establishes that pergolide is *efficacious* as adjunctive therapy to levodopa in the treatment of parkinsonism among subjects with advanced disease.

Cabergoline

One placebo-controlled level I study examined cabergoline-related changes in the UPDRS motor and ADL subscales, as well as reductions in daily levodopa requirements (17). All measures improved on cabergoline, with both UPDRS subscale scores showing significant reductions. Autonomic nervous system side effects and behavioral complications were more frequent in the cabergoline group compared with the placebo-treated subjects. In a level I comparison study between cabergoline and bromocriptine (see above), comparable improvements in UPDRS ADL and motor scores occurred with both drugs and were strongly significant when compared with baseline function (10). Although the body of literature on cabergoline is smaller than that on bromocriptine or pergolide, the results are sufficient to conclude that cabergoline is *efficacious* as an adjunct to levodopa in treating the motor signs of advanced PD.

Pramipexole

Four level I studies, all placebo-controlled and one with an added bromocriptine arm, have established pramipexole efficacy as an adjunctive therapy to levodopa in patients with advanced PD. Lieberman et al. (18) led a large randomized parallel group comparison of 360 patients evaluated with UPDRS ratings in both "on" and "off" states. Using an average of the "on" and "off" ADL scores on the last visit, they documented a significant improvement with pramipexole compared with placebo. Levodopa daily requirements were also significantly reduced at study end compared with placebo treatment. Dyskinesias, orthostatic hypotension, and hallucinations, however, were more frequent among the pramipexole-treated subjects. A smaller study of 69 patients also used the UPDRS as the primary rating tool and found a significant improvement with pramipexole compared with placebo (19). Another study evaluated patients 2 hours after taking medication at study end and documented significant improvement on the UPDRS total scores in the pramipexole group compared with placebo-treated subjects (20). Most other subscales assessed also favored pramipexole over placebo in this adjunctive therapy study of levodopa-treated patients with advanced PD. The final study was designed as a three-arm evaluation of pramipexole, placebo, or bromocriptine addition to levodopa (8). Both bromocriptine (see above) and pramipexole treatment were significantly more effective than placebo in improving UPDRS scores, but between the two drugs, there were no statistically significant differences. Both agents also significantly improved several measures of quality of life. The cumulative data from these placebo-controlled trials using different, but complementary measurement tools, are sufficient to establish that pramipexole is *efficacious* in improving parkinsonian signs in patients with advanced PD.

Other Agonists

Studies of other agonists in levodopa-treated patients with advanced PD have not adequately evaluated changes in the primary elements of parkinsonism. Two level I studies of ropinirole exist, but their outcome measures were "amount of time spent off" (21) or reduction in levodopa dose with no specific regard to detailed reporting on parkinsonian motor scores (22). As such, there are *insufficient data* to conclude on ropinirole efficacy in controlling parkinsonism in patients with advanced disease. Apomorphine, a very short-acting agonist used predominantly in the treatment of motor complications (see below), has not been evaluated with long-duration level I studies, although one 4-day study with an open-label observation over several weeks and another open-label study documented improvements in UPDRS motor scores, Hoehn–Yahr stage, and levodopa requirements (23,24). Several open-label observations support these finding. These consistently positive data permit apomorphine to be classified as *likely efficacious.*

Slow-release Formulations of Levodopa

Historically, the introduction and universal acceptance of levodopa as a treatment for patients with severe motor impairments from PD preceded the standard use of placebo-controlled trials. Furthermore, because the operational definition of advanced PD in this analysis includes current treatment with levodopa, an evaluation of other formulations of levodopa cannot be made with placebo-controlled trials. Comparative trials of slow-release formulations, marketed as Sinemet-CR or Madopar-HBS, have used standard levodopa treatment as the control arm, and the primary focus has been on the amelioration of motor fluctuations (see below). Multiple level I studies in this category, however, monitored parkinsonism using the UPDRS or other standard scales during these trials. Uniformly, they reported equal efficacy on these measures with the two preparations (25–28). One study showed slow-release levodopa to be superior to standard levodopa efficacy in improving parkinsonian disability on the New York University Parkinson's Disease Scale (29). These studies are adequate to conclude that slow-release levodopa is *efficacious* in treating motor signs of parkinsonism in patients with advanced PD.

Other Medications

Amantadine

Two level I studies exist for amantadine, showing that it is *likely efficacious* as adjunctive therapy to levodopa in moderately advanced patients without motor complications. Amantadine, however, has not been specifically studied in patients with advanced PD. Therefore, data are *insufficient* to conclude on its efficacy in the patient population under discussion—that is, those with advanced motor impairment and motor fluctuations.

Catechol-O-Methyltransferase Inhibitors

Two agents are available: tolcapone and entacapone. In patients with advanced PD, tolcapone and entacapone are usually used in conjunction with levodopa to ameliorate motor fluctuations. Some studies, however, have included information on primary motor signs of parkinsonism when these drugs are used. For tolcapone, several level I studies evaluated patients with PD already on levodopa, although some did not concern subjects with advanced disease as defined in the introduction of this chapter. Of those reporting on advanced patients and monitoring drug-induced changes in parkinsonism using UPDRS scores (30–33), three showed no changes in UPDRS scores when tolcapone was added to levodopa. In one, a significant improvement occurred at doses of 600 mg per day, but not at 300 mg per day (33). The study comparing tolcapone with bromocriptine found equivalent improvements in UPDRS scores with both drugs (15). Because of the inconsistency of results, there are *insufficient data* to conclude on the efficacy of tolcapone to improve parkinsonism itself in patients with advanced PD. This drug is currently restricted in many countries because of concerns regarding liver toxicity.

Entacapone was studied in patients with advanced PD in two level I studies that focused primarily on motor fluctuations but assessed changes in parkinsonism using the UPDRS. Both studies showed significant improvement in motor impairment scores on entacapone (34,35). These studies permit a sound conclusion that entacapone is *efficacious* in improving motor signs of parkinsonism in levodopa-treated patients with advanced PD.

Selegiline

Level I studies have tested the utility of selegiline as adjunctive treatment to levodopa in patients with advanced PD. In two, based on objective measurement of parkinsonism, motor scores were unchanged by selegiline addition in one (36) and significantly improved in the other (37). The primary focus of all these studies was change in motor fluctuations (see below). Because of these inconsistent results, there are *insufficient data* to make conclusions on the efficacy of selegiline for the treatment of parkinsonian signs in advanced PD.

Anticholinergics

Several level I studies compared anticholinergic drugs with placebo treatment in patients with parkinsonism, but none focused specifically on levodopa-treated patients with advanced PD. Patient groups were mixed with mild, moderate, and advanced PD cases (38), included other diagnoses like postencephalitic parkinsonism (39), or were methodologically weak and without adequate statistical analysis (40). Nonrandomized level II studies suffered with the same problems for analysis. For these reasons, there are *insufficient data* to conclude on the use of anticholinergic drugs as adjunctive therapy to levodopa in patients with advanced PD.

Surgical Treatments

Pallidotomy

Although an extensive open-label literature exists on various neurosurgical interventions in patients with advanced PD, level I and level II (nonrandomized but controlled comparison) studies are very few. For pallidotomy, de Bie et al. (41) conducted a prospective, randomized single-blind study of 37 subjects who received either unilateral pallidotomy or best medical management. At 6 months, the primary outcome, "off" motor scores on the UPDRS, significantly improved, whereas that of the control group declined. UPDRS ADL measures and Schwab and England ratings significantly improved compared with control patients as well. The most marked effects occurred contralateral to the surgical side. Adverse effects occurred in approximately half the series, and the major ones were dysarthria and altered behavior. Other pallidotomy studies used medically managed comparison groups, but there was no randomization (level II). Perrine et al. (42) examined 28 patients preoperatively and after 1 year, comparing their results with those of 10 subjects who qualified for surgery but did not desire it. The UPDRS motor and ADL scores significantly improved postoperatively in the pallidotomy group, and there was no change in the control group. There was no distinction between "on" and "off" scores in this report. Young et al. (43) compared two different pallidotomy techniques, gamma-knife lesions in 29 patients, and radiofrequency lesions in 22 patients. Both groups improved in their parkinsonian scores compared with baseline, but at short- and long-term (mean, 20.6 months) evaluation, there were no differences between outcomes on UPDRS scores between the two groups (43). These studies, in association with the large volume of open-label observations and long-term follow-up experience, provide sufficient data to conclude that unilateral pallidotomy is *likely efficacious* in improving motor signs of PD, particularly on the contralateral side to the surgery. Side effects, however, are common and include intracerebral hemorrhage, speech impairment, behavioral aberrations, and visual disturbances. There are *insufficient data* to conclude on bilateral pallidotomies.

Other Surgeries

No other lesion or DBS intervention studies include a nonintervention comparison group, either by randomization (level I) or other methods of assignment (level II). Pallidal and subthalamic DBS, however, are *likely efficacious*. The thalamotomy literature includes multiple open-label series with reports of improvement in contralateral tremor, sometimes with improvement in bradykinesia and rigidity (44–46). A level I randomized comparison between thalamotomy and deep brain thalamic stimulation showed statistically equivalent improvement with the two surgeries and slightly better outcome with stimulation and fewer adverse effects (47). Other open-label observations on thalamic DBS, both unilateral and bilateral, report improvement in tremor located contralaterally to the stimulator (48,49). In one report, rigidity and akinesia significantly improved when the stimulator was turned on (50). Although encouraging, these results provide *insufficient data* to conclude on thalamotomy and thalamic DBS as treatments of parkinsonism in advanced PD.

Changes in parkinsonism after subthalamic DBS and pallidal stimulation have been documented in open-label observations and comparative trials with other surgical treatments, but no studies used a medically managed control group. Few of these comparative trials involved the minimal standard of 20 patients used in the criteria of Table 22.1. Burchiel et al. (51) conducted a blind randomized comparison of 10 patients, half assigned bilateral pallidal stimulation and half bilateral subthalamic stimulation. At 12 months after surgery when the stimulators were on, UPDRS scores were equivalent in the two groups. Most of the improvement was due to reduced rigidity in both groups. The patients with subthalamic stimulation, however, reduced their levodopa dose and two of these patients stopped levodopa altogether, whereas those with pallidal stimulation maintained their preoperative doses. Krause et al. (52) conducted a larger study of bilateral pallidal stimulations in 6 patients and bilateral subthalamic stimulation in 12 patients. Best Schwab and England scores 12 months after subthalamic stimulation surgery significantly improved compared with baseline values, whereas this measure did not significantly improve in those with pallidal stimulation. UPDRS scores improved with subthalamic stimulation, but not with pallidal stimulation. In yet another comparative study of pallidal stimulation versus subthalamic stimulation, UPDRS scores when the stimulator was turned on or off improved in both groups compared with baseline values (53).

The Deep Brain Stimulation for Parkinson's Disease Study Group (DBSPDSG) (54) conducted a 35-patient study with level I data on randomized, double-blind crossover assessments of the acute effects of pars interna pallidal stimulation 3 months after bilateral electrode placement. Open-label data comparing baseline values and 6 months of stimulation treatment were also included. The level I study tested acute changes in early morning function without medication when the stimulator was turned on for 2 hours compared with the stimulator being turned off. Subjects and raters were blind to the stimulator settings, and in all patients, both conditions (on→off and off→on) were tested. UPDRS scores with the stimulator on were significantly better than when it was turned off. In the open phase of follow-up, baseline to 6-month scores were compared in four conditions: no medication/stimulator off (no change over 6 months); with medication/stimulator off (no change); no medication/stimulator on (significant improvement compared with preoperative baseline); and with medication/stimulator on (significant improvement compared to preoperative baseline). For subthalamic stimulation, the same group examined 96 subjects with a similar acutely blinded assessment of stimulation and an open-label 6-month follow-up evaluation, showing the same pattern of efficacy seen with pallidal stimulation. The positive results with both pallidal and subthalamic stimulation warrant a designation of *likely efficacious*.

Although there are small series of open-label observations on subthalamotomies in subjects with advanced PD, there are *insufficient data* to permit an accurate assessment of efficacy in control of parkinsonism at the present time (55,56).

Implantation of fetal dopaminergic cells into the striatum of patients with advanced PD has been a controversial area of therapy research. Two level I studies with non-interventional arms of traditional medical therapy as the control group have been conducted. Spencer et al. (57) studied four patients who received cryopreserved fragments of fetal mesencephalic tissue into the right caudate nucleus and compared them 1 year later with three patients who were medically treated over the same period. UPDRS scores on and off medication, Hoehn–Yahr state, and Schwab and England evaluations were not different between the two groups. In a larger double-blind comparison of fetal transplantation versus medical management after a sham operation that involved a burr hole in the skull for the control group, 1 year after surgery, the patients 60 years or younger at the time of enrollment showed a significant improvement in "off" motor scores compared with controls. Among older patients, subjects with fetal transplants were not different from those who received medical management alone (58). In addition, troublesome dyskinesias that did not respond to levodopa reduction occurred in

15% of patients who received fetal transplants, suggesting aberrant reinnervation. A third level I study compared high-dose (three or more fetus transplants) with low-dose transplant and found significant improvement in both groups, with greater improvement among high-dose recipients (59). Although several open-label observations report strong efficacy of fetal transplants because of the small amount of level I data and inconsistent results, currently the data are *insufficient* to conclude on the efficacy of fetal transplantation as an adjunctive therapy to levodopa in patients with advanced PD. For transplantation with other cell sources (60), data are likewise *insufficient* to judge efficacy in treating parkinsonism in patients with advanced PD.

TREATMENT OF MOTOR COMPLICATIONS

Besides disabling parkinsonism, the other cardinal element of advanced PD is motor complications. Motor complications involve various disorders that are a consequence of advanced PD and levodopa therapy (1,2). The "wearing off" of medication effect near the end of each dose, sudden "off" periods in the midst of a medication cycle, and overmedication or undermedication effects such as dyskinesia and dystonia can all be features of motor complications. Because these problems occur throughout the day, physicians base most assessments of motor fluctuations on reports from patients, rather than objective observations. The measurement tools include diaries that patients complete throughout the day and summarize whether they are "on" with a good medication effect, "on" but with dyskinesias, or "off" with poor treatment response in spite of taking their medication. The UPDRS Part IV (UPDRS-IV) has several interview items that summarize stability of medication response to give a composite score that incorporates motor fluctuations, dyskinesias, and painful dystonia. Dyskinesia rating scales also exist for assessing severity, anatomical distribution, patient disability, and phenomenology of involuntary movements. This analysis, therefore, reexamines the studies discussed already, but with a focus specifically on each treatment's efficacy in reducing motor complications. Recognizing that motor complications include both motor fluctuations and dyskinesias, the author has considered a significant improvement in either as an index of efficacy. For each treatment deemed *efficacious,* whether the conclusion is based on improvement in only motor fluctuations, only dyskinesias, or both is indicated (Table 22.3). Using these methods, three agonists (pergolide, pramipexole, and ropinirole); two catechol-*O*-methyltransferase inhibitors (tolcapone and entacapone); and amantadine are *efficacious* in treating motor complications in advanced PD. Other agonists (bromocriptine,

TABLE 22.3. *Efficacy data: treatment of motor complications in levodopa-treated subjects with advanced Parkinson's disease*

	Efficacious	Likely efficacious	Insufficient data
Medications	Pergolide (MF) Pramipexole (MF) Ropinirole (MF) Entacapone (MF) Tolcapone (MF) Amantadine (D)	Bromocriptine (MF) Cabergoline (MF) Apomorphine (MF)	Selegiline Slow release levodopa Anticholinergics Lisuride
Surgical interventions			Pallidotomy Pallidal DBS Subthalamic DBS Thalamic DBS Thalamotomy Subthalamotomy Fetal transplantation

Note: D, dyskinesias; DBS, deep brain stimulation; MF, motor fluctuations.

cabergoline, and apomorphine) are *likely efficacious*. Data on the remaining treatments, including all surgical interventions, are *insufficient* to permit confident conclusions.

Agonists

Bromocriptine

Some placebo-controlled trials document that bromocriptine improves motor complications, including "wearing off," dystonia, and dyskinesia (5–7). In the Hoehn and Elton study (6), reduced "wearing off" occurred in 72% and reduced off-period dystonia occurred in 69% of bromocriptine-treated subjects compared with the placebo group in which no patients improved. Similar changes were documented by Toyokura et al. (7), but they were not statistically significant. These placebo-controlled trials complement a number of comparator trials with other agents used as adjunctive therapy to levodopa in patients with advanced PD. In these, bromocriptine improved motor fluctuations compared with baseline function and was equivalent to that seen with pergolide (11), lisuride (14), cabergoline (10), and tolcapone (15). The positive data are further tempered by a high-quality level I study by Guttman (8), in which bromocriptine did not significantly reduce the amount of time spent "off," as derived from diary cards. Because most, but not all, data support a positive effect, bromocriptine is *likely efficacious* in controlling motor fluctuations.

Pergolide

In the placebo-controlled level I trial conducted by Olanow et al. (16), a significant improvement in hours spent in the "off" phase occurred with pergolide. In the comparator study (11) with bromocriptine, both bromocriptine and pergolide significantly improved wearing off compared with baseline and the two drugs were equivalent. Based on the high-quality placebo-controlled data and absence of inconsistent results, pergolide can be considered *efficacious* in controlling motor complications, specifically motor fluctuations, in levodopa-treated patients with advanced PD.

Cabergoline

Two level I studies examined motor fluctuations in patients with advanced PD (10,17). Cabergoline treatment was associated with significantly less "off" time and significantly more "on" time compared with placebo, although no raw numbers were reported (17). In a comparator trial (10) between cabergoline and bromocriptine, both drugs caused significant improvement in "off" time compared with baseline function. Although these two studies are internally consistent because the placebo-controlled study was weak in reporting methods, the body of evidence permits the conclusion that cabergoline is *likely efficacious* in controlling motor complications.

Pramipexole

Four randomized double-blind level I studies qualified for review (8,18–20). Based on patient diary data, each showed an improvement in "off" time when pramipexole was added to levodopa. In the Guttman study (8), pramipexole significantly improved motor fluctuations compared with that seen with placebo and bromocriptine. In one study (20), dyskinesia ratings were also assessed, and there was no significant change with pramipexole. These studies permit the conclusion that pramipexole is *efficacious* in controlling motor complications, specifically motor fluctuations, in levodopa-treated patients with advanced PD.

Ropinirole

Two level I studies examined motor fluctuations using patient diaries that assessed time spent "off." In the Rascol et al. study (21), which used patient diaries, time spent "off" significantly decreased compared with baseline and end of placebo treatment. Likewise, in the Lieberman et al. study (22), compared with placebo-treated patients, ropinirole-treated subjects had a greater reduction in hours spent "off." The primary endpoint of this study was the number of patients who achieved a 20% or greater reduction in time "off" derived from patient diaries *and* reduced levodopa dose by at least 20%; a significantly greater number of subjects assigned ropinirole met the primary endpoint compared with placebo (35% vs. 13%, respectively; $p < .002$). These data permit the conclusion that ropinirole is *efficacious* in treating motor complications, specifically motor fluctuations. In both studies, dyskinesias increased with ropinirole, but no statistical analysis was provided.

Other Agonists

Apomorphine has primarily been studied for its effects on motor fluctuations, but no level I studies meeting the criteria in Table 22.1 exist for analysis. In a short-term level I evaluation involving 4 days of subcutaneous apomorphine and 4 days of placebo treatment in patients with severe fluctuations, Ostergaard et al. (23) evaluated motor fluctuations with onsite assessment of "on" and "off" periods and severity. Apomorphine significantly reduced both severity and duration of "off" periods. This short-term evaluation was followed by an open-label observation period (level III data) and supported the original observations (23). Several other level III clinical observational series document improved "off" function, both in reduced duration and in reduced severity, with apomorphine (24,61, 62). Apomorphine-induced effects on dyskinesia were variable. The body of data supports apomorphine as *likely efficacious* in controlling motor complications in levodopa-treated patients with advanced PD.

Other agonists have not been extensively studied for their effects on motor fluctuations. Lisuride has no level I placebo-controlled study, although in a comparator trial with bromocriptine, the investigators reported that fluctuations improved in both groups (14). Data are *insufficient* to judge on the efficacy of lisuride in the management of motor fluctuations.

Slow-release Levodopa

Because levodopa is considered important to the pathogenesis of motor complications (1), equivalency of slow-release levodopa to standard levodopa cannot be used as a measure of efficacy because it was with the evaluation of effects on parkinsonism. For testing efficacy of slow-release levodopa, the outcome of superiority to levodopa in substitution trials, however, can be used. The body of data comparing long-duration levodopa with standard formulation levodopa is large but does not give a clear outcome on differential effects on motor complications, either motor fluctuations or dyskinesias. Four show significant improvement with slow-release levodopa, measured as number of patients with improved "on" hours, UPDRS-IV scores, or number of "off" episodes each day (28,29,63, 64). In two, however, other measures of motor fluctuations, dyskinesia, or number of hours "off" showed no improvement or exacerbation (28,63). One study (1) showed a trend toward improvement with slow-release levodopa, but without statistical significance. Others showed no changes (25), and in the evaluation by Jankovic et al. (27), the patients assigned slow-release levodopa actually had more hours "off" and less time "on" without dyskinesias." The body of evidence, therefore, though large in the number of studies and patients enrolled, is *insufficient* to judge on the efficacy of slow-release levodopa in treating motor fluctuations in advanced PD.

Amantadine

The primary aspect of motor fluctuations examined with amantadine has been dyskinesias. Verhagen-Metman et al. (65) conducted a level I study that involved levodopa-treated patients with advanced PD who received either amantadine or placebo for 3 weeks. This study is shorter and had fewer subjects than the criteria outlined in Table 22.1 but is included because of the small number of studies available. On the testing day, patients were admitted to a research unit and received intravenous levodopa at a dose that produced an antiparkinsonian effect. At this dose, those on amantadine demonstrated significantly less dyskinesia than those on placebo treatment. Furthermore, the motor fluctuations, as derived from diary information, significantly improved. In long-term follow-up after chronic treatment with amantadine, the same challenge with intravenous levodopa was performed and those assigned amantadine continued to show reduced dyskinesias compared with the placebo group's scores from the beginning of the study (66). A similarly designed study by Snow et al. (67) of 24 subjects confirmed the same findings and showed reduced dyskinesias, as well as improvement in the UPDRS-IV, which assessed the combined intensity of dyskinesias and other components of motor fluctuations, including painful dystonia and end-of-dose "wearing off." A smaller study with 11 subjects showed that amantadine significantly improved dyskinesia (68). Because of consistent findings of efficacy in ameliorating dyskinesia and one study with adequate size, amantadine is considered *efficacious* as a treatment of motor complications, specifically dyskinesias.

Catechol-O-Methyltransferase Inhibitors

Both tolcapone and entacapone have been well studied for effects on motor fluctuations in levodopa-treated subjects with advanced PD. Five level I studies with placebo-treated control subjects document that tolcapone reduces motor fluctuations with reduced "off" time and/or enhanced "on" time (30–33,69). The usual assessment tool was patient diary, but in the Kurth et al. (69) study, patients were evaluated onsite for more than 10 hours. These well-designed studies and consistent results permit the conclusion that tolcapone is *efficacious* in improving motor complications, specifically fluctuations, in levodopa-treated subjects with advanced PD. Because dyskinesias, however, increased in several tolcapone-treated subjects, this conclusion on efficacy applies only to motor fluctuations.

Three level I studies of entacapone compared with placebo treatment studied motor fluctuations and consistently found significant improvements in "on" time derived from diaries (34,35,70). Based on these findings, entacapone is *efficacious* in improving motor complications, specifically motor fluctuations, in levodopa-treated subjects with advanced PD. Like the tolcapone data, dyskinesias increased with entacapone, so these findings apply to motor fluctuations and not the dyskinetic elements of motor fluctuations.

Selegiline

In the three level I studies that examined motor fluctuations, two showed modest positive results (36,71), although no statistical analysis was provided on diary information in the study by Lees et al. (36). The third study did not find a significant improvement in the number of hours spent "on" (37). Based on these results, data are *insufficient* to conclude on the use of selegiline in controlling motor fluctuations in advanced PD.

Anticholinergics

No studies with anticholinergics adequately evaluated motor fluctuations, so data are *insufficient* to evaluate the effect of anticholinergic drugs on motor complications.

Surgical Treatments

Pallidotomy

Of all results related to pallidotomy, the most consistent reported contribution has been the control of dyskinesias, particularly contralateral to the side of the lesion. However, postoperative medication changes, usually in the form of reduced levodopa doses, confound the interpretation of these studies of motor complications. In the level I study by de Bie et al. (41), the change score in dyskinesias significantly improved with pallidotomy. As an index of motor fluctuations, the amount of time spent "on without dyskinesias" significantly improved and "off" time diminished, although the latter change did not reach statistical significance. Several of the open-label level III observations strongly support this finding. Kondziolka et al. (72) found contralateral dyskinesia scores improved 9 months, with persistence of effects at 18 months in the 21 patients followed for that duration. In the report by Giller et al. (73) using a 0 to 3 severity rating system, they found dyskinesia abated at 2 weeks after surgery and remained improved. The scores were even more dramatic when only the contralateral dyskinesia ratings were considered. Shannon et al. (74) found similar improvements using the UPDRS-based dyskinesia ratings, finding significant improvements in both duration score and severity score. Using different assessment measures, including the UPDRS-IV, the Rush dyskinesia scale, and the Mayo dyskinesia scale, improved dyskinesias have been documented with consistency (75–77). Based on this body of evidence and the post-operative changes in medications, these data are encouraging but still are *insufficient* to conclude on the efficacy of pallidotomy in managing motor complications of advanced PD. Data are also *insufficient* to judge efficacy of bilateral pallidotomy.

For pallidal stimulation, the study by Burchiel et al. (51) examined effects of pallidal stimulation and STN stimulation on dyskinesias. The analysis was confounded by a significant reduction in daily levodopa doses in the subthalamic surgery group. At 12 months, the two groups were not different from each another, although both had improved in comparison to their baseline. In the pallidal stimulation group, the mean baseline dyskinesia score was 9.5 and, at 12 months, was 5.0 (not statistically significant), whereas the group receiving subthalamic stimulation changed significantly from a mean baseline score of 11.6 to 3.8 at 12 months. The 6-month follow-up portion of the DBSPDSG (54) assessed motor complications using diaries to capture on time without dyskinesias and also assessed dyskinesia severity. Significant improvement occurred in both indices when the stimulator was chronically used. Although results are encouraging, they include only a single level I study that lacked a medical control group and open-label evaluations; therefore, there is still *insufficient* evidence to conclude on efficacy of pallidal stimulation on motor complications of advanced PD. The subthalamic stimulation evidence for improvement in motor complications is based primarily on the study by Burchiel et al. (51) but is complimented by level III data, particularly that of the DBSPDSG. In the latter (54), diary rating for "on" time without dyskinesias, dyskinesia severity ratings, and medication doses significantly declined with chronic subthalamic stimulation. The study by Limousin et al. (50) monitored three motor complications of PD: painful dystonia, dyskinesias, and motor fluctuations. Among the 16 patients with painful `off" dystonia before surgery, all improved and 12 experienced full resolution. Levodopa-induced dyskinesias decreased, but the improvements did not reach statistical significant. The motor fluctuation assessment (item 39 from the UPDRS-IV) improved, changing from a mean score before surgery of 2.2 to 0.6 at 1 year. Based on this body of evidence, lack of a level I study with a medical control arm and lack of consistently significant improvement in dyskinesias, the data are *insufficient* to conclude on the efficacy of subthalamic DBS on motor complications of advanced PD.

For thalamotomy and thalamic DBS, as well as subthalamotomy, no level I studies focused on motor fluctuations, so the data are *insufficient* to judge the efficacy of thalamotomy, thalamic DBS, and subthalamotomy on motor complications in advanced PD.

For fetal transplantation, two level I studies showed no improvement in motor fluctuations (57,58). In the other level I study comparing high-dose to low-dose fetal transplantation, subjects assigned to high-dose treatment (three or more fetuses) had significantly less "off" time than the low-dose treatment group (59). Other open-label level III studies with multiple fetuses transplanted likewise reported improved "on" time and reduced "off" time (78,79). In terms of dyskinesia, results are also inconsistent. The study by Freed et al. (58) found choreodystonic dyskinesias in 15% of their sample of patients receiving transplants and cited these cases of exacerbated or new dyskinesias as a likely effect of surgery. This finding was not seen in other studies in which dyskinesia improved, both in severity and in duration (58). Because of these inconsistent findings, there are *insufficient data* to conclude on the effects of fetal transplantation on motor complications of advanced PD. Likewise, the data on other transplant cell sources are *insufficient* to judge efficacy in controlling motor complications in subjects with advanced PD (60).

INTEGRATION OF BOTH INDICES

The treating physician's final choice of agents to treat advanced PD must integrate efficacy data on both the parkinsonism and the motor complications of therapy and disease. In Table 22.4, the treatments that are *efficacious* for each category are designated. The four treatments that meet criteria for *efficacious* in the treatment of parkinsonism and motor complications in subjects with advanced PD are pergolide, pramipexole, and entacapone. No surgical procedure merits this designation.

These results are based on specific methods and analytical techniques. The outcomes depend not only on the actual results but also on the study designs that led to them. Because the science of clinical trial conduct is an evolving one, many of the treatments available are not able to be comprehensively evaluated because of the absence of appropriate data. This limitation is particularly problematic for treatments studied primarily before the 1980s when double-blind placebo-controlled trials were not regularly used. Contemporary high-quality standardized study designs offer the potential to test numerous putative therapies for PD with the same basic efficacy criteria. In this way, several future outcomes can be envisioned for understanding and prioritizing new treatments for patients with advanced PD. First, clinicians will be potentially able to identify more *efficacious* treatments with a clear delineation of the impairments that actually abate. Second, they will be able to identify treatments that are *not efficacious* and thereby can be avoided. Third, wherever data are *insufficient,* clinical researchers can develop additional protocols and thereby determine more definitive efficacy conclusions. Until such added trials are performed, treatments assigned to the limbo of *insufficient data* remain problematic but important to the contemporary clinician who can at least appreciate that data are weak or controversial. This equipoise is essential to incorporate into the final recommendations of practical treatment plans, particularly at a time when patients are increasingly proactive in the choice of their treatments.

TABLE 22.4. *Final integration of treatment of parkinsonism and motor complications*

Treatment	Efficacious parkinsonism	Efficacious motor fluctuations
Bromocriptine	+	
Pergolide	+	
Pramipexole	+	+
Ropinirole		+
Cabergoline	+	
Lisuride		
Apomorphine		
Slow release levodopa	+	
Tolcapone		+
Entacapone	+	+
Anticholinergics		
Amantadine		+
Selegiline		
Pallidotomy	+	+
Pallidal DBS		
Thalamotomy		
Thalamic DBS		
Subthalamotomy		
STN DBS		

DBS, deep brain stimulation; STN, subthalamic nucleus.

REFERENCES

1. Jankovic J, Toloso E, eds. *Parkinson's disease and movement disorders.* Baltimore: Williams & Wilkins, 1998.
2. Lang AE, Lozano AM. Parkinson's disease. *N Engl J Med* 1998;339:1044–1053,1130–1143.
3. Sackett DL, Straus S, Richardson S, et al, eds. *Evidence-based medicine: how to practice and teach EBM,* 2nd ed. Churchill Livingstone, 2000.
4. Goetz CG, Koller WC, Poewe W, et al. Management of Parkinson's disease: an evidence-based review. *Mov Disord* 2002 (in press) .
5. Kartzinel R, Teychenne P, Gillespie MM. Bromocriptine and levodopa (with or without carbidopa) in parkinsonism. *Lancet* 1976;2:272–275.
6. Hoehn MMM, Elton RL. Low dosages of bromocriptine added to levodopa in Parkinson's disease. *Neurology* 1985;35:199–206.
7. Toyokura Y, Mizuno Y, Kase M, et al. Effects of bromocriptine on parkinsonism. A nationwide collaborative double-blind study. *Acta Neurol Scand* 1985;72: 157–170.
8. Guttman M, and the International Pramipexole-Bromocriptine Study Group. Double-blind randomized, placebo-controlled study to compare safety, tolerance and efficacy of pramipexole and bromocriptine in advanced Parkinson's disease. *Neurology* 1997;49: 1060–1065.
9. MacMahon DG, Overstall PW, Marshall T. Simplification of the initiation of bromocriptine in elderly patients with advanced Parkinson's disease. *Age Aging* 1991;20: 146–151.
10. Inzelberg R, Nisipeaunu P, Rabey JM, et al. Double-blind comparison of cabergoline and bromocriptine in Parkinson's disease patients with motor fluctuations. *Neurology* 1996;47:785–788.
11. Mizuno Y, Kondo T, Narabayashi H. Pergolide in the treatment of Parkinson's disease. *Neurology* 1995; 45[Suppl 3]:S13–S21.
12. Pezzoli G, Martignoni E, Pacchetti C, et al. A crossover controlled study comparing pergolide with bromocriptine as an adjunct to levodopa for the treatment of Parkinson's disease. *Neurology* 1995;45[Suppl 3]: S22–S27.
13. Boas J, Worm-Petersen J, Dupont E, et al. The levodopa dose-sparing of pergolide compared with that of bromocriptine in an open-label, crossover study. *Eur J Neurol* 1996;3:44–49.
14. Laihinen A, Rinne UK, Suchy I. Comparison of lisuride and bromocriptine in the treatment of advanced Parkinson's disease. *Acta Neurol Scand* 1992;86:593–595.
15. The Tolcapone Study Group. Efficacy and tolerability of tolcapone compared with bromocriptine in levodopa-treated parkinsonian patients. *Mov Disord* 1999;14: 38–44.
16. Olanow CW, Fahn S, Muenter M, et al. A multicenter double-blind placebo-controlled trial of pergolide as an adjunct to Sinemet in Parkinson's disease. *Mov Disord* 1994;9:40–47.
17. Hutton JT, Koller WC, Ahlskog JE, et al. Multicenter, placebo-controlled trial of cabergoline taken once daily in the treatment of Parkinson's disease. *Neurology* 1996; 46:1062–1065.
18. Lieberman A, Ranhosky A, Korts D. Clinical evaluation of pramipexole in advanced Parkinson's disease: results of a double-blind, placebo-controlled, parallel group study. *Neurology* 1997;49:162–168.
19. Wermuth L, and the Danish Pramipexole Study Group. A double-blind, placebo-controlled, randomized, multicenter study of pramipexole in advanced Parkinson's disease. *Eur J Neurol* 1998;5:235–242.
20. Pinter MM, Pogarell O, Oertel WH. Efficacy, safety, and tolerance of the non-ergoline dopamine agonist pramipexole in the treatment of advanced Parkinson's disease: a double-blind, placebo-controlled, randomized, multicenter study. *J Neurol Neurosurg Psychiatry* 1999;66:436–441.
21. Rascol O, Lees AJ, Senard JM, et al. Ropinirole in the treatment of levodopa-induced motor fluctuations in patients with Parkinson's disease. *Clin Neuropharmacol* 1996;19:234–245.
22. Lieberman A, Olanow CW, Sethi K, et al, and the Ropinirole Study Group. A multicenter trial of ropinirole as adjunct treatment for Parkinson's disease. *Neurology* 1998;51:1057–1062.
23. Ostergaard L, Werdelin L, Odin P, et al. Pen injected apomorphine against off phenomena in late Parkinson's disease: a double-blind, placebo-controlled study. *J Neurol Neurosurg Psychiatry* 1995;58:681–687.
24. Pietz K, Hagell P, Odin P. Subcutaneous apomorphine in late state Parkinson's disease: a long-term follow-up. *J Neurol Neurosurg Psychiatry* 1998;65:709–716.
25. Feldman RG, Mosbach PA, Kelly MR, et al. Double-blind comparison of standard Sinemet and Sinemet CR in patients with mild to moderate Parkinson's disease. *Neurology* 1989;39:96–101.
26. Ahlskog JE, Muenter MD, McManis P, et al. Controlled-release Sinemet (CR-4): a double-blind crossover study in patients with fluctuating Parkinson's disease. *Mayo Clin Proc* 1988;63:876–886.
27. Jankovic J, Schwartz K, Vander Linden C. Comparison of Sinemet CR4 and standard Sinemet: double-blind and long-term open label trial in parkinsonian patients with fluctuations. *Mov Disord* 1989;4:303–309.
28. Lieberman A, Gopinathan G, Miller E, et al. Randomized double-blind crossover study of Sinemet-controlled release (CR4 50/200) versus Sinemet 25/100 in Parkinson's disease. *Eur Neurol* 1990;30:75–78.
29. Wolters EC, Tesselaar HJM, International (NL & UK) Sinemet CR Study Group. International (NL-UK) double-blind study of Sinemet CR and standard Sinemet (25/100) in 170 patients with fluctuating Parkinson's disease. *J Neurol* 1996;243:235–240.
30. Rajput AH, Martin W, Saint-Hilaire MH, et al. Tolcapone improves motor function in parkinsonian patients with the "wearing-off" phenomenon: a double-blind, placebo-controlled, multicenter trial. *Neurology* 1997;49:1066–1071.
31. Myllylä VV, Jackson M, Larsen JP, et al. Efficacy and safety of tolcapone in levodopa-treated Parkinson's disease patients with "wearing-off" phenomenon: a multicenter, double-blind, randomized, placebo-controlled trial. *Eur J Neurol* 1997;4:333–341.
32. Adler CH, Singer C, O'Brien C, et al. Tolcapone Fluctuators Study Group III. Randomized, placebo-controlled study of tolcapone in patients with fluctuating Parkinson disease treated with levodopa-carbidopa. *Arch Neurol* 1998;55(8):1089–1095.
33. Baas H, Beiske AG, Ghika J, et al. Catechol-*O*-methyl-

transferase inhibition with tolcapone reduces the "wearing off" phenomenon and levodopa requirements in fluctuating parkinsonian patients. *J Neurol Neurosurg Psychiatry* 1997;63:421–428.
34. Parkinson Study Group. Entacapone improves motor fluctuations in levodopa-treated Parkinson's disease patients. *Ann Neurol* 1997;42:747–755.
35. Rinne UK, Larsen JP, Siden A, et al, and the Nome-COMT Study Group. Entacapone enhances the response to levodopa in parkinsonian patients with motor fluctuations. *Neurology* 1998;51:1309–1314.
36. Lees AJ, Shaw KM, Kohout LJ. Deprenyl in Parkinson's disease. *Lancet* 1977;2:791–795.
37. Lieberman AN, Gopinathan G, Neophytides AN, et al. Deprenyl vs placebo in Parkinson's disease. *N Y State J Med* 1987;87:646–649.
38. Iivainen M. KR 339 in the treatment of parkinsonian tremor. *Acta Neurol Scand* 1974;50:469–470.
39. Parkes JD, Baxter RC, Marsden CD, et al. Comparative trial of benzhexol, amantadine, and levodopa in the treatment of Parkinson's disease. *J Neurol Neurosurg Psychiatry* 1974;37:422–426.
40. Martin WE, Loewenson RB, Resch JA, et al. A controlled study comparing trihexyphenidyl hydrochloride plus levodopa with placebo plus levodopa in patients with Parkinson's disease. *Neurology* 1974;24:912–919.
41. de Bie RM, de Haan RJ, Nijssen PC, et al. Unilateral pallidotomy in Parkinson's disease: a randomized, single-blind, multicenter trial. *Lancet* 1999;354(9191): 1665–1669.
42. Perrine K, Dogali M, Fazzini E, et al. Cognitive functioning after pallidotomy for refractory Parkinson's disease [see Comments]. *J Neurol Neurosurg Psychiatry* 1998;65:150–154.
43. Young RF, Vermeulen S, Posewitz A, et al. Pallidotomy with the gamma knife: a positive experience. *Stereotact Funct Neurosurg* 1998;70[Suppl 1]:218–228.
44. Duma CM, Jacques DB, Kopyov OV, et al. Gamma knife radiosurgery for thalamotomy in parkinsonian tremor: a five-year experience [see Comments]. *J Neurosurg* 1998;88:1044–1049.
45. Jankovic J, Cardoso F, Grossman RG, et al. Outcome after stereotactic thalamotomy for parkinsonian, essential, and other types of tremor. *Neurosurgery* 1995;37:680–686.
46. Giller CA, Dewey RB, Ginsburg MI, et al. Stereotactic pallidotomy and thalamotomy using individual variations of anatomic landmarks for localization. *Neurosurgery* 1998;42:56–65.
47. Schuurman PR, Bosch DA, Bossuyt PM, et al. A comparison of continuous thalamic stimulation and thalamotomy for suppression of severe tremor. *N Engl J Med* 2000;342(7):461–468.
48. Koller W, Pahwa R, Busenbark K, et al. High frequency unilateral thalamic stimulation in the treatment of essential and parkinsonian tremor. *Ann Neurol* 1997;42: 292–299.
49. Benabid AL, Pollak P, Gao DM, et al. Chronic electrical stimulation of the ventralis intermedius nucleus of the thalamus as a treatment of movement disorders. *J Neurosurg* 1996;84:203–214.
50. Limousin P, Krack P, Pollak P, et al. Electrical stimulation of the subthalamic nucleus in advanced Parkinson's disease. *N Engl J Med* 1998;339(16):1105–1111.
51. Burchiel KJ, Anderson VC, Favre J, et al. Comparison of pallidal and subthalamic nucleus deep brain stimulation for advanced Parkinson's disease: results of a randomized, blinded pilot study. *Neurosurgery* 1999;45(6): 1375–1382.
52. Krause M, Fogel W, Heck A, et al. Deep brain stimulation for the treatment of Parkinson's disease: subthalamic nucleus versus globus pallidus internus. *J Neurol Neurosurg Psychiatry* 2001;70(4):464–470.
53. Katayama Y, Kasai M, Oshima H, et al. Double-blind evaluation of the effects of pallidal and subthalamic nucleus stimulation of daytime activity in advanced Parkinson's disease. *Parkinsonism Related Disord* 2000; 7(1):35–40.
54. Deep Brain Stimulation for Parkinson's Disease Study Group (DBSPDSG). Deep brain stimulation of the subthalamic nucleus or the pars interna of the globus pallidus in Parkinson's disease. *N Engl J Med* 2001;345: 956–963.
55. Alvarez L, Macias R, Guridi J, et al. Dorsal subthalamotomy for Parkinson's disease. *Mov Disord* 2001;16(1): 72–78.
56. Barlas O, Hanağasi HA, Imer M, et al. Do unilateral ablative lesions of the subthalamic nucleus in parkinsonian patients lead to hemiballism? *Mov Disord* 2001;16: 306–310.
57. Spencer DD, Robbins RJ, Naftolin F, et al. Unilateral transplantation of human fetal mesencephalic tissue into the caudate nucleus of patients with Parkinson's disease. *N Engl J Med* 1992;327(22):1541–1558.
58. Freed CR, Breeze RE, Rosenbert NL, et al. Survival of implanted fetal dopamine cells and neurologic improvements 12 to 46 months after transplantation for Parkinson's disease. *N Engl J Med* 1992;327(22):1549–1555.
59. Kopyov OV, Jacques DS, Lieberman A, et al. Outcome following intrastriatal fetal mesencephalic grafts for Parkinson's patients is directly related to the volume of grafted tissue. *Exp Neurol* 1997;146:536–545.
60. Schumacher JM, Ellias SA, Palmer EP, et al. Transplantation of embryonic porcine mesencephalic tissue in patients with PD. *Neurology* 2000;54(5):1042–1050.
61. Hughes AJ, Bishop S, Kleedorfer B, et al. Subcutaneous apomorphine in Parkinson's disease: response to chronic administration for up to five years. *Mov Disord* 1993;8:165–170.
62. Colzi A, Turner K, Lees AJ. Continuous subcutaneous waking day apomorphine in the long-term treatment of levodopa-induced interdose dyskinesias in Parkinson's disease. *J Neurol Neurosurg Psychiatry* 1998;64:573–576.
63. Sage J, Mark M. Comparison of controlled release Sinemet (CR4) and standard Sinemet (25 mg/100 mg) in advanced Parkinson's disease: a double-blind, crossover study. *Clin Neuropharmacol* 1988;11:174–179.
64. Hutton JT, Morris JL, Bush DF, et al. Multicenter controlled study of Sinemet CR vs. Sinemet (25/100) in advanced Parkinson's disease. *Neurology* 1989;39:67–72.
65. Verhagen-Metman L, Del Dotto P, van den Munckhof P, et al. Amantadine as treatment for dyskinesias and motor fluctuations in Parkinson's disease. *Neurology* 1998; 50:1323–1326.
66. Verhagen-Metman L, Del Dotto P, LePoole K, et al. Amantadine for levodopa-induced dyskinesias. A 1-year follow-up study. *Arch Neurol* 1999;56:1383–1386.
67. Snow BJ, MacDonald L, Mcauley D, et al. The effect of amantadine on levodopa-induced dyskinesias in Parkinson's disease: a double-blind, placebo-controlled study. *Clin Neuropharmacol* 2000;23(2):82–85.

68. Luginger E, Wenning GK, Bosch S, et al. Beneficial effects of amantadine on L-dopa–induced dyskinesias in Parkinson's disease. *Mov Disord* 2000;15(5):873–878.
69. Kurth MC, Tetrud JW, Tanner CM, et al. Double-blind, placebo-controlled, crossover study of duodenal infusion of levodopa/carbidopa in Parkinson's disease patients with "on-off" fluctuations. *Neurology* 1993; 43:1698–1703.
70. Ruottinen HM, Rinne UK. Entacapone prolongs levodopa response in a one-month double-blind study in parkinsonian patients with levodopa related fluctuations. *J Neurol Neurosurg Psychiatry* 1996;60:36–40.
71. Golbe LI, Lieberman AN, Muenter MD, et al. Deprenyl in the treatment of symptom fluctuations in advanced Parkinson's disease. *Clin Neuropharmacol* 1988;11: 45–55.
72. Kondziolka D, Bonaroti E, Baser S, et al. Outcomes after stereotactically guided pallidotomy for advanced Parkinson's disease. *J Neurosurg* 1999;90:197–202.
73. Giller CA, Dewey RB, Ginsburg MI, et al. Stereotactic pallidotomy and thalamotomy using individual variations of anatomic landmarks for localization. *Neurosurgery* 1998;42:56–65.
74. Shannon KM, Penn RD, Kroin JS, et al. Stereotactic pallidotomy for the treatment of Parkinson's disease: efficacy and adverse effects at 6-months in 26 patients. *Neurology* 1998;50:434–438.
75. Lang AE, LozanoAM, Montgomery E, et al. Posteroventral medial pallidotomy in advanced Parkinson's disease. *N Engl J Med* 1997;337:1036–1042.
76. Krauss JK, Desaloms JM, Lai EC, et al. Microelectrode-guided posteroventral pallidotomy for treatment of Parkinson's disease: postoperative magnetic resonance imaging analysis [see Comments]. *J Neurosurg* 1997;87:358–367.
77. Kishore A, Turnbull IM, Snow BJ, et al. Efficacy, stability and predictors of outcome of pallidotomy for Parkinson's disease: 6-month follow-up with additional 1-year observations. *Brain* 1997;120:729–737.
78. Hauser RA, Freeman TB, Snow BJ, et al. Long-term evaluation of bilateral fetal nigral transplantation in Parkinson's disease. *Arch Neurol* 1999;56:179–187.
79. Freeman TB, Olanow CW, Hauser RA, et al. Bilateral fetal nigral transplantation into the post-commissural putamen in Parkinson's disease. *Ann Neurol* 1995; 38(3):379–388.

Parkinson's Disease: Advances in Neurology, Vol. 91.
Edited by Ariel Gordin, Seppo Kaakkola,
and Heikki Teräväinen
Lippincott Williams & Wilkins, Philadelphia © 2003

23

Strategies to Modify Levodopa Treatment

Håkan Widner

Department of Clinical Neurosciences, Wallenberg Neuroscience Center, Lund University Hospital, Lund, Sweden

It has been almost five decades, and a Nobel Prize later since Arvid Carlsson demonstrated that levodopa could become an effective treatment of basal ganglia disorders and that dopamine (DA) was critically involved for symptoms related to DA depletion in reserpine-treated rabbits (1). The metabolic pathways (Fig. 23.1) for the catecholamines had been worked out at about the same time, defining the enzymes, the metabolic steps, and the sequential order of synthesis of the catechols, which was awarded with a Nobel Prize to Julius Axelrod (2). The demonstration of profound defects of catecholamines in the brain of parkinsonian patients confirmed the animal predictions of DA being critically important for the symptoms of parkinsonism (3). The logical treatment with levodopa was soon initiated, with brief improvements demonstrated by single levodopa injections (4,5). However, for lasting antiparkinsonian effects, oral treatment turned out to be difficult to maintain, although dramatic improvements could be achieved. The development of various treatment-related side effects and the shear amount of levodopa needed to be taken—5 to 10 g—limited the wider use of this treatment. Cotzias et al. (6) experimented with peripherally acting, but without any action within the brain, aromatic amino acid decarboxylase (or dopa decarboxylase [DDC]) inhibitors such as α-methyldopa, and Papavasiliou et al. (7) demonstrated marked antiparkinsonian effects with drastically lowered dosages. Clinically more relevant inhibitors were discovered, and the combination treatment with a peripherally acting DDC inhibitor and levodopa became the established mode of administering levodopa (8). To this day, levodopa is considered the most effective antiparkinsonian medication (9). The objective of this chapter is to review some aspects on how to optimize levodopa therapy.

ADDITIONAL PLAYERS IN THE LEVODOPA METABOLISM

There are several factors that are involved in the pharmacokinetics of levodopa, both peripherally and centrally acting. The rate-limiting biological structures are the large neutral amino acid (LNAA) transporter, which is located in the intestinal mucosa and in the blood–brain barrier (BBB). The degrading enzymes, DDC, catechol-*O*-methyltransferase (COMT), and monoamine oxidases (MAOs) in the gastrointestinal (GI) tract, and the time for the drug spent in various compartments of the GI tract, for example, in the ventricle or small intestine. Within the central dopaminergic synapse compartment, the DA transporter (DAT) is also of importance for the regulation of levodopa and DA concentrations, in addition to the degrading enzymes. Additional factors that often interfere with the physical absorption of levodopa include delayed gas-

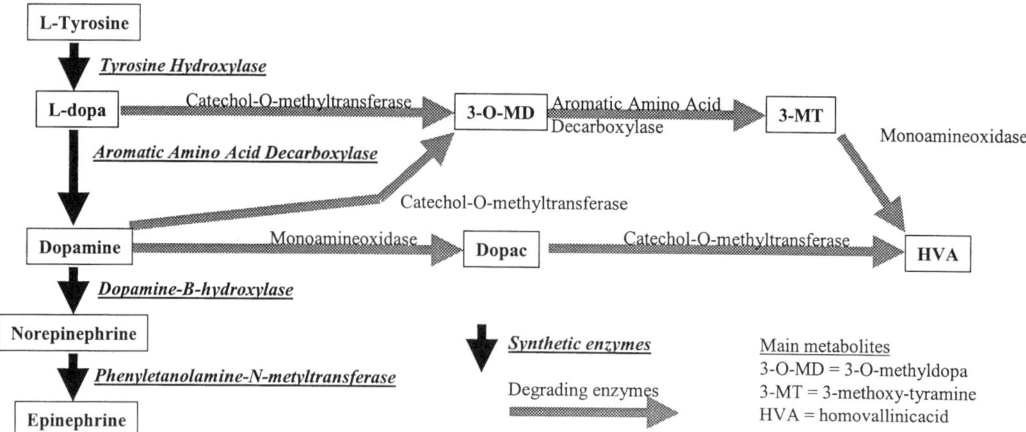

FIGURE 23.1. Chart of some of the steps in catecholamine metabolism.

tric emptying, acidity of the gastric juices, intestinal transportation and metabolism, food intake, physical interaction of absorption with other drugs, peripheral metabolism, BBB transport, and reuptake of DA.

SYMPTOMS AND FINE-TUNING OF LEVODOPA EFFECTS

The conventional description of levodopa effects early in the course of Parkinson's disease (PD) is that all symptoms should improve by the levodopa treatment. However, there are several phases of treatment effects that may be experienced by the astutely observant patient. The first symptoms of parkinsonism may be transient and occur after, for example, an acute illness or various efforts. There is usually good recovery after these symptoms, and the patient usually seeks no medical attention.

During this period of parkinsonism, there is a reduction in DA synthesis and storage capacity, but there is an increased turnover of levodopa and DA and often an upregulation of tyrosine hydroxylase (TH) enzymatic activity, best described in animal models of DA depletion (10). Symptoms of parkinsonism are usually restricted to an anatomical compartment such as a limb, and DA depletion in the terminals in the putamen is further evident by compensatory mechanisms in the neuronal circuits of the basal ganglia, which are somatotopically organized. When levodopa treatment is initiated, there is most often an initial improvement of hypokinesia and rigidity, lasting for several days to weeks, but many patients experience a period of transient deterioration after this initial period. If treatment is continued, most commonly a second phase of improvement occurs, which is sustained. This early course of variability in levodopa effects could be explained by a reduction of TH overactivity and a reduced abnormally high DA turnover rate within the remaining dopaminergic terminals in the regions affected by the disease process. Once the TH levels have been normalized, and the compensatory increased DA turnover rate is reduced, the storage of DA may be more efficient, and a sustained beneficial effect of levodopa may be achieved. As this phase is fulfilled, patients most typically have a very good antiparkinsonism effect of the treatment and can readily eliminate a single dose or multiple doses without reappearance of symptoms of PD. This pattern of responses may be seen regardless of whether a patient is started on levodopa directly or initially started treatment with a DA agonist, followed by levodopa for improvement of the beneficial effects.

INCOMPLETE SYMPTOMATIC RELIEF

Due to the peripheral metabolism and losses along the pathway to the brain and the synaptic storage site for DA, too small a dose of levodopa may be insufficient to result in any functional benefit and may incompletely restore the DA transmission. It is estimated that of a dose of levodopa, taken alone without a DDC inhibitor or other inhibitors of degrading enzymes, only about 1% of levodopa reaches the brain, and this increases to 10% with the addition of a DDC inhibitor (11).

In this case, it is logical to increase the dose of levodopa or to add drugs that could augment the symptomatic effect, either an MAO inhibitor or a DA agonist.

EARLY REAPPEARANCE OF SYMPTOMS

However, as a consequence of the progressive degeneration of the presynaptic dopaminergic terminals, which result in a declining rate of levodopa conversion to endogenous DA and a diminished storage capacity of DA, symptoms of parkinsonism may reappear during parts of day, and the buffering capacity is gradually lost. This is usually first manifested as reappearance of symptoms when the longest time has elapsed from the last drug intake. This may be in the evening or in the late night, commonly manifested as early morning dystonia. Logical treatment options are addition of bedtime medication with a controlled-release (CR) levodopa formulation, and to optimize the duration of this medication, it could be combined with a COMT inhibitor. The initial dose of the CR levodopa could be kept low, and the reduced bioavailability of CR levodopa preparations, due to the prolonged GI tract passage time and the increased time for GI tract metabolism, may be optimized. Longer acting DA agonists may also be beneficial in reducing the nighttime symptoms, although the choice of which treatment to use has not been established in any controlled study. The current treatment recommendation trend to avoid introduction of levodopa treatment as much as possible could, in part, be circumvented by adding a bedtime levodopa/COMT inhibitor medication to replenish the dopaminergic compartment more effectively than by DA agonist monotherapy; this kind of combined treatment may be a gentle way to introduce levodopa. Late evening or early morning dystonia often heralds the advent of additional symptoms of reduced levodopa effects, which may occur before daytime levodopa doses wear off.

DELAYED "ON," MISSED ABSORPTION, AND PHYSICAL DRUG INTERACTIONS

If a patient progresses to the stage in which symptoms may reappear if multiple drugs or a single drug is missed, and if the reappearance of symptoms is not simply a matter of time from last drug intake, the patient should be analyzed for potential factors that may interfere with drug effects. A very commonly appearing problem is delayed "on." This could be due to several factors, and if appearing suddenly after additional medication has been prescribed, drug interactions may be suspected. Chelate formation with oral iron treatment or sometimes aluminum/magnesium-containing antacids may drastically reduce the levodopa bioavailability, as may pyridoxine (vitamin B_6), and certain anti-hypercholesterolemia drugs. Inflammatory cytokines can be suspected to interfere with the drug effects, because it is commonly observed that slight infections and febrile periods result in transient worsening of symptoms; however, there is no firm evidence for any direct link and action with any particular cytokine, and there is no biological function such as interference with the LNAA transport capacity. When closely analyzing the drug intake and subsequent drug effects, Nutt et al. (12) reported that 20% to 30% of all levodopa drugs taken may not result in a beneficial antiparkinsonism effect. Delayed gastric emptying is an important factor that can often be eliminated by instructing the patient to take the medication in sufficient time before meals. Occasionally, the problem remains in spite of separation of medication and meals, and it might be beneficial to reduce any fat intake in relation to medication, but more importantly to eliminate any anticholinergic drugs that slow down the emptying of the stomach, as do high acidity and high doses of levodopa itself and other biogenic amines. The individual dose of levodopa may be important. In this case, addition of domperidone (Motilium) may be beneficial. To reduce hyperacidity, one should avoid buffering drugs and use antihistamines or hydrogen ion pump inhibitors. Lack of drug effects may also be a consequence of interference at the GI tract absorption, particularly when the LNAA transport capacity is overwhelmed (12,13). A meal or drink rich in proteins may severely interfere with the absorption of an oral dose of levodopa, virtually eliminating any plasma effects. In addition, high levels of circulating LNAA in the blood also interfere with the passage of levodopa into the brain, which has been quantified using positron emission tomography (14). As a potential treatment, subcutaneous injection of levodopa methyl ester has been suggested, but the drug is not available (15).

LEVODOPA AND DOPAMINE METABOLITES

Levodopa, given with a DDC inhibitor, results in the production of large amounts of a levodopa metabolite in the periphery, 3-*O*-methyldopa (3-OMD), through the peripheral action of COMT. The biological half-life of this metabolite, which has no biological function, is 15 to 18 hours, compared with the half-life of levodopa of about 60 to 90 minutes. For every levodopa dose given, 3-OMD is increased. Whether this results in accumulated concentrations of 3-OMD is still unknown, but one might presume that this is the case. It has been difficult to correlate 3-OMD as a sole contributor to the development of dyskinesias, but it can certainly contribute to reduced levels of absorption. The failure of CR levodopa preparations to reduce the development of dyskinesias has been puzzling (15–19). The reduced bioavailability and increased 3-OMD production in CR levodopa plus DDC inhibitor formulas may contribute to variations in effective drug concentrations, and thus contribute to pulsatile levodopa effects in spite of the CR function. COMT inhibitors in combination with CR levodopa may be an option to obtain constant blood levels and to reduce the developments of dyskinesias, but there are no studies with any data to demonstrate this.

WEARING OFF

Wearing off of beneficial drug effects is usually defined as a reduced time of action of a given drug, and sometimes a time limit, at least for levodopa, of 4 hours is used. The underlying mechanism is probably mainly related to the reduced number of dopaminergic nerve terminals in the basal ganglia, resulting in reduced storage capacity of DA and an immediate dependency for and DA to be formed, a sufficiently high level of levodopa available. The reappearance of symptoms often occurs after exercise and efforts of various kinds, and symptoms appear in the dominant extremity but are more pronounced than at the beginning of the disease. Water-soluble levodopa, which has a more rapid time of onset, is often prescribed and may be highly efficacious to bridge a temporary lack of levodopa. However, short-acting levodopa effects may precipitate dyskinesias, so this remedy may well be a treatment that causes additional difficulties and should be regarded as an emergency treatment only. The same argument is valid for injection of subcutaneous levodopa ester and for intermittent apomorphine injections. When a pattern of wearing off has been established, and the analysis does not reveal any absorption difficulty or simple drug interference, additional treatment should be initiated.

If a patient is treated with levodopa plus selegiline, it is logical to add a COMT inhibitor to continue the treatment principle of levodopa treatment and try to optimize it. Several controlled studies demonstrate that the strategy of adding a COMT inhibitor is successful (20–23). There are two phases of COMT inhibition. One is immediate and reflects the prolongation of the levodopa effect by reducing the elimination and the increased area under the curve of levodopa. The other phase, which may be observed after a period of treatment, is manifested as a smoothing of the levodopa effects and may reflect the elimination of 3-OMD.

The demands for safety with a drug such as a COMT inhibitor are high because it has no endogenous antiparkinsonism effect itself and acts only to optimize the use and pharmacokinetics of levodopa. Complete lack of COMT enzymatic activity is compatible with a completely normal life span in knockout mice and an apparent normal development (24). However, because COMT inhibitors are adjuncts, the safety margins are more narrow than those for other types of drugs, which, in part, explains why tolcapone was withdrawn from the European market after hepatotoxic events were described (25). There are no indications that there is a class effect for this to appear, and the safety monitoring of entacapone has been favorable.

If a patient is treated with a DA agonist and starts to experience wearing-off symptoms or lack of efficiency, it is logical to add either selegiline or levodopa. Because the patient is not a *de novo* patient and receives levodopa for the first time, it is highly advantageous to initiate levodopa treatment with a COMT inhibitor, to optimize the pharmacokinetics right from the start.

DRUG-INDUCED ABNORMAL INVOLUNTARY MOVEMENTS, DYSKINESIAS

As a consequence of both dopaminergic denervation and the reduced uptake of levodopa in the striatum, which result in very high concentrations of levodopa in the extracellular space, oral levodopa treatment with time results in a very pulsatile stimulation of the receptors. The loss of terminals also leads to the loss of the CR of DA and reduces neuronal conversion of levodopa to DA in favor or conversion by glial cells and nondopaminergic neurons, which further compound the injury of a pulsatile stimulation pattern and delivery of levodopa to the brain. This may result in abnormal involuntary movements and symptoms of dyskinesias (15,16). It is likely that post-DA receptor changes and translation events in the GABAergic projection neurons contribute to the development and manifested primed state of dyskinesias (27). Conversion of a pulsatile receptor stimulation, either with levodopa or with DA agonists, can reduce the development and the degree of dyskinesias. The extent to which levodopa metabolites, such as 3-OMD and 3-*O*-methyltyrosine (3-*O*-MT), contribute to bioavailability and passage of levodopa across the BBB and the development of dyskinesias is not known, but it is likely to be minor.

Strategies to convert a pulsatile levodopa stimulation to a more stable type include adding a COMT inhibitor or an MAO-B inhibitor, reducing levodopa dose by shorter intervals, and using various forms of infusions. Combining levodopa with a COMT inhibitor and then longer acting DA agonists is possible, as well as adding amantadine. Sipping of small amounts of soluble levodopa may be a simple approach to achieve this but requires a diligent patient (28). Further, invasive treatments such as subcutaneous or intravenous treatment with levodopa ester or GI tract infusion of, say, soluble levodopa or more concentrated forms in cellulose preparations (Duodopa) may all be very effective for reducing dyskinesias (29) but are costly and require very committed patients.

There are no controlled studies to demonstrate the superiority of any strategy, and no such study is likely to be initiated due to the complexity of the treatments.

CONCLUSIONS

There are several strategies to modify the peripheral and central pharmacokinetics of levodopa in all phases of the disease and treatment. The suggestions and principle pathways are outlined in Figures. 23.2 and 23.3.

Trouble shooting - Levodopa treatment

Wearing off or no on / lack of drug effect

Gastric emtying difficulites

Consider this when
long delay in response to drug intake
"indigestion" discomfort
high L-dopa dose

Try:
Reduce individual L-dopa dose
Add domperidon (10 - 30 mg/intake)
Reduce hyperacidity
Eliminate anticholinergics
Reduce food intake at time point (reduce fat)
Add COMT-I
In extreme cases consider PEG
for Duodopa infusion in jejunum

Missed absorption

Consider this when
No effect of drug taken
Long delay in response to drug intake
High L-dopa dose, variable effects
Food intake in last 30-120 minutes
Recently added medication

Try:
Drug interaction
reduce oral iron medication
reduce vitamine B6 (pyridoxine)
reduce buffering antacids
Take L-dopa 15 - 30 min. prior to meal
Reduce protein content in food
Add COMT-I to reduce 3-OMD
Future treatment ?
L-dopa methylester injection s.c.

Wearing off

Consider this when
Drug duration less than 4 hours
First sign often after exercise
Commonly manifested as late night dystonia

Try:
Add soluable L-dopa for short time relief
When pattern established:
at bed time add L-dopa CR (with
or without COMT-I)
If on L-dopa only
add COMT-I, selegeline or
dopamine agonist
If on dopamine agonist only
add L-dopa and COMT-I from start

FIGURE 23.2. Troubleshooting scheme for various situations in which failure of a levodopa dose may occur, manifested as lack of drug effect (previously established and regular drug effect) and apparent wearing off and actual wearing off.

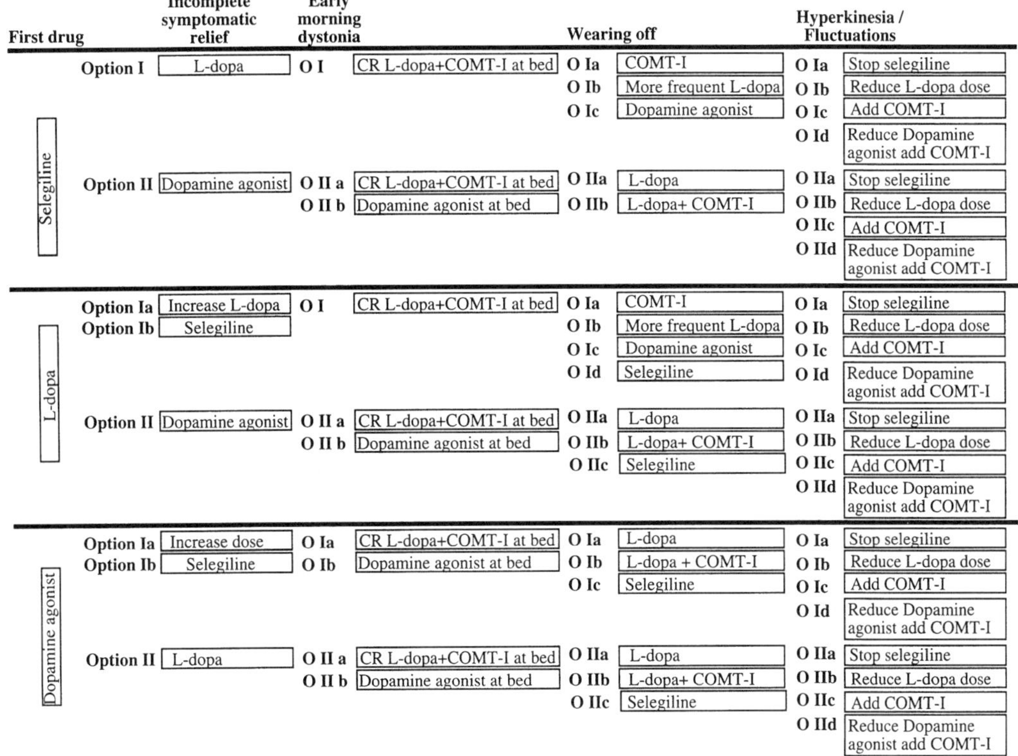

FIGURE 23.3. Various treatment options for symptoms appearing while on treatment. Columns indicate the type of difficulty or new symptoms, and rows indicate, the type of medical treatments the patient is taking on a sequential order. The first medication is either selegiline, levodopa, or dopamine agonist, and dose changes or additions are added sequentially further to the right in the columns. The various options are listed I-II, with subsequent subheading I a-c, etc. The treatment options can be followed throughout, along with the various additional and increasing complications, and are logically connected. Which option to choose depends on individual factors, drug interactions, concomitant diseases, among others.

REFERENCES

1. Carlsson A, Lindquist M, Magnusson T. 3,4-Dihydroxyphenylalanine and 6-hydroxytryptophan as reserpine antagonists. *Nature* 1957;180:1200–1201.
2. Axelrod J, Tomchick R. Enzymatic *O*-methylation of epinephrine and other catechols. *J Biol Chem* 1958;233: 702–705.
3. Ehringer H, Hornykiewicz O. Distribution of noradrenaline and dopamine (3-hydroxytyramine) in the human brain and their behaviour in diseases of the extrapyramidal system. *Wien Klin Wochenschr* 1960;38: 1236–1239.
4. Birkmayer W, Hornykiewicz O. Der L-3,4-dioxyphenylalanine (DOPA) effect beim der Parkinson-Akinese. *Wien Klin Wochenschr* 1961;73:787–788.
5. Barbeau A. L-dopa therapy in Parkinson's disease: a critical review of 9 years' experience. *Can Med Assoc J* 1969;101:791–800.
6. Cotzias GC, Van Woert MH, Schiffer LM. Aromatic amino acids and modification of parkinsonism. *N Engl J Med* 1967;276:374–379.
7. Papavasiliou PS, Cotzias GC, Duby S, et al. Levodopa in parkinsonism: potentiation of central effects with a peripheral inhibitor. *N Engl J Med* 1972;285:814.
8. Buckard WP, Gey KF, Pletscher A. A new inhibitor of decarboxylase of aromatic amino acids. *Experientia* 1962;18:411.
9. Agid Y, Ahlskog E, Albanese A, et al. Levodopa in the treatment of Parkinson's disease: a consensus meeting. *Mov Disord* 1999;16:911–913.
10. Zigmond MJ. Do compensatory process underlie the preclinical phase of neurodegenerative disease? Insights from an animal model of parkinsonism. *Neurobiol Dis* 1997;4:247–253.
11. Nutt JG, Fellman JH. Pharmacokinetics of levodopa. *Clin Neuropharmacol* 1984;7:35–49.
12. Nutt JG, Woodward WR, Hammerstad JP, et al. The

"on-off" phenomenon in Parkinson's disease. Relation to levodopa absorption and transport *N Engl J Med* 1984;310:438–488.

13. Wade DN, Mearrick PT, Morris J. Active transport of L-dopa in the intestine. *Nature* 1973;242:463–465.
14. Leenders KL, Poewe WH, Palmer AJ, et al. Inhibition of I-(^{18}F) fluorodopa uptake into human brain by amino acids demonstrated by positron emission tomography. *Ann Neurol* 1986;20:258–262.
15. Nutt JG, Obeso JA, Stocchi F. Continuous dopamine-receptor stimulation in advanced Parkinson's disease. *Trends Neurosci* 2000;23:S109–S115.
16. Olanow CW, Schapira AHV, Rascol O. Continuous dopamine-receptor stimulation in early Parkinson's disease. *Trends Neurosci* 2000;23:S1117–S1126.
17. Koller WC, Hutton JT, Tolosa E, et al, and the Carbidopa/Levodopa Study Group. Immediate release and controlled-release carbidopa/levodopa in PD: a 5 year randomized multi-center study. *Neurology* 1999;53: 1012–1019.
18. Block G, Liss C, Reines S, et al. Comparison of immediate-release and controlled-release of carbidopa/levodopa in Parkinson's disease: a multi-center 5-year study. *Eur J Neurol* 1997;37:23–27.
19. Dupont E, Andersen A, Boas J, et al. Sustained-release Madopar HBS compared with standard Madopar in the long-term treatment of *de novo* parkinsonian patients. *Acta Neurol Scand* 1996;93:14–20.
20. Nutt JG, Woodward WR, Beckner RM, et al. Effect of peripheral catechol-*O*-methyltransferase (COMT) inhibition on the pharmacokinetics of levodopa in parkinsonian patients. *Neurology* 1994;44:913–919.
21. Parkinson Study Group. Entacapone improves motor fluctuations in levodopa treated Parkinson's disease patients. *Ann Neurol* 1997;42:747–755.
22. Rinne UK, Larsen JP, Siden Å, et al, and the NOMECOMT Study Group. Entacapone enhances the responses to levodopa in parkinsonian patients with motor fluctuations *Neurology* 1998;51:1309–1314.
23. Männistö PT, Kaakkola S. Catechol-*O*-methyltransferase (COMT): biochemistry, molecular biology, pharmacology and clinical efficacy of the new selective COMT inhibitors. *Pharmacol Rev* 1999;51:593–628.
24. Gogos JA, Morgan M, Luine V, et al. Catechol-*O*-methyltransferase–deficient mice exhibit sexually dimorphic changes in catecholamine levels and behavior. *Proc Natl Acad Sci USA* 1998;18:9991–9996.
25. Assal F, Spahr L, Hadengue A, et al. Tolcapone and fulminant hepatitis. *Lancet* 1998;352:958.
26. Andersson M, Hibertsson A, Cenci MA. Striatal *fos*B expression is causally linked with L-dopa–induced abnormal involuntary movements and the associated upregulation of striatal prodynorphin mRNA in a rat model of Parkinson's disease. *Neurobiol Dis* 1999;6:461–474.
27. Pappert EJ, Goetz CG, Niederman F, et al. Liquid levodopa/carbidopa produces significant improvement in motor fluctuations without dyskinesia exacerbation. *Neurology* 1996;47:1493–1495.
28. Bredberg E, Nilsson D, Johansson K, et al. Intraduodenal infusion of water-based levodopa dispersion for optimisation of the therapeutic effect in severe Parkinson's disease. *Eur J Clin Pharmacol* 1993;45:117–122.
29. Roberts J, Waller DG, O'Shea N, et al. The effects of selegiline on the peripheral pharmacokinetics of levodopa in young volunteers. *Br J Clin Pharmacol* 1995;40: 404–406.

Parkinson's Disease: Advances in Neurology, Vol. 91.
Edited by Ariel Gordin, Seppo Kaakkola, and Heikki Teräväinen
Lippincott Williams & Wilkins, Philadelphia © 2003

24

Position of COMT Inhibition in the Treatment of Parkinson's Disease

*Ariel Gordin, †Seppo Kaakkola, and †Heikki Teräväinen

**Research Centre, Orion Pharma, Espoo, Finland; and †Department of Neurology, University of Helsinki, Helsinki, Finland*

Even if levodopa is the most effective symptomatic treatment of Parkinson's disease (PD), it is not an ideal drug. Levodopa treatment is associated with both short-term and long-term problems (Table 24.1). These are related not only to the poor and variable bioavailability of levodopa and its pharmacokinetics, but also to the variable clinical response during long-term treatment. Levodopa undergoes an extensive metabolism in the periphery (gut, liver, circulation), resulting in a short elimination half-life (about 1 to 2 hours) (1,2). Initially, the duration of levodopa effects is apparently independent of the plasma levodopa kinetics. Later, as the disease progresses, the benefit of levodopa becomes dependent on plasma levodopa concentration and the symptoms return even earlier before the intake of the next daily dose, within 4, 3, and even 2 hours or less. This is called the "end-of-dose phenomenon" or "wearing off" (3–5). Controlled-release (CR) or slow-release levodopa preparations were originally developed with the aim of prolonging the clinical effect of levodopa. The different formulations have not fulfilled the expectations of providing a markedly longer clinical benefit compared with standard levodopa preparations. The CR levodopa preparations are often more problematic in clinical use than the standard levodopa preparations (6,7).

TABLE 24.1. *Drawbacks of levodopa therapy in Parkinson's disease*

Immediate drawbacks
- Poor bioavailability
- Irregular gastrointestinal absorption
- Short plasma half-life
- Competition for transport with dietary amino acids

Long-term drawbacks
- Fluctuations in clinical response
- Dyskinesias and dystonias
- Dose failures
- Psychiatric disturbances

The aim of prolonging the effect of levodopa can be achieved by drugs that inhibit the enzyme catechol-*O*-methyltransferase (COMT) (8,9). Levodopa is metabolized mainly by two routes: decarboxylation and *O*-methylation (1,2). When levodopa was introduced in the late 1960s, it was used without inhibitors of decarboxylation. Adding a dopa decarboxylase (DDC) inhibitor could markedly reduce (up to 80%) the daily levodopa dose and avoid most peripheral adverse effects of dopamine (DA), such as nausea, hypotension, and cardiac arrhythmias (10,11). The two original DDC inhibitors, carbidopa and benserazide, are still in use and are part of the current levodopa combination preparations.

Even with this "double therapy" (levodopa/carbidopa or levodopa/benserazide, hereafter called levodopa therapy), only a small proportion of the oral levodopa dose, probably 5% to 10%, reaches the brain, where it is decarboxylated to DA (1,12,13). During "double therapy," the metabolism of levodopa by COMT is increased and the major part of levodopa is inactivated to 3-*O*-methyldopa (3-OMD) (12–15) (Fig. 24.1).

The COMT enzyme is ubiquitous and is abundant, for instance, in the liver, kidneys, and gut (16,17). The biological importance of COMT is both to detoxify exogenous catechol-structured compounds (foodstuffs) and their metabolites and to inactivate endogenous catecholamines (epinephrine, norepinephrine, DA) and their metabolites by methylation. In addition, several drugs are metabolized by COMT, such as levodopa, α-methyldopa, dobutamine, and rimiterol (17).

During the mid-1980s, Orion Pharma and F. Hoffman-La Roche started to develop COMT inhibitors independently of each other. Both companies ended with the same conclusions: that nitrocatechol-structured inhibitors (e.g., entacapone and tolcapone) were extremely potent, being about 1,000 times more effective than the "first-generation" inhibitors of the 1970s (18–21). Both these compounds, apart from being highly specific and reversible inhibitors of COMT, do not affect other aminergic enzyme systems (19,21). Both compounds are poorly lipophilic. Their clinical effect is most probably peripheral only (22,23), even if tolcapone penetrates the blood–brain barrier to some extent in the rat (24), and measurable concentrations have been detected in cere-

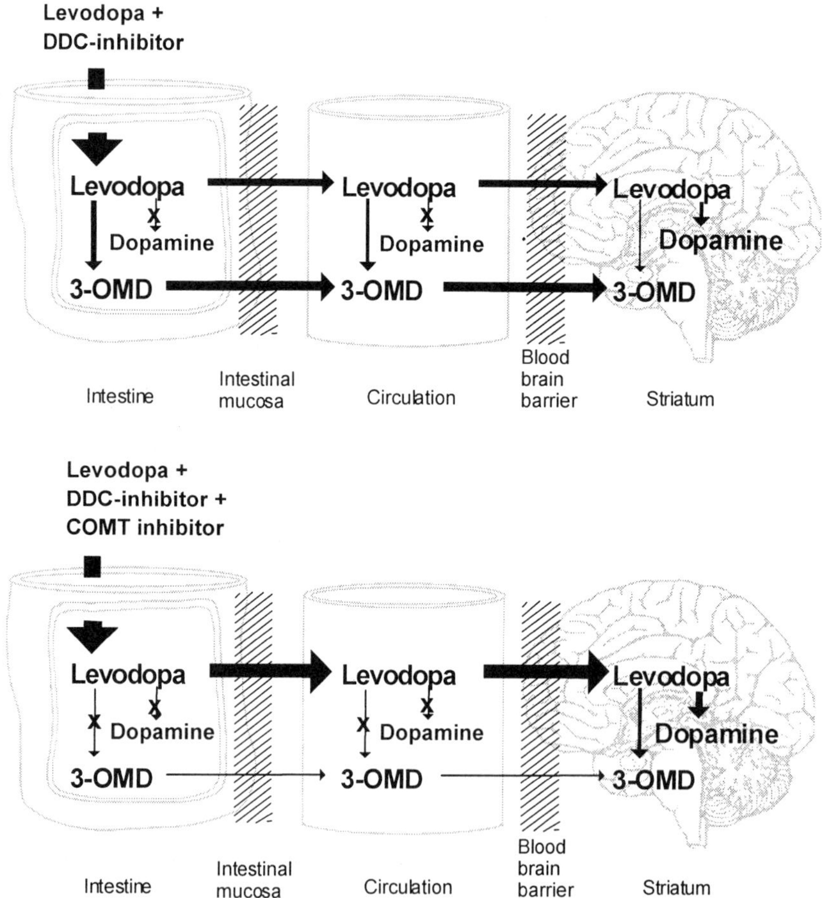

FIGURE 24.1. Principle of catechol-*O*-methyltransferase (COMT) inhibitor treatment using a peripherally acting COMT inhibitor. (DDC, dopa decarboxylase; 3-OMD, 3-*O*-methyldopa.)

brospinal fluid in humans (25). The total content of COMT enzyme in brain is small compared with its contents in the whole body, so central COMT inhibition is of minor, if any, significance in the levodopa metabolism of PD (14,15,22). Recently, as an indication of the actuality of the topic, a new nitrocatechol-structured COMT inhibitor has been described in the literature (26). As far as we know, it has yet to be studied in human.

This chapter deals mostly with entacapone because tolcapone has been suspended in all European countries and Canada and has several restrictions in use in some countries, such as the United States and Switzerland due to liver toxicity (27,28). Thus, the properties of entacapone and tolcapone will be compared in some instances only. Other antiparkinsonian treatment possibilities such as DA agonists or selegiline also are not dealt with in this chapter.

EFFECT OF COMT INHIBITION ON THE PHARMACOKINETICS AND PHARMACODYNAMICS OF LEVODOPA

The pharmacodynamic properties of COMT inhibition can be studied by directly measuring plasma and tissue COMT activity, by assaying plasma concentrations of 3-OMD, by studying the accumulation and metabolism of radioactive fluorodopa in the brain with positron emission tomography (PET), and by studying the pharmacokinetic profile of levodopa in plasma. Only the latter method is of importance concerning the clinical efficacy of COMT inhibition in PD (12,13,23,29) (Fig. 24.1 and Table 24.2).

Both entacapone and tolcapone are rapidly absorbed, with a t_{max} of about 1 hour (30,31). Entacapone is almost totally glucuronized in the liver (32), whereas tolcapone is mainly glucuronized, but also methylated and oxidized to some extent (33). Both metabolites of these COMT inhibitors are eliminated mainly by the kidneys and gut. They may also have an enterohepatic circulation. The main elimination half-life of entacapone is about 1 hour (the beta phase) (30,34) and that of tolcapone 2 to 3 hours (35). Because the half-life of orally administered entacapone is quite similar to that of levodopa (about 1 to 1.5 hours) and because there is a close correlation between the plasma entacapone levels and COMT inhibition in erythrocytes, it is logical to administer entacapone concomitantly with each levodopa dose (29,36). Because tolcapone has a longer half-life, it also has a more prolonged effect on COMT inhibition. This is explained by a twofold greater bioavailability, a twofold smaller volume of distribution, and a sixfold slower clearance, leading to more sustained plasma levels of tolcapone compared with entacapone (13,37). As a result, tolcapone is administered three times a day irrespective of the dosing of levodopa (13,14).

By slowing the elimination of levodopa, both COMT inhibitors prolong the elimination half-life of levodopa and increase its bioavailability (area under the time–concentration curve, [AUC]), without particularly affecting the peak plasma concentrations (C_{max}) or time to reach the peak concentration (t_{max}) (13,23,29). Clinically, however, only the length of time plasma levodopa stays over an optimal therapeutic level is of importance

TABLE 24.2. *Pharmacodynamic actions of COMT inhibitors in levodopa therapy for Parkinson's disease*

Increase the half-life of elimination of levodopa
└→ Longer action of each dose of levodopa
Decrease the plasma levodopa peak-trough variations (continuous dopaminergic stimulation)
└→ Smoothening of the clinical condition due to reduction of off periods
Smaller requirement of levodopa dosing

COMT, catechol-*O*-methyltransferase.

(Fig. 24.2). According to a dose-finding study, the most effective dose of entacapone both pharmacokinetically and clinically is 200 mg (38). Increasing the entacapone dose to 400 mg did not further improve these parameters (38). In other entacapone studies, 200 mg of entacapone has prolonged the half-life of levodopa by 25% to 75% and increased the AUC by 25% to 50% (39–43). Entacapone is effective already after the first dose, and the effect is sustained in repeated long-term use. Quite similar results have been obtained with tolcapone, although a clear dose response has not been demonstrated in all studies (44–46). The pharmacokinetics of levodopa or the effects of COMT inhibition on the pharmacokinetics of levodopa were not influenced by the severity of PD or the age of the patient.

The other pharmacodynamically and clinically important property of COMT inhibition is the "smoothening" effect on plasma levodopa levels. When given with frequent daily levodopa doses, the COMT inhibitors will generally increase the plasma levels of levodopa during the day (23,42). This occurs because the plasma concentration of levodopa at the end of the preceding dose is greater than it would be in the absence of a COMT inhibitor. A consequence is that peak levodopa concentrations increase, but less than the interdose trough concentrations (23). Entacapone decreases the peak-trough variations in the daily plasma levels by some 30% to 50%. This phenomenon has also been seen with tolcapone (47). However, there is no accumulation of either entacapone or levodopa, even in frequent (up to 10 times) daily dosing from one day to another (48).

Entacapone (200 mg) increases the bioavailability of levodopa and prolongs its clinical effect also with CR levodopa preparations to a similar degree as when used with standard levodopa preparations. Unlike its effect with standard levodopa preparations, entacapone may increase the peak levodopa concentration up to 30% with CR levodopa/carbidopa (Sinemet CR) (49,50). This may be of benefit in patients with low plasma levodopa concentrations typical to the slow-release levodopa preparations. Comparable results have been reported with tolcapone (51).

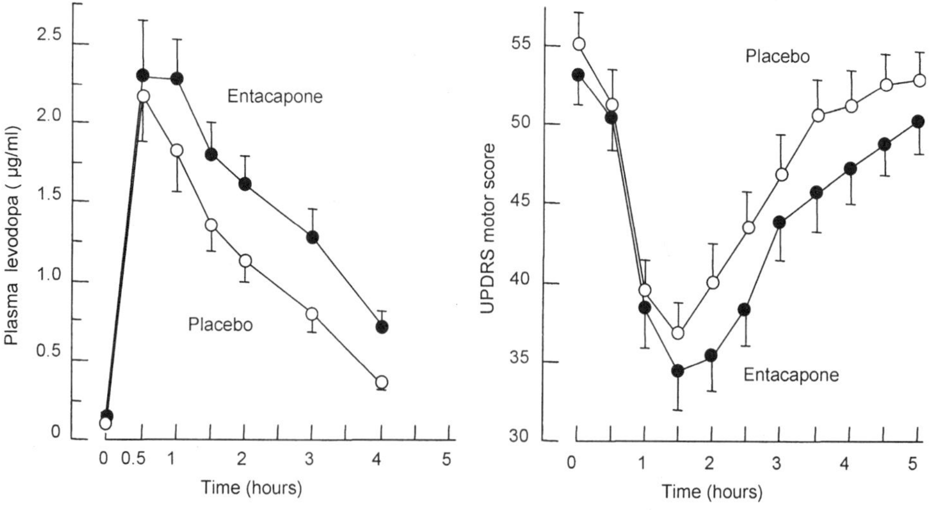

FIGURE 24.2. Plasma levodopa concentrations and corresponding Unified Parkinson's Disease Rating Scale (UPDRS) motor scores during the levodopa test after levodopa/entacapone or levodopa/placebo in patients with Parkinson's disease with end-of-dose–type motor fluctuations. (From Ruottinen HM, Rinne UK. Entacapone prolongs levodopa response in a one month double blind study in parkinsonian patients with levodopa related fluctuations. *J Neurol Neurosurg Psychiatry* 1996;60:36–40, with permission.)

POSITRON EMISSION TOMOGRAPHY STUDIES

PET studies have been used to investigate the effects of COMT inhibitors in the brain with 6-^{18}F-fluorodopa, a radioactive analogue of levodopa, as a marker. A single dose of entacapone increases the availability of fluorodopa in plasma by 30% to 40% (52–55). This is mirrored as better availability also in the striatum, where fluorodopa is decarboxylated and stored as fluorodopamine. The effect of entacapone in healthy volunteers and patients with early PD is seen as a clear increase in the striatal uptake of radioactivity. The response to entacapone in fluorodopa studies is attenuated when the severity of PD increases. This may be due to a marked reduction in the number of dopaminergic neurons, resulting in a smaller capacity to decarboxylate levodopa and store DA (54). However, prolonged (late) imaging for 3.5 hours showed a significantly higher increase in fluorodopa uptake than the standard 1.5 hours (early) of imaging after entacapone, both in age-matched healthy volunteers and in patients with PD (55). Late imaging, thus, shows the storing potential of fluorodopa better than is seen during early fluorodopa PET imaging, even in patients with severe presynaptic dopaminergic hypofunction (55). PET studies excellently illustrate the clinical effect of COMT inhibition.

THE EFFECT OF COMT INHIBITION ON THE CLINICAL RESPONSE TO LEVODOPA

The clinical effect of COMT inhibition is a result of a prolonged elimination of plasma levodopa as a consequence of reduced *O*-methylation of levodopa to 3-OMD, producing a more prolonged availability of levodopa (and DA) in the brain. COMT inhibitors do not have any clinical effects without levodopa in the treatment of PD.

The effect of entacapone has been studied mainly in patients with motor fluctuations, mostly with the wearing-off phenomenon (13,29), because the effect is most obvious in this patient group. All other antiparkinsonian medications have been allowed, except apomorphine. The prolongation of elimination of levodopa is seen clinically as a prolonged positive response of levodopa on "on" time. This has been documented in phase II studies by using both the so-called (single dose) levodopa test and daily home diaries filled by the patients (42,56). In the earlier mentioned dose–response study, the 200-mg entacapone dose used as an adjunct to levodopa was the most effective, both pharmacokinetically and clinically, compared wit placebo (38). The 200-mg entacapone dose prolonged the clinical effect of a single levodopa dose by 20% to 80%, as measured by different methods. The absolute prolongation of the clinical benefit of single levodopa dose has been from 30 to 40 minutes (40–43,56). The mean daily increase in "on" time was 2.1 hours in these 20 patients (entacapone vs. placebo) (56). The effect could be seen already after the first entacapone dose and was unchanged even in long-term treatment. Similar results have been reported in tolcapone studies (14). Entacapone does not markedly affect the magnitude or start of clinical response. This is in accordance with the unchanged peak plasma levodopa concentration (C_{max}) and time to reach it after entacapone administration.

Five placebo-controlled, randomized, double-blind, 6- to 12-month, phase III entacapone studies have been reported in patients with wearing-off symptoms (57–61). The daily "on" time has increased on average by 1 to 2 hours compared with placebo (57,58). The "off" time has decreased correspondingly in patients using standard levodopa preparations. These benefits were considered clinically meaningful in patients already treated with optimized antiparkinsonian therapy. The effect has been sustained over at least 3 years, shown by an open extension study of the controlled studies (62). There have been no marked differences between patients using either levodopa/carbidopa or levodopa/benserazide medications. The effect of entacapone in patients using CR levodopa preparations has been comparable to that seen in patients using standard levodopa preparations in phase III studies (59).

Because entacapone prolongs the "on" time in patients with wearing-off symptoms, it may also prolong preexisting dyskinesias (38,43, 56). In some studies, the severity of these has increased to some extent. Entacapone rarely causes dyskinesias in patients not previously having them (38,42,43,56–58). These findings are in good accordance with the unchanged peak levodopa plasma levels after single doses and the slightly elevated mean daily plasma levodopa concentration after repeated frequent daily dosing of entacapone and levodopa (42).

The knowledge of COMT inhibitors as adjuncts to levodopa in patients without wearing-off symptoms is still limited. In two 6-month randomized, placebo-controlled phase III entacapone studies, the activities of daily living (ADL) subscale of the Unified Parkinson's Disease Rating Scale, Part II (UPDRS-II), score was improved in patients without wearing-off symptoms (59,60). The daily levodopa dose remained unchanged or slightly decreased in the entacapone groups, whereas it was increased in the placebo groups. Quite comparable results have been obtained in one study with tolcapone (63). Further studies are needed in this patient population.

SAFETY OF COMT INHIBITORS

The adverse effects of COMT inhibitors can be classified in two main categories: dopaminergic and nondopaminergic. The dopaminergic adverse effects are due to the pharmacodynamic action of the drugs, the enhanced effect of levodopa. The most common are increased dyskinesias (peak-dose dyskinesias) in previously dyskinetic patients during the first days after introducing a COMT inhibitor. The severity of dyskinesias returns to baseline after levodopa dose reductions (Fig. 24.3). Tolcapone has caused severe dyskinesias in some patients (64,65), possibly related to the increased C_{max} reported in some patients (66). Other dopaminergic adverse effects, such as nausea or vomiting, can also usually be handled by reducing the levodopa dose (57–59). The most common nondopaminergic adverse effects are abdominal pain, loose stools, and diarrhea (61,67,68) (Table 24.3). These have seldom been problematic but have led to discontinuations in 3% to 4% of patients participating in long-term entacapone studies of up to 3 years' duration The use of tolcapone has been connected to more severe diarrhea, described as "explosive" by some patients, leading to discontinuations in about 8% to 10% of the long-term tolcapone patients (64,69,70). Although the

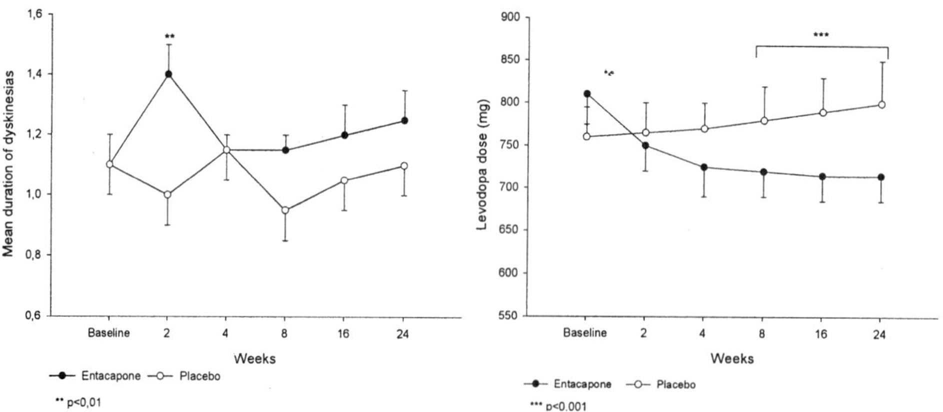

FIGURE 24.3. Mean proportional duration of dyskinesias and mean daily levodopa dose in a United States–Canadian phase III controlled study. (From Haapaniemi H, Reinikainen K, Leinonen M, et al. Tolerability and safety of entacapone in the treatment of Parkinson's disease. *Parkinsonism Related Disord* 2001;7[Suppl 1]:S57, with permission.)

TABLE 24.3. *Adverse events in controlled phase III entacapone studies*

Adverse event	Entacapone (n = 806) (%)	Placebo (n = 497) (%)
Dyskinesia/hyperkinesia	30.4***	17.5
Nausea	13.6***	7.4
Parkinsonism aggravated	13.5	15.3
Urine discoloration	10.8***	0.0
Diarrhea	10.3***	3.8
Dizziness	7.9	5.6
Abdominal pain	7.3*	4.2
Constipation	7.2*	4.2
Hypokinesia	6.9	6.2
Fatigue	6.1*	3.6
Insomnia	5.6	6.8
Pain	5.6	4.6
Tremor	5.5	6.6
Hallucination	4.6	4.0
Back pain	4.5	2.8
Fall	4.3	4.2
Depression	3.7	3.8
Headache	3.7	3.6
Vomiting	3.6**	1.2
Sweating increased	3.2	2.8
Dystonia	2.9	4.4
Hypotension postural	2.5	3.0

*$p < .05$; **$p < .01$; ***$p < .001$.

Source: From Haapaniemi H, Reinikainen K, Leinonen M, et al. Tolerability and safety of entacapone in the treatment of Parkinson's disease. *Parkinsonism Related Disord* 2001;7[Suppl 1]:S57, with permission.

dopaminergic adverse events occur almost immediately, diarrhea starts usually weeks to months after initiating COMT inhibitor treatment. Diarrhea is often quite therapy resistant. Constipation has also been reported as an adverse event with both entacapone and tolcapone. Both drugs may turn the patient's urine dark yellow or red, which is due to the color of the drugs (the nitrocatechol structure) and their metabolites. It is a harmless phenomenon to the health of the patients (57,58, 69,70).

In several studies and in general practice, entacapone has been shown to be hemodynamically safe. It does not markedly affect blood pressure or heart rate, and it does not cause changes in electrocardiographic readings. Entacapone does not affect plasma epinephrine or norepinephrine levels. When the metabolism through the COMT pathway is reduced, these catecholamines are metabolized by the enzyme monoamine oxidase (MAO). Orthostatic hypotension has seldom been problematic in connection with use of entacapone (39,71,72).

Entacapone has been safe with other medications for PD, such as selegiline, DA agonists, anticholinergics, and amantadine, in controlled phase III studies (57–59,61). Formal interaction studies have been performed with the antidepressants imipramine and moclobemide. There have been no hemodynamic or safety interactions with these drugs in healthy volunteers (73,74) or in patients. In clinical use, no meaningful interactions have been reported in patients using antidepressants (75). Because the COMT inhibitors can inhibit the metabolism of catechol-structured drugs, such as isoproterenol (isoprenaline), epinephrine (adrenaline), and norepinephrine (noradrenaline), they can increase or prolong the clinical effect of these drugs and should preferably be avoided (76). Apomorphine is also partly metabolized by COMT, but this combination may even be beneficial.

There is a difference between the effect of entacapone and tolcapone on liver function. Long-term levodopa treatment can, although rarely, cause slight elevations in liver enzymes, usually temporarily. In placebo-con-

TABLE 24.4. *Liver function tests and hepatobiliary adverse events in controlled phase III entacapone studies*

Parameter	Entacapone (double-blind) (n = 806) (%)	Placebo (double-blind) (n = 497) (%)	Entacapone (open long-term safety extension studies) (n = 899) (%)
PCS abnormality			
SGOT/AST (>3 UNL)	0.3	0.2	0.2
SGPT/ALT (>3 UNL)	0.5	0.4	0.3
Alkaline phosphatase (>3 UNL)	0.3	0	0.3
Adverse events			
Liver and biliary systemic disease/all	1.7	1.4	1.9
Hepatitis	0	0	0
Jaundice	0	0	0
Serious adverse events			
Liver and biliary systemic disease/all	0.4[a]	0.2	0.4[b]
Hepatitis	0	0	0
Jaundice	0	0	0
Discontinuations due to adverse hepatic disorders	0	0	0

ALT, alanine aminotransferase; AST, aspartate aminotransferase; SGOT, serum glutamic-oxaloacetic transaminase; SGPT, serum glutamic-pyruvic transaminase; PCS, potentially clinically significant.

[a]3/806 = 0.4%; one patient with hepatic enzymes increased associated to a gallstone attack, two patients underwent elective cholecystectomy operations.

[b]4/899 = 0.4%; three cases of cholelithiasis and one gallbladder disorder with cholecystectomy.

Source: From Haapaniemi H, Reinikainen K, Leinonen M, et al. Tolerability and safety of entacapone in the treatment of Parkinson's disease. *Parkinsonism Related Disord* 2001;7[Suppl 1]:S57, with permission.

trolled, long-term (6 to 12 months), double-blind trials, entacapone has not increased liver transaminase levels more than placebo (68) (Table 24.4). There are no formal requirements to follow liver function tests during entacapone treatment. Unlike entacapone, tolcapone may influence liver function, increasing liver transaminase levels to a clinically relevant level (more than three times the upper reference limit). Discontinuations due to liver problems have been reported in about 3% of patients in clinical trials with tolcapone (63,69,70). At least three cases of deaths have been connected to the use of tolcapone (27,28). The pathological changes in liver function do not seem to be due to COMT inhibition *per se* (77). Other possibilities include differences in metabolism between entacapone and tolcapone (e.g., oxidation) (33) and the property of tolcapone being an uncoupler of oxidative phosphorylation (78).

Abrupt withdrawal of tolcapone has been reported to be connected with malignant neuroleptic syndrome or rhabdomyolysis (13). These phenomena have not been reported with abrupt withdrawal of entacapone in clinical practice or in phase III trials, in more than 800 patients (57,58,61).

LEVODOPA/CARBIDOPA/ ENTACAPONE COMBINATION

Should also the COMT pathway be routinely blocked in levodopa treatment? The main effect of peripheral DDC inhibition is to increase the absorption of levodopa from the gut (Fig. 1). This is seen as markedly increased bioavailability and an increase in the peak concentration of plasma levodopa (Table 24.5). The oral dose of levodopa could be reduced by some 50 to 80%, and most peripheral dopaminergic adverse events could be avoided (10). COMT inhibitors mainly prolong the elimination of levodopa, thus, increasing its bioavailability (42). This is seen as a prolongation of the clinical benefit of levodopa. DDC and COMT inhibitors have different mechanisms of action, which, in fact, are complementary (Table 24.5). It is,

TABLE 24.5. *Effects of DDC and COMT inhibition on the pharmacokinetics of levodopa*[a]

	DDC inhibition	COMT inhibition
C_{max}	↑	↔
t_{max}	↔	↔
Area under the curve	↑	↑
Elimination	↔	↑

COMT, catechol-*O*-methyltransferase; DDC, dopa decarboxylase.

[a]*Conclusion:* DDC inhibitors increase primarily absorption, and COMT inhibitors decrease primarily elimination of levodopa.

thus, logical to add both a DDC and a COMT inhibitor to levodopa treatment.

Levodopa/carbidopa/entacapone tablets are under development at Orion Pharma. Such "triple-combination" tablets will reduce the number of tablets used and, thus, most probably increase compliance. Several tablet strengths may be needed, due to the need of flexibility in the levodopa medication. The tablets under development contain different amounts of levodopa, but always 200 mg of entacapone. The "triple-combination" formulation will probably be on the market in the next few years.

PRACTICAL USE OF COMT INHIBITORS IN PARKINSON'S DISEASE

PET studies have shown that the effect of entacapone in the brain depends on the capacity of the presynaptic dopaminergic system (54,55). With entacapone, the best PET and clinical response occurs in the early or moderate stages of the shortening of duration of response to levodopa (wearing off). The response to COMT inhibitors may be less evident in patients with sudden on-offs and/or freezing.

Several articles have been published on the positioning of COMT inhibition in the treatment of PD. They all are subjective and present one or a few authors' opinion only. However, all include COMT inhibition as an option to treat patients with wearing off. COMT inhibition thus has an established and accepted position in the treatment of patients with wearing off (79–81). We have treated patients with PD with COMT inhibitors, first in various clinical studies since 1987 and in clinical practice later. Our opinion is also subjective, however, because objective studies have not been performed in minority patient groups, for example, in those becoming dyskinetic with 50 mg of levodopa.

We will limit our discussion to COMT inhibitors. Other treatment alternatives have been given by Nutt (15) and by Widner (see Chapter 23). These include increasing the levodopa dose, increasing the dosing frequency of levodopa, changing standard levodopa to CR levodopa, and adding a DA agonist or the MAO-B inhibitor selegiline if these have not been used earlier.

General Aspects

Concomitant administrations of entacapone (200 mg) with each levodopa dose give the best benefit and may improve the compliance of entacapone treatment. No separate dose titration is needed with entacapone. Entacapone is recommended to be taken, and the best results are probably achieved when taken with each levodopa dose. Tolcapone has two tablet strengths, 100 and 200 mg, and the therapy is started with a dose of 100 mg three times a day. The recommendation is not to increase the dose to 200 mg but in exceptional cases, due to possibility of liver toxicity. Thus, even if most clinical phase III studies were performed with the higher 200-mg dose. The first tolcapone dose is taken concomitantly with the first levodopa dose, the second and third with 6-hour intervals.

Informing the patient of the effects of entacapone or tolcapone before starting the therapy is very important because these usually cause marked and rapid changes in the levodopa response, possibly in dopaminergic adverse events and a need to adjust the levodopa medication. Patients should also be told that their urine may be stained dark yellow or orange.

Entacapone treatment does not require follow-up of any laboratory tests. In countries where tolcapone is in use, there are restrictions in its indications, and liver function tests have to be followed up regularly. Tolcapone has to be discontinued if the values of transaminases exceed the upper limit of reference at any phase of the medication.

Levodopa Nonresponders

If a patient does not clinically respond to levodopa, it is unlikely that the addition of a COMT inhibitor is of benefit. However, if a poor levodopa bioavailability is suspected, a COMT inhibitor may be tried, because the response, whether positive or not, is seen within a few days.

Levodopa-naive Patients

Almost all patients with PD respond positively to initiation of levodopa treatment and this improvement is usually sustained for the first 1 to 2 years. In most cases, there is no apparent need for COMT inhibitors in these patients with early PD without symptoms of wearing off.

Could nonfluctuating patients benefit from a COMT inhibitor added to the levodopa medication? It is generally considered that patients without fluctuations treated with either small doses of levodopa or DA agonists are practically symptom free, but this is probably not the case in many instances. Subjectively stable patients have fluctuations in motor function when they are monitored closely enough through the day (82). In a population-based study, Larsen et al. (83) showed that the severity of motor disability and nonmotor manifestations were almost as common in nonfluctuators as in fluctuators. The general quality of life in these patients with PD was markedly poorer than in an age- and sex-matched general population (83). There is preliminary evidence that the quality of life is improved by entacapone in such patients (59,60). Further studies are needed to prove this concept.

It has been suggested that treatment with a COMT inhibitor should be started concomitantly with the initiation of levodopa therapy (84). Because COMT inhibition prolongs the effect of levodopa, it also leads to less fluctuating levodopa levels than levodopa alone and helps to keep the daily levodopa dose at a lower level than without entacapone. It has been proven that continuous dopaminergic stimulation, for example, with long-term continuous levodopa infusion or apomorphine infusion, can prevent and even reverse motor fluctuations and dyskinesias, and even the therapeutic plasma levodopa window may be widened (85). The use of COMT inhibitors helps to stabilize levodopa plasma levels and lets patients use lower daily levodopa dosages. Whether this could reduce or postpone the emergence of fluctuations and/or dyskinesias should be adequately studied in *de novo* or early stage parkinsonian patients (84).

Incomplete Relief

In most cases, one has to consider increasing the levodopa dose or adding a DA agonist. Adding a COMT inhibitor to levodopa treatment in patients with significant parkinsonian signs is not likely to change considerably the magnitude of the levodopa effect in patients using standard levodopa formulations, but the duration of benefit is likely to increase. However, in patients using CR levodopa, both the magnitude and the duration of the effect is likely to increase. This is also true in patients using simultaneously standard and CR preparations. This is due to the fact that COMT inhibition does not affect the maximum levodopa plasma concentration with immediate-release formulations but does increase it by some 30% with CR preparations.

Short Duration of Improvement—Simple Fluctuations

Buffering capacity of the dopaminergic system is progressively decreasing during years, and consequently, the patient will start to experience symptoms of parkinsonism a few hours after initial improvement from a single levodopa dose. Treatment with entacapone can be started as soon as the duration of action of levodopa begins to be shortened. Because entacapone acts through levodopa, one has to choose between increasing the dosing frequency of levodopa and adding entacapone. Adding a COMT inhibitor has the advantage of prolonging the effect of levodopa without increasing the dosing frequency or daily dose of levodopa. Eventually, with the progress of the disease, both alternatives usually have to be combined.

Patients with Dyskinesias

When a COMT inhibitor treatment is initiated, the dose of levodopa should, in principle, be kept unchanged at first; however, in patients with dyskinesias, the levodopa dose can be decreased at the time of initiating the inhibitor. The patients should be informed that possible initial "adverse events" are a result of enhanced response to levodopa and are a sign of the efficacy of the medication. In patients using CR preparations and with a significant tendency to manifest dyskinesias before initiation of COMT inhibitor, it is advisable to decrease the levodopa dose from the first dose. Even in patients with only clinically insignificant dyskinesias, these may become more intense, particularly toward the end of the day because the plasma levodopa level has a tendency to increase during repeated dosing. In these cases, one could either prolong the interdose interval or decrease individual levodopa doses. It may be best to try to reduce the individual doses first, and if this does not lead to an acceptable result, prolong the time between individual doses by 30 to 60 minutes.

In our hands, COMT inhibition has not been particularly beneficial in most patients with a very low threshold for dyskinesias—for example, those taking very small single levodopa doses (50 mg or less) every 1 to 1.5 hours.

Missed or Delayed "On"

Both missed and delayed improvements after a single levodopa dose are common in patients with advanced disease, more frequently seen in patients using relatively small individual doses (e.g., 100 mg) of CR levodopa formulations than with immediate-release formulations. Various reasons for this are discussed in Chapter 23. Adding a COMT inhibitor to the treatment may significantly improve the reliability of each levodopa dose.

CONCLUSIONS

COMT inhibitors offer a new mechanism of action in the treatment of PD. Current clinical evidence relates their benefit in levodopa treatment, particularly in patients with wearing-off symptoms. Entacapone has a good risk/benefit ratio, whereas tolcapone is hampered by the risk of liver toxicity. The "triple-combination" therapy—levodopa/carbidopa/entacapone—may become a feasible alternative in long-term treatment of PD.

REFERENCES

1. Nutt JG, Fellman JH. Pharmacokinetics of levodopa. *Clin Neuropharmacol* 1984;7:35–49.
2. Cedarbaum JM. Clinical pharmacokinetics of antiparkinsonian drugs. *Clin Pharmacokin* 1987;13:141–178.
3. Rinne UK. Treatment of Parkinson's disease: problems with a progressing disease. *J Neural Transm* 1981;51:161–174.
4. Lees AJ. The on-off phenomenon. *J Neurol Neurosurg Psychiatry* 1989;52[Suppl]:29–37.
5. Marsden CD. Problems with long-term levodopa therapy for Parkinson's disease. *Clin Neuropharmacol* 1994;17[Suppl 2]:S32–S44.
6. MacMahon DG, Sachdev D, Boddie HG, et al. A comparison of the effects of controlled-release levodopa (Madopar CR) with conventional levodopa in late Parkinson's disease. *J Neurol Neurosurg Psychiatry* 1990;53:220–223.
7. Koller WC, Pahwa R. Treating motor fluctuations with controlled-release levodopa preparations. *Neurology* 1994;44[Suppl 6]:S23–S28.
8. Männistö PT, Kaakkola S. New selective COMT inhibitors: useful adjuncts for Parkinson's disease? *Trends Pharmacol Sci* 1989;10:54–56.
9. Männistö PT, Kaakkola S. Rationale for selective COMT inhibitors as adjuncts in the drug treatment of Parkinson's disease. *Pharmacol Toxicol* 1990;66:317–323.
10. Cotzias GC, van Woert MH, Schiffer LM. Aromatic amino acids and modification of parkinsonism. *N Engl J Med* 1967;276:374–379.
11. Cotzias GC, Papavasiliou PS, Gellene R. Modification

of parkinsonism—chronic treatment with L-dopa. *N Engl J Med* 1969;280:337–345.
12. Kaakkola S, Gordin A, Männistö PT. General properties and clinical possibilities of new selective inhibitors of catechol *O*-methyltransferase. *Gen Pharmacol* 1994;25: 813–824.
13. Kaakkola S. Clinical pharmacology, therapeutic use and potential of COMT inhibitors in Parkinson's disease. *Drugs* 2000;59:1233–1250.
14. Dingemanse J. Catechol-*O*-methyltransferase inhibitors: clinical potential in the treatment of Parkinson's disease. *Drug Dev Res* 1997;42:1–25.
15. Nutt JG. Catechol-*O*-methyltransferase inhibitors for treatment of Parkinson's disease. *Lancet* 1998;351: 1221–1222.
16. Nissinen E, Tuominen R, Perhoniemi V, et al. Catechol-*O*-methyltransferase activity in human and rat small intestine. *Life Sci* 1988;42:2609–2614.
17. Männistö PT, Kaakkola S. Catechol-*O*-methyltransferase (COMT): biochemistry, molecular biology, pharmacology, and clinical efficacy of the new selective COMT inhibitors. *Pharmacol Rev* 1999;51: 593–628.
18. Männistö PT, Kaakkola S, Nissinen E, et al. Properties of novel effective and highly selective inhibitors of catechol-*O*-methyltransferase. *Life Sci* 1988;43:1465–1471.
19. Zürcher G, Keller HH, Kettler R, et al. Ro 40-7592, a novel, very potent, and orally active inhibitor of catechol-*O*-methyltransferase: a pharmacological study in rats. *Adv Neurol* 1990;53:497–503.
20. Männistö PT, Ulmanen I, Taskinen J, et al. Catechol-*O*-methyltransferase (COMT) and COMT inhibitors. In: Sandler M, Smith J, eds. *Design of enzyme inhibitors as drugs.* Oxford: Oxford University Press, 1993:623–646.
21. Nissinen E, Linden IB, Schultz E, et al. Biochemical and pharmacological properties of a peripherally acting catechol-*O*-methyltransferase inhibitor entacapone. *Naunyn Schmiedebergs Arch Pharmacol* 1992;346: 262–266.
22. Troconiz IF, Naukkarinen TH, Ruottinen HM, et al. Population pharmacodynamic modeling of levodopa in patients with Parkinson's disease receiving entacapone. *Clin Pharmacol Ther* 1998;64:106–116.
23. Nutt JG. Effect of COMT inhibition on the pharmacokinetics and pharmacodynamics of levodopa in parkinsonian patients. *Neurology* 2000;55[Suppl 4]:S33–S37.
24. Da Prada M, Borgulya J, Napolitano A, et al. Improved therapy of Parkinson's disease with tolcapone, a central and peripheral COMT inhibitor with an *S*-adenosyl-L-methionine-sparing effect. *Clin Neuropharmacol* 1995; 17[Suppl 3]:S26–S37.
25. Russ H, Müller T, Woitalla D, et al. Detection of tolcapone in the cerebrospinal fluid of parkinsonian subjects. *Naunyn Schmiedebergs Arch Pharmacol* 1999; 360:719–720.
26. Parada A, Loureiro AI, Vieira-Coelho MA, et al. BIA 3-202, a novel catechol-*O*-methyltransferase inhibitor, enhances the availability of L-DOPA to the brain and reduces its *O*-methylation. *Eur J Pharmacol* 2001;420: 27–32.
27. Assal F, Spahr L, Hadengue A, et al. Tolcapone and fulminant hepatitis. *Lancet* 1998;352:958.
28. Colosimo C. The rise and fall of tolcapone. *J Neurol* 1999;246:880–882.
29. Ruottinen HM, Rinne UK. COMT inhibition in the treatment of Parkinson's disease. *J Neurol* 1998;245: 25–34.
30. Keränen T, Gordin A, Karlsson M, et al. Inhibition of soluble catechol-*O*-methyltransferase and single-dose pharmacokinetics after oral and intravenous administration of entacapone. *Eur J Clin Pharmacol* 1994;46: 151–157.
31. Dingemanse J, Jorga KM, Schmitt M, et al. Integrated pharmacokinetics and pharmacodynamics of the novel catechol-*O*-methyltransferase inhibitor tolcapone during first administration to humans. *Clin Pharmacol Ther* 1995;57:508–517.
32. Wikberg T, Vuorela A, Ottoila P, et al. Identification of major metabolites of the catechol-*O*-methyltransferase inhibitor entacapone in rats and humans. *Drug Metab Dispos* 1993;21:81–92.
33. Jorga K, Fotteler B, Heizmann P, et al. Metabolism and excretion of tolcapone, a novel inhibitor of catechol-*O*-methyltransferase. *Br J Clin Pharmacol* 1999;48: 513–520.
34. Heikkinen H, Saraheimo M, Antila S, et al. Pharmacokinetics of entacapone, a peripherally acting catechol-*O*-methyltransferase inhibitor, in man—a study using a stable isotope technique. *Eur J Clin Pharmacol* 2001; 56:821–826.
35. Jorga KM. Pharmacokinetics, pharmacodynamics, and tolerability of tolcapone: a review of early studies in volunteers. *Neurology* 1998;50[Suppl 5]:S31–S38.
36. Keränen T, Gordin A, Harjola VP, et al. The effect of catechol-*O*-methyltransferase inhibition by entacapone on the pharmacokinetics and metabolism of levodopa in healthy volunteers. *Clin Neuropharmacol* 1993;16: 145–156.
37. Jorga KM, Fotteler B, Heizmann P, et al. Pharmacokinetics and pharmacodynamics after oral and intravenous administration of tolcapone, a novel adjunct to Parkinson's disease therapy. *Eur J Clin Pharmacol* 1998;54:443–447.
38. Ruottinen HM, Rinne UK. A double-blind pharmacokinetic and clinical dose-response study of entacapone as an adjuvant to levodopa therapy in advanced Parkinson's disease. *Clin Neuropharmacol* 1996;19:283–296.
39. Myllylä VV, Sotaniemi KA, Illi A, et al. Effect of entacapone, a COMT inhibitor, on the pharmacokinetics of levodopa and on cardiovascular responses in patients with Parkinson's disease. *Eur J Clin Pharmacol* 1993; 45:419–423.
40. Kaakkola S, Teräväinen H, Ahtila S, et al. Effect of entacapone, a COMT inhibitor, on clinical disability and levodopa metabolism in parkinsonian patients. *Neurology* 1994;44:77–80.
41. Merello M, Lees AJ, Webster R, et al. Effect of entacapone, a peripherally acting catechol-*O*-methyltransferase inhibitor, on the motor response to acute treatment with levodopa in patients with Parkinson's disease. *J Neurol Neurosurg Psychiatry* 1994;57: 186–189.
42. Nutt JG, Woodward WR, Beckner RM, et al. Effect of peripheral catechol-*O*-methyltransferase inhibition on the pharmacokinetics and pharmacodynamics of levodopa in parkinsonian patients. *Neurology* 1994;44: 913–919.
43. Ruottinen HM, Rinne UK. Effect of one month's treatment with peripherally acting catechol-*O*-methyltransferase inhibitor, entacapone, on pharmacokinetics and

motor response to levodopa in advanced parkinsonian patients. *Clin Neuropharmacol* 1996;19:222–233.

44. Limousin P, Pollak P, Pfefen JP, et al. Acute administration of levodopa-benserazide and tolcapone, a COMT inhibitor, in Parkinson's disease. *Clin Neuropharmacol* 1995;18:258–265.
45. Davis TL, Roznoski M, Burns RS. Acute effects of COMT inhibition on L-DOPA pharmacokinetics in patients treated with carbidopa and selegiline. *Clin Neuropharmacol* 1995;18:333–337.
46. Napolitano A, Del Dotto P, Petrozzi L, et al. Pharmacokinetics and pharmacodynamics of L-Dopa after acute and 6-week tolcapone administration in patients with Parkinson's disease. *Clin Neuropharmacol* 1999;22: 24–29.
47. Jorga K, Banken L, Fotteler B, et al. Population pharmacokinetics of levodopa in patients with Parkinson's disease treated with tolcapone. *Clin Pharmacol Ther* 2000;67:610–620.
48. Rouru J, Gordin A, Huupponen R, et al. Pharmacokinetics of oral entacapone after frequent multiple dosing and effects on levodopa disposition. *Eur J Clin Pharmacol* 1999;55:461–467.
49. Kaakkola S, Teräväinen H, Ahtila S, et al. Entacapone in combination with standard or controlled-release levodopa/carbidopa: a clinical and pharmacokinetic study in patients with Parkinson's disease. *Eur J Neurol* 1995; 2:341–347.
50. Piccini P, Brooks DJ, Korpela K, et al. The catechol-*O*-methyltransferase (COMT) inhibitor entacapone enhances the pharmacokinetic and clinical response to Sinemet CR in Parkinson's disease. *J Neurol Neurosurg Psychiatry* 2000;68:589–594.
51. Jorga K, Fotteler B, Sedek G, et al. The effect of tolcapone on levodopa pharmacokinetics is independent of levodopa/carbidopa formulation. *J Neurol* 1998;245: 223–230.
52. Sawle GV, Burn DJ, Morrish PK, et al. The effect of entacapone (OR-611) on brain [^{18}F]-6-L-fluorodopa metabolism: implications for levodopa therapy of Parkinson's disease. *Neurology* 1994;44:1292–1297.
53. Ruottinen HM, Rinne JO, Ruotsalainen UH, et al. Striatal [^{18}F]fluorodopa utilization after COMT inhibition with entacapone studied with PET in advanced Parkinson's disease. *J Neural Transm Parkinson Dis Dementia Sect* 1995;10:91–106.
54. Ruottinen HM, Rinne JO, Oikonen VJ, et al. Striatal 6-[^{18}F]fluorodopa accumulation after combined inhibition of peripheral catechol-*O*-methyltransferase and monoamine oxidase type B: differing response in relation to presynaptic dopaminergic dysfunction. *Synapse* 1997;27:336–346.
55. Ruottinen HM, Niinivirta M, Bergman J, et al. Detection of response to COMT inhibition in FDOPA PET in advanced Parkinson's disease requires prolonged imaging. *Synapse* 2001;40:19–26.
56. Ruottinen HM, Rinne UK. Entacapone prolongs levodopa response in a one month double blind study in parkinsonian patients with levodopa related fluctuations. *J Neurol Neurosurg Psychiatry* 1996;60:36–40.
57. Parkinson Study Group. Entacapone improves motor fluctuations in levodopa-treated Parkinson's disease patients. *Ann Neurol* 1997;42:747–755.
58. Rinne UK, Larsen JP, Siden A, et al, and the NOMECOMT Study Group. Entacapone enhances the response to levodopa in parkinsonian patients with motor fluctuations. *Neurology* 1998;51:1309–1314.
59. Poewe W, Deuschl G, Gordin A, et al, and the Celomen Study Group. Efficacy and safety of entacapone in Parkinson's disease patients with suboptimal levodopa response. *Acta Neurol Scand* 2002;105:245–255.
60. Sagar H, Brooks D, the UK-Irish Entacapone Study Group. The UK-Irish double-blind study of entacapone in Parkinson's disease. *Mov Disord* 2000;15[Suppl 3]: S135.
61. Myllylä VV, Kultalahti ER, Haapaniemi H, et al. Twelve-month safety of entacapone in patients with Parkinson's disease. *Eur J Neurol* 2001;8:53–60.
62. Larsen JP, Siden Å, Worm-Petersen J, et al. Long-term efficacy and safety of entacapone in parkinsonian patients with motor fluctuations. An open study of 3 years duration. *Parkinsonism Related Disord* 2001;7[Suppl 1]:S61.
63. Waters CH, Kurth M, Bailey P, and the Tolcapone in stable Parkinson's disease: efficacy and safety of long-term treatment. The Tolcapone Stable Study Group. *Neurology* 1997;49:665–671.
64. Kurth MC, Adler CH, St. Hilaire M, et al. Tolcapone improves motor function and reduces levodopa requirement in patients with Parkinson's disease experiencing motor fluctuations: a multicenter, double-blind, randomized, placebo-controlled trial. *Neurology* 1997;48: 81–87.
65. Myllylä VV, Jackson M, Larsen JP, et al. Efficacy and safety of tolcapone in levodopa-treated Parkinson's disease patients with "wearing-off" phenomenon: a multicentre, double-blind, randomized, placebo-controlled study. *Eur J Neurol* 1997;4:333–341.
66. Müller T, Woitalla D, Schulz D, et al. Tolcapone increases maximum concentration of levodopa. *J Neural Transm* 2000;107:113–119.
67. *Comtess Product Monograph.* Espoo, Finland: Orion Corp, 1999.
68. Haapaniemi H, Reinikainen K, Leinonen M, et al. Tolerability and safety of entacapone in the treatment of Parkinson's disease. *Parkinsonism Related Disord* 2001; 7[Suppl 1]:S57.
69. Baas H, Beiske AG, Ghika J, et al. Catechol-*O*-methyltransferase inhibition with tolcapone reduces the "wearing off" phenomenon and levodopa requirements in fluctuating parkinsonian patients. *J Neurol Neurosurg Psychiatry* 1997;63:421–428.
70. Rajput AH, Martin W, Saint-Hilaire MH, et al. Tolcapone improves motor function in parkinsonian patients with the "wearing-off" phenomenon: a double-blind, placebo-controlled, multicenter trial. *Neurology* 1997;49:1066–1071.
71. Illi A, Sundberg S, Koulu M, et al. COMT inhibition by high-dose entacapone does not affect hemodynamics but changes catecholamine metabolism in healthy volunteers at rest and during exercise. *Int J Clin Pharmacol Ther* 1994;32:582–588.
72. Lyytinen J, Sovijärvi A, Kaakkola S, et al. The effect of catechol-*O*-methyltransferase inhibition with entacapone on cardiovascular autonomic responses in L-dopa–treated patients with Parkinson's disease. *Clin Neuropharmacol* 2001;24:50–57.
73. Illi A, Sundberg S, Ojala-Karlsson P, et al. Simultaneous inhibition of catechol-*O*-methyltransferase and monoamine oxidase A: effects on hemodynamics and

catecholamine metabolism in healthy volunteers. *Clin Pharmacol Ther* 1996;59:450–457.
74. Illi A, Sundberg S, Ojala-Karlsson P, et al. Simultaneous inhibition of catecholamine-*O*-methylation by entacapone and neuronal uptake by imipramine: lack of interactions. *Eur J Clin Pharmacol* 1996;51:273–276.
75. Reinikainen K, Karonen T, Haapaniemi H, et al. No indication for interactions between entacapone and antidepressants. *Parkinsonism Related Disord* 2001; 7[Suppl 1]:S67.
76. Illi A, Sundberg S, Ojala-Karlsson P, et al. The effect of entacapone on the disposition and hemodynamic effects of intravenous isoproterenol and epinephrine. *Clin Pharmacol Ther* 1995;58:221–227.
77. Watkins P. COMT inhibitors and liver toxicity. *Neurology* 2000;55[Suppl 4]:S51–S52.
78. Nissinen E, Kaheinen P, Penttilä KE, et al. Entacapone, a novel catechol-*O*-methyltransferase inhibitor for Parkinson's disease, does not impair mitochondrial energy production. *Eur J Pharmacol* 1997; 340:287–294.
79. Schapira AHV, Obeso JA, Olanow CW. The place of COMT inhibitors in the armamentarium of drugs for the treatment of Parkinson's disease. *Neurology* 2000; 55[Suppl 4]:S65–S68.
80. Waters C. Practical issues with COMT inhibitors in Parkinson's disease. *Neurology* 2000;55[Suppl 4]: S57–S59.
81. Olanow CW, Obeso JA. Pulsatile stimulation of dopamine receptors and levodopa-induced motor complications in Parkinson's disease: implications for the early use of COMT inhibitors. *Neurology* 2000; 55[Suppl 4]:S72–S77.
82. Nutt JG, Woodward WR, Carter JH, et al. Effect of long-term therapy on the pharmacodynamics of levodopa. Relation to on-off phenomenon. *Arch Neurol* 1992;49:1123–1130.
83. Larsen JP, Karlsen K, Tandberg E. Clinical problems in non-fluctuating patients with Parkinson's disease: a community-based study. *Mov Disord* 2000;15:826–829.
84. Olanow CW, Schapira AHV, Rascol O. Continuous dopamine-receptor stimulation in early Parkinson's disease. *Trends Neurosci* 2000;23[Suppl]:S117–S126.
85. Nutt JG, Obeso JA, Stocchi F. Continuous dopamine-receptor stimulation in advanced Parkinson's disease. *Trends Neurosci* 2000;23[Suppl]:S109–S115.

Parkinson's Disease: Advances in Neurology, Vol. 91.
Edited by Ariel Gordin, Seppo Kaakkola, and Heikki Teräväinen
Lippincott Williams & Wilkins, Philadelphia © 2003

25

Renaissance of Amantadine in the Treatment of Parkinson's Disease

*†Pierre J. Blanchet, *‡Leo Verhagen Metman, and *Thomas N. Chase

**Experimental Therapeutics Branch, National Institute of Neurological Disorders and Stroke, National Institutes of Health, Bethesda, Maryland; †Faculty of Dentistry, University of Montreal, Montreal, Quebec, Canada; and ‡Department of Neurology, Rush-Presbytarian-St. Luke's Medical Center, Chicago, Illinois*

First introduced as an antiviral agent for influenza, amantadine hydrochloride was serendipitously found in April 1968 to relieve parkinsonian symptoms in a single patient treated for influenza prophylaxis, and then was shown to produce a variable degree of improvement in two thirds of 163 patients (1). These results were soon confirmed (2). The parkinsonian triad symptoms responded to the drug (1,3,4), although rigidity (2) and tremor (5) appeared to be less sensitive in some reports. Adverse events were minor and affected up to 22% of cases (1). Although clinical results were favorable in most patients, the improvement was often deemed modest (5,6) and some questioned the effectiveness of prolonged treatment (1,6,7). A synergistic but transient beneficial effect averaging 5.7 months was also reported in combination with levodopa (8). The mechanism of action in Parkinson's disease (PD) was obscure and attributed to prodopaminergic and anticholinergic activities (9). Renewed enthusiasm about the therapeutic effects of amantadine in PD grew in light of findings concerning the antiglutamatergic action of 1-amino-adamantanes and the implication of the glutamatergic system in levodopa-related motor response complications observed in most patients with PD.

MECHANISM OF ACTION OF AMANTADINE

The antiparkinsonian action of amantadine was long thought to be related to its capacity to directly inhibit dopamine (DA) reuptake at nigrostriatal terminals (10), but other investigators later proposed that this effect was observed only at supratherapeutic dosing (11). Nondopaminergic activities at GABAergic, glycinergic, and glutamatergic receptors were eventually explored. The 1-amino-adamantanes were shown to interfere with glutamatergic *N*-methyl-D-aspartate (NMDA) receptor transmission, with amantadine displaying no functionally significant anti-GABAergic or antiglycinergic effect (12). The NMDA antagonistic effect was thought to be exerted at the Zn^{2+} site until Kornhuber et al. (13) demonstrated amantadine's affinity at the glutamatergic NMDA receptor coupled ion channel based on the displacement of the noncompetitive antagonist MK-801 within therapeutic concentrations in the human cortex. In accordance with this, amantadine inhibits in a noncompetitive way the NMDA-evoked release of acetylcholine in rat neostriatal tissue slices at low micromolar concentrations, an effect that could account in part for its clinical efficacy (14). The antagonism of NMDA receptors may also constitute the basis for indirect effects on the nigrostriatal dopaminergic system by stimulating dopa decarboxylase (DDC) activity and DA synthesis in the human brain, as positron emission tomography results suggest (15). Thus, amantadine displays complex direct and indirect effects in the brain that appear largely attributable to antagonism at glutamatergic NMDA receptors.

GLUTAMATE- AND LEVODOPA-RELATED MOTOR RESPONSE COMPLICATIONS

The renaissance of amantadine stemmed not only from the recognition of its noncompetitive antagonism of NMDA receptors but also from important advances made about the anatomical and physiological role of glutamate in the basal ganglia circuitry and contribution to disease states such as PD (16). Prominent glutamatergic afferents to the basal ganglia largely originate from the cerebral cortex, intralaminar thalamic, subthalamic, and pedunculopontine nuclei. NMDA receptors are found in all basal ganglial nuclei, particularly in the striatum (17). The NMDA receptor is a heteromeric complex made of the combination of at least four subunits, mainly divided in two families: NR1 and NR2. The NR1 subunits exist in eight alternatively spliced isoforms encoded by a single gene and are necessary for function. Four different NR2 subunits have been identified that are encoded by different genes and are expressed in a distinct regional pattern. High levels of both NR2A and NR2B subunit expression are found in the striatum. Lower levels of NR2B subunit expression are also detected in the substantia nigra pars compacta (SNpc) and the subthalamic nucleus. Significant NR2C expression is found in the SNpc, and NR2D subunit expression is significant in the pallidum and subthalamic nucleus, and at lower levels in the SNpc. These regional differences offer the potential for the development of pharmacological agents with targeted action and fewer adverse effects. Other glutamate receptors (kainate, α-amino-3-hydroxy-5-methyl-4-isoxazole propionic acid, metabotropic) are also present in the basal ganglia. There is an unresolved controversy regarding the regulation of NMDA receptors in PD. Although a relation between dyskinesias and upregulated striatal glutamate receptor binding in 1-methyl-4-phenyl-1,2,3,6-tetrahydropyridine (MPTP)-lesioned parkinsonian monkeys remains possible (18), postmortem PD brain studies have yielded variable results. In one report, NMDA-sensitive ^{3}H-glutamate binding was reduced by two thirds in the striatum, but NMDA NR1 messenger RNA levels were unchanged, perhaps reflecting the loss of NMDA receptors localized on degenerated presynaptic nigrostriatal projections (19).

Experimental evidence in support of the contribution of glutamatergic mechanisms to the development of motor response complications in levodopa-treated patients with PD has been gathered in recent years (20–21). In 6-hydroxydopamine (OHDA)–lesioned rats, apomorphine "priming" or sensitization of D_2 receptor–mediated rotational behavior and striatal *Fos* expression are dependent on NMDA receptor stimulation and attenuated by pretreatment with NMDA antagonists (22). In the same model, systemic and intrastriatal injections of NMDA antagonists reversed (23,24) and even prevented (25) the changes in response that take place during sustained levodopa treatment, suggesting that NMDA receptor sensitization plays an important role in the development of this complication. In addition, NMDA NR2B subunits, and NR2A subunits to a lesser extent, showed enhanced tyrosine phosphorylation in the striatum in 6-OHDA rats with a shortened response to levodopa (26). The intrastriatal injection of the tyrosine kinase inhibitor genistein also normalized the pharmacological response and attenuated the phosphorylation increase in NR2 subunits. A potent, competitive, non–subunit selective NMDA receptor antagonist reduced the severity of levodopa-induced choreic dyskinesias by 68% in nonhuman primates with MPTP parkinsonism (27). Thus, important physiological changes underlying the development of levodopa-related motor response complications take place at the level of the medium spiny output neurons in the striatum, where

NMDA antagonists may have a strategic role to play in therapy. At the moment, it is unclear whether glutamate antagonists mediate a "pharmacological pallidotomy" (28); "pharmacological striatal depriming" might be a better term, but caution should be used not to prematurely exclude other NMDA sites affecting basal ganglionic–thalamocortical transmission that may contribute to the pharmacological effects of these drugs.

These advances prompted us to evaluate the antidyskinetic effect of amantadine in four nonhuman primates with MPTP parkinsonism, displaying consistent levodopa-induced dyskinesias (29). Amantadine (2.5 mg/kg twice daily for 3 to 6 days) nearly suppressed choreic dyskinesias and reduced by 35% dystonic dyskinesias produced by a low effective dose (mean 47.5 mg subcutaneously) of levodopa methyl ester (with benserazide), at the expense of a 50% reduction in motor benefit. In combination with a high dose (mean, 110 mg subcutaneously) of levodopa methyl ester, amantadine still reduced dyskinesias by nearly 40% while sparing the antiparkinsonian response (Fig. 25.1). These results cannot be interpreted on the basis of prodopaminergic or anticholinergic pharmacological effects

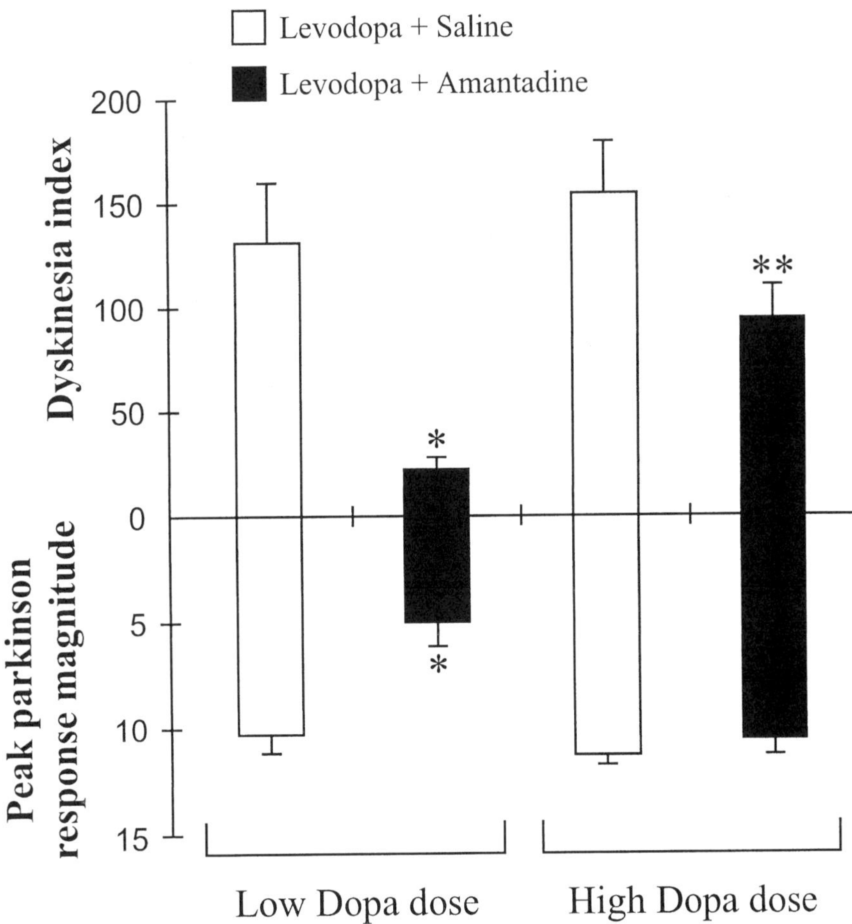

FIGURE 25.1. Mean (±SEM) dyskinesia severity index ([sum of all dyskinesia scores]/[duration of antiparkinsonian effect] × 500) and peak antiparkinsonian response magnitude of four parkinsonian monkeys administered two effective subcutaneous (s.c.) doses of levodopa/benserazide combined with amantadine (2.5 mg/kg s.c. twice daily for 3 to 6 days) or saline. (*$p < .05$ vs. low dopa dose + saline; **$p < .05$ vs. high dopa dose + saline.)

but implicate NMDA receptors in the production of levodopa-induced dyskinesias. They also indicate that inadequate dosing and/or other factors may potentially interfere with the overall benefit derived from amantadine.

We have previously attempted to use the subunit selectivity profile and affinity of different experimental glutamate antagonists for diheteromeric NMDA receptor subunit combinations (NR1A/NR2A, NR1A/NR2B, NR1A/NR2C) expressed in *Xenopus laevis* oocytes to predict their behavioral outcome in MPTP monkeys with dyskinesias (30). The electrophysiological effects of the drugs on these cloned binary NMDA subtypes were assayed by measuring inhibition of membrane current responses elicited by fixed concentrations of the coagonists glutamate and glycine. The glutamate site antagonist LY 235959 inhibited agonist-evoked currents with IC_{50} values between 0.3 and 0.5 μmol/L, depending on the subunit combination. Converting IC_{50} values into apparent affinity constants (K_b values) demonstrated no apparent selectivity across the subunit combinations tested. The allosteric site antagonist Co 101244 inhibited agonist-evoked currents at NR1A/NR2B, with IC_{50} values of 0.026 μmol/L but was inactive at the other subunit combinations (about 10,000-fold selectivity for the NR1A/NR2B subunit combination). The noncompetitive NMDA receptor–coupled ionic channel antagonist amantadine inhibited agonist-evoked currents with IC_{50} values between 14 and 29 μmol/L across the different subunit combinations and displayed no selectivity (E. R. Whittemore, *personal communication,* 1997). All three drugs demonstrated antidyskinetic activity regardless of their selectivity for the different NMDA subunits present in the basal ganglia (27,29,30). Nonetheless, the affinity and selectivity of glutamate antagonists for the different NMDA subunits are likely to affect their therapeutic index.

CLINICAL IMPACT OF AMANTADINE ON DYSKINESIA

In a retrospective chart review, amantadine (200 to 300 mg per day) afforded sustained (more than 9 months) benefit in four fluctuating patients with PD and dyskinesias (31). In a brief account of the benefit of amantadine on dyskinesias in 42 patients with PD, 27 cases were kept on a stable drug regimen by the time amantadine (200 to 300 mg per day) was initiated. In this subgroup, 70% reported improvement of at least 25% in dyskinesia duration and severity (32). All types of dyskinesias were ameliorated. Nearly half of the patients who benefited also noticed better antiparkinsonian symptomatic control. A little less than half of these patients noticed sustained benefit from the drug at the last follow-up visit (8 to 28 months after initiation). The antidyskinetic effect was carefully quantitated in 18 patients with advanced PD and dyskinesias (33) randomized to take amantadine (300 to 400 mg per day) or placebo capsules orally for 3 weeks, each in a double-blind crossover design. On the last days of each study arm, subjects were admitted to the hospital to evaluate their motor and dyskinetic response to a constant intravenous levodopa infusion in combination with oral amantadine or placebo. Plasma amantadine concentration was measured 3 hours after dosing. Fourteen patients completed the study. Dyskinesias were objectively reduced by 60% during amantadine treatment while the antiparkinsonian response to intravenous levodopa was unaffected (Fig. 25.2). The antidyskinetic efficacy was significantly related to the plasma amantadine concentration (between 7 to 14 μmol/L in most cases). Home diaries disclosed reduction in dyskinesia duration and severity and in daily "off" time. In a follow-up study, the benefit of amantadine on dyskinesia was shown to extend to at least 1 year (34).

Since then, several short-term, double-blind, placebo-controlled studies using validated rating scales have confirmed the potential of amantadine to relieve levodopa-induced dyskinesias (Table 25.1). The impact on dyskinesia is variable but consistently positive, and no reduction in motor benefit is observed. The long-term outcome of this effect should be reevaluated because it is apparent that patients with PD, even late in the disease, still benefit from amantadine (39).

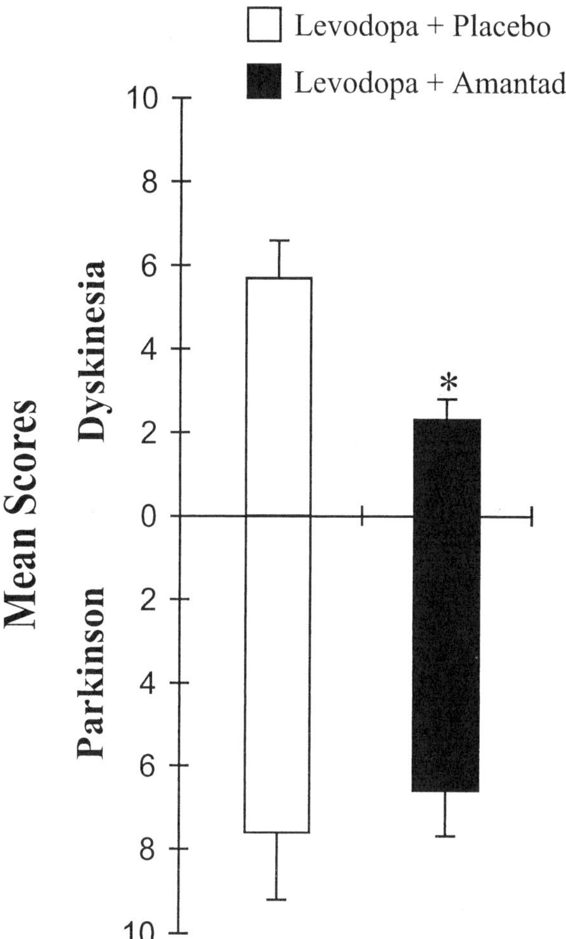

FIGURE 25.2. Mean (±SEM) modified Abnormal Involuntary Movement Scale (dyskinesia) and abbreviated Unified Parkinson's Disease Rating Scale (parkinsonian) scores of 14 patients under continuous intravenous levodopa perfusion (66 ± 6 mg per hour) combined with oral amantadine (300 to 400 mg per day) or placebo. (*p = .001.)

In addition to the body of literature related to the contribution of striatal NMDA receptors to levodopa-induced motor response alterations, the "weak excitotoxic hypothesis" (glutamate as one contributing factor to a final common pathway leading to cell death) also generated hope that NMDA antagonists might also interfere with ongoing nigral cell damage in PD. Indeed, the severe degeneration of the dopaminergic nigrostriatal system in PD has profound effects on glutamatergic pathways, leading to overactivity in subthala-

TABLE 25.1. *Recent double-blind, placebo-controlled clinical studies on the antidyskinetic effect of AH and AS in Parkinson's disease*

Drug	Daily dose	No. of patients	Duration of active treatment	Dyskinesia relief	Reference
AH	300–400 mg orally	14	3 wk	–60%	33
AH	200 mg orally	24	3 wk	–24%	35
AS	300 mg orally	11	2 wk	–52%	36
AS	400 mg intravenously	21	1 wk	–33% (trend) (AIMS)	37
	300–600 mg orally		2 wk	–40% (UPDRS-IV)	
				–48% (diaries)	
AS	200 mg intravenously	9	Single dosing	–50%	38

AH, amantadine hydrochloride; AS, amantadine sulphate; UPDRS-IV, Unified Parkinson's Disease Rating Scale, section four; AIMS, abnormal involuntary movement scale.

mic projections (notably to the pallidum and SNpc) and corticostriatal projections in particular (16). This excessive glutamatergic activity may impair vital cellular functions and may be toxic for compromised or healthy neurons. *In vitro,* adamantanes (memantine and amantadine) have been shown to ameliorate NMDA-induced excitotoxicity (40) and amantadine reduced the toxic effects of MPTP *in vivo* in mice (41). Other NMDA antagonists have provided neuroprotection in animal models of parkinsonism (42,43). Interestingly, an apparent improvement in survival has been observed with amantadine treatment in patients with PD (44), but no random treatment assignment was used, and the result has not been replicated. The mechanism of action underlying this finding remains to be elucidated.

CONCLUSIONS

The search for more effective glutamate antagonists in the treatment of PD is certainly worth pursuing. In the meantime, given the favorable therapeutic index of the drug and its low cost, all patients with PD experiencing disabling dyskinesias should be given a trial on amantadine before a stereotaxic neurosurgical intervention is contemplated.

REFERENCES

1. Schwab RS, England AC Jr, Poskanzer DC, et al. Amantadine in the treatment of Parkinson's disease. *JAMA* 1969;208:1168–1170.
2. Parkes JD, Zilkha KJ, Calver DM, et al. Controlled trial of amantadine hydrochloride in Parkinson's disease. *Lancet* 1970;1:259–262.
3. Zeldowicz LR, Huberman J. Long-term therapy of Parkinson's disease with amantadine, alone and combined with levodopa. *Can Med Assoc J* 1973;109: 588–593.
4. Bauer RB, McHenry JT. Comparison of amantadine, placebo, and levodopa in Parkinson's disease. *Neurology* 1974;24:715–720.
5. Dallos V, Heathfield K, Stone P, et al. Use of amantadine in Parkinson's disease. Results of a double-blind trial. *Br Med J* 1970;4:24–26.
6. Hunter KR, Stern GM, Laurence DR, et al. Amantadine in parkinsonism. *Lancet* 1970;1:1127–1129.
7. Yahr MD, Duvoisin RC. Drug therapy of parkinsonism. *N Engl J Med* 1972;287:20–24.
8. Shannon KM, Goetz CG, Carroll VS, et al. Amantadine and motor fluctuations in chronic Parkinson's disease. *Clin Neuropharmacol* 1987;10:522–526.
9. Kulisevsky J, Tolosa E. Amantadine in Parkinson's disease. In: Koller WC, Paulson G, eds. *Therapy of Parkinson's disease.* New York: Marcel Dekker Inc, 1990: 143–160.
10. Fletcher EA, Redfern PH. The effect of amantadine on the uptake of dopamine and noradrenaline by rat brain homogenates. *J Pharm Pharmacol* 1970;22:957–959.
11. Jackisch R, Link T, Neufang B, et al. Studies on the mechanism of action of the antiparkinsonian drugs memantine and amantadine: no evidence for direct dopaminomimetic or antimuscarinic properties. *Arch Int Pharmacodyn* 1992;320:21–42.
12. Vamvakidès A. Action mechanism of the adamantanes: do their activity on the glutamatergic (NMDA) receptors operate in the expression of their pharmacological profile? *Ann Pharm Fr* 1991;49:249–257.
13. Kornhuber J, Bormann J, Hübers M, et al. Effects of the 1-amino-adamantanes at the MK-801–binding site of the NMDA-receptor–gated ion channel: a human postmortem brain study. *Eur J Pharmacol Mol Pharmacol Sect* 1991;206:297–300.
14. Stoof JC, Booij J, Drukarch B, et al. The anti-parkinsonian drug amantadine inhibits the *N*-methyl-D-aspartic acid–evoked release of acetylcholine from rat neostriatum in a non-competitive way. *Eur J Pharmacol* 1992;213:439–443.
15. Deep P, Dagher A, Sadikot A, et al. Stimulation of dopa decarboxylase activity in striatum of healthy human brain secondary to NMDA receptor antagonism with a low dose of amantadine. *Synapse* 1999;34: 313–318.
16. Greenamyre JT. Glutamatergic influences on the basal ganglia. *Clin Neuropharmacol* 2001;24:65–70.
17. Ravenscroft P, Brotchie J. NMDA receptors in the basal ganglia. *J Anat* 2000;196:577–585.
18. Calon F, Morissette M, Ghribi O, et al. Alteration of glutamate receptors in the striatum of dyskinetic 1-methyl-4-phenyl-1,2,3,6-tetrahydropyridine–treated monkeys following dopamine agonist treatment. *Progr Neuropsychopharmacol Biol Psychiatry* 2001;26:1–12.
19. Meoni P, Bunnemann BH, Kingsbury AE, et al. NMDA NR1 subunit mRNA and glutamate NMDA-sensitive binding are differentially affected in the striatum and pre-frontal cortex of Parkinson's disease patients. *Neuropharmacology* 1999;38:625–633.
20. Chase TN, Oh JD, Blanchet PJ. Neostriatal mechanisms in Parkinson's disease. *Neurology* 1998;51[Suppl]: S30–S35.
21. Chase TN, Oh JD. Striatal dopamine- and glutamate-mediated dysregulation in experimental parkinsonism. *Trends Neurosci* 2000;23[Suppl]:S86–S91.
22. Pollack AE, Strauss JB. Time dependence and role of *N*-methyl-D-aspartate glutamate receptors in the priming of D2-mediated rotational behavior and striatal *Fos* expression in 6-hydroxydopamine lesioned rats. *Brain Res* 1999;827:160–168.
23. Engber TM, Papa SM, Boldry RC, et al. NMDA receptor blockade reverses motor response alterations induced by levodopa. *NeuroReport* 1994;5:2586–2588.
24. Papa SM, Boldry RC, Engber TM, et al. Reversal of levodopa-induced motor fluctuations in experimental parkinsonism by NMDA receptor blockade. *Brain Res* 1995;701:13–18.

25. Marin C, Papa SM, Engber TM, et al. MK801 prevents levodopa-induced motor response alterations in parkinsonian rats. *Brain Res* 1996;736:202–205.
26. Oh JD, Russell D, Vaughan CL, et al. Enhanced tyrosine phosphorylation of striatal NMDA receptor subunits: effect of dopaminergic denervation and L-DOPA administration. *Brain Res* 1998;813:150–159.
27. Papa SM, Chase TN. Levodopa-induced dyskinesias improved by a glutamate antagonist in parkinsonian monkeys. *Ann Neurol* 1996;39:574–578.
28. Greenamyre JT. Pharmacological pallidotomy with glutamate antagonists? *Ann Neurol* 1996;39:557–558.
29. Blanchet PJ, Konitsiotis S, Chase TN. Amantadine reduces levodopa-induced dyskinesias in parkinsonian monkeys. *Mov Disord* 1998;13:798–802.
30. Blanchet PJ, Konitsiotis S, Whittemore ER, et al. Differing effects of *N*-methyl-D-aspartate receptor subtype selective antagonists on dyskinesias in levodopa-treated 1-methyl-4-phenyl-1,2,3,6-tetrahydropyridine monkeys. *J Pharmacol Exp Ther* 1999;290:1034–1040.
31. Adler CH, Stern MB, Vernon G, et al. Amantadine in advanced Parkinson's disease: good use of an old drug. *J Neurol* 1997;244:336–337.
32. Rajput AH, Rajput A, Lang AE, et al. New use for an old drug: amantadine benefits levodopa-induced dyskinesia. *Mov Disord* 1998;13:851.
33. Verhagen Metman L, Del Dotto P, van den Munckhof P, et al. Amantadine as treatment for dyskinesias and motor fluctuations in Parkinson's disease. *Neurology* 1998; 50:1323–1326.
34. Verhagen Metman L, Del Dotto P, LePoole K, et al. Amantadine for levodopa-induced dyskinesias. A 1-year follow-up study. *Arch Neurol* 1999;56:1383–1386.
35. Snow BJ, Macdonald L, Mcauley D, et al. The effect of amantadine on levodopa-induced dyskinesias in Parkinson's disease: a double-blind, placebo-controlled study. *Clin Neuropharmacol* 2000;23:82–85.
36. Luginger E, Wenning GK, Bösch S, et al. Beneficial effects of amantadine on L-dopa–induced dyskinesias in Parkinson's disease. *Mov Disord* 2000;15:873–878.
37. Ruzicka E, Streitová H, Jech R, et al. Amantadine infusion in treatment of motor fluctuations and dyskinesias in Parkinson's disease. *J Neural Transm* 2000;107: 1297–1306.
38. Del Dotto P, Pavese N, Gambaccini G, et al. Intravenous amantadine improves levodopa-induced dyskinesias: an acute double-blind placebo-controlled study. *Mov Disord* 2001;16:515–520.
39. Factor SA, Molho ES, Brown DL. Acute delirium after withdrawal of amantadine in Parkinson's disease. *Neurology* 1998;50:1456–1458.
40. Chen H-S V, Pellegrini JW, Aggarwal SK, et al. Open-channel block of *N*-methyl-D-aspartate (NMDA) responses by memantine: therapeutic advantage against NMDA receptor–mediated neurotoxicity. *J Neurosci* 1992;12:4427–4436.
41. Rojas P, Altagracia M, Kravzov J, et al. Amantadine increases striatal dopamine turnover in MPTP-treated mice. *Drug Dev Res* 1993;29:222–226.
42. Turski L, Bressler K, Löschmann P, et al. Protection of substantia nigra from MPP^+ neurotoxicity by *N*-methyl-D-aspartate antagonists. *Nature* 1991;349:414–418.
43. Bezard E, Stutzmann J-M, Imbert C, et al. Riluzole delayed the appearance of parkinsonian motor abnormalities in a chronic MPTP monkey model. *Eur J Pharmacol* 1998;356:101–104.
44. Uitti RJ, Rajput AH, Ahlskog JE, et al. Amantadine treatment is an independent predictor of improved survival in Parkinson's disease. *Neurology* 1996;46: 1551–1556.

Parkinson's Disease: Advances in Neurology, Vol. 91.
Edited by Ariel Gordin, Seppo Kaakkola, and Heikki Teräväinen
Lippincott Williams & Wilkins, Philadelphia © 2003

26

Are There Clinically Significant Differences between Dopamine Agonists

Fabrizio Stocchi, Laura Vacca and Marco Onofrj*

Institute of Neurology IRCCS "Neuromed" (Is) and University "La Sapienza", Rome, Italy;
**Department of Oncology and Neurosciences, University "GD'annunzio", Chieti, Italy*

Given the limitations of levodopa in the long-term management of Parkinson's disease (PD), dopamine (DA) receptor agonists were introduced in the treatment of this disease in the early 1970s. These agents have diverse physical and chemical properties but share the capacity to stimulate DA receptors and to provide an antiparkinsonian effect.

DA agonists were initially introduced as adjuncts to levodopa for patients with advanced PD (1). Several studies have demonstrated the capacity of these drugs to improve motor fluctuations and to reduce dyskinesia in levodopa-treated parkinsonian patients (2). Moreover, DA agonists provide a levodopa-sparing effect (3,4). However, DA agonists have also been reported as having a clear symptomatic effect when used as monotherapy in patients with *de novo* PD (i.e., patients who had only recently been diagnosed and who had not received any other treatment for the disease) (5). Recently, however, the therapeutic approach to PD has begun to change, and the role of DA agonists has become more prominent (6). Animal and human data have shown that a lower incidence of motor adverse effects is induced by DA agonists compared with levodopa. As a result, the use of DA agonists in early treatment (e.g., use as monotherapy and as an adjuvant to levodopa in patients who have not previously received any other dopaminergic treatment for PD) has been considered.

Today, there are a number of DA agonists on the market, and the question is if there are clinically significant differences between these drugs.

AVAILABLE DOPAMINE AGONISTS

There are currently two general classes of DA agonists available: ergot and non-ergot agents.

Ergot Derivatives

Bromocriptine is the DA agonist that has been in use the longest for the treatment of PD and is still available worldwide. It is a D_2/D_3 receptor agonist, as well as a D_1 receptor and serotonin 5-HT_2 receptor antagonist (7). Pergolide has D_1 and D_2 receptor agonistic properties and no affinity for 5-HT_2 receptors (7,8). Cabergoline is a D_1 and D_2 receptor agonist that is characterized by a very long elimination half-life (24 to 65 hours). Lisuride is a potent ergoline D_2 and D_3 receptor agonist but is only available in Europe and in South America.

Non-ergot Derivatives

The non-ergot DA agonists were developed with the hope that they would have a decreased liability for the toxic effects (e.g., pulmonary and retroperitoneal fibrosis and peripheral vascular effects) that are associated with the ergoline structure. Apomorphine is the oldest DA agonist. It is a potent, short-acting, non-ergoline derivative that is active at D_1 and D_2 receptors. Ropinirole and pramipexole are newer non-ergot derivatives. Ropinirole is a D_2 receptor agonist that also has strong affinity for D_3 receptors. It has negligible affinity for central 5-HT, and 5-HT_2, benzodiazepine, and γ-aminobutyric acid (GABA) receptors, as well as for α and β adrenoceptors (9). Pramipexole has a higher affinity (approximately sevenfold) for D_3 than for D_2 receptors. It also has a low affinity for adrenoceptors, serotonin receptors, and D_4 receptors (10,11).

PHARMACOLOGICAL PROPERTIES

DA agonists act directly on striatal DA receptors. Unlike levodopa, they do not require metabolic conversion to exert their antiparkinsonian effects, so their effects are to a greater extent independent of the degenerative state of the dopaminergic terminals (7, 12,13). Furthermore, DA agonists do not compete with circulating plasma amino acids for absorption and transport into the brain. DA agonists share the capacity to stimulate DA receptors, but they have different affinity for the different receptors. From this point of view, apomorphine differs from all the others for its capacity to stimulate D_1 receptors. Pramipexole has the strongest affinity for D_3 receptors, whereas pergolide shows a weak affinity for D_1 receptors. Table 26.1 outlines the affinity of available agents for DA receptors.

PHARMACOKINETIC PROPERTIES

The pharmacokinetic characteristics of different DA agonists may be an item to differentiate these drugs. The most important factor is the half-life, which varies from the 2 hours of lisuride to the 68 hours of cabergoline. Animal studies have shown that levodopa induces dyskinesias in monkeys treated with the neurotoxin methylphenyltetrahydropyridine (MPTP) more frequently than the DA agonist bromocriptine (14). Both levodopa and bromocriptine provided comparable behavioral benefits in these monkeys. However, all levodopa-treated monkeys rapidly developed dyskinesias, whereas this complication was seen in only one of the bromocriptine-treated animals. Similar observations have been made by other authors in MPTP-treated common marmosets (15). They noted that dyskinesias were much less severe in the animals treated with bromocriptine or ropinirole compared with those treated with levodopa. Dyskinesias developed within 1 to 2 days after treatment with levodopa but were hardly seen in animals treated with bromocriptine or ropinirole. Again, motor benefits were comparable in all groups.

It is likely that this potential to protect against the development of dyskinesia is, at least to some extent, dependent on the elimination half-life of DA agonists because it is only seen with DA agonists that have a relatively long half-life, such as bromocriptine and ropinirole, and is not seen with short-acting DA agonists such as naxagolide or quinpirole (14). This phenomenon is not related solely to the stimulation of D_2 receptors, as dyskinesias can be induced by short-acting D_1 receptor selective DA agonists (CY-208243 and SKF-82958) but does not occur with

TABLE 26.1. *Dopamine receptor affinity of dopamine agonists*

	D_1	D_2	D_3	D_4	D_5
Bromocriptine	–	++	++	+	+
Lisuride	+	+++	+++	?	?
Pergolide	+	+++	+++	?	+
Cabergoline	+	+++	?	?	?
Ropinirole	–	+++	+++	+	–
Pramipexole	–	++	++++	++	?

TABLE 26.2. *Pharmacokinetic characteristics of dopamine agonists*

	Bromocriptine	Lisuride	Pergolide	Pramipexole	Ropinirole	Cabergoline
Usual daily dose	15–60 mg	1–5 mg	1.5–5.0 mg	1.5–4.5 mg	3–24 mg	0.5–6.0 mg
Starting dose	1.25 mg t.i.d.	0.1 mg t.i.d.	0.05 mg t.i.d.	0.125 mg t.i.d.	0.25 mg t.i.d.	0.5 mg q.d.
T_{max} (hr)	1.3–3.0	0.5–1.0	1–2	1–2	1–2	2
$T_{½}$ (hr)	3–7	2	7	8	6	68
Route of elimination	Biliary/fecal	Biliary/fecal	Biliary/fecal	Renal	Hepatic/ renal	Biliary/ fecal

q.d., every day; t.i.d., three times daily.

long-acting D_1 receptor–selective agonists (SKF-38393) (14,15).

The route of elimination is similar for most of the agonists; only pramipexole and partially ropinirole are excreted through the kidneys (Table 26.2).

PHARMACODYNAMICS OF DA AGONISTS: THE LONG-DURATION RESPONSE

As soon as levodopa was introduced into clinical practice for the treatment of PD, it was recognized that the drug had both a short-duration immediate effect (1 to 4 hours) and a long-duration slower action (3 to 5 days) (16,17). In a recent study, we demonstrated that in patients with *de novo* PD, the long-duration action of levodopa may last up to 12 days (18). Thus, despite the short elimination half-life of the drug, patients with PD do not experience fluctuations in motor performance for many years, despite taking two or four daily doses of levodopa. So far, this phenomenon bas been attributed to presynaptic storage and release of DA (16).

We also studied the effect of withdrawal of treatment with the directly acting D_2 receptor agonists in patients with *de novo* PD. After stopping ropinirole, patients deteriorated back to baseline states over 4 to 8 days (18). We repeated the experiment using lisuride, the DA agonist with a very short half-life, in a group of six patients with *de novo* PD (19). When the patients were receiving a stable dose and achieving maximum symptomatic benefit, lisuride was substituted with placebo and the change in symptoms was scored. Both the patients and the neurologist performing the scoring were blind to the treatment. Once on placebo, the patients deteriorated back to baseline state over 7 to 12 days (mean ± SD, 9.0 ± 1.9 days). Recently, we repeated the same experiment using cabergoline, the DA agonist with the longest half-life, in a different group of six *de novo* parkinsonian patients with similar clinical characteristics of the previous group. When patients were switched from cabergoline to placebo, they deteriorated back to baseline states over 5 to 9 days (mean, 6.6 ± 1.36 days). Cabergoline induces a shorter long-duration response compared with lisuride. This may be due to a reduced postsynaptic hypersensitivity induced by this long-acting drug (20) (Fig. 26.1).

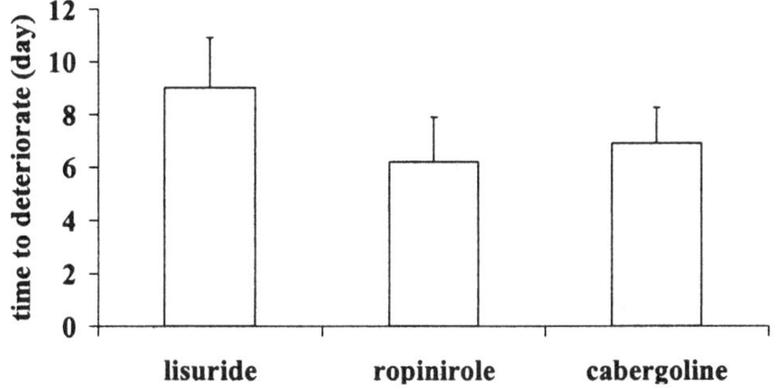

FIGURE 26.1. Dopamine agonists and the long-duration effect: time to deteriorate back to baseline after stopping the drugs (mean ±SD).

From these results it can be concluded that DA agonists have long-duration effects that are similar to the effects of levodopa. Thus, this phenomenon may be due to postsynaptic effects and not only to a change in the presynaptic storage compartment. As a consequence of this phenomenon, the absolute elimination half-lives of the different DA agonists may not be relevant when the drugs are used in patients with early parkinsonism, but it may influence the length of the long-duration response.

INCIDENCE OF MOTOR COMPLICATIONS

Clinical Studies

The available laboratory observations suggest that DA agonists may be less likely to induce motor complications in patients with PD than levodopa. Indeed, clinical information is available to suggest that this is the case.

Montastruc et al. (5) performed a pilot study to compare the occurrence of long-term motor complications in patients with PD when the introduction of levodopa was delayed by an initial treatment with high doses of bromocriptine alone. The trial was a prospective, randomized, controlled study comparing 31 patients with *de novo* PD who were initially treated with bromocriptine alone and later switched to a bromocriptine/levodopa combination (B/L group) with 29 other *de novo* patients who were treated with levodopa alone from treatment initiation (L group). The endpoint was the occurrence of the first motor complication (wearing off or dyskinesia). The patients in the B/L group remained on bromocriptine monotherapy for a mean of 2.7 years, after which time levodopa was added. Motor complications and dyskinesias were less severe and appeared later in the B/L group than in the L group (56% of the patients in this group after 4.9 ± 0.5 years of treatment vs. 90% after 2.7 ± 0.5 years). Peak-dose dyskinesias were less frequent in the B/L group of patients (3 vs. 14 cases). Despite their clinical relevance, these studies were neither double blind nor prospective.

The *056 study* (21) was the first prospective, randomized, double-blind, parallel-group study to compare the long-term efficacy and safety of early treatment with a DA agonist with that of levodopa in *de novo* patients. The study involved 268 patients who were treated for 5 years with ropinirole or levodopa. It was completed in January 1999. Patients requiring dopaminergic therapy were randomized to receive either ropinirole or levodopa in a ratio of 2 : 1. Patients with insufficient therapeutic benefit could supplement the double-blind medication with open use of adjunct levodopa and continue in the study. Efficacy and complications of therapy were assessed using the Unified Parkinson's Disease Rating Scale (UPDRS) and adverse experience information. Forty-seven percent of ropinirole and 51% of levodopa-treated patients completed all 5 years of the study. Of these, 34% of ropinirole-treated and 64% of levodopa-treated patients did so on monotherapy, although overall more ropinirole-treated patients (51%) than levodopa-treated patients (35%) were given adjunct open levodopa at any point during the 5 years. The incidence of dyskinesias before administration of any adjunct open levodopa was 5% in those receiving ropinirole and 36% in those receiving levodopa (odds ratio [OR], 15.2; 95% confidence interval [CI], 6.2–36.9; $p < .0001$). The incidence of dyskinesias in the ropinirole and levodopa groups, regardless of whether or not adjunct open levodopa was used, was 20% and 46%, respectively (OR, 3.8; 95% CI, 2.1–6.9; $p < .0001$). The mean activities of daily living (ADL) scores (UPDRS Part II) remained similar in both groups at each time during the study. In those patients completing all 5 years, the mean ADL scores were 9.1 ± 5.8 with ropinirole and 7.2 ± 5 with levodopa.

After the *056 study,* other DA agonists have shown a reduced incidence of dyskinesias compared with levodopa in different trials. The Parkinson Study Group reported the results of a multicenter, parallel-group, double-blind, randomized controlled trial to compare the development of motor complication after initial treatment of early PD with pramipexole versus levodopa (CALM-PD) (22). There were

TABLE 26.3. *Design of controlled studies comparing long-term efficacy and safety of a dopamine agonist and levodopa in* de novo *patients*

	Pramipexole CALM-PD	Cabergoline study 09	Ropinirole study 056
Duration (yr)	2	5	5
Randomization	1:1	1:1	2:1
Patient sample	127 (PX) 131 (LD)	211 (CB) 208 (LD)	179 (RP) 89 (LD)
Dosing of experimental drug	No increase after titration	No increase after titration	Increases allowed all along the study
Concomitant anti-PD drug	Allowed at unchanged doses	Not allowed	Allowed at unchanged doses
Assessment	All motor complications	All motor complications	Only dyskinesias
Imaging	SPECT	NO	NO

CALM-PD, CALM-PD study; CB, cabergoline group; LD, levodopa group; PD, Parkinson's disease; PX, pramipexole group; RP, ropinirole group; SPECT, single-photon emission computed tomography; NO, no imaging study.

301 patients enrolled: 151 received pramipexole and 150 levodopa. At the end of the 3-year study, 128 patients in the pramipexole group and 131 in the levodopa group completed the trial. Initial pramipexole treatment resulted in significantly less development of motor fluctuations (28%) compared with levodopa (51%) (hazard ratio, 0.45; 95% CI, 0.30–0.66; $p < .001$). Similar results were obtained in a 5-year prospective trial with cabergoline versus levodopa and in a shorter study with pergolide (Tables 26.3 and 26.4). The results of these large multinational trials conclusively show that patients with early PD can be successfully managed on DA agonists alone or with a low dose of adjunct levodopa added later for up to many years. Most importantly, the risk of developing dyskinesias was substantially reduced in patients receiving DA agonists, either as monotherapy for the entire study period or in conjunction with a low dose of adjunct levodopa in the latter part of the study, compared with those treated with levodopa from the onset.

Comparison of these studies does not emerge elements that can help differentiate the DA agonists studied—all of them being less likely to induce motor complications than levodopa.

Comparative Studies

Only two comparative studies using DA agonists have been performed. The *053 study,* a prospective, double-blind, parallel-group study, compared the long-term efficacy and safety of ropinirole with bromocriptine over 3 years in patients with early PD with limited or no previous dopaminergic therapy. This study randomized 335 patients; 60% of ropinirole-

TABLE 26.4. *Results of controlled studies comparing long-term efficacy and safety of a dopamine agonist and levodopa in* de novo *patients*

	Pramipexole CALM-PD	Cabergoline study 09	Ropinirole study 056
% reduction in all motor complications	45% (From 51% to 28%)	33% (From 33% to 22%)	Not assessed
% reduction in dyskinesias	70% (From 31% to 10%)	57% (From 21% to 9%)	56% (From 46% to 20%)
UPDRS motor	PX: 3.5 LD: 7 Difference 3.5	CB: 8 LD: 12 Difference 4	RP: 1 LD: 5 Difference 4
UPDRS ADL	PX: 1 LD: 2 Difference 1	CB: 1.5 LD: 3 Difference 1.5	RP: 1 LD: 2.5 Difference 1.5

PD, Parkinson's disease; LD, levodopa group; PX, pramipexole group; CB, cabergoline group; RP, ropinirole group; D, difference between end of study score versus baseline score; UPDRS, Unified Parkinson's Disease Rating Scale; ADL, activities of daily living.

treated and 53% of bromocriptine-treated patients completed the study on the DA agonist alone. Occurrence of adverse experiences in both groups was similar, and both treatments induced marked improvements in the UPDRS scores (ADL and motor score) over the first 12 weeks, which were maintained during the study. After 3 years, patients in the ropinirole group had a mean improvement in motor score of 31% compared with 22% in the bromocriptine group and a significantly better ADL score (23). In a short-term, single-blind, controlled crossover study, the efficacy and safety of pergolide and bromocriptine were compared in 57 patients with a declining response to levodopa therapy, for 12 plus 12 weeks. A significantly greater efficacy was demonstrated by both drugs as adjunctive therapy to levodopa compared with previous treatment of levodopa alone. Pergolide was slightly more effective than bromocriptine according to the score (p = .02) and motor scores (p = .038); there were no differences in dyskinesias, dystonias, or psychoses (24).

Side-effects Profile

The authors reviewed the side effects reported in all the controlled trials published and there was not a significant difference in the side-effects profile between the DA agonists. The only difference was the incidence of swelling of legs, which is associated mostly with the ergot derivatives, and somnolence, which is very rarely associated with cabergoline. However, somnolence deserves a more accurate analysis.

Somnolence and Dopaminergic Drugs

Frucht et al. (25) reported eight cases of "sleep attacks" in parkinsonian patients who had an accident while driving a car. The authors identified the DA agonists (pramipexole and ropinirole) they were taking as the cause of the accidents. Recently, "sleep attacks" have also been described with pergolide, bromocriptine, and levodopa (26,27). However, the term "sleep attack" should not be used because it is not recognized in the sleep disturbance classifications. Sudden-onset somnolence or irresistible somnolence would be more appropriate to define these events, which may be a consequence of excessive daytime sleepiness (EDS). Sleep disturbances are present in 74% to 98% of parkinsonian patients. EDS is common, being present in about 52% of patients. Somnolence is a well-known adverse effect of dopaminergic drugs and may become irresistible in some individuals. We analyzed sleep disturbances in 100 healthy subjects and in 200 parkinsonian patients: 62% of patients experienced EDS (20% alone and 42% associated with nocturnal insomnia) compared with 31% of controls (12% alone and 19% with insomnia). In the group of 39 patients who had experienced EDS only, we analyzed their parkinsonian therapy with particular reference to DA agonists: 23% of patients had levodopa monotherapy, 15% DA agonist monotherapy, and 62% levodopa-plus-agonist–associated therapy. Patients receiving DA agonist therapy (alone or with associated levodopa) experienced EDS with the same percentage (28). Sanjiv et al. (29) studied daytime sleepiness in 160 patients with PD and 40 healthy subjects, comparing the prevalence of EDS in those who were taking levodopa alone, levodopa with bromocriptine, levodopa with ropinirole, and levodopa with pramipexole (40 patients in each group). EDS was significantly lower in the control group of healthy subjects, but no significant differences among the parkinsonian groups were found. The authors concluded that all antiparkinsonian drugs can cause EDS, with no difference in the risks for each drug.

CONCLUSIONS

DA agonists are very effective drugs for the treatment of PD. They improve the quality of life of the patients and delay motor fluctuations when used early in the disease. It is difficult to establish if one agonist is superior to another in terms of clinical efficacy. Indeed, all of them have to be used at the optimal dosage to express their best effectiveness. Three controlled long-term clinical trials have shown that agonist monotherapy delays motor complications. The agonists used in these trials were ropinirole, pramipexole, and cabergoline; therefore, these are the agonists that should be used as a first approach for treatment of parkinsonian patients. In terms of side effects, ergot alkaloid derivatives can cause typical side effects such as fibrosis and more easily induce swelling of legs. The pharmacokinetic profile appears to be an important factor, and agonists with a long half-life are less likely to induce dyskinesias than the ones with a short half-life, with 3 hours being probably the minimum half-life.

All dopaminergic drugs induce somnolence, so the agonists cannot be differentiated according to this effect. From clinical practice, it appears clear that patients tolerate one agonist better than another, and this can influence the clinical response. Therefore, the more agonists are available, the more chances patients have to improve their condition. Moreover, the combination between different agonists still must be explored.

REFERENCES

1. Calne DB, Teychenne PF, Claveria LE, et al. Bromocriptine in parkinsonism. *Br Med J* 1974;4:442–444.
2. Rinne UK. Combined bromocriptine-levodopa therapy early in Parkinson's disease. *Neurology* 1985;35:1196–1198.
3. Olsson JE, and the European Multicentre Trial Group. Bromocriptine and levodopa in early combination in Parkinson's disease: first results of the Collaborative European Multicentre Trial. *Adv Neurol* 1990;53:421–423.
4. Factor SA, Weiner WJ. Early combination therapy with bromocriptine and levodopa in Parkinson's disease. *Mov Disord* 1993;8:257–262.
5. Montastruc JL, Rascol O, Rascol A. A randomized controlled study of bromocriptine versus levodopa in previously untreated parkinsonian patients: a 3 year follow-up. *J Neurol Neurosurg Psychiatry* 1989;52:773–775.
6. Calne DB. Treatment of Parkinson's disease. *N Engl J Med* 1993;329:1021–1027.
7. Goetz GG, Diederich NJ. Dopaminergic agonists for the treatment of Parkinson's disease. *Neurol Clin* 1992;10:527–540.
8. Langtry HD, Clissold SP. Pergolide: a review of its pharmacological properties and therapeutic potential in Parkinson's disease. *Drugs* 1990;39:491–506.
9. Eden RJ, Costall B, Domeney AM, et al. Preclinical pharmacology of ropinirole (SKF 101468-A), a novel D_2 agonist. *Pharmacol Biochem Behav* 1991;38:147–154.
10. Mierau J, Schneider FJ, Ensinger HA, et al. Pramipexole binding and activation of cloned and expressed dopamine D_2, D_3 and D_4 receptors. *Eur J Pharmacol* 1995;290:29–36.
11. Mierau J. Pramipexole: a dopamine-receptor agonist for treatment of Parkinson's disease. *Clin Neuropharmacol* 1995:18[Suppl 1]:195–206.
12. Montastruc JL, Rascol O, Senard JM. Current status of dopamine agonists in Parkinson's disease management. *Drugs* 1993;46:384–393.
13. Uitti RJ, Ahlskog JE. Comparative review of dopamine receptor agonists in Parkinson's disease. *CNS Drugs* 1996;5:369–388.
14. Bedard PJ, DiPaolo T, Falardeau P, et al. Chronic treatment with levodopa but not bromocriptine induces dyskinesia in MPTP-parkinsonian monkeys. Correlation with ^{3}H spiperone binding. *Brain Res* 1986;379:294–299.
15. Jenner P, Tulloch I. The preclinical pharmacology of ropinirole–receptor interactions, antiparkinsonian activity and potential to induce dyskinesia. In: Olanow CW, Obeso JA, eds. *Dopamine agonists in early Parkinson's disease. Beyond the decade of the brain,* vol 2. United Kingdom: Wells Medical Limited, 1997:115–128.
16. Muenter MD, Tyce GM. L-Dopa therapy of Parkinson's disease. Plasma L-dopa concentration, therapeutic response, and side effects. *Mayo Clin Proc* 1971;46:231–239.
17. Kaye JA, Feldman RG. The role of L-dopa holiday in the long term management of Parkinson's disease. *Clin Neuropharmacol* 1986;9:1–13.
18. Barbato L, Stocchi F, Monge A, et al. The long-duration action of levodopa may be due to a post-synaptic effect. *Clin Neuropharmacol* 1997;20:394–401.
19. Stocchi F, Vacca L, Berardelli A, et al. The long-lasting effect and the postsynaptic compartment: a study using a dopamine agonist with a short half-life *Mov Disord* 2001;16:301–305.
20. Stocchi F, Vacca L, Berardelli A, et al. Dopamine agonists and the long duration effect. *Parkinsonism Related Disord* 2001;7[Suppl]:S70.
21. Rascol O, Brooks DJ, Korczyn AD, et al. A five-year study of the incidence of dyskinesia in patients with early Parkinson's disease who were treated with ropinirole or levodopa. *N Engl J Med* 2000;18:1484–1491.
22. Parkinson Study Group. Pramipexole vs levodopa as initial treatment for Parkinson disease: a randomized controlled trial. Parkinson Study Group. *JAMA* 2000;284:1931–1938.
23. Korczyn AD, Brunt ER, Larsen JP, et al. A 3-year randomized trial of ropinirole and bromocriptine in early Parkinson's disease. The 053 Study Group. *Neurology* 1999;53:364–370.
24. Pezzoli G, Martignoni E, Pacchetti C, et al. Pergolide compared with bromocriptine in Parkinson's disease: a multicenter, crossover, controlled study. *Mov Disord* 1994;9:431–436.

25. Frucht S, Rogers JD, Greene PE, et al. Falling asleep at the wheel: motor vehicle mishaps in persons taking pramipexole and ropinirole. *Neurology* 1999;52: 1908–1910.
26. Ferreira JJ, Galitzky M, Montastrouc JL, et al. Sleep attacks and Parkinson's disease treatment. *Lancet* 2000; 355:1333–1334.
27. Shapira AH. Sleep attacks (sleep episodes) with pergolide. *Lancet* 2000:355:132–133.
28. Stocchi F, Vacca L, Valente M, et al. Sleep disorders in Parkinson's disease. *Adv Neurol* 2001;86:289–293.
29. Sanjiv CC, Schulzer M, Mark E, et al. Daytime somnolence in patients with Parkinson's disease. *Parkinsonism Related Disord* 2001;7:283–286.

Parkinson's Disease: Advances in Neurology, Vol. 91.
Edited by Ariel Gordin, Seppo Kaakkola, and Heikki Teräväinen
Lippincott Williams & Wilkins, Philadelphia © 2003

27

Dopaminergic Drugs in Development for Parkinson's Disease

Amos D. Korczyn

Sieratzki Chair of Neurology, Tel-Aviv University Medical School, Ramat-Aviv, Israel

Although deficiencies in several neurotransmitters have been identified in Parkinson's disease (PD), undoubtedly the main one relates to the dopaminergic system. Dopamine (DA) loss occurs predominantly in the nigrostriatal system, and the degree of reduction in other systems (particularly the mesolimbic) and its clinical significance are still not well understood.

Levodopa remains the "gold standard" of PD therapy. It is the most potent antiparkinsonian drug available. The miraculous effects of levodopa in PD are based on the following facts:

1. Substantia nigra neurons release DA tonically, rather than in a phasic manner.
2. After degeneration of the nigrostriatal system, there is little change in postsynaptic sensitivity of DA receptors (1).
3. Levodopa crosses the blood–brain barrier through an efficient carrier-mediated mechanism.

Although levodopa is extremely effective at the early and intermediate stages of PD, clearly the main drug effects are on the motor system, but even these are limited, affecting bradykinesia and rigidity with a lesser effect on tremor and freezing, even less (and sometimes detrimental) effects on affective, autonomic, and cognitive changes accompanying the disease from its onset. As the disease advances, these limitations are highlighted. Although levodopa maintains its effect, higher doses are required to compensate for the increasing loss of endogenous DA.

Several problems emanate relating to the use of levodopa at the advanced stage:

1. Higher doses affect nonmotor systems, possibly precipitating hallucinations and other psychotic reactions (2).
2. Because of the need for higher doses, the transporting system across the blood–brain barrier approaches its maximal capacity, and this is particularly relevant regarding drug–food interactions. Several amino acids use the same transporter and may compete with levodopa access, for example, after a high-protein meal.
3. Arguably, levodopa itself may be toxic to remaining dopaminergic neurons through the oxidative formation of reactive metabolites.
4. The most significant problems in the motor control of patients with advanced PD are related to the shortening of the duration of the effects of single doses and the appearance of fluctuations and dyskinesias.

Levodopa has a relatively short biological half-life, about 2 to 4 hours. Its much longer clinical effect is due to its absorption into remaining dopaminergic neurons, where it is transformed to DA and stored in vesicles until being released. As the disease advances, this buffering capacity is progressively lost, and DA concentrations at the receptors reflect serum levels of levodopa. Long-term use of levodopa therapy often leads to complications later in the disease, with wearing off, dyskinesias, freezing episodes, and the unpredictable "on-off" fluctuations being the most problematic (1,3). Therefore, patients develop motor fluctuations, converting from "off" to "on" states after drug administration. Later, however, the fluctuations become more complex and lose their relationship to peripheral drug levels. The pathogenesis of these fluctuations is still unclear.

The shortening of the effects of individual doses is partly addressed by prolonging the biological half-life of levodopa, which is coadministered with L-amino acid decarboxylase (dopa decarboxylase) inhibitor and lately with catechol-*O*-methyltransferase (COMT) inhibitors. These agents limit the conversion of levodopa in the periphery, and thus, the effect of the synthesized DA is maintained for 3 to 4 hours or more. However, these agents do not have such a beneficial effect on the later-occurring unpredictable fluctuations, and particularly on the dyskinesias.

The alternative (or complementary) approach to the treatment of these troublesome late complications of the disease is to use direct-acting DA agonists. These agents do not depend on metabolism or carrier systems for absorption from the gastrointestinal tract or through the brain and, thus, should be superior to levodopa. In clinical practice, however, their advantage is marginal, and although motor fluctuations will be reduced, they will rarely be completely suppressed when DA agonists are added to partly replace levodopa. This limited effect is not related to pharmacokinetic factors because even cabergoline, with a half-life of several days, is only slightly better than bromocriptine (4).

Alternatives that delay or reduce the exposure to levodopa have been explored; this trend will probably continue. The main advantage of DA agonists at the early stages of the disease relates to their ability to prevent or at least markedly delay the appearance of dyskinesias (5).

DA agonists are, at present, the most widely used adjunct therapies to levodopa (6). Similar to levodopa, they stimulate DA receptors, albeit with variations in their affinity toward receptor subtypes. Consequently, they can be used to reduce the levodopa dose or to replace levodopa altogether, thereby limiting or abolishing altogether its unwanted effects (7,8). Indeed, there is a heated controversy regarding the preferred initial therapy; the use of DA agonist monotherapy as first-line therapy for PD is increasingly advocated, sparing levodopa for later stages of the disease (5,9–11).

Apomorphine is the most potent DA agonist and the only one that stimulates effectively both D_1 and D_2 receptors (as does DA itself). However, its therapeutic effect is hampered by its complex interindividual pharmacokinetics and pharmacodynamic variability and its narrow therapeutic range. To overcome these difficulties, several attempts to create individualized controlled delivery systems for apomorphine are being explored, such as transdermal iontophoresis (12) and sublingual delivery of apomorphine, for a fast effect to control fluctuations (13,14). In a recent study, carboxymethylcellulose powder of apomorphine was tested as an intranasal sustained-release formulation (15). These newer delivery systems would hopefully enhance its use as a rescue medication in severe cases.

Currently used DA agonists include the "ergot-derived" or "ergoline" DA agonists bromocriptine, cabergoline, lisuride, and pergolide, with chemical structures based on ergot, a plant alkaloid. The newer "non-ergoline" DA agonists including synthetic medications, pramipexole and ropinirole—chemically unrelated to ergot—are being promoted vigorously.

Side effects typical of all DA agonists and levodopa include nausea, vomiting, dizziness, and orthostatic hypotension (16,17). At higher doses, DA agonists may induce confusion, hallucinations, or psychosis (18–20). Sedation and insomnia are other reported side effects of some DA agonists, as well as of levodopa (21,22), and are probably not associated with any specific agonist. Events of compelling urge to sleep (so-called "sleep attacks") of patients treated with DA agonists have been observed (23–25). This is a serious side effect that may cause driving accidents.

Some of the side effects specifically linked to the ergot derivatives include digital or coronary vasospasm, as well as pleuropulmonary and retroperitoneal fibrosis (26). These are not associated with the newer and safer "non-ergoline" DA agonist ropinirole and pramipexole (27).

In addition, novel delivery systems are being tested, to overcome the devastating "on-off" fluctuations and dyskinesias, such as implanted pumps that release a continuous supply of levodopa (28).

Schwarz Pharma and Discovery Therapeutics are developing a transdermal formulation of the experimental D_2 selective agonist rotigotine (29). It was found to reduce daily levodopa doses by 30% in a multicenter phase IIb trial in mild to severe PD. A phase II efficacy trial also gave encouraging results (30). Levodopa methyl ester and levodopa ethylester—new, highly soluble prodrugs of levodopa—are being evaluated in clinical trials as rescue therapies for severe fluctuations in advanced PD (31,32).

The efficacy of the DA agonists is primarily attributed to their interaction with the D_2 subtype DA receptors, and less, if at all, to the D_1 stimulation. Nevertheless, some interest in pure D_1 agonists still exists, for example, in ABT-431 (33) and BAM-1110 (34), as well as in dinapsoline, which is being developed by Bristol-Myers-Squibb (35,36). The results may direct future research efforts toward developing a combination of D_1 and D_2 agonists.

Table 27.1 summarizes DA agonists currently under development, along with other novel PD therapies.

In addition to drugs acting directly on DA receptors, various agents that could potentially prolong the effects of endogenous DA are being studied. In addition to enzyme inhibitors (specific and nonspecific monoamine oxidase inhibitors and COMT inhibitors), an attempt to block the reuptake of DA into terminals (e.g., brasofensive) has been made. This cocaine-like agent interacts with the DA transporter that is specific to these monoaminergic terminals. However, as these neurons degenerate, the effects of the drug are expected to diminish, so it is doubtful if this approach will lead to a significant clinical benefit.

Several subtypes of DA agonists have been identified. The main antiparkinsonian effect resides with D_2 postsynaptic actions, which are common to all currently marketed agonists. Stimulation of D_1 receptors may also contribute to the antiparkinsonian action (33). The most efficacious DA agonist, apomorphine, has potent D_1 agonist activity, not just D_2. It is, therefore, likely that efforts will continue to use this drug and others.

TABLE 27.1. *Drugs for Parkinson's disease in clinical development*

Name	Phase	Originator
Apomorphine sublingual	Phase III	
CHF 1301 (levodopa ethylester, levodopa prodrug)	Registered in Italy	Chiesi
TV 1203 (levodopa ethylester dopamine agonist, levodopa Pharmaceuticals pro-drug)	Phase II	Teva
Rotigotine (N 0923, SP 962) transdermal formulation D_2 agonist Therapeutics/Schwarz	Phase III	Discovery Pharma
PNU 95666 D_2 agonist	Phase II	Pharmacia
Sumarinole D_2 agonist	Phase II	
Talipexole α_2 adrenoreceptor agonist, D_2 agonist	Launched in Japan	Boehringer Ingelheim

D_2-type receptors include, in addition to D_2 itself, D_3 and D_4 subtypes. Their function is still unknown. Several of the DA agonists are known to interact with these receptors (although no assay exists that will say whether this is an agonist or antagonist) (37). This point may be of major importance, if claims of neuroprotective effects of D_3 agonism are confirmed (37,38).

With the progressive loss of dopaminergic neurons, a greater burden is placed on remaining ones, which may, in turn, cause them to degenerate further, perhaps through the production of excessive amounts of DA, which in turn metabolizes intracellularly into toxic products. Treatment with direct-acting DA agonists reduces the need for the release of endogenous DA. The agonist interacts with presynaptic D_2 auto-receptors on dopaminergic terminals, which inhibit DA release. This probably underlies the "neuroprotective" effect of DA. It is still unclear, however, whether there are any special attributes to these auto-receptors. If such will be discovered (and these could be either qualitative or quantitative vs. the postsynaptic DA receptors), this will lead to attempts to stimulate these receptors selectively.

A basic issue is whether PD is indeed one disease. Because its pathogenesis is unknown, it should be viewed as a group of disorders with common manifestations (clinical and pathological) (39). For example, sporadic, toxic, and genetic patients develop the disease through different mechanisms. Although it is still not clear whether this reflects on disease therapy, it may well be that the elucidation of specific diseases, presently grouped as "Parkinson's diseases" will lead to a more targeted therapeutic strategy.

REFERENCES

1. Korczyn AD. Pathophysiology of drug-induced dyskinesias. *Neuropharmacology* 1973;11:601–607.
2. Korczyn AD. Hallucinations in Parkinson's disease. *Lancet* 2001;358:1031–1032.
3. Giladi N, Nisipeanu P, Rabey JM, et al. Freezing of gait in patients with advanced Parkinson's disease. *J Neural Transm* 2001;108:53–61.
4. Inzelberg R, Nisipeanu P, Rabey JM, et al. Double-blind comparison of cabergoline and bromocriptine in Parkinson's disease patients with motor fluctuations. *Neurology* 1996;47:785–788.
5. Rascol O, Brooks DJ, Korczyn A, et al. A five-year study of the incidence of dyskinesia in patients with early Parkinson's disease who were treated with ropinirole or levodopa. *N Engl J Med* 2000;342:1484–1491.
6. Korczyn AD, Nisipeanu P. Newer therapies for Parkinson's disease. *Neurol Neurochir Pol* 1996;30[Suppl 2]: 105–111.
7. Jenner P. The rationale for the use of dopamine agonists in Parkinson's disease. *Neurology* 1995;45[Suppl]:S6–S12.
8. Watts RL. The role of dopamine agonists in early Parkinson's disease. *Neurology* 1997;49[Suppl]:S34–S48.
9. Montastruc JL, Rascol O, Senard JM. Treatment of Parkinson's disease should begin with a dopamine agonist. *Mov Disord* 1999;14:725–730.
10. Hubble JP, Koller WG, Gutler NR, et al. Pramipexole in patients with early Parkinson's disease. *Clin Neuropharmacol* 1995;18:338–370.
11. Korczyn AD, Brunt ER, Larsen A, et al. A 3-year randomized trial of ropinirole and bromocriptine in early Parkinson's disease. *Neurology* 1999;53:364–370.
12. Danhof M, Van der Geest R, VanLaar T, et al. An integrated pharmacokinetic-pharmacodynamic approach to optimization of R-apomorphine delivery in Parkinson's disease. *Adv Drug Deliv Rev* 1998;33:253–263.
13. Ondo W, Hunter G, Almaguer M, et al. A novel sublingual apomorphine treatment for patients with fluctuating Parkinson's disease. *Mov Disord* 1999;14:664–668.
14. Montastruc JL, Rascol O, Senard JM, et al. Sublingual apomorphine: a new pharmacological approach in Parkinson's disease? *J Neural Transm* 1995;45[Suppl]:157–161.
15. Ikechukwu Ugwoke M, Kaufman M, Verbeke N, et al. Intranasal bioavailability of apomorphine from carboxymethylcellulose-based drug delivery systems. *Int J Pharm* 2000;202:125–131.
16. Korczyn AD. Autonomic nervous system disturbances in Parkinson's disease. *Adv Neurol* 1990;53:463–468.
17. Kujawa KA, Leurgans S, Raman R, et al. Dopamine agonists and orthostatic hypotension in Parkinson's disease. *Neurology* 1999;52[Suppl 2]:A407.
18. Moskovitz C, Moses H, Klawans HL. Levodopa-induced psychosis: a kindling phenomenon. *Am J Psychiatry* 1978;135:669–675.
19. Saint-Cyr JA, Taylor AE, Lang AE. Neuropsychological and psychiatric side effects in the treatment of Parkinson's disease. *Neurology* 1993;43[Suppl 6]:S47–S52.
20. Goetz CG, Vogel G, Tanner CM, et al. Early dopaminergic drug-induced hallucinations in parkinsonian patients. *Neurology* 1998;51:811–814.
21. Nausieda PA, Weiner WJ, Kaplan LR, et al. Sleep disruption in the course of chronic levodopa therapy: an early feature of the levodopa psychosis. *Clin Neuropharmacol* 1982;5:183–194.
22. Ferreira JJ, Thalamas G, Montastruc JL, et al. Levodopa monotherapy can induce "sleep attacks" in Parkinson's disease patients. *J Neurol* 2001;248:426–427.
23. Frucht S, Rogers JD, Greene PE, et al. Falling asleep at the wheel: motor vehicle mishaps in persons taking pramipexole and ropinirole. *Neurology* 1995;52: 1908–1910.
24. Olanow CW, Schapira AH, Roth T. Waking up to sleep episodes in Parkinson's disease. *Mov Disord* 2000;15: 212–215.
25. Ryan M, Slevin JT, Wells A. Non-ergot dopamine ago-

nists-induced sleep attacks. *Pharmacotherapy* 2000;6: 724–726.

26. Ling LH, Ahlskog JE, Munger TM, et al. Constrictive pericarditis and pleuropulmonary disease linked to ergot dopamine agonist therapy (cabergoline) for Parkinson's disease. *Mayo Clin Proc* 1999;74:371–375.
27. Bressman SB, Shulman LM, Tanner CM, et al. Long-term safety and efficacy of pramipexole in early Parkinson's disease. *Neurology* 1999;52[Suppl 2]:A261.
28. Trugman JM, Hubbard CA, Bennett JP. Dose-related effects of continuous levodopa infusion in rats with unilateral lesions of the substantia nigra. *Brain Res* 1996; 725:177–183.
29. Roberts JW, et al. D_2 agonist N-0923 treatment of Parkinson's disease. *Neurology* 1994;44[Suppl 2]:244.
30. Hutton JT, Chase T, Verhage L, et al. Transdermal dopamine D_2 receptor agonist therapy with N-0923 TDS in Parkinson's disease: a double-blind, placebo-controlled study. *Mov Disord* 1998;13[Suppl 2]:62.
31. Djaldetti R, Melamed E. Levodopa ethylester: a novel rescue therapy for response fluctuations in Parkinson's disease. *Ann Neurol* 1996;39:400–404.
32. Djaldetti R, Giladi N, Peretz-Aharon Y, et al. Oral levodopa ethylester (LDEE) for treatment of response fluctuations in patients with advanced Parkinson's disease: results of a double-blind controlled study. *Mov Disord* 1998;13[Suppl 2]:58.
33. Rascol O, Blin O, Thalamas G, et al. ABT-431, a D_1 receptor agonist prodrug has efficacy in Parkinson's disease. *Ann Neurol* 1999;45:736–741.
34. Uchiumi M, Ochiai K, Nakano T, et al. Phase I study of BAM-1110: single and repeated administration. *Mov Disord* 1996;11[Suppl 1]:163.
35. Doll MK, Nichols DE, Kilts JD, et al. Synthesis and dopaminergic properties of benzo-fused analogues of quinpirole and quinelorane. *J Med Chem* 1999;42: 935–940.
36. Ghosh D, Snyder SE, Watts VJ, et al. 9-Dihydroxy-2,3,7,11b-tetrahydro-1H-naph[1,2,3-de]isoquinoline: a potent full dopamine D_1 agonist containing a rigid-beta-phenyldopamine pharmacophore. *J Med Chem* 1996; 39:549–555.
37. Guttman M, Jaskolka J. The use of pramipexole in Parkinson's disease: are its actions D_3 mediated? *Parkinsonism Related Disord* 2001;7:231–234.
38. Carvey PM, McGuire SO, Ling ZD. Neuroprotective effects of D_3 dopamine receptor agonists. *Parkinsonism Related Disord* 2001;7:213–223.
39. Korczyn AD. Parkinson's disease: one disease entity or many? *J Neural Transm* 1999;56:107–111.

Parkinson's Disease: Advances in Neurology, Vol. 91.
Edited by Ariel Gordin, Seppo Kaakkola, and Heikki Teräväinen
Lippincott Williams & Wilkins, Philadelphia © 2003

28

Potential Nondopaminergic Drugs for Parkinson's Disease

*Monty A. Silverdale, †S. H. Fox, ‡A. R. Crossman, and ‡J. M. Brotchie

**Manchester Movement Disorder Laboratory, Division of Neuroscience, School of Biological Sciences, University of Manchester, Manchester, United Kingdom; †Motac Neuroscience Ltd., Manchester, United Kingdom; and ‡Walton Centre for Neurology and Neurosurgery, Fazakerley, Liverpool, United Kingdom*

Parkinson's disease (PD) is a common neurological condition affecting 0.1% of the general population (1). The treatment of PD was revolutionized when it was shown that PD is caused by degeneration of the dopaminergic nigrostriatal pathway, leading to a loss of dopamine (DA) in the striatum (2,3). This led to the development of DA-based treatments for PD, initially using the DA precursor, levodopa (4), and subsequently with DA receptor agonists (5,6). DA-replacement therapy with levodopa dramatically improves the symptoms of PD, but after several years of treatment, virtually all patients develop motor fluctuations including "wearing off," "on-off" fluctuations, and in particular involuntary movements termed dyskinesias (1,7–9). Although DA receptor agonists have a lower propensity than levodopa to cause dyskinesia (5,10,11), the addition of levodopa to maintain efficacy is generally required, and resulting from this, motor complications, as described, eventually emerge (1,12). In addition, cognitive problems that are exacerbated by dopaminergic drugs may emerge in endstage PD (13,14). These side effects of dopaminergic therapy can be more disabling than the underlying PD itself. Alternative nondopaminergic approaches to the treatment of PD have, therefore, been considered. Furthermore, although DA receptor agonists (DA) have been suggested as being neuroprotective (15), to date, there is no evidence that current therapies can modify the progression of the disease in humans. Novel neuroprotective strategies would therefore dramatically alter the approach to treating PD, were such therapies available. There is emerging evidence that nondopaminergic neurotransmitter and neuromodulatory systems are involved in basal ganglia function and may have a role in the pathophysiology of PD, and in particular the development of dyskinesia. Thus, the use of nondopaminergic therapies as treatments for PD has been increasingly investigated.

Nondopaminergic treatments for PD could have value either as (a) symptomatic treatment, that is, to be given instead of or to supplement levodopa to treat the symptoms of PD without causing motor fluctuations; as (b) adjuvant treatment, that is, given with levodopa to alleviate motor fluctuations, in particular dyskinesia; or as (c) neuroprotectants, to reduce or halt ongoing loss of dopaminergic neurons within the substantia nigra pars compacta (SNpc).

BASAL GANGLIA FUNCTIONAL ANATOMY

To appreciate the rationale underpinning the development of nondopaminergic treatments for PD, one must understand the functional anatomy of the basal ganglia, and how this (a) is affected by DA depletion after nigrostriatal degeneration, (b) is affected by repeated DA replacement in PD leading to dyskinesia, and (c) is involved in the progression of neurodegeneration in PD. A simplified view of the functional anatomy of the basal ganglia is shown in Figure 28.1A.

The basal ganglia is a group of subcortical nuclei. They consist of the striatum (containing the caudate nucleus and the putamen), the globus pallidus (which is divided into a medial or internal segment [GPm or GPi]) and a lateral or external segment (GPi or GPe), the subthalamic nucleus (STN), and the substantia nigra (the SNpc and the substantia nigra pars reticulata [SNpr]) (Fig. 28.1). The striatum is the main input region of the basal ganglia and it receives dopaminergic afferents from the SNpc (the nigrostriatal pathway) (16) and glutamatergic afferents from the cerebral cortex (the corticostriatal pathway) (17). The output regions of the basal ganglia are the SNpr and the GPi. These project to non–basal ganglia regions involved in the control of movement, such as the thalamus and the pedunculopontine nucleus (18,19). More than 90% of the neurons in the striatum are medium spiny projection neurons, which are inhibitory neurons using the neurotransmitter γ-aminobutyric acid (GABA) (20). Medium spiny neurons expressing predominantly the D_1 receptor project to the output regions of the basal ganglia (the SNpr and the GPi) (21). This pathway has been termed the direct pathway. Medium spiny neurons expressing predominantly the D_2 receptor project to the GPe (21). The GPe sends an inhibitory GABAergic projection to the STN, which in turn sends an excitatory projection to both the output nuclei (the GPi and the SNpr) and the SNpc. The pathway (striatum–GPe–STN–GPi/SNpr) is termed the indirect pathway (22). The basal ganglia output projections inhibit excitatory thalamocortical projections, thereby inhibiting movement (23–27).

This relatively simple model of basal ganglia function has been the subject of some criticism and debate over the past few years (28,29). There are four main criticisms of the model: First, it is clearly an oversimplification because it ignores several other potentially important pathways in the basal ganglia (27); second, there are some medium spiny neurons that express both D_1 and D_2 receptors (30); third, it ignores the pattern of firing in the basal ganglia nuclei because it is now becoming evident that the basal ganglia codes information not simply in firing rate, but also in firing pattern (31); and fourth, it ignores extrastriatal DA (32). More detailed reviews of basal ganglia functional anatomy are provided elsewhere (27,33,34). However, with these reservations in mind, it is clear that the simplified model provides an excellent framework for the understanding of basal ganglia functional anatomy. It has been invaluable to the development of nondopaminergic treatments for PD and will therefore be used throughout the rest of this chapter to illustrate

FIGURE 28.1. A: Functional anatomy of the basal ganglia. (STR, striatum; GPe, external segment of the globus pallidus; STN, subthalamic nucleus; GPi, internal segment of the globus pallidus; SNpr, substantia nigra pars reticulata; SNpc, substantia nigra pars compacta; Th, thalamus.) **B:** Functional anatomy of the basal ganglia in parkinsonism. The activity of the pathways is represented by the thickness of the arrows. Dopamine depletion leads to overactivity of the indirect pathway and underactivity of the direct pathway. Both of these effects lead to overactivity of the basal ganglia output nuclei (GPi and SNpr), which inhibit thalamocortical projections, thereby inhibiting movement. **C:** Functional anatomy of the basal ganglia in dyskinesia. The activity of the pathways is represented by the thickness of the arrows. Dopaminergic stimulation of the "primed" basal ganglia leads to underactivity of the indirect pathway and overactivity of the direct pathway. Both of these effects lead to underactivity of the basal ganglia output nuclei (GPi and SNpr), which disinhibit the thalamocortical projections, thereby potentiating movement.

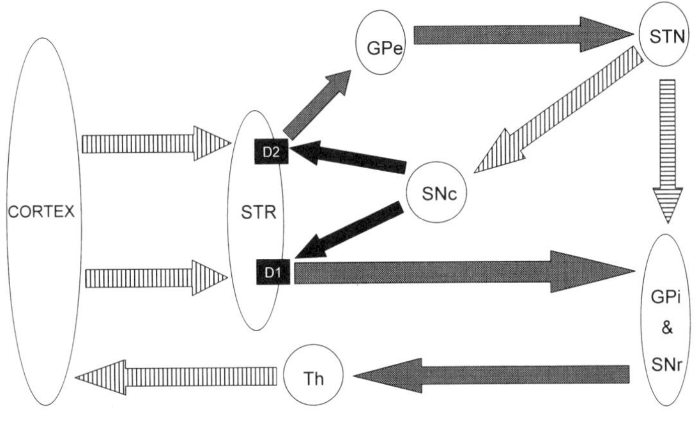

Dopamine

GABA (inhibitory)

A Glutamate (excitatory)

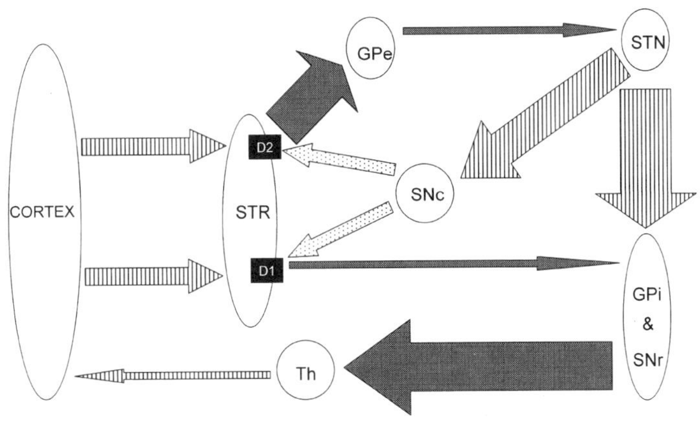

Degenerating dopamine neurons

GABA (inhibitory)

B Glutamate (excitatory)

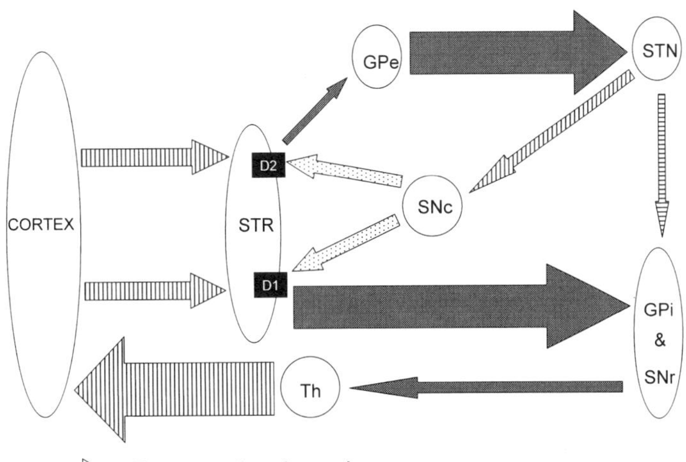

Degenerating dopamine neurons

GABA (inhibitory)

C Glutamate (excitatory)

the rationale underpinning the use of novel therapeutic agents.

Figure 28.1B illustrates an overview of basal ganglia functional anatomy accompanying DA depletion in PD; that is, it defines the proposed pathophysiology of the generation of symptoms in PD. Although the precise role of DA in the basal ganglia is unclear, there is now a great deal of biochemical and electrophysiological evidence that after DA depletion, the D_1 receptor–expressing direct pathway becomes underactive, and the D_2 receptor–expressing indirect pathway becomes overactive (25,35). As shown in Figure 28.1B, underactivity of the direct pathway leads to reduced inhibition of the output nuclei of the basal ganglia, which therefore becomes overactive (23). Overactivity of the indirect striatal GPe pathway reduces the activity of the inhibitory GPe–STN projection. This leads to overactivity of the STN. Overactivity of the excitatory glutamatergic projection from the STN to the output nuclei leads to further overactivity of the output nuclei (23,25,36). Thus, both underactivity of the direct pathway and overactivity of the indirect pathway lead to overactivity of the basal ganglia output nuclei. As these output nuclei inhibit the thalamocortical projections, their overactivity leads to a reduction in thalamocortical activity and a resultant reduction in movement. Reduced thalamocortical activity is thought to be the cause of bradykinesia in PD (24,37). As discussed, the STN is overactive in PD. In the early stages of PD, overactivity of STN inputs to the SNpc may compensate for the loss of dopaminergic neurons by excitation of remaining dopaminergic neurons (38). In the later stages of PD, when there has been a complete loss of dopaminergic neurons in the SNpc, this pathway is likely to be of little functional importance. The putative role of this pathway in neuroprotection is discussed later in this chapter.

When levodopa is first given to a parkinsonian patient, normal movement is essentially restored. However, long-term levodopa treatment in PD leads to a supersensitivity of the basal ganglia called "priming" (39–42). When a primed patient is in the untreated "off" state, the functional anatomy of the basal ganglia still resembles that shown in Fig. 28.1B. However, when levodopa is given to a primed patient, a supersensitive response is elicited, as illustrated in Figure 28.1C, where there is overactivity of the direct pathway and underactivity of the indirect pathway (43). Both of these changes lead to underactivity of the inhibitory basal ganglia output nuclei projections to the thalamus (31,44,45). This leads to overactivity of the excitatory thalamocortical projections, which is thought to be the cause of dyskinesia (46).

The pathogenesis of dyskinesia does not appear to involve changes in DA receptors, as has been reviewed elsewhere (33). However, there is increasing evidence that nondopaminergic neurotransmitters may be involved in the pathophysiology of levodopa-induced dyskinesia (33,47). Thus, abnormalities in glutamate, adenosine, serotonin, opioid, cannabinoid, adrenergic, and cholinergic signaling may be involved in the pathophysiology of parkinsonism and dyskinesia. The neural mechanisms underlying the pathophysiology of PD and levodopa-induced dyskinesia in relation to each of these neurotransmitter systems is discussed here.

As stated, the glutamatergic pathway from the STN to the SNpc becomes overactive in PD (Fig. 28.1B) (38,48). It is known that overactive glutamate transmission can lead to cell death in the postsynaptic neuron via a calcium-dependent mechanism termed excitotoxicity (49). It has, therefore, been hypothesized that overactive glutamatergic STN input to the SNpc in PD may contribute to neuronal cell death in the DA-containing SNpc neurons (48). In fact, the STN is overactive before the appearance of symptoms, and as described already, such overactivity may compensate for lost DA in the early stages of the disease (38). Thus, although the initial insult damaging the SNpc neurons is not well understood, once DA cell loss is initiated, the resultant overactivity of the indirect pathway could establish a vicious cycle

(Fig. 28.2), whereby SNpc degeneration leads (via overactivation of the indirect pathway) to overactivity of the STN and further damage to the SNpc. In support of this, there is evidence from animal studies that glutamate antagonists are neuroprotective (50,51). Indeed, any pharmacological strategy that reduces the activity of STN output to the SNpc could be expected to be neuroprotective by disrupting this vicious cycle (52).

From the above description, it is apparent that abnormalities in nondopaminergic systems contribute to the mechanisms generating parkinsonian symptoms, side effects of current treatment, and the neurodegenerative process itself. Several classes of compounds have potential as drugs to modulate these systems. In the remainder of this chapter, the approaches that currently show the most promise are discussed in turn. Given the nature of the drug-development process, information relating to the stage of development or the interest within a particular pharmaceutical company of a potential product is often not in the public domain. Here, we discuss data available in the public domain, relating to specific compounds, and highlight the pharmaceutical company responsible for the development of such compounds. In so doing, we are not suggesting that such a compound is necessarily still being actively pursued as an antiparkinsonian drug, but we are illustrating recent interest within a company in developing antiparkinsonian agents based on a particular class of drug. Where companies have merged since the conduct of experiments described, the interest of the new entity is highlighted. Second, if a compound has been on license, the company that presently holds an interest in that compound is noted.

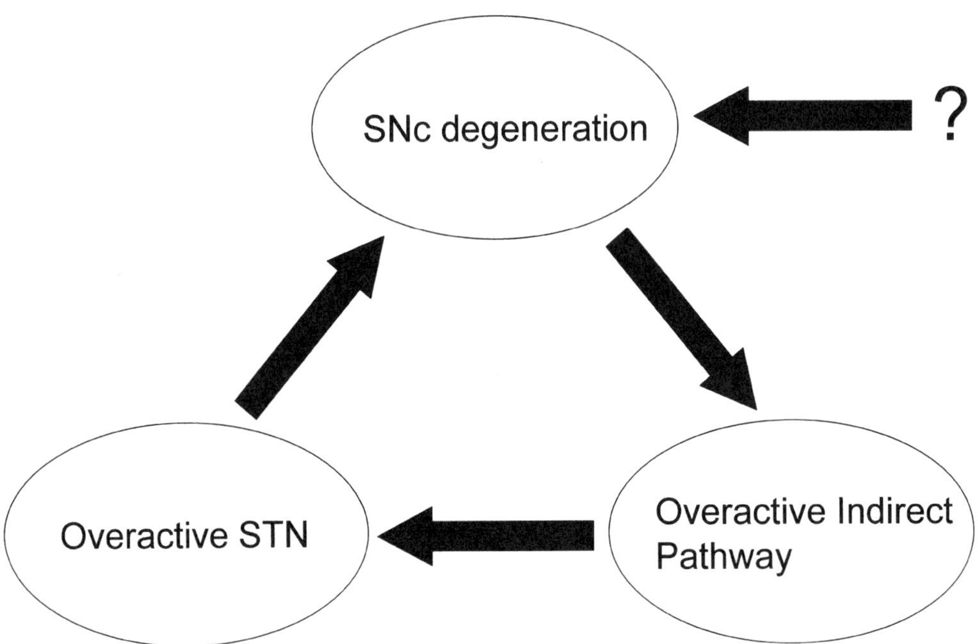

FIGURE 28.2. The "vicious cycle" leading to neurodegeneration in Parkinson's disease. The initial stimulus leading to substantia nigra pars compacta (SNpc) degeneration is unknown and probably represents a range and combination of events. However, as a result of this, the indirect pathway becomes overactive, leading to overactive glutamatergic input from the subthalamic nucleus (STN) to the SNpc. This may lead to excitotoxic damage in the SNpc and further increase the activity of the STN, thereby starting a vicious cycle leading to progressive neurodegeneration.

GLUTAMATE RECEPTOR ANTAGONISTS AND AGENTS ATTENUATING GLUTAMATERGIC TRANSMISSION

Glutamate is the main excitatory neurotransmitter in the brain (53). Glutamate acts on several subtypes of receptors including the inotropic receptors *N*-methyl-D-aspartate (NMDA), α-amino-3-hydroxy-5-methyl-4-isoxazole-propionate (AMPA), and kainate receptors, which are coupled to ion channels (54), as well as the metabotropic receptors (mGluR1 through mGluR8), which are coupled to G proteins (55).

Symptomatic Treatment

Within the basal ganglia, there are two major glutamatergic projections: the cortical input to the striatum and the STN output to the globus pallidus and substantia nigra (Fig. 28.1A). There are also several other potentially important glutamatergic pathways not shown on Figure 28.1A, including thalamic input to the striatum and cortical inputs to the STN (27). In PD, the indirect pathway is overactive. Current models of basal ganglia function predict that the drive for this overactivity comes from the corticostriatal input to the D_2 receptor–expressing striatal neurons (Fig. 28.1). There is evidence that the corticostriatal pathway is not itself overactive but that after DA depletion the D_2 receptor–expressing striatal neurons become hypersensitive to a "normal" glutamate input (23,56,57). This does not appear to be related to changes in glutamate receptor levels (56,58,59) but may be caused by changes in glutamate receptor phosphorylation in these neurons (60,41). In addition, overactivity of the glutamatergic STN projection to the output regions of the basal ganglia, caused by underactivity of the pallidosubthalamic pathway or overactivity of the corticosubthalamic pathway, also contributes to the symptoms of PD (23,36). These observations have led to the development of glutamate receptor antagonists as possible novel therapeutic treatments of PD.

NMDA receptor antagonists exhibit antiparkinsonian effects in several animal models of PD (61–63). However, side effects of NMDA receptor antagonists typically include sedation, memory problems, and ataxia (61,64). The development of glutamate receptor antagonists to treat PD is likely to require selective targeting to those areas of the basal ganglia where there is overactive glutamate neurotransmission, thus avoiding side effects that are thought to arise from areas outside the striatum. There are many subtypes of the NMDA receptor distributed throughout the brain (65). Subtypes are generated by different receptor subunits combining to form the functional receptor. Thus, NMDA receptors are composed of mixtures of two subunit families: NR1 (NR1a through NR1h) and NR2 (NR2A through NR2D) (66). The predominant NMDA receptor expressed on the striatal output neurons contains NR2B subunits (67). Thus, subtype selective NR2B receptor antagonists might be predicted to have an antiparkinsonian action and have minimal side effects, because they would not block transmission at receptors that do not contain NR2B subunits. The NR2B selective NMDA antagonists ifenprodil (Sanofi-Synthelabo) (68) and Ro 25-6981 (Roche) (69) have antiparkinsonian actions equivalent to those of levodopa without causing side effects such as ataxia at therapeutic doses. However, the NR2B selective antagonists Co 101244 (Pfizer) (70) and CI-1041 (Pfizer) (71) do not have antiparkinsonian actions in the methylphenyltetrahydropyridine (MPTP)-lesioned primate. Both ifenprodil and Ro 25-6981 are activity-dependent NMDA receptors antagonists; that is, their ability to block NMDA receptors is related to the level of NMDA receptor activity (72,73). Because striatal NMDA receptor transmission is thought to be overactive in PD (41,74), it is possible that the antiparkinsonian actions of ifenprodil and Ro 25-6981 are related not only to their selectivity for NR2B subunits, but also to their ability to selectively target the overactive striatal NMDA receptors.

The NMDA antagonist MDL 100,453 (Aventis) has a fivefold to tenfold selectivity for NR2A receptors over NR2B (70). It has antiparkinsonian actions in the MPTP primate model, although this may be related to an action outside the striatum, possibly in the output nuclei (70).

AMPA receptor antagonists, including NBQX (Novo Nordisk) (75) and LY 300164 (talampanel, IVAX) (76) also have been claimed to have antiparkinsonian actions in several animal models, although the magnitude of this effect is less than that with levodopa. It has not yet proved possible to develop AMPA receptor antagonists selective for the striatum, as is the case with NMDA antagonists, although such anatomical targeting might not be as necessary for AMPA antagonists because they have been associated with a more acceptable side-effect profile in comparison to NMDA antagonists (77).

As stated, there are eight known metabotropic receptor subtypes (mGluR1 through mGluR8). In rodent models, direct injection of the mGluR2 agonist DCG-IV into the output nuclei has an antiparkinsonian action (78), which may occur through the reduction of glutamate release (79). Although the development of antiparkinsonian agents acting through the metabotropic receptors is at a very early stage, some pharmaceutical companies including Novartis have shown interest in such an approach (80). A greatly increased understanding of the role of metabotropic glutamate receptors in the control of movement is needed before metabotropic agents can be developed as novel therapeutic agents for PD (81).

As yet, only a few glutamate antagonists have been tested in parkinsonian patients. Remacemide (Astra Zeneca) is used in the treatment of epilepsy (82). It is an NMDA receptor antagonist, probably acting within the NMDA receptor ion channel (82). In the reserpine-treated rat model, remacemide had little effect on its own but potentiated the antiakinetic actions of levodopa (83). In the MPTP-lesioned primate, remacemide also potentiated the effects of levodopa (83). A phase II trial in 33 parkinsonian patients showed a nonsignificant trend toward improvement in Unified Parkinson's Disease Rating Scale (UPDRS) motor scores (84). Two large phase II clinical studies have been performed on parkinsonian patients. One trial was performed on patients with early PD who had yet to receive any symptomatic treatment (85). This trial involved 200 patients followed up for 5 weeks. Remacemide was generally well tolerated. Side effects reported included dizziness, nausea, vomiting, somnolence, insomnia, and postural hypotension; 85% of these patients were able to complete the trial, although some required dosage adjustment. The main aim of this trial was to assess tolerability. No symptomatic benefit was seen, in keeping with animal studies, in which remacemide does not have an antiparkinsonian action unless given with levodopa (83). The second trial involved 279 patients with motor fluctuations followed for 7 weeks (64). Remacemide was well tolerated, with similar side effects to those seen in the previous study. A trend toward improvement in UPDRS motor scores and percentage of "on" time was seen, although this did not reach significance. However, it is not clear whether remacemide will progress further in clinical development.

Riluzole (Aventis) is currently used in the treatment of amyotrophic lateral sclerosis (86). Although its mechanism of action is not fully understood, it is known to inhibit glutamate release (87). Riluzole has demonstrated antiparkinsonian actions in animal models (88). A phase II trial to assess the symptomatic benefit of riluzole is underway, but its status remains unclear. The weak NMDA antagonist memantine (Merz) has antiparkinsonian actions in animal models and in patients with PD (89). Amantadine (Merz), which is a weak NMDA antagonist, has been widely used as an antiparkinsonian agent (90). However, such actions are not at a level equivalent to DA-replacement therapy and may be related to an ability to release DA (at least in the early stages of PD), rather than an NMDA receptor–mediated effect (91). The effects of ifenprodil have been tested in a small clinical study, at low doses, but did not show any therapeutic benefit (92). In conclusion, well-tolerated agents, attenuating glutamate transmission have been used in humans but with, at best, moderate antiparkinsonian efficacy. Subtype-selective NMDA or AMPA receptor antagonists show more promise in the preclinical field and are now entering clinical trials.

Antidyskinetic Treatment

In levodopa-induced dyskinesia, the direct striatopallidal pathway is overactive (Fig. 28.1C). According to current concepts of basal ganglia functional anatomy (Fig. 28.1), the drive for this overactivity comes from the corticostriatal input to the D_1-expressing striatal neurons, although the corticostriatal pathway is not itself overactive (43,56). As with the situation with the D_2-expressing striatal neurons in parkinsonism, it is thought that in dyskinesia, the D_1-expressing direct pathway striatal neurons become hypersensitive to a "normal" glutamate input from the cortex. This hypersensitivity may be related to increased glutamate receptor levels, although this has not been reported in all studies (56,58,59,93). Changes in glutamate receptor phosphorylation are more likely to be the cause of this hypersensitivity (42,60). This is reviewed in this volume and elsewhere (41). Since glutamate receptors are thought to become hypersensitive in dyskinesia, the potential antidyskinetic actions of glutamate antagonists have been studied. NMDA antagonists have antidyskinetic actions in animal models, reducing dyskinesia by up to 70% (70,94,95). The AMPA receptor antagonist LY 300164 (talampanel, IVAX) (76) and amantadine (Merz), which is a weak NMDA receptor antagonist (70,90), have both been shown to have antidyskinetic actions when administered in combination with levodopa in the MPTP-lesioned primate model. Concerning NMDA subtype selectivity, the selective NR2B antagonists Co 101244 (70) and CI-1041 (71) have an antidyskinetic action, whereas the NMDA antagonist MDL 100,453 (which shows partial selectivity for the NR2A receptor) exacerbates dyskinesia (70). The antidyskinetic actions of the NR2B selective antagonists are likely to be mediated through an action in the striatum where NR2B receptors are concentrated (67). Antagonizing glutamatergic cortical input to the direct pathway in the striatum would be expected to reduce the activity of the direct pathway, thereby reducing dyskinesia (Fig. 28.1). It is tempting to speculate that the actions of MDL 100,453 may be in the output nuclei (70). Antagonizing the glutamatergic STN input to the output nuclei would be expected to worsen dyskinesia by further reducing the activity of the output nuclei (Fig. 28.1C).

Concerning studies in parkinsonian patients, amantadine is already being used clinically as a treatment for dyskinesia (96). In a small study of six parkinsonian patients, riluzole was well tolerated and patients showed a 30% reduction in dyskinesia (97). Remacemide has been employed in a small phase II study of 33 parkinsonian patients. A trend toward improvement in dyskinesia scores was seen (84). A further larger study investigating the potential antidyskinetic actions of remacemide is currently underway. Ifenprodil has been used, at low doses, in a small study, but patients did not show any reductions in dyskinesia (92).

Neuroprotection

As discussed already, there is increasing evidence that glutamate antagonists may be neuroprotective by blocking the vicious cycle leading to progressive neurodegeneration in the SNpc (Fig. 28.2) (48,50).

Riluzole has been demonstrated to have neuroprotective effects in animal models of PD (51,98). A phase III trial was commenced, though may not be completed, to assess the putative neuroprotective actions of riluzole using single-photon emission computed tomography scans to assess dopaminergic neuron survival.

Thus, glutamate receptor antagonists have potential antiparkinsonian, antidyskinetic, and neuroprotective effects. Several glutamate antagonists are now in development for PD. As noted, subtype-selective glutamate receptor antagonists may be needed to minimize side effects. At present, most glutamatergic drugs in development are nonsubtype selective, although their mechanism of action is such that there is an expectation that they would be associated with a better side-effect profile than most glutamate receptor antagonists.

Several other glutamate antagonists are in development and may have applications in PD. These include ARL-15896AR (Astra Arcus), CNS-1237 (CeNeS), conantokins (Cognetix), and serine racemase (Guilford). (This information is from www.pdindex.com, www.biospace.com, www.clinicaltrials.gov, www.parkinson.org, and www.veritasmedicine.com.)

ADENOSINE A_{2A} RECEPTOR ANTAGONISTS

Symptomatic Treatment

Adenosine A_{2a} receptors are located predominantly on striatal neurons of the indirect pathway (99). Adenosine A_{2a} agonists stimulate the indirect pathway, causing increased GABA release in the GPe, whereas adenosine A_{2a} antagonists inhibit the indirect pathway, reducing GABA release in the GPe (100). Overactive stimulation of NMDA receptors on the indirect pathway occurs in PD (41) (Fig. 28.1B). NMDA receptor stimulation on the indirect pathway has been hypothesized to lead to adenosine release in the striatum and stimulation of A_{2a} receptors with further activation of the indirect pathway (57). Thus, overactivity of the indirect pathway is, in part, due to stimulation of adenosine A_{2a} receptors, and A_{2a} antagonists would therefore be predicted to have an antiparkinsonian action. Several adenosine A_{2a} antagonists have been shown to have antiparkinsonian actions in animal models, including SCH 58261 (Schering–Plough) (101) and DMPX (102). In the MPTP-lesioned primate model, the adenosine A_{2a} receptor antagonist KW-6002 (Kyowa) has an antiparkinsonian effect, inducing motor activity similar to that seen in normal animals (unlike levodopa, which at supraoptimal levels can cause motor activity much higher than that seen in normal animals). Repeated KW-6002 treatment has a sustained benefit without inducing dyskinesia (103). A phase II study investigating the symptomatic benefits of KW-6002 is currently underway. Vernalis is also developing a series of adenosine A_{2a} antagonists for use in PD (www.vernalis.com).

Neuroprotection

Adenosine A_{2a} receptor antagonists may indirectly reduce the activity of the potentially excitotoxic STN–SNpc pathway, by reducing the activity of the indirect pathway (Fig. 28.2). Such an action may be predicted to be neuroprotective (48). Indeed, in the MPTP-lesioned mouse model of PD, the A_{2a} antagonists KW-6002, SCH 58261, and DMPX were all shown to slow neurodegeneration (52). Interestingly, caffeine at doses similar to those found in one cup of coffee was also shown to slow neurodegeneration (52). Caffeine is an adenosine antagonist (104), and this may explain why coffee drinkers have a lower incidence of PD (105).

SEROTONERGIC DRUGS

Symptomatic Treatment

The basal ganglia receives a serotonergic (5-HT) input from the brainstem dorsal raphe nucleus. This projection innervates the striatum and the output regions of the basal ganglia, the SNpr and the globus pallidus. This latter projection is particularly large and of great interest, given that overactivity of the SNpr and the GPi occurs in PD (Fig. 28.1B). Within the SNpr, there are three predominant 5-HT receptors, $5\text{-}HT_{1B}$, $5\text{-}HT_{2C}$ and $5\text{-}HT_4$. Within the central nervous system, the $5\text{-}HT_{2C}$ receptor is located with its highest concentration in the GPi and SNpr (106). Thus, selective targeting of serotonin neurotransmission within the output regions of the basal ganglia might be achievable by targeting the 5-HT_{2C} receptor and may influence motor control without causing side effects. Increased 5-HT_{2C} receptor binding has been demonstrated in the SNpr in postmortem brain tissue from parkinsonian patients (107). No change in 5-HT_{1B} or 5-HT_4 receptors has been demonstrated in postmortem brain tissue from parkinsonian patients (108,109). That antagonism of 5-HT_{2C} receptors may form the basis of a treatment for PD, is suggested by findings that the 5-HT_{2C} receptor knockout mouse displays spontaneous hyperlocomotion (110). Furthermore, selective 5-HT_{2C} receptor antagonists have been shown to potentiate the antiparkinsonian action of D_1 and D_2 receptor agonists in rodent models of parkinsonism via an action in the SNpr (111–113), whereas the selective 5-HT_{2C} receptor antagonist SB-228357 has been shown to reduce haloperidol-induced catalepsy (114). To date, no selective 5-HT_{2C} receptor antagonists are in development for the symptomatic treatment of PD, although this is a target that should attract significant attention.

Although selective 5-HT_{2C} compounds are not available, a number of "atypical" neuroleptic agents are used in the treatment of psychotic symptoms in PD. As well as being antagonists at D_2 and D_4 receptors, these agents act as 5-HT_{2A} receptor antagonists, and the relatively high 5-HT compared with D_2 antagonist properties is thought to underlie the lack of extrapyramidal side effects (115). A metabolite of clozapine, normethylclozapine, is a 5-HT_{2C} receptor antagonist (116), so blockade of 5-HT_{2C} receptors may account for the reduced potential to exacerbate parkinsonism with clozapine unlike that seen with other so-called atypical neuroleptics (e.g., olanzapine), which are not 5-HT_{2C} antagonists (117,118).

Antidyskinetic Treatment

The selective serotonin reuptake inhibitor (SSRI) fluoxetine has been shown to reduce apomorphine-induced dyskinesia in PD (119). This would suggest that stimulation of 5-HT receptors may reduce levodopa-induced dyskinesia. However, the site of such actions is not clear. SSRI administration results in 5-HT release in striatum and forebrain regions (120,121). 5-HT_{1A} receptor levels are increased in the putamen in the MPTP primate (122). The 5-HT_{1A} receptor agonist sarizotan (EMD 128130, Merck) has been shown to be antidyskinetic in the MPTP-lesioned primate (123) and phase II clinical trials in PD are underway (www.biospace.com).

In addition to its role in parkinsonism, as described already, the 5-HT_{2C} receptor has also been implicated in dyskinesia. Evidence from normal rodents has demonstrated that 5-HT_{2C} receptor agonists induce oral dyskinesia via an action in the STN, an effect blocked by 5-HT_{2C} receptor antagonists (124). Thus, 5-HT_{2C} antagonists may have potential as antidyskinetic and antiparkinsonian agents. As noted, a metabolite of the atypical neuroleptic, clozapine, is a 5-HT_{2C} receptor antagonist. Open-label studies have demonstrated clozapine as effective in reducing levodopa-induced dyskinesia without exacerbating parkinsonism (125,126). Further clinical trials are underway.

The 5-HT_{2A} receptor has also been implicated in dyskinesia. 5-HT_{2A} receptors are localized on medium spiny neurons in the striatum (127). As noted, the atypical neuroleptics clozapine and quetiapine are both 5-HT_{2A} receptor antagonists (115). Quetiapine has been shown to reduce levodopa-induced dyskinesia in the MPTP-lesioned primate (128), and the antidyskinetic actions of clozapine may involve 5-HT_{2A} receptor antagonism. The mechanism of action of these atypical neuroleptics probably involves a combination of relative activity at 5-HT and DA receptors. Further work is required to delineate the precise subtype and site of action.

OPIOID RECEPTOR ANTAGONISTS

Opioid peptides are involved in many aspects of basal ganglia function (129). The striatopallidal GABAergic projection neurons are segregated with respect to the opioid peptides used as co-transmitters. Thus, the striatal neurons of the indirect pathway, projecting to the GPe, express enkephalins derived from the high-molecular-weight precursor, preproenkephalin A (PPE-A). In contrast, the striatal neurons of the direct pathway, projecting to the output neurons of the basal ganglia (GPi and SNpr), use opioid peptides including dynorphin, derived from preproenkephalin B (PPE-B) (129,130).

Symptomatic Treatment

Increased PPE-A production by the indirect pathway occurs after DA depletion (21,131). Recently, it has been suggested that increased PPE-A synthesis represents one of the mechanisms that compensates for the loss of DA during the period of the progressive neurodegenerative process when there is significant DA loss, but symptoms are not apparent (131). Efforts to enhance opioid transmission, specifically by stimulating δ-opioid receptors with the selective agonist SNC 80 (132), have been shown to attenuate parkinsonian symptoms in rodent and primate models of PD. It is unclear whether such agents are currently under development for PD, but some pharmaceutical industry activity has been demonstrated in rodent models of PD (Astra Zeneca) (133).

Antidyskinetic Treatment

In animal models of levodopa-induced dyskinesia, there is increased expression of PPE-A and PPE-B within the striatum (134). In addition, in humans, positron emission tomography has demonstrated increased opioid neuropeptide transmission in the basal ganglia of patients with PD with levodopa-induced dyskinesia when compared with nondyskinetic levodopa-treated patients (135). These findings would suggest that increased opioid neurotransmission may be involved in the neural mechanisms underlying levodopa-induced dyskinesia. Increased release of enkephalin from terminals of the indirect pathway neurons in the GPe reduces GABA release via Δ-opioid receptors (136). Increased release of opioid peptides from terminals of the direct pathway neurons in the output nuclei (GPi and SNpr) may increase GABA release via activation of the μ-opioid receptor (137). Both of these actions would be expected to reduce the activity of the basal ganglia output neurons, contributing to the mechanisms of dyskinesia (Fig. 28.1C). Thus, opioid receptor antagonists have been studied as potential novel treatments of dyskinesia. Indeed, opioid receptor antagonists reduce levodopa-induced dyskinesia in the MPTP-lesioned primate (138). This effect was seen with μ-opioid and δ-opioid receptor antagonists, rather than κ receptor antagonists. In patients, beneficial effects have been seen in some, but not all, studies. Two open-label studies have reported an antidyskinetic action of the nonsubtype-selective opioid receptor antagonist, naloxone (139,140). However, oral administration of naltrexone, a longer acting analogue of naloxone, was ineffective or had minimal effect in alleviating levodopa- or apomorphine-induced dyskinesias (141,142). These negative results may be related to insufficient plasma levels of the drugs and/or lack of subtype selectivity.

A phase II "proof of principle," double-blind, placebo-controlled trial of the efficacy of nonsubtype-selective opioid antagonists is underway. This study is using intravenous naloxone at sufficient dose to block neuronal opioid receptors, to determine whether opioid receptor antagonists can reduce levodopa-induced dyskinesia in parkinsonian patients.

CANNABINOIDS

The basal ganglia contain the highest concentrations of endogenous cannabinoids (endocannabinoids) and cannabinoid receptors within the brain (143,144). Cannabinoids are thought to act as neuromodulators and have been implicated in diverse functions such as movement, cognition, pain, and immunomodulation (145). Within the basal ganglia, endocannabinoids are released by neurons of both the direct and the indirect pathway (144).

Symptomatic Treatment

Stimulation of cannabinoid receptors has been shown to block GABA reuptake, thereby potentiating the effects of GABA (146,147). Cannabinoid receptor stimulation also reduces GABA release in the output nuclei of the basal ganglia (148) and glutamate release in the striatum (149) and has a range of other neuromodulatory effects (145,150). Cannabinoids are released in response to depolarization and calcium influx in an activity-dependent manner (151). In PD, the indirect pathway is overactive, so one would expect increased endocannabinoid release from the indirect pathway terminals in the GPe. Recent studies have provided evidence for both increased release of endocannabinoids (146) and increased stimulation of cannabinoid receptors in the GPe (152) in the reserpine-treated rat model of PD. One potential effect of activating cannabinoid receptors in PD would be potentiating GABA transmission in the GPe. Increased release of endocannabinoids would thus be expected to contribute to the symptoms of PD (Fig. 28.1B). Cannabinoid receptor antagonists could, therefore, be predicted to have an antiparkinsonian action. In fact, the selective cannabinoid receptor antagonist SR141716A (Sanofi-Synthelabo) has an antiparkinsonian action in the reserpine-treated rat model of PD (144).

Antidyskinetic Treatment

In levodopa-induced dyskinesia, the direct pathway is thought to be overactive, so there may be increased endocannabinoid release in the output nuclei. Potentiation of GABA transmission, by reducing GABA reuptake in the output nuclei, would reduce the activity of the SNpr and GPi, and thus could contribute to the generation of dyskinesia. The cannabinoid receptor antagonist SR141716A significantly reduces levodopa-induced dyskinesia in the MPTP-lesioned primate model (153).

However, the effects of cannabinoids in the basal ganglia are much more complicated than simply reducing GABA uptake in the GPe and GPi. It is likely that targeting several cannabinoid-mediated processes would be beneficial in PD. Indeed, it appears that although antagonists such as SR141716A can have antiparkinsonian and antidyskinetic actions, cannabinoid agonists may also be useful. Thus, the synthetic cannabinoid nabilone significantly reduces levodopa-induced dyskinesia in the MPTP-lesioned primate model of PD (154). This finding has recently been extended to patients, in whom nabilone reduced levodopa-induced dyskinesia in a study on nine patients with PD (155). At antidyskinetic doses, there was no exacerbating effect on parkinsonism in either study. The role of endocannabinoids and cannabinoid receptors in basal ganglia function remains unclear. Further understanding of the role of cannabinoids in basal ganglia function is needed before the development of cannabinoid-based treatments for PD can be realistically achieved. Such an understanding would be of value, because there is much interest within the pharmaceutical industry in using the cannabinoid system as a therapeutic target, for example, HU-211 (Pharmos), tetrahydrocannabinol (GW Pharma), and nabilone (Cambridge Laboratories).

α_2 NORADRENERGIC RECEPTOR ANTAGONISTS

The role of noradrenaline and adrenergic receptors within the basal ganglia remains unclear. However, noradrenergic terminals have been demonstrated within the striatum (156) and postmortem studies have measured noradrenaline in the striatum (157). Lesion studies of noradrenergic pathways result in a reduction in noradrenaline in the nucleus accumbens and substantia nigra (157,158). A functional role for noradrenaline within the striatum is demonstrated by the identification of striatal neurons that alter their firing rates in response to noradrenaline (159). Furthermore, α_{2c}-adrenoceptor agonists reduce striatal cyclic adenosine monophosphate levels (160). However, to date, there are no conclusive studies defining α_2 adrenoceptor subtype changes within the basal ganglia in PD or in patients with levodopa-induced dyskinesias.

Symptomatic Treatment

Even in the absence of a clear understanding of the role of α_2 receptors in basal ganglia function, the selective α_2 receptor antagonist idazoxan (Pierre Fabre) (161) has been shown to extend the antiparkinsonian action of levodopa in MPTP-lesioned primates. There have been two phase IIa studies investigating the actions of idazoxan in parkinsonian patients. In one study, the effect of idazoxan on a levodopa challenge was assessed in 20 parkinsonian patients (162). In the other study, the effect of idazoxan on an apomorphine challenge was assessed in eight patients, although only four patients completed the study due to side effects, including headache, nausea, and vomiting (163). Neither of these studies provided supportive evidence for an extension of "on" time or an antiparkinsonian action with idazoxan. It is thus not clear whether the actions of α_2 antagonists to extend "on" time, observed in nonhuman primates, can be transferred to the clinic.

Antidyskinetic Treatment

The nonselective α_2 adrenoceptor antagonist yohimbine can reduce levodopa-induced dyskinesia in the MPTP-lesioned primate model of PD (164). Similarly, the selective α_2 receptor antagonists idazoxan (161) and JP-1730 (Juvantia Pharma) (165) have antidyskinetic actions in the MPTP-lesioned primate. How this relates to basal ganglia functional anatomy is not yet known, but it may involve an interaction with the direct pathway (166). In the MPTP-lesioned primate, idazoxan reduces the dyskinesia induced by levodopa, but not by apomorphine (167). This suggests either that levodopa acts on α_2 noradrenergic receptors or that the conversion of levodopa to noradrenaline or to another metabolite that can activate α_2 receptors may be involved in the prodyskinetic actions of levodopa. In this respect, the nonhuman primate studies have been predictive of actions in humans. In the two clinical studies mentioned, there was evidence for antidyskinetic properties of idazoxan in combination with levodopa (162), but not with apomorphine (163). Thus, α_2 receptors are an effective target for PD therapy, but a major issue in the development of α_2 receptor antagonists will be tolerability, particularly regarding cardiovascular side effects. Thus, in the study of the effects of idazoxan on apomorphine-induced dyskinesia, 50% of patients failed to complete the trial. Further work is needed to develop the possibility of using α_2 adrenergic receptor antagonists as treatments for dyskinesia. One attractive approach may involve using antagonists selective for the α_{2c} subtype of adrenergic receptors. The basal ganglia has a high concentration of α_{2c} receptors (168), whereas other brain regions, including those responsible for the control of the cardiovascular system, express other α_2 adrenergic receptor subtypes (169).

NICOTINIC RECEPTOR AGONISTS

Nicotinic acetylcholine receptors (nAChRs) are widely distributed throughout the brain. There are particularly high levels in the substantia nigra, thalamus, and cortex (170). Lower levels are seen in the striatum (170). Neuronal nAChRs receptors are ligand-gated ion channels and contain five subunits inserted in the plasma membrane (171). There are a large number of subunit types, including alpha subunits (α_2 through α_7) and beta subunits (β_2 through β_4) (172). nAChRs exist either as homopentamers (containing only one type of alpha subunit) or as heteropentamers (containing at least one type of alpha subunit and one type of beta subunit) (171,172).

Symptomatic Treatment

Postmortem studies in human brain tissue suggest a substantial loss of cholinergic transmission in PD (173). Such reductions may contribute to both the motor and the cognitive symptoms of the disease (174). Nicotinic receptor agonists elicit DA release from the rat striatum (175), suggesting that they may offer symptomatic relief at least in the early stages of the disease where some dopaminergic transmission remains and can be enhanced. In support of this concept, the nicotinic receptor agonist SIB-1765F (MSD) has a mild antiparkinsonian action on its own and potentiates the effects of levodopa in the reserpine-treated rat (176). The nicotinic receptor agonist SIB-1508Y (MSD) has antiparkinsonian actions in the MPTP-lesioned primate (177–178). Nicotine itself has been demonstrated to improve motor and cognitive function in patients with PD (174). However, in a separate study, transdermal nicotine did not affect the motor or affective symptoms of PD (178).

Neuroprotection

Epidemiological studies demonstrate that cigarette smokers have a lower incidence of PD than nonsmokers (179,180). This has led to the suggestion that nicotine may be neuroprotective (181). Nicotinic receptor agonists have been shown to be neuroprotective in several animal models by a poorly understood mechanism that may involve the stimulation of neurotrophic factors (181–183). Targacept in collaboration with Aventis are actively developing nAChR-targeted treatments for PD (www.targacept.com).

CONCLUSIONS

Several novel nondopaminergic compounds are in development for PD. It is now clear that PD is not solely a disease of DA transmission. Although DA replacement has formed the basis of PD therapies for more than three decades, it is unlikely that it will remain the sole target in the coming years.

ACKNOWLEDGMENTS

The authors would like to thank the Medical Research Council (United Kingdom) and the Parkinson Disease Society for their financial support. M. A. Silverdale is supported by a Medical Research Council Clinical Training Fellowship.

REFERENCES

1. Marsden CD. Parkinson's disease. *J Neurol Neurosurg Psychiatry* 1994;57:672–681.
2. Carlsson A, Lindquist M, Magnusson T. 3,4-Dihydroxyphenylalanine and 5-hydroxytryptophan as reserpine antagonists. *Nature* 1957;180:1200.
3. Hornykiewicz O. Dopamine (3-hydroxytyramine) and brain function. *Pharmacol Rev* 1966;18:925–964.
4. Cotzias GC, Van Woert MH, Schiffer LM. Aromatic amino acids and modification of parkinsonism. *N Engl J Med* 1967;276:374–379.
5. Rascol O, Brooks DJ, Korczyn AD, et al. A five-year study of the incidence of dyskinesia in patients with early Parkinson's disease who were treated with ropinirole or levodopa. *N Engl J Med* 2000;342:1484–1491.
6. Montastruc JL, Rascol O, Senard JM. Current status of dopamine agonists in Parkinson's disease management. *Drugs* 1993;46:384–393.
7. Fahn S. "On-off" phenomenon with levodopa therapy in parkinsonism. Clinical and pharmacologic correlations and the effect of intramuscular pyridoxine. *Neurology* 1974;24:431–441.
8. Duvoisin RC. Variations in the "on-off" phenomenon. *Adv Neurol* 1974;5:339–340.
9. Vidailhet M, Bonnet AM, Marconi R, et al. The phenomenology of L-dopa–induced dyskinesias in Parkinson's disease. *Mov Disord* 1999;14[Suppl 1]:13–18.
10. Blanchet P, Bedard PJ, Britton DR, et al. Differential effect of selective D-1 and D-2 dopamine receptor agonists on levodopa-induced dyskinesia in 1-methyl-4-phenyl-1,2,3,6-tetrahydropyridine. *J Pharmacol Exp Ther* 1993;267:275–279.
11. Jenner P. Factors influencing the onset and persistence of dyskinesia in MPTP-treated primates. *Ann Neurol* 2000;47[Suppl 1]:S90–S99.
12. Nutt JG, Obeso JA, Stocchi F. Continuous dopamine-receptor stimulation in advanced Parkinson's disease. *Trends Neurosci* 2000;23[Suppl]:S109–S115.
13. Damasio AR, Lobo-Antunes J, Macedo C. Psychiatric aspects in parkinsonism treated with L-dopa. *J Neurol Neurosurg Psychiatry* 1971;34:502–507.
14. Waters CH. Managing the late complications of Parkinson's disease. *Neurology* 1997;49[Suppl 1]: S49–S57.
15. Olanow CW, Jenner P, Brooks D. Dopamine agonists and neuroprotection in Parkinson's disease. *Ann Neurol* 1998;44[Suppl 1]:S167–S174.
16. Fallon JH, Moore RY. Catecholamine innervation of the basal forebrain, IV: topography of the dopamine projection to the basal forebrain and neostriatum. *J Comp Neurol* 1978;180:545–580.
17. Kunzle H. Bilateral projections from precentral motor cortex to the putamen and other parts of the basal gan-

glia. An autoradiographic study in Macaca fascicularis. *Brain Res* 1975;88:195–209.
18. Parent A, Hazrati LN. Functional anatomy of the basal ganglia, I: the cortico–basal ganglia–thalamocortical loop. *Brain Res Rev* 1995;20:91–127.
19. Alexander GE, Crutcher MD. Functional architecture of basal ganglia circuits: neural substrates of parallel processing. *Trends Neurosci* 1990;13:266–271.
20. Kita H, Kitai ST. Glutamate decarboxylase immunoreactive neurons in rat neostriatum: their morphological types and populations. *Brain Res* 1988;447:346–352.
21. Gerfen CR, Engber TM, Mahan LC, et al. D_1 and D_2 dopamine receptor–regulated gene expression of striatonigral and striatopallidal neurons. *Science* 1990;250: 1429–1432.
22. Gerfen CR. The neostriatal mosaic: multiple levels of compartmental organization. *Trends Neurosci* 1992; 15:133–139.
23. Mitchell IJ, Clarke CE, Boyce S, et al. Neural mechanisms underlying parkinsonian symptoms based upon regional uptake of 2-deoxyglucose in monkeys exposed to 1-methyl-4-phenyl-1,2,3,6-tetrahydropyridine. *Neuroscience* 1989;32:213–226.
24. Rascol O, Sabatini U, Chollet F, et al. Supplementary and primary sensory motor area activity in Parkinson's disease. Regional cerebral blood flow changes during finger movements and effects of apomorphine. *Arch Neurol* 1992;49:144–148.
25. DeLong MR. Primate models of movement disorders of basal ganglia origin. *Trends Neurosci* 1990;13: 281–285.
26. Albin RL, Young AB, Penney JB. The functional anatomy of basal ganglia disorders. *Trends Neurosci* 1989;12:366–375.
27. Bolam JP, Hanley JJ, Booth PA, et al. Synaptic organisation of the basal ganglia. *J Anat* 2000;196:527–542.
28. Chesselet MF, Delfs JM. Basal ganglia and movement disorders: an update. *Trends Neurosci* 1996;19: 417–422.
29. Levy R, Hazrati LN, Herrero MT, et al. Re-evaluation of the functional anatomy of the basal ganglia in normal and parkinsonian states. *Neuroscience* 1997;76: 335–343.
30. Surmeier DJ, Song WJ, Yan Z. Coordinated expression of dopamine receptors in neostriatal medium spiny neurons. *J Neurosci* 1996;16:6579–6591.
31. Boraud T, Bezard E, Bioulac B, et al. Dopamine agonist–induced dyskinesias are correlated to both firing pattern and frequency alterations of pallidal neurones in the MPTP-treated monkey. *Brain* 2001;124: 546–557.
32. Smith Y, Kieval JZ. Anatomy of the dopamine system in the basal ganglia. *Trends Neurosci* 2000;23[Suppl]: S28–S33.
33. Bezard E, Brotchie JM, Gross CE. Pathophysiology of levodopa-induced dyskinesia: potential for new therapies. *Nat Rev Neurosci* 2001;2:577–588.
34. Obeso JA, Rodriguez-Oroz MC, Rodriguez M, et al. Pathophysiology of levodopa-induced dyskinesias in Parkinson's disease: problems with the current model. *Ann Neurol* 2000;47[Suppl 1]:S22–S32.
35. Pan HS, Penney JB, Young AB. Gamma-aminobutyric acid and benzodiazepine receptor changes induced by unilateral 6-hydroxydopamine lesions of the medial forebrain bundle. *J Neurochem* 1985;45:1396–1404.
36. Bergman H, Wichmann T, DeLong MR. Reversal of experimental parkinsonism by lesions of the subthalamic nucleus. *Science* 1990;249:1436–1438.
37. Bezard E, Crossman AR, Gross CE, et al. Structures outside the basal ganglia may compensate for dopamine loss in the presymptomatic stages of Parkinson's disease. *FASEB J* 2001;15:1092–1094.
38. Bezard E, Boraud T, Bioulac B, et al. Compensatory effects of glutamatergic inputs to the substantia nigra pars compacta in experimental parkinsonism. *Neuroscience* 1997;81:399–404.
39. Jenner P. Pathophysiology and biochemistry of dyskinesia: clues for the development of non-dopaminergic treatments. *J Neurol* 2000;247[Suppl 2]:II43–II50.
40. Henry B, Crossman AR, Brotchie JM. Characterization of a rodent model in which to investigate the molecular and cellular mechanisms underlying the pathophysiology of L-dopa–induced dyskinesia. *Adv Neurol* 1998;78:53–61.
41. Chase TN, Oh JD. Striatal mechanisms and pathogenesis of parkinsonian signs and motor complications. *Ann Neurol* 2000;47[Suppl 1]:S122–S129.
42. Oh JD, Vaughan CL, Chase TN. Effect of dopamine denervation and dopamine agonist administration on serine phosphorylation of striatal NMDA receptor subunits. *Brain Res* 1999;821:433–442.
43. Mitchell IJ, Boyce S, Sambrook MA, et al. A 2-deoxyglucose study of the effects of dopamine agonists on the parkinsonian primate brain. Implications for the neural mechanisms that mediate dopamine agonist–induced dyskinesia. *Brain* 1992;115:809–824.
44. Papa SM, Desimone R, Fiorani M, et al. Internal globus pallidus discharge is nearly suppressed during levodopa-induced dyskinesias. *Ann Neurol* 1999;46: 732–738.
45. Vitek JL, Chockkan V, Zhang JY, et al. Neuronal activity in the basal ganglia in patients with generalized dystonia and hemiballismus. *Ann Neurol* 1999;46:22–35.
46. Rascol O, Sabatini U, Brefel C, et al. Cortical motor overactivation in parkinsonian patients with L-dopa–induced peak-dose dyskinesia. *Brain* 1998;121: 527–533.
47. Brotchie JM. Adjuncts to dopamine replacement: a pragmatic approach to reducing the problem of dyskinesia in Parkinson's disease. *Mov Disord* 1998;13: 871–876.
48. Rodriguez MC, Obeso JA, Olanow CW. Subthalamic nucleus-mediated excitotoxicity in Parkinson's disease: a target for neuroprotection. *Ann Neurol* 1998; 44[Suppl 1]:S175–S188.
49. Sattler R, Tymianski M. Molecular mechanisms of calcium-dependent excitotoxicity. *J Mol Med* 2000; 78:3–13.
50. Lange KW, Loschmann PA, Sofic E, et al. The competitive NMDA antagonist CPP protects substantia nigra neurons from MPTP-induced degeneration in primates. *Naunyn Schmiedebergs Arch Pharmacol* 1993; 348:586–592.
51. Bezard E, Stutzmann JM, Imbert C, et al. Riluzole delayed appearance of parkinsonian motor abnormalities in a chronic MPTP monkey model. *Eur J Pharmacol* 1998;356:101–104.
52. Chen JF, Xu K, Petzer JP, et al. Neuroprotection by caffeine and A_{2a} adenosine receptor inactivation in a model of Parkinson's disease. *J Neurosci* 2001;21:RC143.

53. Curtis DR, Phillis JW, Watkins JC. Chemical excitation of spinal neurones. *Nature* 1959;183:611–612.
54. Barnard EA. Inotropic glutamate receptors: new types and new concepts. *Trends Pharmacol Sci* 1997;18: 141–148.
55. Pin JP, De Colle C, Bessis AS, et al. New perspectives for the development of selective metabotropic glutamate receptor ligands. *Eur J Neurol* 1999;375:277–294.
56. Calon F, Morissette M, Ghribi O, et al. Striatal glutamate receptors in dyskinetic MPTP monkeys. *Soc Neurosci Abstracts* 2000;26:1291.
57. Nash JE, Brotchie JM. A common signaling pathway for striatal NMDA and adenosine A_{2a} receptors: implications for the treatment of Parkinson's disease. *J Neurosci* 2000;20:7782–7789.
58. Ravenscroft P, Henry B, Brotchie JM. Striatal NR2B NMDA receptor subunit expression is elevated in the 6-OHDA–lesioned rat model of L-DOPA–induced dyskinesia. *Soc Neurosci Abstracts* 1999;25:1718.
59. Silverdale MA, Crossman AR, Brotchie JM. Striatal AMPA receptor binding is unaltered in the MPTP-lesioned macaque model of Parkinson's disease and dyskinesia. *Exp Neurol* 2001;174:21–28 .
60. Dunah AW, Wang Y, Yasuda RP, et al. Alterations in subunit expression, composition, and phosphorylation of striatal *N*-methyl-D-aspartate glutamate receptors in a rat 6-hydroxydopamine model of Parkinson's disease. *Mol Pharmacol* 2000;57:342–352.
61. Mitchell IJ, Carroll CB. Reversal of parkinsonian symptoms in primates by antagonism of excitatory amino acid transmission: potential mechanisms of action. *Neurosci Biobehav Rev* 1997;21:469–475.
62. Klockgether T, Turski L. NMDA antagonists potentiate antiparkinsonian actions of L-dopa in monoamine-depleted rats. *Ann Neurol* 1990;28:539–546.
63. Nash JE, Hill MP, Brotchie JM. Antiparkinsonian actions of blockade of NR2B-containing NMDA receptors in the reserpine-treated rat. *Exp Neurol* 1999; 155:42–48.
64. Parkinson Study Group. A randomized, controlled trial of remacemide for motor fluctuations in Parkinson's disease. *Neurology* 2001;56:455–462.
65. Cull-Candy S, Brickley S, Farrant M. NMDA receptor subunits: diversity, development and disease. *Curr Opin Neurobiol* 2001;11:327–335.
66. Dingledine R, Borges K, Bowie D, et al. The glutamate receptor ion channels. *Pharmacol Rev* 1999;51:7–61.
67. Standaert DG, Testa CM, Young AB, et al. Organization of *N*-methyl-D-aspartate glutamate receptor gene expression in the basal ganglia of the rat. *J Comp Neurol* 1994;343:1–16.
68. Nash JE, Fox SH, Henry B, et al. Antiparkinsonian actions of ifenprodil in the MPTP-lesioned marmoset model of Parkinson's disease. *Exp Neurol* 2000;165: 136–142.
69. Loschmann PA. The NMDA 2B antagonist Ro 25-6981 is an anti-parkinsonian agent. *Mov Disord* 1997; 15[Suppl]:A525.
70. Blanchet PJ, Konitsiotis S, Whittemore ER, et al. Differing effects of *N*-methyl-D-aspartate receptor subtype selective antagonists on dyskinesias in levodopa-treated 1-methyl-4-phenyl-tetrahydropyridine monkeys. *J Pharmacol Exp Ther* 1999;290:1034–1040.
71. Christoffersen CL, Wright JL, Kesten SR, et al. Effects of CI-1041, a selective NMDA 1A/2B receptor antagonist in MPTP-treated monkeys. *Soc Neurosci Abstracts* 2000;26:A1409.
72. Kew JN, Trube G, Kemp JA. A novel mechanism of activity-dependent NMDA receptor antagonism describes the effect of ifenprodil in rat cultured cortical neurones. *J Physiol* 1996;497:761–772.
73. Fischer G, Mutel V, Trube G, et al. Ro 25-6981, a highly potent and selective blocker of *N*-methyl-D-aspartate receptors containing the NR2B subunit. Characterization *in vitro. J Pharmacol Exp Ther* 1997;283: 1285–1292.
74. Dunah AW, Wang Y, Yasuda RP, et al. Alterations in subunit expression, composition, and phosphorylation of striatal *N*-methyl-D-aspartate glutamate receptors in a rat 6-hydroxydopamine model of Parkinson's disease. *Mol Pharmacol* 2000;57:342–352.
75. Klockgether T, Turski L, Honore T, et al. The AMPA receptor antagonist NBQX has antiparkinsonian effects in monoamine-depleted rats and MPTP-treated monkeys. *Ann Neurol* 1991;30:717–723.
76. Konitsiotis S, Blanchet PJ, Verhagen L, et al. AMPA receptor blockade improves levodopa-induced dyskinesia in MPTP monkeys. *Neurology* 2000;54: 1589–1595.
77. Lees GJ. Pharmacology of AMPA/kainate receptor ligands and their therapeutic potential in neurological and psychiatric disorders. *Drugs* 2000;59:33–78.
78. Dawson L, Chadha A, Megalou M, et al. The group II metabotropic glutamate receptor agonist, DCG-IV, alleviates akinesia following intranigral or intraventricular administration in the reserpine-treated rat. *Br J Pharmacol* 2000;129:541–546.
79. East SJ, Hill MP, Brotchie JM. Metabotropic glutamate receptor agonists inhibit endogenous glutamate release from rat striatal synaptosomes. *Eur J Pharmacol* 1995; 277:117–121.
80. Spooren WP, Gasparini F, Bergmann R, et al. Effects of the prototypical mGlu(5) receptor antagonist 2-methyl-6-(phenylethynyl)-pyridine on rotarod, locomotor activity and rotational responses in unilateral 6-OHDA–lesioned rats. *Eur J Pharmacol* 2000;406: 403–410.
81. Rouse ST, Marino MJ, Bradley SR, et al. Distribution and roles of metabotropic glutamate receptors in the basal ganglia motor circuit: implications for treatment of Parkinson's disease and related disorders. *Pharmacol Ther* 2000;88:427–435.
82. Davies JA. Remacemide hydrochloride: a novel antiepileptic agent. *Gen Pharmacol* 1997;28:499–502.
83. Greenamyre JT, Eller RV, Zhang Z, et al. Antiparkinsonian effects of remacemide hydrochloride, a glutamate antagonist, in rodent and primate models of Parkinson's disease. *Ann Neurol* 1994;35:655–661.
84. Clarke CE, Cooper JA, Holdich TA. A randomized, double-blind, placebo-controlled, ascending-dose tolerability and safety study of remacemide as adjuvant therapy in Parkinson's disease with response fluctuations. *Clin Neuropharmacol* 2001;24:133–138.
85. Parkinson Study Group. A multicenter randomized controlled trial of remacemide hydrochloride as monotherapy for PD. *Neurology* 2000;54:1583–1588.
86. Lacomblez L, Bensimon G, Leigh PN, et al. Dose-ranging study of riluzole in amyotrophic lateral sclerosis. Amyotrophic Lateral Sclerosis/Riluzole Study Group II. *Lancet* 1996;347:1425–1431.

87. Doble A. The pharmacology and mechanism of action of riluzole. *Neurology* 1996;47[Suppl 4]:S233–S241.
88. Starr MS, Starr BS, Kaur S. Stimulation of basal and L-DOPA–induced motor activity by glutamate antagonists in animal models of Parkinson's disease.*Neurosci Biobehav Rev* 1997;21:437–446.
89. Parsons CG, Danysz W, Quack G. Memantine is a clinically well tolerated *N*-methyl-D-aspartate (NMDA) receptor antagonist—a review of preclinical data. *Neuropharmacology* 1999;38:735–767.
90. Stoof JC, Booij J, Drukarch B, et al. The anti-parkinsonian drug amantadine inhibits the *N*-methyl-D-aspartic acid–evoked release of acetylcholine from rat neostriatum in a non-competitive way. *Eur J Pharmacol* 1992;213:439–443.
91. Bailey EV, Stone TW. The mechanism of action of amantadine in parkinsonism: a review. *Arch Int Pharmacodyn Ther* 1975;216:246–262.
92. Montastruc JL, Rascol O, Senard JM, et al. A pilot study of *N*-methyl-D-aspartate (NMDA) antagonist in Parkinson's disease. *J Neurol Neurosurg Psychiatry* 1992;55:630–631.
93. Ulas J, Weihmuller FB, Brunner LC, et al. Selective increase of NMDA-sensitive glutamate binding in the striatum of Parkinson's disease, Alzheimer's disease, and mixed Parkinson's disease/Alzheimer's disease patients: an autoradiographic study. *J Neurosci* 1994;14: 6317–6324.
94. Papa SM, Chase TN. Levodopa-induced dyskinesias improved by a glutamate antagonist in parkinsonian monkeys. *Ann Neurol* 1996;39:574–578.
95. Pollack AE, Strauss JB. Time dependence and role of *N*-methyl-D-aspartate glutamate receptors in the priming of D_2-mediated rotational behavior and striatal *Fos* expression in 6-hydroxydopamine lesioned rats. *Brain Res* 1999;827:160–168.
96. Metman LV, Del Dotto P, LePoole K, et al. Amantadine for levodopa-induced dyskinesias: a 1-year follow-up study. *Arch Neurol* 1999;56:1383–1386.
97. Merims D, Ziv I, Djaldetti R, et al. Riluzole for levodopa-induced dyskinesias in advanced Parkinson's disease. *Lancet* 1999;353:1764–1765.
98. Araki T, Muramatsu Y, Tanaka K, et al. Riluzole (2-amino-6-trifluoromethoxy benzothiazole) attenuates MPTP (1-methyl-4-phenyl-1,2,3,6-tetrahydropyridine) neurotoxicity in mice. *Neurosci Lett* 2001;312:50–54.
99. Schiffmann SN, Jacobs O, Vanderhaeghen JJ. Striatal restricted adenosine A_2 receptor (RDC8) is expressed by enkephalin but not by substance P neurons: an *in situ* hybridization histochemistry study. *J Neurochem* 1991;57:1062–1067.
100. Ochi M, Koga K, Kurokawa M, et al. Systemic administration of adenosine A_{2A} receptor antagonist reverses increased GABA release in the globus pallidus of unilateral 6-hydroxydopamine-lesioned rats: a microdialysis study. *Neuroscience* 2000;100:53–62.
101. Fenu S, Pinna A, Ongini E, et al. Adenosine A_{2A} receptor antagonism potentiates L-DOPA–induced turning behaviour and *c-fos* expression in 6-hydroxydopamine–lesioned rats. *Eur J Pharmacol* 1997;321: 143–147.
102. Jiang H, Jackson-Lewis V, Muthane U, et al. Adenosine receptor antagonists potentiate dopamine receptor agonist-induced rotational behavior in 6-hydroxydopamine-lesioned rats. *Brain Res* 1993;613:347–351.
103. Kanda T, Jackson MJ, Smith LA, et al. Adenosine A_{2A} antagonist: a novel antiparkinsonian agent that does not provoke dyskinesia in parkinsonian monkeys. *Ann Neurol* 1998;43:507–513.
104. Fredholm BB, Battig K, Holmen J, et al. Actions of caffeine in the brain with special reference to factors that contribute to its widespread use. *Pharmacol Rev* 1999;51:83–133.
105. Ross GW, Abbott RD, Petrovitch H, et al. Association of coffee and caffeine intake with the risk of Parkinson's disease. *JAMA* 2000;283:2674–2679.
106. Julius D, MacDermott AB, Axel R, et al. Molecular characterization of a functional cDNA encoding the serotonin 1c receptor. *Science* 1988;241:558–564.
107. Fox SH, Brotchie JM. 5-HT_{2C} receptor binding is increased in the substantia nigra pars reticulata in Parkinson's disease. *Mov Disord* 2000;15:1064–1069.
108. Waeber C, Palacios JM. Serotonin-1 receptor binding sites in the human basal ganglia are decreased in Huntington's chorea but not in Parkinson's disease: a quantitative *in vitro* autoradiography study. *Neuroscience* 1989;32:337–347.
109. Reynolds GP, Mason SL, Meldrum A, et al. 5-Hydroxytryptamine (5-HT) 4 receptors in post mortem human brain tissue: distribution, pharmacology and effects of neurodegenerative diseases. *Br J Pharmacol* 1995; 114:993–998.
110. Tecott LH, Sun LM, Akana SF, et al. Eating disorder and epilepsy in mice lacking 5-HT_{2c} serotonin receptors. *Nature* 1995;374:542–546.
111. Fox SH, Brotchie JM. 5-HT_{2C} receptor antagonists enhance the behavioural response to dopamine D_1 receptor agonists in the 6-hydroxydopamine–lesioned rat. *Eur J Pharmacol* 2000;398:59–64.
112. Fox SH, Moser B, Brotchie JM. Behavioral effects of 5-HT_{2C} receptor antagonism in the substantia nigra zona reticulata of the 6-hydroxydopamine–lesioned rat model of Parkinson's disease. *Exp Neurol* 1998; 151:35–49.
113. Fox S, Brotchie J. Normethylclozapine potentiates the action of quinpirole in the 6-hydroxydopamine lesioned rat. *Eur J Pharmacol* 1996;301:27–30.
114. Reavill C, Kettle A, Holland V, et al. Attenuation of haloperidol-induced catalepsy by a 5-HT_{2C} receptor antagonist. *Br J Pharmacol* 1999;126:572–574.
115. Meltzer HY. The importance of serotonin-dopamine interactions in the action of clozapine. *Br J Psychiatry* 1992;160[Suppl]:22–29.
116. Kuoppamäki M, Syvälahti E, Hietala J. Clozapine and *N*-desmethylclozapine are potent 5-HT_{1C} receptor antagonists. *Eur J Pharmacol* 1993;245:179–182.
117. Goetz CG, Blasucci LM, Leurgans S, et al. Olanzapine and clozapine: comparative effects on motor function in hallucinating PD patients. *Neurology* 2000;55: 789–794.
118. Friedman JH, Factor SA. Atypical antipsychotics in the treatment of drug-induced psychosis in Parkinson's disease. *Mov Disord* 2000;15:201–211.
119. Durif F, Vidailhet M, Bonnet AM, et al. Levodopa-induced dyskinesias are improved by fluoxetine. *Neurology* 1995;45:1855–1858.
120. Perry KW, Fuller RW. Effect of fluoxetine on serotonin and dopamine concentration in microdialysis fluid from rat striatum. *Life Sci* 1992;50:1683–1690.
121. Rutter JJ, Auerbach SB. Acute uptake inhibition in-

creases extracellular serotonin in the rat forebrain. *J Pharmacol Exp Ther* 1993;265:1319–1324.
122. Frechilla D, Cobreros A, Saldise L, et al. Serotonin 5-HT_{1A} receptor expression is selectively enhanced in the striosomal compartment of chronic parkinsonian monkeys. *Synapse* 2001;39:288–296.
123. Bibbiani F, Oh JD, Chase TN. Serotonin 5-HT_{1A} agonist improves motor complications in rodent and primate parkinsonian models. *Neurology* 2001;57:1829–1834.
124. Eberle-Wang K, Lucki I, Chesselet MF. A role for the subthalamic nucleus in 5-HT_{2C}–induced oral dyskinesia. *Neuroscience* 1996;72:117–128.
125. Bennett JP Jr, Landow ER, Dietrich S, et al. Suppression of dyskinesias in advanced Parkinson's disease: moderate daily clozapine doses provide long-term dyskinesia reduction. *Mov Disord* 1994;9:409–414.
126. Pierelli F, Adipietro A, Soldati G, et al. Low dosage clozapine effects on L-dopa induced dyskinesias in parkinsonian patients. *Acta Neurol Scand* 1998;97: 295–299.
127. Rodriguez JJ, Garcia DR, Pickel VM. Subcellular distribution of 5-hydroxytryptamine 2A and *N*-methyl-D-aspartate receptors within single neurons in rat motor and limbic striatum. *J Comp Neurol* 1999;413:219–231.
128. Oh JD, Bibbiani F, Sarsoza FM, et al. Serotonin 5-HT_{2A} antagonist attenuates levodopa-induced motor response alterations in rodent and primate parkinsonian models. *Soc Neurosci* 2001;27[Suppl]:A966.
129. Beckstead RM, Kersey KS. Immunohistochemical demonstration of differential substance P-, met-enkephalin-, and glutamic-acid-decarboxylase–containing cell body and axon distributions in the corpus striatum of the cat. *J Comp Neurol* 1985;232:481–498.
130. Gerfen CR, Young WS III. Distribution of striatonigral and striatopallidal peptidergic neurons in both patch and matrix compartments: an *in situ* hybridization histochemistry and fluorescent retrograde tracing study. *Brain Res* 1988;460:161–167.
131. Bezard E, Ravenscroft P, Gross CE, et al. Upregulation of striatal preproenkephalin gene expression occurs before the appearance of parkinsonian signs in 1-methyl-4-phenyl-1,2,3,6-tetrahydropyridine–lesioned macaque model of Parkinson's disease. *Neurobiol Dis* 2001;8:343–350.
132. Hille CJ, Fox SH, Maneuf YP, et al. Antiparkinsonian action of a delta opioid agonist in rodent and primate models of Parkinson's disease. *Exp Neurol* 2001;172: 189–198.
133. Macdonald, Hudzik TJ, Cross AJ. Antiparkinsonian potential of opioid delta receptor agonists. *Soc Neurosci* 1998;24[Suppl]:1723.
134. Henry B, Crossman AR, Brotchie JM. Effect of repeated L-DOPA, bromocriptine, or lisuride administration on preproenkephalin A and preproenkephalin B mRNA levels in the striatum of the 6-hydroxydopamine–lesioned rat. *Exp Neurol* 1999;155:204–220.
135. Piccini P, Weeks RA, Brooks DJ. Alterations in opioid receptor binding in Parkinson's disease patients with levodopa-induced dyskinesias. *Ann Neurol* 1997;42: 720–726.
136. Maneuf YP, Mitchell IJ, Crossman AR, et al. On the role of enkephalin cotransmission in the GABAergic striatal efferents to the globus pallidus. *Exp Neurol* 1994;125:65–71.
137. You ZB, Herrera-Marschitz M, Nylander I, et al. Effect of morphine on dynorphin B and GABA release in the basal ganglia of rats. *Brain Res* 1996;710:241–248.
138. Henry B, Fox SH, Crossman AR, et al. μ- and δ-opioid receptor antagonists reduce levodopa-induced dyskinesia in the MPTP-lesioned primate model of Parkinson's disease. *Exp Neurol* 2001;171:139–146.
139. Trabucchi M, Bassi S, Frattola L. Effect of naloxone on the "on-off" syndrome in patients receiving long-term levodopa therapy. *Arch Neurol* 1982;39:120–121.
140. Sandyk R, Snider SR. Naloxone treatment of L-dopa–induced dyskinesias in Parkinson's disease. *Am J Psychiatry* 1986;143:118.
141. Rascol O, Fabre N, Blin O, et al. Naltrexone, an opiate antagonist, fails to modify motor symptoms in patients with Parkinson's disease. *Mov Disord* 1994;9: 437–440.
142. Manson AJ, Katzenschlager R, Hobart J, et al. High dose naltrexone for dyskinesias induced by levodopa. *J Neurol Neurosurg Psychiatry* 2001;70:554–556.
143. Mailleux P, Vanderhaeghen J. Distribution of neuronal cannabinoid receptor in the adult rat brain: a comparative receptor binding radioautography and *in situ* hybridization histochemistry. *Neuroscience* 1992;48: 655–668.
144. Di MV, Hill MP, Bisogno T, et al. Enhanced levels of endogenous cannabinoids in the globus pallidus are associated with a reduction in movement in an animal model of Parkinson's disease. *FASEB J* 2000;14:1432–1438.
145. Di Marzo V, Melck D, Bisogno T, et al. Endocannabinoids: endogenous cannabinoid receptor ligands with neuromodulatory action. *Trends Neurosci* 1998;21: 521–528.
146. Banerjee SP, Snyder SH, Mechoulam R. Cannabinoids: influence on neurotransmitter uptake in rat brain synaptosomes. *J Pharmacol Exp Ther* 1975;194:74–81.
147. Maneuf YP, Nash JE, Crossman AR, et al. Activation of the cannabinoid receptor by delta 9 tetrahydrocannabinol reduces gamma aminobutyric acid uptake in the globus pallidus. *Eur J Pharmacol* 1996;308:161–164.
148. Chan PK, Chan SC, Yung WH. Presynaptic inhibition of GABAergic inputs to rat substantia nigra pars reticulata neurones by a cannabinoid agonist. *NeuroReport* 1998;9:671–675.
149. Gerdeman G, Lovinger DM. CB1 cannabinoid receptor inhibits synaptic release of glutamate in rat dorsolateral striatum. *J Neurophysiol* 2001;85:468–471.
150. Glass M, Brotchie JM, Maneuf YP. Modulation of neurotransmission by cannabinoids in the basal ganglia. *Eur J Neurosci* 1997;9:199–203.
151. Di Marzo V, Fontana A, Cadas H, et al. Formation and inactivation of endogenous cannabinoid anandamide in central neurons. *Nature* 1994;372:686–691.
152. Silverdale MA, McGuire S, McInnes A, et al. Striatal cannabinoid CB1 receptor mRNA expression is decreased in the reserpine-treated rat model of Parkinson's disease. *Exp Neurol* 2001;169:400–406.
153. Fox SH, Hill MP, Crossman AR, et al. On the role of endocannabinoids in L-Dopa induced dyskinesia. *Soc Neurosci Abstracts* 1999;25:1462.
154. Fox SH, Kobylecki C, Begum S, et al. A role of cannabinoid receptor stimulation in the treatment of L-DOPA–induced dyskinesia in Parkinson's disease. *Mov Disord* 1998;13[Suppl 2]:A32.
155. Sieradzan KA, Fox SH, Dick JPR, et al. The cannabinoid receptor agonist nabilone reduces levodopa-in-

duced dyskinesia in Parkinson's disease. *Neurology* 2001;57(11):2108–2111.

156. Lindvall O, Björklund A. The organization of the ascending catecholamine neuron systems in the rat brain as revealed by the glyoxylic acid fluorescence method. *Acta Physiol Scand* 1974;412[Suppl]:1–48.
157. Jenner P, Sheehy M, Marsden CD. Noradrenaline and 5-hydroxytryptamine modulation of brain dopamine function: implications for the treatment of Parkinson's disease. *Br J Clin Pharmacol* 1983;15[Suppl 2]: S277–S289.
158. Donaldson IM, Dolphin AC, Jenner P, et al. Rotational behaviour produced in rats by unilateral electrolytic lesions of the ascending noradrenergic bundles. *Brain Res* 1977;138:487–509.
159. York DH. Possible dopaminergic pathway from substantia nigra to putamen. *Brain Res* 1970;20:233–249.
160. Lu L, Ordway GA. Alpha 2C-adrenoceptors mediate inhibition of forskolin-stimulated cAMP production in rat striatum. *Mol Brain Res* 1997;52:228–234.
161. Henry B, Fox SH, Peggs D, et al. The alpha 2-adrenergic receptor antagonist idazoxan reduces dyskinesia and enhances anti-parkinsonian actions of L-dopa in the MPTP-lesioned primate model of Parkinson's disease. *Mov Disord* 1999;14:744–753.
162. Rascol O, Arnulf I, Peyro-Saint PH, et al. Idazoxan, an alpha-2 antagonist, and L-DOPA–induced dyskinesias in patients with Parkinson's disease. *Mov Disord* 2001; 16:708–713.
163. Manson AJ, Iakovidou E, Lees AJ. Idazoxan is ineffective for levodopa-induced dyskinesias in Parkinson's disease. *Mov Disord* 2000;15:336–337.
164. Gomez-Mancilla B, Bedard PJ. Effect of nondopaminergic drugs on L-dopa–induced dyskinesias in MPTP-treated monkeys. *Clin Neuropharmacol* 1993;16: 418–427.
165. Merivuori H, Brotchie JM, Crossman AR, et al. JP-1730, a selective alpha-2 adrenergic receptor antagonist, reduces L-dopa–induced dyskinesia in the MPTP-lesioned primate. *Parkinsonism Related Disord* 2001; 63[Suppl]:A7.
166. Hill MP, Brotchie JM. The adrenergic receptor agonist, clonidine, potentiates the anti-parkinsonian action of the selective kappa-opioid receptor agonist, enadoline, in the monoamine-depleted rat. *Br J Pharmacol* 1999; 128:1577–1585.
167. Fox SH, Henry B, Hill MP, et al. Neural mechanisms underlying peak-dose dyskinesia induced by levodopa and apomorphine are distinct: evidence from the effects of the alpha (2) adrenoceptor antagonist idazoxan. *Mov Disord* 2001;16:642–650.
168. Holmberg M, Scheinin M, Kurose H, et al. Adrenergic alpha 2C-receptors reside in rat striatal GABAergic projection neurons: comparison of radioligand binding and immunohistochemistry. *Neuroscience* 1999;93: 1323–1333.
169. MacMillan LB, Hein L, Smith MS, et al. Central hypotensive effects of the alpha 2a-adrenergic receptor subtype. *Science* 1996;273:801–803.
170. Han ZY, Le Novere N, Zoli M, et al. Localization of nAChR subunit mRNAs in the brain of Macaca mulatta. *Eur J Neurosci* 2000;12:3664–3674.
171. Weiland S, Bertrand D, Leonard S. Neuronal nicotinic acetylcholine receptors: from the gene to the disease. *Behav Brain Res* 2000;113:43–56.
172. Sargent PB. The diversity of neuronal nicotinic acetylcholine receptors. *Annu Rev Neurosci* 1993;16: 403–443.
173. Court JA, Piggott MA, Lloyd S, et al. Nicotine binding in human striatum: elevation in schizophrenia and reductions in dementia with Lewy bodies, Parkinson's disease and Alzheimer's disease and in relation to neuroleptic medication. *Neuroscience* 2000;98:79–87.
174. Rusted JM, Newhouse PA, Levin ED. Nicotinic treatment for degenerative neuropsychiatric disorders such as Alzheimer's disease and Parkinson's disease. *Behav Brain Res* 2000;113:121–129.
175. Sacaan AI, Dunlop JL, Lloyd GK. Pharmacological characterization of neuronal acetylcholine gated ion channel receptor-mediated hippocampal norepinephrine and striatal dopamine release from rat brain slices. *J Pharmacol Exp Ther* 1995;274:224–230.
176. Menzaghi F, Whelan KT, Risbrough VB, et al. Interactions between a novel cholinergic ion channel agonist, SIB-1765F and L-DOPA in the reserpine model of Parkinson's disease in rats. *J Pharmacol Exp Ther* 1997;280:393–401.
177. Schneider JS, Pope-Coleman A, Van Velson M, et al. Effects of SIB-1508Y, a novel neuronal nicotinic acetylcholine receptor agonist, on motor behavior in parkinsonian monkeys. *Mov Disord* 1998;13:637–642.
178. Vieregge A, Sieberer M, Jacobs H, et al. Transdermal nicotine in PD: a randomized, double-blind, placebo-controlled study. *Neurology* 2001;57:1032–1035.
179. Gorell JM, Rybicki BA, Johnson CC, et al. Smoking and Parkinson's disease: a dose–response relationship. *Neurology* 1999;52:115–119.
180. Fratiglioni L, Wang HX. Smoking and Parkinson's and Alzheimer's disease: review of the epidemiological studies. *Behav Brain Res* 2000;113:117–120.
181. Belluardo N, Mudo G, Blum M, et al. Central nicotinic receptors, neurotrophic factors and neuroprotection. *Behav Brain Res* 2000;113:21–34.
182. Costa G, Abin-Carriquiry JA, Dajas F. Nicotine prevents striatal dopamine loss produced by 6-hydroxydopamine lesion in the substantia nigra. *Brain Res* 2001;888:336–342.
183. Janson AM, Fuxe K, Sundström E, et al. Chronic nicotine treatment partly protects against the 1-methyl-4-phenyl-2,3,6-tetrahydropyridine–induced degeneration of nigrostriatal dopamine neurons in the black mouse. *Acta Physiol Scand* 1988;132:589–591.

Parkinson's Disease: Advances in Neurology, Vol. 91.
Edited by Ariel Gordin, Seppo Kaakkola, and Heikki Teräväinen
Lippincott Williams & Wilkins, Philadelphia © 2003

29

Deep Brain Stimulation: What Does It Offer?

Alim-Louis Benabid, Laurent Vercucil, Abdelhamid Benazzouz, Adnan Koudsie, Stephan Chabardes, Lorella Minotti, Philippe Kahane, Michèle Gentil, *Doris Lenartz, *Christian Andressen, Paul Krack, and *Pierre Pollak

*Department of Clinical Neurosciences, University Joseph Fourier, Grenoble, France; and *University of Köln, Köln, Germany*

Electrical stimulation has been used for a long time, initially to elicit responses from excitable tissues including neurons, muscle, and glands. This started in the early days of the first century, when the nature of electricity was not yet understood and when empirically electrical discharges from electrical fish such as the torpedo were used in ancient Rome to treat pain from rheumatism. When the nature of electricity was starting to be understood, in the sixteenth century, static electricity coming from the friction of an ebonite rod with a cat skin was used mainly as an entertainment at the French court by Mesmer. At the end of the nineteenth century, coming essentially from the work of Lapicque, electrical devices were used either for diagnostic purposes measuring chronaxy and rheobase of excitable elements and of human nerves or for therapeutic reasons using either electrical discharges inducing contraction or the thermal effects of electricity called "diathermia." However, in Bologna, in the beginning of the nineteenth century (1804), experiments were done in humans using Volta batteries to elicit responses that described the sensory and motor responses. Therefore, since the very beginning, the reciprocal relationships between electricity and biology were observed, the biological tissues being able to generate electricity (as in the electrical organ of fish) or to respond to electricity (such as contractions elicited in frog muscles by voltaic batteries). It is interesting to note that except in lightning, the only origin of electricity is biological. The birth of neurobiology is contemporaneous of the use of electricity, which for several decades has been used through single shocks or relatively short trains, to induce neural events while triggering recording devices, ink recorder initially and later oscilloscopes. As soon as functional neurosurgery using stereotaxy was born, electrical stimulation was used for the same purposes of diagnosis and study of reactions. Based on the observed phenomenon, which soon became a principle that electrical shocks were excitatory, therapeutic applications were made when equipment became available through implanted generators, receiving their energy using either transcutaneous electrical coupling with antennas or later totally implantable stimulators, bearing their own source of energy as a battery and also being externally programmable. Based on this, cardiac pacing was the most widespread and used application, and at the same time, stimulation of the nervous system, either peripherally or centrally, was attempted. Treatments of pain, epilepsy, and some movement disorders were reported, which demonstrated the efficiency of the method but did not last, essentially because of the poor medical evaluation of the results and because of the explosion of pharmacology that provided a huge amount of drugs to treat the same diseases. More recently, in the late 1980s, we clearly established that stimulation at high frequency could mimic the effects of lesioning, and although the mechanism is poorly understood, stimulation at high frequency has been applied to movement disorders in various targets (the ventral intermediate [VIM] nucleus of the thalamus, the internal segment of the globus pallidus [GPi], and the centromedian parafascicular (CmPf) nucleus of the thalamus, and subthalamic nucleus [STN]). The efficiency of these methods, their low morbidity, and their adaptability have led to trial application of high-frequency stimulation (HFS) to other diseases such as epilepsy, obsessive-compulsive disorders (OCDs), and pain, again with the introduction of a new site for stimulation, which is the premotor cortex. As these methods of HFS are becoming more developed, and as the stability of the effects provides us with long-term follow-ups, which are about or longer than 10 years, it becomes clear that we almost know nothing about the biology, the physiology, the physics, and the biophysics of living tissues in situations of long-term chronic stimulation. This opens a new field of research and potentially of applications, probably not only to nervous diseases, but also to other cellular and organ dysfunctions.

ESTABLISHMENT OF THE SPECIFIC EFFECT OF HIGH-FREQUENCY STIMULATION

The retrospective analysis of literature shows that nothing is totally new (1–14). It has been reported on various occasions that stimulation, instead of exciting nervous tissue, would be able to induce effects opposite to those expected from excitation and more likely to mimic the effects of lesioning. These reports are apparently nonsystematic, essentially because the conditions of stimulation were not consistently reported, and when they were, the conditions were not directly related to the effect in terms of frequency. When this was established, it allowed physicians to use it as a method *per se* and to start replacing ablative surgery such as thalamotomy by HFS of the thalamic target, mainly the VIM nucleus (15). Quite quickly, this was extended to the pallidum on the same basis of the analogy with pallidotomy (16,17). As quickly, the knowledge brought by experimental research (18) could be used for therapeutic purposes because it was also known that the adaptability of stimulation could modulate the intensity of this mimicry of lesioning, allowing us to obtain the effects expected from ablative surgery without the side effects or complications, or at least in a reversible manner if they happened.

GENERAL METHOD OF DEEP BRAIN STIMULATION AT HIGH FREQUENCY

Independently of the target, the methodology that is used by the various teams engaged in this type of therapy starts to be rather homogeneous around the world. Deep brain stimulation (DBS) is performed using stereotactic implantation of electrodes. These electrodes, which were initially unipolar, are currently tetrapolar with a spacing that has been recently reduced, to provide a better spatial discrimination of the rather small targets that are used, never larger than the 7.5 mm of the new reduced space electrode (Medtronic 3389). Targeting to implant these electrodes is based on a combination of radiological and physiological methods, which may vary from one team to another (19–28). Radiology can use unique ventriculography, which shows the third ventricle, the features of which are the basis of most atlases, or computed tomography scanning, which provides easier although less precise visualization of the third ventricle and of the gross limits of structures such as the thalamus or possibly the pallidum, but not the STN or the subdivisions of these nuclei. Magnetic resonance imaging is, of course, the most frequently used and the most precise radiological method to delineate the targets. However, because of the possible distortions brought by those methods and because it is becoming clear that even in small targets such as the STN there might be a functional somatotopy, it is more and more commonly admitted that in addition to this radiological pretargeting, it is necessary to ascertain the final choice of the position of the electrode using the functional investigation in the operating room. As a matter of fact, this is a unique opportunity to simulate what will be the final result, because these effects can be seen during the operation, using electrical stimulation in the place and with the parameters that will be used in the chronic situation. The stimulation during surgery using the electrodes is a powerful adjunct to radiology to improve the efficiency of these DBS methods. When this is available, including the availability of the equipment and the expertise of the team, microrecording of electrical activities provides the signature of the nucleus, allowing the surgical team to recognize precisely what is the structure that is being investigated. This exploration may be done using several parallel subsequent or simultaneous tracks, which increase the functional precision of the electrode placement. These electrodes are then secured to the skull and connected immediately or a few days later to an implantable programmable single-channel or multichannel generator, generally in the subcutaneous subclavicular area through a connector that is passed under the skin from the head to the chest.

POSTOPERATIVE PERIOD

The morbidity and mortality rates are extremely low and depend on the learning curve of the team. When there are side effects, most generally, they are transient and reversible, and their intensity is adjustable through the adaptation of the parameters mainly of the amplitude. There is currently no proof that multiple microelectrode recording induces more side effects than single-track approaches.

The immediate postoperative period can also be marked by a significant spontaneous improvement of the symptoms due to the mechanical lesioning effect of the introduction of the exploratory and chronic electrodes, but this, which proves that the procedure has involved the right place, usually does not last for long, at least not at the level that would be sufficient to avoid the connection to the stimulator. Moreover, some side effects such as dyskinesias, when they are observed after STN surgery, are good predictors of a good benefit.

The postoperative period is essentially the time when the stimulator is tuned, which is the role of the neurological team, which must do this using knowledge of movement disorders and their therapy, as well as the subtleties of the symptoms to reach the proper setting. This setting, particularly in the STN, must be reached progressively, to avoid premature appearance of side effects such as dyskinesias. At the same time, a drug regimen must be concomitantly decreased, to prevent the appearance of dyskinesias. The attention paid to postoperative tuning plays a major role in the efficiency of the method. Actually, it is not as complicated as initially stated; the multiple combinations of contacts, polarities, and parameters may not necessarily be used together. Usually, putting the case of the generator positive and one of the four contacts negative each at its turn and setting the frequency at 130 Hz and the pulse width at 60 ms allows for an initial prechecking of each of the four electrodes, showing quickly which ones are unusable due to side effects seen before any clinical improvement. More time is needed to correctly set up the parameters for the few electrodes (usually not more than two) that will be used in chronic situations. Periodic rechecking is necessary at 3 weeks, 3 months, and after 6 months. Usually, the parameters are rather stable if the placement is correct. In case of incorrect placement, it is still possible to reoperate on the patient and reposition the electrode in a more efficient place, as we have done it several times.

INDICATIONS AND RESULTS OF DEEP BRAIN STIMULATION AT HIGH FREQUENCY

Movement Disorders

Currently, HFS on patients with movement disorders and mainly Parkinson's disease (PD) has been the most extensively used and validated indication. The first indication was for tremor, to replace thalamotomy (29–32). Although this is still a subject of discussion, it might be stated (for the sake of simplicity) that all the symptoms of PD can be satisfactorily compensated by high-frequency DBS of the STN (33–44). Rest tremor, akinesia, rigidity, and midline symptoms are strongly influenced by high-frequency DBS, providing an average improvement of about 65% of these symptoms and allowing to decrease the drug regimen by an average of 70%; 30% of the patients being without drug. The stability of the effect is remarkable in the on-stimulation stage and in the off-stimulation stage, where the background scores of the patient are not significantly changed after several years of continuous stimulation. The pallidal target for some teams is still considered a valid target and provides comparable benefits (45–51). By far, the best effect is on dyskinesias, which are totally suppressed as in pallidotomy, then unilateral and focal dystonias (52–55). There are recent reports that bilateral GPi stimulation could improve severe cervical spasmodic torticollis. The thalamic target has been used before the pallidal target and has provided significant improvement in the daily life of patients, although it is not that clear on neurological scales and has never reached the magnitude of improvement obtained with pallidal stimulation. Similarly, the use of other targets, such as the STN, is currently being investigated, and preliminary data on Hallervorden–Spatz disease are being observed without the possibility to make any conclusions. It seems that the effect of STN stimulation in these cases would be performed at low frequency, instead of high frequency, in the pallidum. This might have important consequences in terms of understanding the mechanism, as well as in economical aspects, with stimulation at 10 Hz being logically ten times cheaper than stimulation at about 100 Hz. The particular aspect of DBS (and ablative surgery) is the delayed appearance of the beneficial effects, which are extremely rarely observed during surgery but are established progressively in days, weeks, and months after surgery in the progressive return to a normal distribution of the muscle tone and disappearance of joint distortion, making clear that orthopedic surgery should not be performed in those patients in whom the deformities are always reversible because it has been also observed in cases of orthopedic deformities after a prolonged coma stage.

Other movement disorders have also been targeted for stimulation and for ablative surgery. The atypical forms of PD are thus far not considered good indications. The motor components of the symptoms are usually improved, but there is no effect on joint symptoms such as a gaze disturbance in progressive supranuclear palsy and various forms of dementia, which might even be impaired by bilateral surgeries. This is more the part of evolution, which is insensitive to stimulation, that makes a contraindication as in a relatively short-term beneficial effect that might be observed on motor components or motor symptoms, is jeopardized by the rest of the evolution. There are various reports that DBS is efficient on patients with Tourette's syndrome (56) and poststroke, postoperative, or posttraumatic tremors, but the quality of the improvement does not justify the use of these methods.

WHAT DOES DEEP BRAIN STIMULATION PROMISE?

Because of the reversibility of the method, the lower morbidity rate, the reversibility of either beneficial effects or side effects, and the possibility to turn "off" stimulation if a new treatment were to appear for a given disease, the extension of DBS to other functional neurosurgical targets can be envisioned legitimately. Considering either the data coming from basic research or the observation made during previous ablative surgeries, there are several other fields that are currently under investigation and might potentially be new indications.

EPILEPSY

For a long time, epilepsy has been approached using stimulation methods, starting with the stimulation of the cerebellum by Cooper et al. (57–60) and others (61–66). These results are still debated but have not been convincing enough to become routine method. Similarly, although it is totally different, vagus nerve stimulation is another indication that epilepsy could be sensitive to stimulation methods.

NIGRAL CONTROL OF EPILEPSY

There is a large body of evidence from experimental work (67,68) that manipulation of the nigral system by agonists of γ-aminobutyric acid (GABA) receptors or *N*-methyl-D-aspartate antagonists is able to control seizures in various animal models of epilepsy. Based on this, we have performed experimental work in GAERS rats, showing that manipulation of the STN, either by lesioning or stimulation, is able to improve the seizure occurrence (69). The results of this experimental study in rats have been convincing enough to allow us to start a clinical trial in humans. Today, we have implanted four patients with unilateral (in one case) and bilateral (in three cases) implantation of the STN, with the longest follow-up being 32 months. The results are extremely encouraging. The improvement of the seizure rate has been varying from 90% to 50% depending on the cases. Different from what was expected from experimental studies, in which we could think that the effect would be better with intermittent stimulation rather than continuous stimulation, the continuous stimulation in patients has provided a rather stable effect. Preliminary trials with intermittent stimulation have not demonstrated that the improvement is increased by this protocol. However, it could be suggested from experimental studies that stimulation triggered by the onset of seizures would be a solution at least interesting in economic terms, because the stimulation battery would be used only when the seizure starts.

Besides STN stimulation, other sites have been proposed and are under current investigation in other centers: The anterior nucleus of the thalamus has been suggested by various studies including preliminary work by Fisher et al. (61). The intralaminar nuclei are also potentially interesting. Current data provided by the Mexican group of Velasco (63,65) suggest that stimulation into the focus could be able to control seizures and, moreover, to modify the epileptogenic properties of the focus, after continuous stimulation. There is no doubt that DBS will be an important tool in the armamentarium for epilepsy treatment, although several experimental and clinical studies must be performed before we reach the status of a routine application of these methods. It is important to state that, as is the case for PD and other movement disorders, the reversibility of the method is a strong argument in favor of its use in these difficult cases because if a new medical treatment becomes available, one could shut down the stimulators and replace DBS with more efficient drug therapy. This looks like the case for severe myoclonic epilepsy, a disease that we operated on in one case and that seems (in light of recent data) to be highly sensitive to the new drug topiramate.

PSYCHIATRIC DISEASES

Although psychosurgery is not currently widely used in Western countries (70), it has specific indications and lesioning methods using various targets—either in the cingulum or in the anterior capsule—that could significantly improve OCD. Recent attempts to perform stimulation of the anterior capsule have been made (71). Although our current understanding assumes that HFS induces inhibition in various nuclei from the thalamus to the pallidum and the STN independently of the frequency excitation of the fibers, which could be a predictor that HFS could not mimic the effect of lesioning in white-matter bundles such as those in the anterior capsule, preliminary results have been encouraging. Recent attempts (Sturm, et al., *unpublished data,* 2002) to aim at more cellular targets such as the nucleus accumbens seem to be even more efficient. In this indication, as in epilepsy, there is now evidence that DBS could be one possible additional tool for the treatment of these disorders. However, a large amount of fundamental research and the development of animal models and controlled clinical studies must be done before a clear statement can be issued and before this method could become of routine application.

FOOD-INTAKE CONTROL

Experimental results in our laboratory have proven that electrical stimulation of the ventromedial hypothalamus (VMH) and of the lateral hypothalamic (LH) nuclei can modify the feeding behavior of animals. In the VMH, low-frequency stimulation (LFS) inhibits the feeding behavior in fasted animals, and HFS induces compulsory feeding behavior in already-fed animals. This replicates the well-known data of lesioning and LFS experiments performed decades ago in animals, inducing either obesity or cachexy (72). These results have been obtained only in acute experiments, and the effect of chronic stimulation on the weight of animals is not yet established. These data are obviously too experimental and too preliminary to allow their application to clinical situations, and we must be careful before these methods are applied to people having weight problems or, even more, to patients with anorexia nervosa, the limits of which with psychosurgery are unclear.

NEUROPROTECTION

We now have enough evidence from experimental data and preliminary evidence from long-term follow-up parkinsonian patients to suggest that STN stimulation has a potential neuroprotective effect on the neurodegeneration of dopaminergic cells. This is based on the assumption that HFS shuts down the output of the STN using the glutamate output of the STN (glutamate being a well-known excitotoxic amino acid). If this can be further demonstrated, this would obviously profoundly modify the indications of surgery in PD and would suggest that much earlier operations should be considered before the patient has reached a too-advanced stage in its evolution. The principle of long-term modification induced by chronic stimulation, which is suggested by this hypothesis and its preliminary confirmations, would have a larger implication and would suggest that chronic stimulation on various targets could be used not only to acutely suppress symptoms of various diseases, but also in the long-term to modify the networks toward a better functional stage. This concept of long-term modification of networks by chronic stimulation has some current support, with the observation of the disappearance of the tendency of parkinsonian patients to develop levodopa-induced dyskinesias with time, which has also been observed when patients are submitted to continuous infusion of apomorphine or lisuride. Thus, the establishment of a stable regimen of activity at the level of the postsynaptic striatal dopaminergic receptors could induce a return to a stage of normal reactivity to agonists, instead of the "on-off" fluctuations, which are characteristics of the late stages of PD under levodopa treatment. Further support of the hypothesis of long-term modification is provided by the observed effect of chronic stimulation in dystonia. It is noteworthy that different from in PD, the improvement of those patients is rather delayed, and it takes days, weeks, or months before the full benefit of stimulation is obtained, suggesting also here that the effect would be by resetting normal function in the network of neurons responsible for the control of muscle tone. One may also find support for this hypothesis in the reported observations that thalamic stimulation in hemiballisms of various origins, which are acutely controlled by thalamic stimulation, could be efficient with time to such an extent that stopping the stimulation after 1 year would correspond to the nonreappearance of these ballistic movements (73). Therefore, extension of this concept to various neurological situations using various targets and various parameters of stimulation could be a potential important future application.

EXPECTABLE APPLICATIONS COMING FROM THE UNDERSTANDING OF THE MECHANISM

Although both experimental and clinical aspects tend to suggest that HFS could act as an inhibitory mechanism, this is too far to definitely establish. Coming from various ongoing studies at the moment, a large amount of data are not always totally coherent, and there is no clear scheme of the mechanism induced by DBS at high frequency currently consensually accepted. This means that we can expect ongoing studies to provide an important understanding of this mechanism, which necessarily will open new avenues and suggest new ideas and new approaches. It is too early to describe the list of the potential applications that may come from better knowledge of the mechanisms.

CONCLUSIONS: TOWARD A PHYSIOLOGY OF THE STIMULATED STATE

As mentioned already, a totally new area of research has been opened: Besides pathological studies showing that the brain locally well tolerates the presence of electrodes (74–77), there are no data about how the nervous tissue and its complex organization are going to evolve after years of continuously being subjected to an "extreme condition," which is brought by chronic stimulation. This means that investigations from the molecular level to the behavioral level must be started, and they necessarily will provide extremely interesting data, opening by themselves new avenues and new ideas. It can even be suggested and expected that HFS of nonnervous tissues such as glandular tissues could also be of importance and might have possible applications to the treatment of other neurological diseases. How do cells respond to chronic stimulation? How is the intermediate metabolism affected? How is protein production of nervous and glandular cells influenced? How is synaptology of networks modified by chronic stimulation? How is receptor affinity modified? How is axonal conduction altered? How is the vascular field itself modified? Contraction of vessels? Is there a dilatation? Behavior of blood protein? Hormonal levels?

Just ahead lies a very exciting and promising future, and the now long follow-up results of chronic brain stimulation in PD have established the consistency and the validity of this method and support the enthusiasm to engage in these new fields of research.

Since 1987, high-frequency DBS has been used to produce the same inhibitory effects than ablative lesions. DBS is reversible, adaptable, and the low surgical morbidity allows bilateral procedures in one session. The VIM nucleus of the thalamus is efficient for tremors in PD, essential tremors, and multiple sclerosis. The pallidal target GPi controls levodopa-induced dyskinesias (LIDs) and improves akinesia and rigidity. The STN improves tremor, akinesia, rigidity, and to a lesser extent midline symptoms and speech. Effect on LIDs is indirect, due to the decrease in drug dosage. Whereas VIM and GPi DBS resulted from serendipity, STN DBS came from basic research showing its importance in motor control, and the low morbidity associated with DBS prevented the expected hemiballism. GPi DBS improves progressively but spectacularly primary generalizes dystonias. Secondary dystonias are less responsive than DYT1-related dystonias, but their quality of life is improved. STN DBS seems to be efficient at low frequency. The mechanism of DBS, still unknown, could involve jamming of functional circuits, membrane depolarization, blockade of ion channels, stimulation of inhibitory GABAergic terminals, or a combination of several of these mechanisms. Based on theoretical considerations, the method could be neuroprotective, and animal experiments and human results may support this hypothesis, which however needs further demonstration. Experimental data suggested to apply the STN DBS in epilepsy. Three cases have been followed up for 1 to 2 years, and the strongly encouraging results further support the hypothesis of control by STN DBS in epilepsy. Application to other nuclei, such as the VMH might be useful in the control of pathologically disturbed food intake. Further applications of DBS to various diseases, such as psychiatric disorders (OCD and Tourette's syndrome), are currently being tried, as well as to gene transfer by electroporation. Combination of LFS and HFS of multiple targets opens new perspectives.

REFERENCES

1. Bartholow R. Experimental investigations into the functions of the human brain. *Am J Med Sci* 1874; 67:305–313.
2. Bartholow R. *Br Med J* 1874;3:727.
3. Fritsch G, Hitzig E. On the electrical excitability of the cerebrum. In: Bonin GV, ed. *Some papers on the cerebral cortex.* Springfield, IL: Charles C. Thomas Publisher, 1960:73–96.
4. Hassler R, Riechert TFM. Physiological observations in stereotaxic operations in extrapyramidal motor disturbances. *Brain* 1960;83:337–350.
5. Hassler R. Thalamic regulation of muscle tone and the speed of movements. In: Purpura DP, Yahr MD, eds. *The thalamus.* New York: Columbia University Press, 1966: 419–438.
6. Heath R. *Studies in schizophrenia: a multidisciplinary approach to mind–brain relationships.* Cambridge, MA: Harvard University Press, 1954.
7. Heath R, Mickle W. Evaluation of 7 years' experience with depth electrode studies in human patients. In: Ramey E, O'Doherty D, eds. *Electrical studies in unanesthetized brain.* New York: Harper & Brothers, 1960:214–217.
8. Morgan JP. The first reported case of electrical stimulation of the human brain. *J Hist Med Allied Sci* 1982; 37:51–64.
9. Sheer DE. *Electrical stimulation of the brain.* Austin, TX: University of Texas Press, 1961.
10. Spiegel EA, Wycis HT, Marks M, et al. Stereotaxic apparatus for operations on the human brain. *Science* 1947;106:349–350.
11. Spiegel EA, Wycis HT, Baird HW, et al. Physiopathologic observations on the basal ganglia. In: Ramey E, O'Doherty DS, eds. *Electrical studies on the unanesthetized brain.* New York: Harper & Brothers, 1960: 192–213.
12. Spiegel EA, Wycis HT. Chronic implantation of intracerebral electrodes in humans. In: Sheer DE, eds. *Electrical stimulation of the brain.* Austin, TX: University of Texas Press, 1961:37–44.
13. Thomas RK, Young CD. A note on the early history of electrical stimulation of the human brain. *J Gen Psychol* 1993;120:73–81.
14. Zimmermann M. Electrical stimulation of the human brain. *Hum Neurobiol* 1982;1:227–229.
15. Benabid AL, Pollak P, Louveau A, et al. Combined (thalamotomy and stimulation) stereotactic surgery of the VIM thalamic nucleus for bilateral Parkinson's disease. *Appl Neurophysiol* 1987;50:344–346.
16. Siegfried J, Lippitz B. Bilateral continuous electrostimulation of ventroposterolateral pallidum: a new therapeutical approach for alleviating all parkinsonian symptoms. *Neurosurgery* 1994;35:1126–1130.
17. Siegfried J, Lippitz B. Chronic electrical stimulation of the VL-VPL complex and of the pallidum in the treatment of extrapyramidal and cerebellar disorders. *Stereotact Funct Neurosurg* 1994;62:71–75.
18. Bergman H, Wichmann T, DeLong MR. Reversal of experimental parkinsonism by lesions of the subthalamic nucleus. *Science* 1990;249:1436–1438.
19. Alterman RL, Kall BA, Cohen H, et al. Stereotactic ventrolateral thalamotomy: is ventriculography necessary? *Neurosurgery* 1995;37:717–722.
20. Bejjani BP, Dormont D, Pidoux B, et al. Bilateral subthalamic stimulation for Parkinson's disease by using three-dimensional stereotactic magnetic resonance imaging and electrophysiological guidance. *J Neurosurg* 2000;92:615–625.
21. Carlson JD, Iacono RP. Electrophysiological versus image-based targeting in the posteroventral pallidotomy. *Comput Aided Surg* 1999;4:93–100.
22. Hariz MI, Fodstad H. Do microelectrode techniques increase accuracy or decrease risks in pallidotomy and deep brain stimulation? A critical review of the literature. *Stereotact Funct Neurosurg* 1999;72:157–169.
23. Holtzheimer PE, Roberts DW, Darcey TM. Magnetic resonance imaging versus computed tomography for target localization in functional stereotactic neurosurgery. *Neurosurgery* 1999;45:290–298.
24. Kelly PJ, Derome P, Guiot G. Thalamic spatial variability and the surgical results of lesions placed with neurophysiologic control. *Surg Neurol* 1978;9:307–315.
25. Lozano AM, Hutchison WD, Dostrovsky JO. Microelectrode monitoring of cortical and subcortical structures during stereotactic surgery. *Acta Neurochir* 1995; 64[Suppl]:30–34.
26. Schuurman PR, de Bie RM, Majoie CB, et al. A prospective comparison between three-dimensional magnetic resonance imaging and ventriculography for target-coordinate determination in frame-based functional stereotactic neurosurgery. *J Neurosurg* 1999;91: 911–914.
27. Starr PA, Vitek JL, DeLong M, et al. Magnetic resonance imaging-based stereotactic localization of the

globus pallidus and subthalamic nucleus. *Neurosurgery* 1999;44:303–314.
28. Zonenshayn M, Rezai AR, Mogilner AY, et al. Comparison of anatomic and neurophysiological methods for subthalamic nucleus targeting. *Neurosurgery* 2000;47: 282–294.
29. Benabid AL, Pollak P, Gao D, et al. Chronic electrical stimulation of the ventralis intermedius nucleus of the thalamus as a treatment of movement disorders. *J Neurosurg* 1996;84:203–214.
30. Koller W, Pahwa R, Busenbark K, et al. High-frequency unilateral thalamic stimulation in the treatment of essential and parkinsonian tremor. *Ann Neurol* 1997;42: 292–299.
31. Limousin P, Speelman JD, Gielen F, et al. Multicentre European study of thalamic stimulation in parkinsonian and essential tremor. *J Neurol Neurosurg Psychiatry* 1999;66:289–296.
32. Schuurman PR, Bosch DA, Bossuyt PM, et al. A comparison of continuous thalamic stimulation and thalamotomy for suppression of severe tremor. *N Engl J Med* 2000;342:461–468.
33. Benabid AL, Pollak P, Gross C, et al. Acute and long-term effects of subthalamic nucleus stimulation in Parkinson's disease. *Stereotact Funct Neurosurg* 1994;62:76–84.
34. Krack P, Pollak P, Limousin P, et al. Stimulation of subthalamic nucleus alleviates tremor in Parkinson's disease. *Lancet* 1997;350:1675.
35. Krack P, Limousin P, Benabid AL, et al. Chronic stimulation of subthalamic nucleus improves levodopa-induced dyskinesias in Parkinson's disease. *Lancet* 1997; 350:1676.
36. Kumar R, Lozano AM, Kim YJ, et al. Double-blind evaluation of subthalamic nucleus deep brain stimulation in advanced Parkinson's disease. *Neurology* 1998; 51:850–855.
37. Limousin P, Pollak P, Benazzouz A, et al. Bilateral subthalamic nucleus stimulation for severe Parkinson's disease. *Mov Disord* 1995;10:672–674.
38. Limousin P, Pollak P, Benazzouz A, et al. Effect of parkinsonian signs and symptoms of bilateral subthalamic nucleus stimulation. *Lancet* 1995;345:91–95.
39. Limousin P, Krack P, Pollak P, et al. Electrical stimulation of the subthalamic nucleus in advanced Parkinson's disease. *N Engl J Med* 1998;339:1105–1111.
40. Moro E, Scerrati M, Romito LM, et al. Chronic subthalamic nucleus stimulation reduces medication requirements in Parkinson's disease. *Neurology* 1999;53:85–90.
41. Pollak P, Benabid AL, Gross C, et al. Effects of the stimulation of the subthalamic nucleus in Parkinson disease [in French]. *Rev Neurol* 1993;149:175–176.
42. Pollak P, Benabid AL, Limousin P, et al. Subthalamic nucleus stimulation alleviates akinesia and rigidity in parkinsonian patients. *Adv Neurol* 1996;69:591–594.
43. Rodriguez MC, Guridi OJ, Alvarez L, et al. The subthalamic nucleus and tremor in Parkinson's disease. *Mov Disord* 1998;13:111–118.
44. Yokoyama T, Sugiyama K, Nishizawa S, et al. Subthalamic nucleus stimulation for gait disturbance in Parkinson's disease. *Neurosurgery* 1999;45:41–49.
45. Ardouin C, Pillon B, Peiffer E, et al. Bilateral subthalamic or pallidal stimulation for Parkinson's disease affects neither memory nor executive functions: a consecutive series of 62 patients. *Ann Neurol* 1999;46:217–223.
46. Bejjani B, Damier P, Arnulf I, et al. Pallidal stimulation for Parkinson's disease. Two targets? *Neurology* 1997; 49:1564–1569.
47. Benabid AL, Benazzouz A, Hoffmann D, et al. Long-term electrical inhibition of deep brain targets in movement disorders. *Mov Disord* 1998;13:119–125.
48. Durif F, Lemaire JJ, Debilly B, et al. Acute and chronic effects of anteromedial globus pallidus stimulation in Parkinson's disease. *J Neurol Neurosurg Psychiatry* 1999;67:315–322.
49. Ghika J, Villemure JG, Fankhauser H, et al. Efficiency and safety of bilateral contemporaneous pallidal stimulation (deep brain stimulation) in levodopa-responsive patients with Parkinson's disease with severe motor fluctuations: a 2-year follow-up review. *J Neurosurg* 1998;89:713–718.
50. Krack P, Pollak P, Limousin P, et al. Opposite motor effects of pallidal stimulation in Parkinson's disease. *Ann Neurol* 1998;43:180–192.
51. Volkmann J, Sturm V, Weiss P, et al. Bilateral high-frequency stimulation of the internal globus pallidus in advanced Parkinson's disease. *Ann Neurol* 1998;44: 953–961.
52. Krauss JK, Pohle T, Weber S, et al. Bilateral stimulation of globus pallidus internus for treatment of cervical dystonia. *Lancet* 1999;354:837–838.
53. Kumar R, Dagher A, Hutchison WD, et al. Globus pallidus deep brain stimulation for generalized dystonia: clinical and PET investigation. *Neurology* 1999;53: 871–874.
54. Lozano AM, Kumar R, Gross RE, et al. Globus pallidus internus pallidotomy for generalized dystonia. *Mov Disord* 1997;12:865–870.
55. Tronnier VM, Fogel W. Pallidal stimulation for generalized dystonia. Report of three cases. *J Neurosurg* 2000; 92:453–456.
56. Vandewalle V, van der Linden C, Groenewegen HJ, et al. Stereotactic treatment of Gilles de la Tourette syndrome by high frequency stimulation of thalamus. *Lancet* 1999;353:724.
57. Cooper IS, Amin I, Gilman S, et al. The effect of chronic stimulation of cerebellar cortex on epilepsy in man. In: Cooper IS, Riklan M, Snider RS, eds. *The cerebellum, epilepsy, and behavior.* New York: Plenum Publishing, 1974:122.
58. Cooper IS, Amin I, Riklan M, et al. Chronic cerebellar stimulation in epilepsy. *Arch Neurol* 1976;33:559–570.
59. Cooper IS, Amin I, Gilman S. The effect of chronic cerebellar stimulation upon epilepsy in man. *Trans Am Neurol Assoc* 1978;98:192–196.
60. Cooper IS, Upton AR. Therapeutic implications of modulation of metabolism and functional activity of cerebral cortex by chronic stimulation of cerebellum and thalamus. *Biol Psychiatry* 1985;20:811–813.
61. Fisher RS, Uematsu S, Krauss GL, et al. Placebo-controlled pilot study of centromedian thalamic stimulation in treatment of intractable seizures. *Epilepsia* 1992;33: 841–851.
62. Van Buren JM, Wood JH, Oakley J, et al. Preliminary evaluation of cerebellar stimulation by double-blind stimulation and biological criteria in the treatment of epilepsy. *J Neurosurg* 1978;48:407–416.
63. Velasco F, Velasco M, Ogarrio C, et al. Electrical stimulation of the centromedian thalamic nucleus in the treatment of convulsive seizures: a preliminary report. *Epilepsia* 1987;28:421–430.

64. Velasco F, Velasco M, Velasco AL, et al. Electrical stimulation of the centromedian thalamic nucleus in control of seizures: long-term studies. *Epilepsia* 1995;36:63–71.
65. Velasco F, Velasco M, Jimenez F, et al. Predictors in the treatment of difficult-to-control seizures by electrical stimulation of the centromedian thalamic nucleus. *Neurosurgery* 2000;47:295–305.
66. Wright G, McLellan D, Brice A. A double-blind trial of chronic cerebellar stimulation in twelve patients with epilepsy. *J Neurol Neurosurg Psychiatry* 1984;47: 769–774.
67. Deransart C, Le BT, Marescaux C, et al. Role of the subthalamo-nigral input in the control of amygdala-kindled seizures in the rat. *Brain Res* 1998;807:78–83.
68. Deransart C, Vercueil L, Marescaux C, et al. The role of basal ganglia in the control of generalized absence seizures. *Epilepsy Res* 1998;32:213–223.
69. Vercueil L, Benazzouz A, Deransart C, et al. High-frequency stimulation of the subthalamic nucleus suppresses absence seizures in the rat: comparison with neurotoxic lesions. *Epilepsy Res* 1998;31:39–46.
70. Pool JL. Psychosurgery in older people. *J Am Geriatr Soc* 1954;2:456–465.
71. Nuttin B, Cosyns P, Demeulemeester H, et al. Electrical stimulation in anterior limbs of internal capsules in patients with obsessive-compulsive disorder. *Lancet* 1999; 354:1526.
72. Quaade F, Vaernet K, Larsson S. Stereotaxic stimulation and electrocoagulation of the lateral hypothalamus in obese humans. *Acta Neurochir* 1974;30:111–117.
73. Katayama Y, Fukaya C, Yamamoto T. Control of post-stroke involuntary and voluntary movement disorders with deep brain or epidural cortical stimulation. *Stereotact Funct Neurosurg* 1997;69:73–79.
74. Caparros-Lefebvre D, Ruchoux MM, Blond S, et al. Long-term thalamic stimulation in Parkinson's disease: postmortem anatomoclinical study. *Neurology* 1994;44: 1856–1860.
75. Gybels J, Dom R, Cosyns P. Electrical stimulation of the central gray for pain relief in human: autopsy data. *Acta Neurochir* 1980;30[Suppl]:259–268.
76. Haberler C, Alesch F, Mazal PR, et al. No tissue damage by chronic deep brain stimulation in Parkinson's disease. *Ann Neurol* 2000;48:372–376.
77. Kuroda R, Nakatani J, Yamada Y, et al. Location of a DBS-electrode in lateral thalamus for deafferentation pain. An autopsy case report. *Acta Neurochir* 1991; 52[Suppl]:140–142.

Parkinson's Disease: Advances in Neurology, Vol. 91.
Edited by Ariel Gordin, Seppo Kaakkola, and Heikki Teräväinen
Lippincott Williams & Wilkins, Philadelphia © 2003

30

Surgery for Parkinson's Disease, the Five *W*'s: Why, Who, What, Where, and When

Andres M. Lozano

Toronto Western Hospital, University of Toronto, Toronto, Ontario, Canada

There has been a tremendous increase in the use of stereotactic functional neurosurgery in the treatment of Parkinson's disease (PD) (1). There are various reasons for this. First, in many instances, despite the best available medical therapy, patients with advanced PD continue to be disabled. In these patients, drugs provide insufficient benefit or are associated with significant side effects, particularly the development of drug-induced involuntary movements or dyskinesias. When patients reach this point, then alternative strategies, including functional neurosurgery, are important considerations. Perhaps the most important reason functional neurosurgery has made a return is that there is now, for the first time, a scientific rationale for targeting specific basal ganglia structures in the treatment of PD (2). Fundamental observations in the animal models of PD have highlighted the striking abnormalities in the activity of the basal ganglia output nuclei, in particular the internal segment of the globus pallidus (GPi) and the subthalamic nucleus (STN) in parkinsonian states (3,4). It is thought that the pathological outflow from the basal ganglia output structures to the targets in the thalamus and brainstem causes a disruption in motor function. Surgical procedures, thus, aim to cancel or neutralize this pathological outflow. This is accomplished either by lesioning or by the application of deep brain stimulation (DBS). One of the paradoxes that remains is why it is better to have reduced or no information outflow from the basal ganglia, as occurs when the motor pallidum is destroyed with a pallidotomy, for example, rather than the misinformation that is characteristic of the parkinsonian state?

WHY SURGERY?

There are several reasons to consider surgery: first, to provide symptomatic treatment when there is insufficient sustained benefit with parkinsonian medication; second, to diminish the adverse effects associated with medical treatment; and third, to prevent the loss of opportunity that exists despite medical treatment. PD affects patients in subtle ways. They are often underemployed and withdrawn from social situations. The issues of the diminished quality of life and the loss of opportunity that these patients face are becoming appreciated.

Surgery has several effects on the various manifestations of PD. Procedures directed at either the pallidum or the STN have influenced the major motor manifestations of the disease differentially (5–11). The symptoms that are most responsive to surgical interventions are levodopa-induced dyskinesias, which diminish on the order of 80% to 90%, followed by reductions in tremor on the order of 80%, rigidity and akinesia on the order of 60%, and gait and postural disturbances, which benefit on the order of 40% with bilateral procedures. In contrast, parkinsonian symptoms that are resistant to levodopa also tend to be resistant to surgical interventions. These include bladder dysfunction, constipation, speech difficulties, sexual dysfunction, psychological difficulties, seborrhea, and other autonomical disturbances.

TABLE 30.1. *Reasons for turning down patients for neurosurgical procedure for Parkinson's disease*

Inadequate medical trial
Insufficient disability
Cognitive disturbance
Predominant surgically unresponsive symptoms
Does not have Parkinson's disease
Unrealistic expectations of patient or family
Unable to follow or tolerate presurgical/surgical/postsurgical demands for treatment

WHO SHOULD BE OPERATED ON?

Patient selection is one of the most important aspects of surgery for movement disorders. Choosing the best patients is essential because of the potential for surgical morbidity and mortality. It is important to identify patients who will obtain the greatest benefit with surgery and who will maintain benefit for the longest period. It is also important to identify patients who are physically, cognitively, and emotionally able to tolerate surgery and postoperative care.

In the patient selection process, an important attribute and predictor of benefit is the degree to which the patient's symptoms respond to levodopa. Patients can be investigated "off" their drugs and then given a levodopa challenge. In the practically defined "off" condition, after overnight withdrawal of their medications, they are given one to one-half times their regular morning dose of levodopa. As a rule of thumb, the benefit with this levodopa challenge should approximate the benefits attainable with surgery for bilateral movement disorders either in the pallidum or in the STN. The levodopa challenge test not only predicts the potential benefit of surgery but also is important for educating the patient and family as to what the surgery is designed to accomplish and what disability is likely to persist despite surgery.

Other predictors of benefit with surgery include the extent to which the disability is related to motor complications. There has also been a correlation between the degree of pallidal hypermetabolism, as seen in fluorodeoxyglucose testing and the benefits with pallidal surgery interventions (12,13). With respect to age, it is not clear whether patients who are younger show greater benefit and whether this is related to the higher incidence of levodopa-resistant symptoms in the older population, or whether it could be related to the cognitive disturbances or coincident medical conditions. Younger patients may also better tolerate the surgical procedures and their associated adverse effects.

It is also important to stress that many patients who are referred to functional neurosurgical centers for potential surgery for PD are turned down. The main reasons for turning down patients are outlined in Table 30.1.

SURGICAL OPTIONS

Among the options and current usage are lesioning of the thalamic, GPi, or STN or the application of chronic DBS electrodes.

Lesions may continue to have a role, particularly when social and economic factors make the use of chronic DBS impractical. The use of lesions may also be considered when the patient's disability is predominantly unilateral. The main difficulty with the lesioning procedures is when bilateral procedures are required to treat bilateral or axial symptoms. It is under these circumstances that the incidence of side effects rises dramatically and where the application of DBS, a reversible procedure, has certain advantages, as shown in Table 30.2.

TABLE 30.2. *Lesions versus deep brain stimulation*

Lesions	Deep brain stimulation
Irreversible	Reversible
Nonadjustable	Adjustable
The risks are taken "upfront," have a low "upfront" cost	Risk amortized over the lifetime of the patients and the stimulating hardware
Low maintenance	
The safety of bilateral surgery is in question	High "upfront" cost
	High maintenance
	Bilateral surgery may be safer

TARGET SELECTION

Over the course of time, various targets have been chosen for PD. In 1985, a survey by Laitinen (14), of 16 functional neurosurgeons, identified 16 different targets in the thalamus, pallidal fugal pathways, and subthalamic area that were in use. Today, the main targets are the thalamus in tremor-dominant parkinsonism and the GPi and STN in akinetic rigid and dyskinetic forms of PD.

The thalamic target appears to have benefit for tremor, but not for the other cardinal manifestations of PD. The preferred target is moving toward the GPi and STN because they provide benefits not only to tremor but also with the other cardinal manifestations of PD including the rigidity, bradykinesia, gait, and levodopa-induced dyskinesias.

Today, the STN and its adjacent area appear to be a favorite target. The reasons for this are not entirely clear but may include that the STN projects to both output nuclei GPi and the substantia nigra pars reticulata (SNpr) and is, thus, in a position to influence the entire outflow of the basal ganglia. In addition, there have been variable clinical effects of bilateral GPi DBS, related perhaps to the large size and the segregation of motor subcircuits within the GPi (15,16) in contrast to the relatively smaller size of the STN. There is, in addition, general inexperience with pallidal surgery and a lack of incentive for groups doing STN surgery to reconsider their target. Although the STN is the target that may be preferred today, few data suggest that this target is better in terms of efficacy or adverse effects related to other targets. There is, to date, no blinded study comparing the two targets and there is no blinded or randomized study comparing the relative attributes of the two targets. A recent paper in the *New England Journal of Medicine* (11), which included patients from multiple institutions, suggests that both the GPi and the STN can provide significant functional benefit. In this analysis, STN DBS provided a greater degree of motor benefit and was associated with a reduction in drug requirements. GPi and STN targets, however, provided similar increases in "on" periods in the day with associated reductions of "off" periods and "on" periods of dyskinesias.

The relative profile of benefits and adverse effects with surgical procedures is also a function of the experience of each functional neurosurgical center with the target and the location within the target. There is also a great need for experience with case management and the complex interactions between the need to reduce dopaminergic drugs and to increase the stimulation parameters.

One of the important issues today is how DBS works and whether the beneficial effects seen with GPi and STN or thalamic surgery are related to cellular effects or effects on the axonal projections to and from the nucleus. In particular, there is increasing evidence that the large fiber systems surrounding the STN and GPi may be involved in some of the therapeutic benefit (17–19). Working out the mechanisms through which DBS exerts its benefits in patients with PD is one of the future research priorities.

WHEN TO OPERATE?

The issue of when to operate on patients with PD is associated with considerable controversy. In theory, the potential points of intervention include the presymptomatic state, when patients have symptoms but no disability, when patients have disability, or in advanced disease states.

Because there is no evidence that surgical procedure alters the natural history of progression of the disease, there is little rationale at this stage to offer surgery to patients who do not have significant motor disability. As the surgical procedures become safer and safer, there will be greater enthusiasm to offer surgery earlier in the course of the disease, particularly if it is felt that surgery could reduce the requirement for medications. In current usage, surgery should be offered after patients have had an adequate drug trial and should not be offered for patients to prevent motor complications. On the other hand, surgery should not be delayed until patients lose their employment, their responsibilities to their family and society, or their independence. The development of markers for who will continue to respond well to medication and who is destined to have major problems with response fluctuations may provide a rationale for when to operate early. In addition, once response fluctuations develop to a mild extent, knowing who will be relatively easy to treat and who will experience pronounced disability will be important in deciding the timing of surgery. Finally, those who will develop significant problems with drug-resistant symptoms and those who are not the best candidates for surgery at this time would also be useful in determining the ideal candidates.

There are several important future considerations in movement disorder surgery for PD. Does surgery change the natural history of PD? Does it provide neuroprotection, or is there any evidence of neuroplasticity in motor circuits with longstanding changes in function after a prolonged period of stimulation? Another important future consideration is whether there may be beneficial effects of levodopa sparing by introducing surgery at an earlier time. The use of surgery on patients who are not ideal candidates—for example, those who have a mild degree of cognitive deficit or who have a mixture of dopa-responsive and non-dopa–responsive symptoms—is important.

What is clear is that functional neurosurgery for PD will take on an increasingly important role because of the increasing incidence of PD with the demographics of our aging population. The development in molecular biology, imaging, and the further understanding of motor and nonmotor neurological function and dysfunction will provide a strong rationale and will drive the scientific use of these surgical procedures. This will mean an expansion of indications, and perhaps offering surgery earlier and to a greater number of patients.

ACKNOWLEDGMENTS

I thank Dr. A. E. Lang for his ongoing ideas, criticisms, and collaboration. The author receives research funding from the Canadian Institute of Health Research, the National Institutes of Health, and the R. R. Tasker Chair in Functional Neurosurgery at the Toronto Western Hospital and University of Toronto.

REFERENCES

1. Lozano AM, Lang AE. Pallidotomy for Parkinson's disease. *Neurosurg Clin North Am* 1998;9:325–336.
2. DeLong MR. Primate models of movement disorders of basal ganglia origin. *TINS* 1990;13:281–285.
3. Lang AE, Lozano AM. Parkinson's disease. First of two parts. *N Engl J Med* 1998;339:1044–1053.
4. Lang AE, Lozano AM. Parkinson's disease. Second of two parts. *N Engl J Med* 1998;339:1130–1143.
5. Lozano AM, Lang AE, Galvez-Jimenez N, et al. Effect of GPi pallidotomy on motor function in Parkinson's disease. *Lancet* 1995;346:1383–1387.
6. Limousin P, Krack P, Pollak P, et al. Electrical stimulation of the subthalamic nucleus in advanced Parkinson's disease. *N Engl J Med* 1998;339:1105–1111.
7. Limousin P, Speelman JD, Gielen F, et al. Multicentre European study of thalamic stimulation in parkinsonian

and essential tremor. *J Neurol Neurosurg Psychiatry* 1999;66:289–296.
8. Kumar R, Lang AE, Rodriguez-Oroz MC, et al. Deep brain stimulation of the globus pallidus pars interna in advanced Parkinson's disease. *Neurology* 2000;55: S34–S39.
9. Kumar R, Lozano AM, Kim YJ, et al. Double-blind evaluation of subthalamic nucleus deep brain stimulation in advanced Parkinson's disease. *Neurology* 1998; 51:850–855.
10. Kumar R, Lozano AM, Sime E, et al. Comparative effects of unilateral and bilateral subthalamic nucleus deep brain stimulation. *Neurology* 1999;53:561–566.
11. Deep-brain stimulation of the subthalamic nucleus or the pars interna of the globus pallidus in Parkinson's disease. *N Engl J Med* 2001;345:956–963.
12. Eidelberg D, Moeller JR, Ishikawa T, et al. Regional metabolic correlates of surgical outcome following unilateral pallidotomy for Parkinson's disease. *Ann Neurol* 1996;39:450–459.
13. Eidelberg D, Moeller JR, Kazumata K, et al. Metabolic correlates of pallidal neuronal activity in Parkinson's disease. *Brain* 1997;120:1315–1324.
14. Laitinen LV. Brain targets in surgery for Parkinson's disease. Results of a survey of neurosurgeons. *J Neurosurg* 1985;62:349–351.
15. Hoover JE, Strick PL. Multiple output channels in the basal ganglia. *Science* 1993;259:819–821.
16. Gross RE, Lombardi WJ, Lang AE, et al. Relationship of lesion location to clinical outcome following microelectrode-guided pallidotomy for Parkinson's disease. *Brain* 1999;122:405–416.
17. Ashby P, Rothwell JC. Neurophysiologic aspects of deep brain stimulation. *Neurology* 2000;55[Suppl 6]: S17–S20.
18. Ashby P, Kim YJ, Kumar R, et al. Neurophysiological effects of stimulation through electrodes in the human subthalamic nucleus. *Brain* 1999;122:1919–1931.
19. Ashby P, Strafella A, Dostrovsky JO, et al. Immediate motor effects of stimulation through electrodes implanted in the human globus pallidus. *Stereotact Funct Neurosurg* 1998;70:1–18.

Parkinson's Disease: Advances in Neurology, Vol. 91.
Edited by Ariel Gordin, Seppo Kaakkola, and Heikki Teräväinen
Lippincott Williams & Wilkins, Philadelphia © 2003

31

Preclinical Versus Clinical Neuroprotection

*Edna Grünblatt, *Robert Schlößer, †Manfred Gerlach, and *Peter Riederer

**Department of Neurochemistry, the Clinic and Polyclinic of Psychiatry and Psychotherapy, Bayerische Julius-Maximilians-University of Würzburg, Würzburg, Germany; and †Department of Clinical Neurochemistry, University Clinic and Health Center for Children and Youth Psychiatry and Psychotherapy, Würzburg, Germany*

Although the etiology and pathogenesis of Parkinson's disease (PD) are still unknown, some studies demonstrate the importance of family associated genetic factors. Frequently, these genetic alterations are connected with an early onset of the disease. Despite the fact of increasing knowledge, symptomatic treatment to substitute the loss of dopamine (DA) or antagonizing increased *N*-methyl-D-aspartate (NMDA) receptor activity is still the strategy to improve patients symptoms.

Neuroprotective therapies are interventions that produce enduring benefits by favorably influencing underlying etiology or pathogenesis of neurodegenerative disorders. Although preclinical neuroprotection is clearly shown for various DA agonists, monoamine oxidase B (MAO-B) inhibitors, and NMDA receptor antagonists, clinical neuroprotection is assumed at best for ropinirole, pramipexole, pergolide, selegiline, and amantadine in mostly unselected groups of PD. Until now, clinical neuroprotection remains an unachieved goal of experimental therapeutics. Therefore, it is essential to evaluate genetic markers for homogenous subgroups.

The weakness of all our current clinical trials is related to the scientific rigidity of the design of these studies and the current definition of the success of such clinical trials. Such limitations can be avoided by pharmacogenetic studies because they will not only demonstrate clinical effectiveness but also show who the drug will benefit.

PD is one of the major neurodegenerative disorders of middle and old age that was originally described by James Parkinson in 1817 (1). It is characterized by the triad of cardinal symptoms—muscle rigidity, tremor, and bradykinesia—but can also involve postural deficits and impaired gait, as well as psychiatric and autonomous symptoms in a significant minority of patients.

Although idiopathic PD is usually sporadic, it has long been recognized that there is a genetic component to the disease. Case–control studies have typically indicated a twofold to fourfold increase in incidence in close relatives of patients with PD (2). Nevertheless, in sporadic PD, environmental factors have been emphasized (3). The mechanisms involved in the progressive degeneration of nigral dopaminergic neurons in PD are the subject of intense studies (4). Although the proximal causes have not been defined, various mechanisms have been implicated (5) in the more distal pathogenesis of PD (Table 31.1).

Putative propagating factors include oxidative stress (OS), excitatory neurotoxicity, free radical generation, disturbance of mitochondrial respiratory chain activity, calcium homeostasis, nitric oxide (NO) toxicity, immune processes, and apoptosis. These pathogenetic mechanisms may be accelerated by iron and other transitional metals. Levodopa metabolism can generate toxic oxidative metabolites that might accelerate neuronal degeneration in PD (6,7). Levodopa can be converted to

TABLE 31.1. *Possible molecular mechanisms of dopaminergic cell death in Parkinson's disease*

The hypothesized mechanism	Possible processes causing the cascade	Possible neuroprotective strategies
Oxidative stress Neurotoxic effects of oxygen-derived free radicals, such as hydroxyl superoxide, and nitric oxide radicals	1. Metabolism of catecholamines and endogenous or exogenous neurotoxins 2. Impaired free radical scavenging systems 3. Altered brain iron metabolism 4. Inflammatory cytokine-induced gliosis	Antioxidative strategies using iron chelator, radical scavengers, monoamine oxidase inhibitors, and antiinflammatory drugs
Excitotoxic mechanism Excitatory amino acid receptor–mediated influx of cations gives rise to neurotoxic effects	1. Abnormal glutamate accumulation 2. Exogenous excitotoxins (e.g., domoic acid)	Glutamate receptor antagonists and calcium-channel blockers
Disturbance in mitochondrial energy metabolism: Diminished or completely ceased adenosine triphosphate synthesis	1. Mitochondrial toxins (e.g., MPP^+, paraquat, TaClo) 2. Glutamate-induced processes 3. Disturbance of calcium homeostasis	Supplementation of mitochondrial energy metabolism, glutamate receptor antagonists, and calcium-channel blockers
Apoptosis Programmed cell death of the neurons	1. Oxidative stress 2. High glutamate levels 3. Excitotoxins 4. Disturbance of calcium homeostasis 5. Impaired growth factor levels	Antioxidants, *N*-methyl-D-aspartate antagonists, calcium-channel blockers, and growth factors
Cell-cycle arrest Entering the cell cycle without termination	1. Oxidative stress 2. Inflammatory process 3. Impaired growth factor levels	Antioxidants, antiinflammatory drugs, and growth factors

Source: From Gerlach M, Riederer P, Youdim MB. Neuroprotective therapeutic strategies. Comparison of experimental and clinical results. *Biochem Pharmacol* 1995;50:1–16, with permission.

DA, which, when metabolized either enzymatically or by autooxidation, can yield reactive oxygen species (ROS) such as hydrogen peroxide and hydroxyl radicals. Considerable evidence indicates that the substantia nigra pars compacta (SNpc) is under OS in PD (8, 9). This is reflected by increased iron, which promotes OS, and decreased glutathione (GSH), the primary defense mechanism in the brain against OS. Biochemical markers of oxidative damage to proteins, lipids, and DNA are evident in the SNpc of patients with PD. Defects in mitochondrial respiratory functions and in the DA transporter system have been identified as potential sites of nigrostriatal dysfunction. In experimental models, the pathogenetic processes are amenable to experimental treatments and are potentially reversible (4,10).

Much of our knowledge about dopaminergic neurodegeneration has come from studies with two neurotoxins that produce animal models for OS and parkinsonism syndrome in rodents, primates, and other species. Neurotoxins 6-hydroxydopamine (6-OHDA) (11) and 1-methyl-4-phenyl-1,2,3,6-tetrahydropyridine (MPTP) (12,13) cause the degeneration of nigrostriatal dopaminergic neurons with the subsequent loss of striatal DA. The ability of the antiparkinsonian drug, selegiline (previously named L-deprenyl), an irreversible MAO-B inhibitor, to prevent MPTP-induced parkinsonism in mice and nonhuman primates was the first example of possible neuroprotection for PD (14). The mechanism of this process has been explained by the inhibition of MAO-B by selegiline, thus preventing the metabolism of the neurotoxin to the reactive metabolite 1-methyl-4-phenylpyridine (MPP^+) by the enzyme and the formation of hydrogen peroxide. This explanation appears to be too simple because selegiline was shown to prevent and rescue cultured nigral neurons from the induced oxidative damage caused by the reactive metabolite MPP^+ (15). Moreover, other drugs not having MAO-B inhibitory action can also exert neuroprotection in this model. So far, iron chelators (e.g., desferrioxamine) (16–18); antioxidants (vitamin E) (18–20); DA agonists such as apomorphine, bromocriptine, and pramipexole (21–25); GSH analogues (26); and NO synthase inhibitors (7NI but not L-NAME) (27,28) have been described to have the same effect (Table 31.2).

Unfortunately, there is still no clear-cut evidence in the clinic for neuroprotection by either of the drugs used. This may be a consequence of experimental design or interpretation of the outcomes, which are controversial. Traditional endpoints that respond to enhanced dopaminergic activity may not be suitable for distinguishing symptomatic from neuroprotective effects. This chapter aims to review and compare preclinical findings for neuroprotection versus clinical trials and to discuss the difficulties accounted in clinics to achieve neuroprotection.

TABLE 31.2. *Drugs demonstrating neuroprotective properties in experimental models for Parkinson's disease*

Functional group	Chemical drug name	Neuroprotective against			
		MPTP	6-Hydroxy-dopamine	Methamphetamine	Others
Antioxidants	Coenzyme Q/ nicotinamide	+	n.t.	n.t.	
	Cysteamine	+	n.t.	n.t.	
	Ginkgo biloba	+	n.t.	n.t.	
	Salicylic acid				
	Aspirin	+	n.t.	n.t.	
	Vitamin C	+/–	n.t.	n.t.	
	Vitamin E	+/–	+	n.t.	
Iron chelators	Desferrioxamine	n.t.	+	n.t.	
	Cytisine	+	n.t.	n.t.	
	Scavestrogene	n.t.	n.t.	n.t.	Hydroxyl radicals
NOS inhibitors	7-Nitroindazole	+	n.t.	+	
MAO-B inhibitors	Selegiline	+	+	n.t.	DSP-4
	Rasagiline	+	n.t.	n.t.	
Dopamine receptor agonists	Apomorphine	+	+	+	
	Bromocriptine	+	+	n.t.	L-dopa toxicity
	Cabergoline	n.t.	+	n.t.	
	αDHEC	+	n.t.	n.t.	Glutamate
	Lisuride	n.t.	+	n.t.	L-dopa toxicity
	Pergolide	–	+	n.t.	MPP^+
	Pramipexole	+	n.t.	+	L-dopa toxicity MPP^+
	Ropinirole	n.t.	+	n.t.	
Excitatory amino acid receptor inhibitors	Budipine	n.t.	n.t.	n.t.	MPP^+
	Memantine	n.t.	n.t.	n.t.	Glutamate, NMDA
	MK-801	–	n.t.	+	MPP^+
Calcium-channel blockers	Nimodipine	+	–	n.t.	NMDA

DSP-4, *N*-(2-chlorethyl)-*N*-ethyl-2-brombenzylamine; MAO-B, monoamine oxidase B; NMDA, *N*-methyl D-aspartate; NOS, nitric oxide synthase; n.t., not tested; –, no neuroprotection seen; +, neuroprotection.

Source: From Gerlach M, Reichmann H, Riederer P. *Die Parkinson-Krankheit. Grundlagen, Klinik, Therapie,* 2nd ed. Vienna, Austria: Springer-Verlag, 2001, with permission.

PRECLINICAL EXPERIMENTS PRESENTING NEUROPROTECTION

Vitamins C and E as Antioxidants

Vitamins C and E are natural antioxidants used by our body to prevent the OS produced by radicals.

Vitamin C (ascorbic acid) is one of the important water-soluble cytosolic antioxidants. Human brain consists of a high concentration of vitamin C (281 to 331 mg/g of tissue). Ascorbic acid has a strong reduction ability, which in contact to free radical turns to semidehydroascorbic acid. This, in turn, metabolizes back to ascorbic acid through enzymatic reactions.

Membrane-bound vitamin E is an important lipophilic antioxidant. Similar to vitamin C, it cannot be synthesized by the human organism. Vitamin E consists of eight natural molecules, which consist of α, β, γ and Δ-tocopherol.

In some early studies using vitamin C and E in the MPTP mouse model, it was found to induce a partial neuroprotective effect against the neurodegeneration of the dopaminergic neurons (13). However, these effects could not be reproduced. In several studies of nonhuman primates, no neuroprotective effect was seen (30): Even a high dose of vitamin C (100 mg/kg per day) and vitamin E (2,350 mg/kg per day) for 52 days did not affect the DA levels in the striatum of MPTP-treated marmosets. In more recent studies conducted by Offen et al. (31), DA-induced death in pheochromocytoma cells (PC12) could be inhibited by antioxidants such as reduced GSH, *N*-acetylcysteine, and dithiothreitol, whereas vitamins C and E had less effect. The cytoplasmic thiol antioxidants and vitamin C, but not the membrane-bound vitamin E, prevented DA autooxidation and production of DA melanin. Similar findings were reported by Zilkha-Falb et al. (32). In contrast, Iacovitti and Stull (33) demonstrated that the vitamin E analogue Trolox was capable of rescuing striatal neurons from cell death. These results indicate that different antioxidants behave differently in various systems and that H compounds, being cytosolically active, seem to be more effective in preventing toxicity, at least in acute experiments.

DOPAMINE AGONISTS AND NEUROPROTECTION IN PD

There are several possible mechanisms whereby DA agonists might provide neuroprotection in PD. Use of DA agonists decreases the cumulative dose of levodopa that a patient with PD takes over the course of the illness (34,35), so it reduces the number of levodopa molecules undergoing oxidative metabolism, thereby reducing the formation of ROS. Stimulation of D_2 auto-receptors on dopaminergic neurons decreases DA synthesis, release, and metabolism, as well as the formation of ROS. It has recently been suggested that stimulation of D_2 receptors may be associated with apoptosis. D_2 receptor knockout mice developed hyperplasia and increased numbers of lactotrophs within the pituitary gland (36,37). This suggests an antiproliferative function for DA and DA agonists that is regulated through D_2 receptor activation. In addition, a direct antioxidant effect of the DA agonists has been suggested for many of the substances, such as bromocriptine (38,39) and apomorphine (40–42), which showed to be an effective hydroxyl and superoxide radical scavenger *in vitro,* as well as inhibit hydroxyl radical formation and lipid peroxidation *in vivo* (38). Pergolide can also scavenge NO radicals *per se* (43) and induces an increase in basal ganglia levels of superoxide dismutase (SOD) (44). The hydroxylated benzyl ring structure within most DA agonists may bestow free radical scavenger properties of these molecules.

R-apomorphine is a D_1-D_2 receptor agonist, acting both presynaptically and postsynaptically (45). Apomorphine reduces the oxidation of polyunsaturated fatty acids (41), scavenges free radicals, chelates iron (42), and protects PC12 cells in culture from the cytotoxic action of ROS generated by hydrogen peroxide and 6-OHDA (46). These properties are directly linked to its ability to inhibit brain mitochondrial lipid peroxidation and protein oxidation (42). Furthermore, it has also been shown that apomorphine promotes neurite outgrowth in PC12 cells and mesencephalic cell cultures (47). Recently, it was established that *in vivo* both apomorphine enantiomers exert neuroprotective properties in the MPTP mouse model of PD (22,23) and in the methamphetamine rat model (48). The neuroprotective properties of apomorphine may depend in part on its catechol structure because this attribute has repeatedly been shown to confer radical-scavenging ability (49, 50). Both DA and apomorphine have been shown to be radical scavengers, but apomorphine is 20 times more potent (42).

Bromocriptine is a widely used antiparkinsonian drug with potent D_2 agonistic and mild D_1 receptor antagonistic actions (51). Bromocriptine has been shown to possess strong free radical–scavenging action in *in vitro* (38,39) and *in vivo* (52) studies. Studies using the *in vitro* neurotoxicity of glutamate (53) or levodopa (54) for dopaminergic neurons from rat mesencephalic neurons show neuroprotective properties of bromocriptine, which are mediated not only by the inhibition of DA turnover but also by D_2 receptor stimulation and the subsequent synthesis of proteins that scavenge free radicals. Additionally, bromocriptine could be protective against methamphetamine-induced DA depletion (52), 6-OHDA (38), NO (43), and MPTP-induced dopaminergic toxicity *in vivo* in mice (24). Bromocriptine administration in combination with levodopa suppressed the elevation of DA turnover in the striatum of hemiparkinsonism rats (55). Moreover, behavioral effects after administration of MPTP have been shown to be reversed in monkeys (56,57) and mice (58).

Cabergoline is a tetracyclic ergoline compound with a long plasma half-life. It is a selective D_2 receptor agonist with no substantial affinity for D_1 receptors (59). In recent studies, cabergoline was shown to decrease basal lipid peroxidation levels in the hippocampus and striatum of rats and to decrease stimulated lipid peroxidation (60). *In vivo,* acute and prolonged administration of cabergoline reversed the parkinsonian-like symptoms in MPTP-treated monkeys (61). In addition, chronic administration of cabergoline has reversed levodopa-induced dyskinesias in MPTP-treated monkeys (62).

α-Dihydroergocryptine is a hydrogenated derivative of α-ergocryptine, acting as an agonist of D_2 receptors and as a partial agonist of D_1 receptors (63,64). Besides the documented dopaminergic activity, recent studies have found evidence of a neuroprotective effect of α-dihydroergocryptine against free radical damage (65–67). It was reported that α-dihydroergocryptine protects cultured rat cerebellar granule cells against age-dependent and glutamate-induced neurotoxicity presumably by exerting a scavenger action (68). In the MPTP-treated monkeys, α-dihydroergocryptine administration induced a restoration of the unstimulated malondialdehyde values to control levels (66,69). The neuroprotective activity of α-dihydroergocryptine is related to its peculiar activity on antioxidative enzymes of the GSH system and reduction of lipid peroxide–induced cellular degeneration.

Lisuride is a potent ergoline D_2 and D_3 receptor agonist, but it has also some β_2 adrenergic and serotonergic activity (29). This agonist is only available in Europe and South America. Lisuride has also been suggested to be neuroprotective. In primary mouse mesencephalic cultures, lisuride has been shown to protect dopaminergic neurons against levodopa- and MPP^+-induced toxicity (Table 31.2). The metabolism of both of these substances is associated with the production of ROS, suggesting that lisuride might scavenge free radical species and, thus, protect against oxidative damage. Alternatively, or simultaneously, lisuride might increase cell survival by reducing DA turnover via the activation of auto-receptors or by supporting aerobic metabolic pathways. A current study in rats (K. Double, M. Gerlach, *unpublished data*) suggests that lisuride can attenuate iron-induced dopaminergic cell loss and thus may be neuroprotective in PD.

Pergolide, a semisynthetic ergoline derivative, is a potent D_1/D_2 receptor agonist currently used almost exclusively as an adjunct to levodopa therapy to slow the clinical progression of the disease or prevent the serious adverse effects arising during long-term treatment with levodopa (70,71). It was demonstrated that pergolide scavenges both hydroxyl and NO free radicals *in vitro* and inhibits lipid peroxidation in rat brain homogenates (43,72). Chronic administration of pergolide has been shown to be neuroprotective, preserving the integrity of nigrostriatal neurons in the aging rat brain (73). *In vivo* studies have demonstrated that pergolide provides complete protection against 6-OHDA–induced dopaminergic dysfunction and normalizes low DA levels in mice striata (74). In MPTP-treated monkeys, pergolide demonstrated an antiparkinsonian effect (56).

Pramipexole is an amino benzothiazole–type DA agonist. It binds to presynaptic and postsynaptic D_2 and D_3 receptor subtypes. It appears to have little or no activity at the D_1 receptor site. A potential free radical–scavenging ability of pramipexole has been observed in a preliminary *in vitro* study: Pramipexole was susceptible to oxidation at a relatively low electrochemical potential, suggesting that it may have antioxidant properties (75). In tissue culture, pramipexole has been shown to prevent the DA neuronal loss produced by levodopa, DA (76), hydrogen peroxide and 6-OHDA, as well as the neurotoxic metabolite of MPTP MPP^+ (25,77–79), independent of DA receptor activation. Furthermore, intraperitoneal pramipexole administration to MPTP-treated mice significantly inhibited the MPTP-induced striatal DA neuronal loss and protected against the decrease in DA levels (80). Moreover, methamphetamine-induced loss of nigrostriatal neurons was attenuated from 40% to 8% by oral pramipexole in mice (75).

Ropinirole is a selective non-ergoline D_2 receptor agonist that is primarily used for the treatment of idiopathic PD. Ropinirole demonstrated free radical–scavenging and antioxidant activity *in vitro* and neuroprotective effect in mice (81). Ropinirole scavenged hydroxyl free radicals and NO in a concentration-dependent manner but had lower scavenging activity than other DA agonists such as pergolide or bromocriptine. In an *ex vivo* study using striatal tissue, intraperitoneal ropinirole increased levels of antioxidant defense mechanisms such as GSH, catalase, and SOD (81). Pretreatment with ropinirole has shown neuroprotective properties against 6-OHDA–induced neurotoxicity in mice (81).

MONOAMINE OXIDASE B INHIBITORS AND PRECLINICAL NEUROPROTECTION

MAO catalyzes the oxidative deamination of monoamine neurotransmitters and neuromodulators such as DA, noradrenaline, serotonin (5-hydroxytyramine), and β-phenylethylamine (PEA), as well as some exogenous bioactive monoamines. Two types of MAO exist in mammalian tissues, MAO-A and MAO-B, with different substrate and inhibitor specificity (82). MAO-A deaminates preferentially serotonin and is sensitive to selective inhibitors, such as clorgyline. MAO-B deaminates preferentially PEA and is sensitive to MAO-B inhibitors, such as selegiline. Inhibitors of MAO-A have proven to be effective antidepressants, whereas MAO-B blockers have been emphasized in the treatment of PD.

MAO-B constitutes about 80% of the total MAO activity in the human brain (83,84) and is the predominant form of the enzyme in the striatum (85).

Selegiline: Deprenyl irreversibly inhibits MAO-B, and its (−)-isomer (selegiline) is a more potent inhibitor than its (+)-enantiomer (86). The neuroprotective action of selegiline is multifold. There are at least four accepted mechanisms by which selegiline could prevent neurodegeneration (87). First, it may decrease the free radical formation (generation of hydrogen peroxide) from normal metabolism of the biogenic amines, mainly DA, by inhibition of MAO-B in the central nervous systems (CNS) (88). In the presence of the Fe^{2+} ion, hydrogen peroxide metabolizes through the Fenton reaction and generates hydroxyl radicals, which causes membrane and DNA destruction. It is well known that MAO-

B activity increases with age, which leads to the rise in hydrogen peroxide formation (89,90). In addition to the OS caused by age-dependent increase of MAO-B activity, further reactions between endogenous amines and aldehydes formed by MAO-B can play a role in neurodegeneration (91). Second, according to some authors, selegiline may increase the free radical–scavenging capacity of the brain by elevation of SOD activity (92,93), but others failed to observe any increase in SOD function (94). Third, due to MAO-B inhibition, selegiline may prevent the activation of the environmental pretoxins (95). Finally, due to the uptake inhibitory properties of the nerve endings, thereby obviating the neuronal damage, the metabolites of selegiline ([–]-methyl-amphetamine and [–]-amphetamine) are even more potent than the parent compound (96).

The neuroprotective properties of the MAO-B inhibitor, selegiline, which may influence the progress of the disease, has been extensively investigated (97–112), as summarized in Table 31.3.

Rasagiline (*N*-propargyl-1[R]-aminoindan) is a propargylamine-related compound that possesses a selective irreversible inhibitory effect on MAO-B. *In vivo* studies demonstrated that rasagiline is up to ten times more active as an MAO-B inhibitor than selegiline (113). Its neuroprotective activity has been examined in several *in vitro, in vivo,* and cell culture studies (114–116). It was found to

TABLE 31.3. *Evidence for the neuroprotective properties of monoamine oxidase B inhibition by selegiline in preclinical animal models and clinical studies*

Study	Details	References
Protection against neurotoxins	1. Selegiline protected against the neurotoxicity of MPTP by inhibition of the convertion of MPTP to MPP^+. 2. In animal models, selegiline, protected against the toxic damage of MPTP, 6-OHDA, haloperidol and noradrenergic neurotoxin DSP-4.	88,97–99
Protection against free radicals formation	1. Selegiline inhibited dopamine metabolism by MAO-B, which generates hydrogen peroxide. 2. It inhibited hydroxyl radical formation induced by a more toxic 2′-methyl analog of MPTP. 3. It suppressed hydroxyl radical formation induced by MPP^+. 4.It suppressed dopamine melanin synthesis mediated by nonenzymatic autoxidation of dopamine *in vitro.* 5. Long-term treatment with selegiline increased activities of SOD and catalase in the striatum of animals.	100–102
Effects on neurotrophic factors	1. Treatment of cultured mouse astrocytes with selegiline up-regulated the NGF, BDNF, and GDNF synthesis.	103
Protection against apoptosis	1. Selegiline and other propargylamines protected dopaminergic neurons from apoptosis induced by reactive oxygen species.	104
In longevity studies	1. Selegiline have demonstrated to be useful in longevity studies in rats.	101
In PD clinical studies	2. Selegiline delays the emergence of disability in untreated patients with early PD and slows the progression of some cognitive deficits in AD. 3. Selegiline increases life expectancy in PD. 4. Selegiline delays the need for levodopa in newly diagnosed patients. 5. Subjects with early, mild PD, treated with selegiline did not show protection against oxidative stress measured by CSF HVA levels.	101,105–112

AD, Alzheimer's disease; BDNF, brain-derived neurotrophic factor; CSF, cerebrospinal fluid; DSP-4, *N*-(2-chlorethyl-*N*-ethyl-2-brombenzylamine); GDNF, glia-cell derived neurotrophic factor; HVA, homovanillic acid; 6-OHDA, 6-hydroxydopamine; MPP^+, 1-methyl-4-phenylpyridine; MPTP, 1-methyl-4-phenyl-1,2,3,6-tetrahydropyridine; NGF, nerve growth factor; PD, Parkinson's disease; SOD, superoxide dismutase.

prevent cell death caused by apoptosis (117). Rasagiline preserved the mitochondrial membrane potential, $\Delta\psi m$, which was proved also in isolated mitochondria and completely suppressed the activation of caspase-3 and DNA fragmentation (118). In addition, TV1022, the optical (S)-isomer of rasagiline, devoid of MAO-A and MAO-B inhibitory actions, has shown similar neuroprotective antiapoptotic activity as rasagiline (114, 119). The Western blot measurements have shown that both drugs prevent the decrease in Bcl-2 and Cu/Zn-SOD1 during serum and nerve growth factor withdrawal in partially neuronally differentiated PC12 cells. Furthermore, chronic treatment with rasagiline *in vivo* induces the increase of SOD and catalase in brain and other tissues of rats (120). Using neuronal cell lines, rasagiline was shown to be 15% to 20% more effective as a neuronal survival agent than selegiline, increasing the survival of dopaminergic neurons with no statistically significant increase in survival of GABAergic neurons (121).

NMDA RECEPTOR ANTAGONISTS AND PRECLINICAL NEUROPROTECTION

There are a number of interactions between the glutamatergic and dopaminergic pathways in the basal ganglia. The neurons on which DA provides an inhibitory input have an excitatory input from corticostriatal glutamatergic neurons (122–125). Parkinsonian rigidity is produced, in part, by activation of NMDA receptors in the anterior striatum or after activation of non-NMDA receptors in the subthalamic nucleus (STN), internal segment of the globus pallidus or substantia nigra pars reticulata (126). Therefore, pharmacological manipulations that reduce glutamatergic transmission within either the striatum or the medial segment of the globus pallidus will reduce parkinsonian symptoms.

Extensive toxicological studies have demonstrated that excessive NMDA receptor–mediated glutamatergic neurotransmission can result in excitotoxic death of neurons (127). Accordingly, NMDA receptor antagonists have been shown to protect neurons from this process (128).

Amantadine, the antiviral agent (1-aminoadamantane), is a synthetic tricyclic amine with antiparkinsonian effects that were discovered incidentally (129). Amantadine was first synthesized more than 40 years ago and was initially introduced for prophylaxis of influenza (130). Its precise mode of action is unclear, but at pharmacological doses, it includes anticholinergic effects (131) and release of DA from and blockade of DA reuptake into presynaptic nerve endings (132). However, changes in postsynaptic receptor function and glutamatergic NMDA receptor antagonism have been suggested to be relevant in clinical doses (123). Amantadine prevented retinal ganglion cell death in high concentrations (133). Similarly, amantadine protected cultured rat cortical neurons against NMDA-induced toxicity (134).

In the MPTP animal model of PD, amantadine had partially protective effects (135), suggesting that aminoadamantanes may not only ameliorate the motor manifestations of reduced nigrostriatal transmission but also attenuate disease progression. Clearly, further studies to clarify this question are required.

CLINICAL STUDIES FOR NEUROPROTECTION

Prospective controlled clinical studies for neuroprotection in parkinsonian patients (136–150) are listed in Table 31.4.

Selegiline was one of the first drugs tested to prove possible neuroprotective effects in humans. The reasons for this choice were two: (a) the neuroprotective effect of selegiline seen in the MPTP model and (b) the finding of Birkmayer et al. (151), in which patients receiving levodopa combined with selegiline lived longer than those receiving levodopa alone.

Although it was possible to show neuroprotective features of several drugs in preclinical studies by *in vitro* and *in vivo* studies, avail-

TABLE 31.4. *Prospective controlled clinical studies for neuroprotection in parkinsonian patients*

Study group/authors	Objective	Drugs tested	Effect
Tetrud and Langston (111)	Whether selegiline would delay the need for levodopa therapy	Selegiline	Early selegiline therapy delays in about 9 months the requirement for levodopa
The Parkinson Study Group (DATATOP) (106,107,136,137)	Whether selegiline would delay the need for levodopa therapy	Selegiline	Early selegiline therapy delays in about 6–9 months the requirement for levodopa
		α-Tocopherol	No effect
Olanow et al. (34)	Whether pergolide mesylate would delay the need of levodopa therapy	Pergolide	Pergolide provides clinical improvement while permitting a reduction in levodopa dose
PRADO Study (138,139)	Whether bromocriptine would delay the need for levodopa therapy	Bromocriptine	Bromocriptine lessened severity and the occurrence of levodopa-related motor complications
Ropinirole Study Group (140,141)	Whether ropinirole would delay levodopa fluctuations	Ropinirole	Ropinirole reduces levodopa dose with clinical benefit for parkinsonian patients with motor fluctuations
O53 Study Group (142)	To compare the efficacy and safety of ropinirole with or without selegiline	Ropinirole	In absence of selegiline, ropinirole is effective and superior to bromocriptine; selegiline does not affect the response in patients treated with ropinirole
The Parkinson Study Group (143–145)	Whether lazabemide influences the progression of disability in untreated PD	Lazabemide	The effects of lazabemide therapy are similar to DATATOP study
Norwegian-Danish Study Group (146,147)	Study the effects of selegiline on levodopa treatment and parkinsonian disability	Selegiline	Combination of selegiline and levodopa therapy lessens severity and requires lower doses of levodopa
SELEDO (112)	The time point when levodopa dose should be increased by 50%	Selegiline	Early selegiline therapy lowers the levodopa doses required in time
Ahlskog et al. (148)	β-CIT SPECT imaging of dopamine agonist therapy effect on DAT	Pergolide	Pergolide therapy did not significantly affect ^{123}I-β-CIT SPECT imaging
Guttman et al. (149)	Whether levodopa or pramipexole might regulate striatal DAT binding as measured by PET	Pramipexole	Short-term therapy with levodopa and, to a lesser extent, pramipexole, can modestly downregulate striatal DAT in patients with early PD
Linazasoro et al. (150)	Modification of dopamine D_2 receptor activity by pergolide studied with PET	Pergolide	Pergolide therapy caused a slight reduction in the specific striatal ^{11}C-raclopride uptake index

Note: DAT, dopamine transporter; DATATOP, deprenyl and tocopherol antioxidative therapy of Parkinson's disease; PET, positron emission tomography; PRADO, PRA videll + DO-pa; SELEDO, selegiline and levodopa-long-time trial; SPECT, single-photon emission computed tomography.

Source: From Gerlach M, Reichmann H, Riederer P. *Die Parkinson-Krankheit. Grundlagen, Klinik, Therapie,* 2nd ed. Vienna, Austria: Springer-Verlag, 2001, with permission.

able data on clinical trials are not convincing. Due to fundamental problems in study designs and the current definition of the success of such clinical trials, results are discussed controversially.

It is assumed that OS mechanisms are some of the major contributing factors in the pathogenesis of PD (152). For this reason, antioxidative strategies have been the focus of clinical trials for neuroprotection in PD so far.

Selegiline

Selegiline has been proposed to be a possible neuroprotective substance, due to its MAO-B–inhibiting properties and the consequential reduction of hydrogen peroxide and toxic DA metabolites (3,153). In addition to these properties, some other possible neuroprotective actions have been discovered, such as induction of the antioxidant enzymes (Cu/Zn-SOD, Mn-SOD) in patients with PD (154), as well as antiapoptotic and trophic effects in preclinical studies (155). Furthermore, a neuropathological study on nigral degeneration has shown that selegiline reduces the severity of neuronal loss in the lateral tier of the SNpc in PD (156); however, this study is still under discussion.

Clinical Trials with Selegiline

In 1985, a retrospective, uncontrolled long-term study (9 years) by Birkmayer et al. (151) showed a significant increase of life expectancy in a group of patients treated with a combination of levodopa/benserazide (Madopar) and the MAO-B inhibitor selegiline (n = 564), compared with levodopa/benserazide treatment alone (n = 377). A large clinical trial on the neuroprotective effects of selegiline and α-tocopherol was then initiated in 1987 by the Parkinson Study Group of the United States (136). The Deprenyl and Tocopherol Antioxidative Therapy of Parkinsonism (DATATOP) study included 800 *de novo* patients with typical features of idiopathic PD who were not receiving levodopa therapy or other antiparkinsonian medication. They were receiving placebo, α-tocopherol, selegiline (10 mg per day), or a combination of the two drugs. The primary endpoint of this trial was when in the judgment of an investigator, a subject reached a level of functional disability sufficient to necessitate the initiation of levodopa therapy. After a mean of 12 ± 5 months, endpoint events had occurred in only 24% of the selegiline group, but in 43% of the nonselegiline–treated subjects. The onset of disability requiring levodopa therapy was approximately delayed by 9 months in the selegiline group. This highly significant difference was the crucial factor for the decision of an independent committee to switch patients receiving the (selegiline) placebo to the active drug.

However, the clinical advantages seen in this first short period of the trial have not been enduring as measured by sustained functional benefits, complications of levodopa therapy, or duration of life (107,157,158). Unfortunately, the study was designed under the assumption that neither selegiline nor tocopherol produced a short-term amelioration of parkinsonian signs and symptoms. Selegiline, in fact, was found to produce a modest but clear-cut improvement of 1.9 points on the Unified Parkinson's Disease Rate Scale (UPDRS), already after 1 and 3 months of treatment (107).

It remains unclear whether the results found are due to this confounding symptomatic effect or the probable neuroprotective features of selegiline (159–168). In the same trial, measures of the cerebrospinal fluid (CSF) homovanillic acid (HVA), the major CSF metabolite of DA, were not able to support a protective role of selegiline (108). A decline in CSF HVA in subjects assigned to receive selegiline was measurable. However, no significant differences between the selegiline treatment group and the controls were seen after withdrawal of this medication. In case of neuroprotection, levels of HVA in the selegiline groups should not have decreased compared with the placebo group. Interestingly enough, a newer extended analysis of the DATATOP trials has suggested that selegiline may forestall the onset of freezing of gait, a symptom that is likely to be distinct from bradykinesia (164). Freezing of gait, in fact, could be a measure that might not be influenced by dopaminergic effects.

In a 5-year follow-up study by Lees (165), levodopa in combination with selegiline seemed to confer no clinical benefit over levodopa alone in treating patients with early mild PD. Moreover, levodopa doses could be decreased as the duration of the study increased, indicating a beneficial effect of selegiline on disease severity. In several long-term clinical trials as the SINDEPAR, the Scandinavian studies, and the SELEDO study, both prospective 5-year trials, the early combination of selegiline and levodopa proved to be clearly superior to levodopa monotherapy (112).

Selegiline and Clinical Washout Phases

Major criticism of the data arising from the DATATOP study suggested that the washout phase was too short and that MAO-B inhibition was still operative, so interpretation of beneficial effects of selegiline was regarded only to be symptomatic. A basis for this assumption arises from ^{14}C-selegiline imaging studies, showing a half-life of 40 days for cerebral MAO-B.

Other and important more recent data, however, demonstrate that this might not be the case: The work by Green et al. (166) clearly demonstrates that the amine concentrations only increase after a minimum inhibition of MAO of 70% or more. This means that recovery of the enzyme after withdrawal of the inhibitor by only about 30% would lower the amine concentrations to basal levels. As a clinical consequence, no symptomatic effects could be expected. More recent data by measuring PEA concentration in urine demonstrate that only 2 to 3 days after withdrawal of selegiline, significant enzyme proteins must have been resynthesized.

These studies clearly demonstrate that the washout phases in the DATATOP study—and all other trials—are sufficient for a timely re-expression of the enzyme. Therefore, the beneficial effects of selegiline shown in these trials seem not to be due to symptomatic effects. Therefore, disease-slowing processes must be taken into consideration.

Dopamine Agonists

DA agonists provide antiparkinsonian effects by stimulating DA receptors. Possible toxicity of levodopa to susceptible neurons in patients with PD (167) and the hereby probable induction of motor complications are the rationale for the use of DA agonists, both as monotherapy in the early stages of the disease and as adjunct therapy to levodopa. These substances have been demonstrated to protect against the development of levodopa-related motor complications (168). A neuroprotective effect is assumed to be derived from (a) a levodopa-sparing effect, (b) stimulation of DA auto-receptors, (c) direct antioxidant effects, and (d) restoration of dopaminergic tone to suppress excitotoxic effects due to overactivity of the STN (169).

Few clinical studies, however, addressed the potential of DA agonists to provide neuroprotection in PD. A prospective controlled clinical trial, the PRADO study, showed decreased mortality in the group randomized to bromocriptine (plus supplemental levodopa if necessary) compared with the patients randomized to levodopa alone (138). Additionally, a number of clinical studies showed the potential to decrease the levodopa dosage with the DA agonists—for example, a double-blind placebo-controlled study with pramipexole (170,171); a randomized, double-blind multicenter study with ropinirole (141,171); and a double-blind trial with lisuride (172). A double-blind randomized monotherapy study with pergolide showed significant improvement in UPDRS scores and a greater percent of responders than with placebo (173). Long-term studies of patients with PD in the late stages of disease showed that combined therapy of levodopa and the DA agonists—α-dihydroergocryptine (174,175); bromocriptine (139); cabergoline (176); lisuride (177); and ropinirole (140)—had great benefits such as lower levodopa doses.

A new way of visualizing and proving neuroprotective effects is *in vivo* imaging studies, which are performed with different markers to evaluate the function of the nigrostriatal system. Three longitudinal ^{18}F-dopa positron emission tomography (PET) or ^{123}I-β-CIT single-photon emission computed tomography studies found a trend for a slower progression rate in patients with PD treated with either ropinirole (178) or pramipexole (179) and pergolide (173) in comparison with patients treated with levodopa. Results of these studies, however, should be considered with caution because a selection bias might be confounding to the results (178) (patients who can stay on ropinirole monotherapy have a more benign disease). However, a large follow-up study with ropinirole, designed to demonstrate reduction of disease progression in comparison to levodopa, seems to demonstrate exactly this effect (179a).

In general, the methods used so far require a more careful review, due to the findings of Guttman et al. (149), who observed a significant increase in DA transporter binding during the course of a short-term PET study caused either by levodopa or by pramipexole. This effect could also influence longitudinal imaging studies on disease progression and the efficacy of neuroprotective agents.

a-Tocopherol

An uncontrolled clinical study had suggested that high-dose supplementation with vitamin E might slow the worsening of PD in otherwise unmedicated patients (180). In the DATATOP trial, however, no beneficial effect of α-tocopherol or any interaction between tocopherol and selegiline could be detected (dose, 2,000 IU per day) (136), although a significant increase in CSF α-tocopherol concentration could be measured (181).

Amantadine

Clinical observations have suggested several beneficial effects in PD, including a decrease in levodopa-induced motor complications and neuroprotection. In a controlled study for the benefits of amantadine, about two thirds of patients have shown improvement in akinesia, rigidity, and tremor (182). These benefits were confirmed in placebo-controlled studies irrespective of administration as monotherapy or as a levodopa adjunct (183–187). Recent evidence from placebo-controlled studies has shown the beneficial effects of amantadine on motor response complications, such as the wearing-off phenomenon of levodopa (188–190).

The response of amantadine is modest in comparison with that of levodopa. Nevertheless, amantadine showed continued benefit after 12 years of treatment (191) and is used frequently, at least in Europe, for the treatment of akinetic crisis by using the sulphate salt of amantadine (192). More recently, it has been suggested to be neuroprotective in both preclinical (193) and clinical trials (194,195). A retrospective clinical study by Uitti et al. (194,195) demonstrates that long-term amantadine treatment has improved survival, suggesting a neuroprotective potential of this drug. In addition, several clinical placebo-controlled studies clearly indicate an antidyskinetic efficacy of amantadine (189).

DIFFICULTIES IN DEMONSTRATING CLINICAL NEUROPROTECTION

In contrast to experimental designs, the assessment of clinical trials is far more difficult, due to multiple transmitter deficits and underlying multifactorial processes. Another problem is to find the optimum dose of the tested drugs. The used dose of selegiline (10 mg per day), for instance, was suggested to be inadequate to prevent oxidative deamination of DA, as shown in the DATATOP trial (108) and in a study of patients with Alzheimer's disease (196).

It remains unclear whether the dose of vitamin E (2,000 IU) used in these trials was able to produce a significant increase in CNS antioxidative defense, although it was shown that the concentration of CSF α-tocopherol increased significantly after treatment (181). Other unsolved problems are the transport of a substance across the blood–brain barrier and confounding effects of accompanying medications, particularly levodopa.

Late Appearance of Symptoms

A further general problem regarding the attempt to show neuroprotection in PD is the observation that parkinsonian symptoms do not appear before nigral cell loss reaches a certain critical threshold—possibly more than 50% (197,198). Recent neuroimaging and autopsy data indicate a preclinical period of 4 to 5 years before the onset of symptoms, with a more rapid development of underlying pathological features in the early stages of the disease measured as cell loss in the substantia nigra or decline of dopaminergic function in the striatum by *in vivo* imaging, respectively (199).

Due to the lack of a PD marker, possible neuroprotective agents cannot be administered in the asymptomatic phase of the disease—the time when their beneficial actions would be most effective. Indeed, detection of early asymptomatic PD via ^{18}F-dopa PET imaging could make it possible to begin neuroprotective interventions during the preclinical phase. This process, however, cannot be applied in general. The discovery of an easily accessible biochemical marker would crucially change this situation.

Nevertheless, the therapeutic rationale for employing neuroprotective drugs in PD therapy is possible protection of the remaining surviving neurons from the degenerative processes. The decline in clinical measures in this later stage of the disease, however, could more likely represent a failure of compensatory mechanisms, such as increased DA turnover, than the rate of further cell loss.

Subgroups

It is assumed that the underlying pathological processes of PD comprise multifactorial and multigenetic disturbances. Several subtypes have been identified: the equivalence type (akinesia, rigidity, and tremor); the akinetic-rigidity type; the tremor-dominant type; the toxin (MPTP)-induced type; and different genetic types.

It is also known that the different features of the disease (bradykinesia, rigidity, tremor, postural instability, autonomic problems, and psychotic symptoms) progress at different rates in different individuals (200). As a consequence, a sufficient number of individuals is needed to avoid selection bias in prospective clinical trials. The different patients groups must be carefully matched for the predominant symptoms or signs as well. In addition, it is essential for future trials to evaluate genetic markers for homogenous subgroups—for example, the allelic variation of the serotonin transporter found in a subgroup of patients with PD suffering depression (201,202). These markers make it possible for pharmacogenetic studies to demonstrate clinical effectiveness and those subjects in whom the drug bring benefit.

Wrong Diagnosis

There are other neurodegenerative disorders distinguishable from idiopathic PD, which develop "parkinsonism" (multiple system atrophy, olivopontocerebellar atrophy, progressive supranuclear palsy, corticobasal degeneration, and others). Studying the pathology of 100 patients diagnosed prospectively as having PD by consultant neurologists showed that only 76% had nigral Lewy bodies (203). Consequentially, about a 20% diagnostic error rate must be considered in any clinical trial.

Endpoints

It is also questionable whether the traditionally used endpoints are suitable for distinguishing symptomatic from neuroprotective effects. The most widely accepted rating scale is the UPDRS (204). The disadvantage of it is its emphasis on bradykinesia. Although bradykinesia appears to be the best clinical correlate of nigrostriatal dysfunction in PD, as measured by fluorodopa PET (205), the antibradykinetic effects of an experimental treatment may be the result of short-term enhancement of dopaminergic activity, rather than a sustained slowing of nigral degeneration—a fact that may have severely confounded the DATATOP trial. It is noteworthy that not only the DA agonists have a symptomatic effect, but also selegiline.

Other clinical endpoints, not amenable to dopaminergic treatments, could improve neuroprotective inferences in clinical trials. Progressive postural instability and intellectual impairment (dementia) represent two major unmet therapeutic needs. An extended analysis of the DATATOP trial has suggested that selegiline may forestall the onset of freezing of gait in levodopa-treated patients (164).

CONCLUSIONS

Recent advances in our understanding of cellular and molecular processes of PD have led to new perspectives on the disease process and the identification of new pharmacological, neuroprotective, and neurorestorative approaches to therapy. But still, controlled clinical trials achieve incremental gains by resolving important uncertainties about the risks and benefits of therapeutic interventions (206). Clinical trials are usually slow, labor intensive, and expensive. Barring a quantum therapeutic advancement that would completely prevent illness onset or progression, controlled clinical trials will be required to ultimately define neuroprotective therapy for PD.

The prospects for successful neuroprotective therapy in PD would be enhanced by greater knowledge of the etiology and pathogenesis, which would, in turn, lead to more promising and specific interventions. This can be achieved via gene expression techniques in PD models and in patients with PD, which may reveal the whole mechanism of events that cause and develop the progress of the disease. The true aim of therapy for PD must ultimately be to identify the disease process long before symptoms arise, so therapy can be given early enough to forestall the neuronal destruction that underlies patients' discomfort and disability.

REFERENCES

1. Parkinson J. *An essay on the shaking palsy.* London: Sherwood Neely and Jones, 1817.
2. Gasser T. Genetics of Parkinson's disease. *Ann Neurol* 1998;44[Suppl 1]:S53–S57.
3. Langston JW. Epidemiology versus genetics in Parkinson's disease: progress in resolving an age-old debate. *Ann Neurol* 1998;44[Suppl 1]:S45–S52.
4. Olanow C, Jenner P, Youdim M. *Neurodegeneration and neuroprotection in Parkinson's disease.* London: Academic Press, 1996.
5. Gerlach M, Riederer P, Youdim MB. Neuroprotective therapeutic strategies. Comparison of experimental and clinical results. *Biochem Pharmacol* 1995;50: 1–16.
6. Olanow CW. Oxidation reactions in Parkinson's disease. *Neurology* 1990;40[Suppl]:S32–S37.
7. Gutteridge JM, Halliwell B. Free radicals and antioxidants in the year 2000. A historical look to the future. *Ann N Y Acad Sci* 2000;899:136–147.
8. Jenner P, Olanow CW. Oxidative stress and the pathogenesis of Parkinson's disease. *Neurology* 1996; 47[Suppl 3]:S161–S170.
9. Riederer P, Reichmann H, Janetzky B, et al. Neural degeneration in Parkinson's disease. *Adv Neurol* 2001; 86:125–136.
10. Riederer P, Sian J, Gerlach M. Is there neuroprotection in Parkinson syndrome? *J Neurol* 2000;247:8–11.
11. Kostrzewa RM, Jacobowitz DM. Pharmacological actions of 6-hydroxydopamine. *Pharmacol Rev* 1974;26: 199–288.
12. Burns RS, Chiueh CC, Markey SP, et al. A primate model of parkinsonism: selective destruction of dopaminergic neurons in the pars compacta of the substantia nigra by *N*-methyl-4-phenyl-1,2,3,6-tetrahydropyridine. *Proc Natl Acad Sci USA* 1983;80: 4546–4550.
13. Gerlach M, Riederer P. Animal models of Parkinson's disease: an empirical comparison with the phenomenology of the disease in man. *J Neural Transm* 1996; 103:987–1041.
14. Heikkila RE, Manzino L, Cabbat FS, et al. Protection against the dopaminergic neurotoxicity of 1-methyl-4-phenyl-1,2,5,6-tetrahydropyridine by monoamine oxidase inhibitors. *Nature* 1984;311:467–469.
15. Tatton WG. Selegiline can mediate neuronal rescue rather than neuronal protection. *Mov Disord* 1993; 8[Suppl]:S20–S30.
16. Santiago M, Matarredona ER, Granero L, et al. Neuroprotective effect of the iron chelator desferrioxamine against MPP^+ toxicity on striatal dopaminergic terminals. *J Neurochem* 1997;68:732–738.
17. Matarredona ER, Santiago M, Cano J, et al. Involvement of iron in MPP^+ toxicity in substantia nigra: protection by desferrioxamine. *Brain Res* 1997;773: 76–81.
18. Lan J, Jiang DH. Excessive iron accumulation in the brain: a possible potential risk of neurodegeneration in Parkinson's disease. *J Neural Transm* 1997;104: 649–660.
19. Cadet JL, Katz M, Jackson-Lewis V, et al. Vitamin E attenuates the toxic effects of intrastriatal injection of 6-hydroxydopamine (6-OHDA) in rats: behavioral and biochemical evidence. *Brain Res* 1989;476:10–15.
20. Perumal AS, Gopal VB, Tordzro WK, et al. Vitamin E attenuates the toxic effects of 6-hydroxydopamine on free radical scavenging systems in rat brain. *Brain Res Bull* 1992;29:699–701.
21. Gassen M, Pinchasi B, Youdim MB. Apomorphine is a potent radical scavenger and protects cultured pheochromocytoma cells from 6-OHDA and H_2O_2-induced cell death. *Adv Pharmacol* 1998;42: 320–324.
22. Grünblatt E, Mandel S, Berkuzki T, et al. Apomorphine protects against MPTP-induced neurotoxicity in mice. *Mov Disord* 1999;14:612–618.
23. Grünblatt E, Mandel S, Maor G, et al. Effects of R- and S-apomorphine on MPTP-induced nigro-striatal dopamine neuronal loss. *J Neurochem* 2001;77: 146–156.
24. Muralikrishnan D, Mohanakumar KP. Neuroprotection by bromocriptine against 1-methyl-4-phenyl-1,2,3,6-tetrahydropyridine-induced neurotoxicity in mice. *FASEB J* 1998;12:905–912.
25. Zou L, Jankovic J, Rowe DB, et al. Neuroprotection by

pramipexole against dopamine- and levodopa-induced cytotoxicity. *Life Sci* 1999;64:1275–1285.
26. Di Monte D, Sandy MS, Smith MT. Increased efflux rather than oxidation is the mechanism of glutathione depletion by 1-methyl-4-phenyl-1,2,3,6-tetrahydropyridine (MPTP). *Biochem Biophys Res Commun*1987; 148:153–160.
27. Przedborski S, Jackson-Lewis V, Yokoyama R, et al. Role of neuronal nitric oxide in 1-methyl-4-phenyl-1,2,3,6-tetrahydropyridine (MPTP)–induced dopaminergic neurotoxicity. *Proc Natl Acad Sci U S A* 1996;93: 4565–4571.
28. Schulz JB, Matthews RT, Beal MF. Role of nitric oxide in neurodegenerative diseases. *Curr Opin Neurol* 1995;8:480–486.
29. Gerlach M, Reichmann H, Riederer P. *Die Parkinson-Krankheit. Grundlagen, Klinik, Therapie,* 2nd ed. Vienna, Austria: Springer-Verlag, 2001.
30. Mihatsch W, Russ H, Gerlach M, et al. Treatment with antioxidants does not prevent loss of dopamine in the striatum of MPTP-treated common marmosets: preliminary observations. *J Neural Transm Parkinson Dis Dementia Sect* 1991;3:73–78.
31. Offen D, Ziv I, Sternin H, et al. Prevention of dopamine-induced cell death by thiol antioxidant: possible implications for treatment for Parkinson's disease. *Exp Neurol* 1996;141:32–39.
32. Zilkha-Falb R, Ziv I, Nardi N, et al. Monoamine-induced apoptotic neuronal cell death. *Mol Cell Neurobiol* 1997;17:101–118.
33. Iacovitti L, Stull ND, Mishizen A. Neurotransmitters, KCl and antioxidants rescue striatal neurons from apoptotic cell death in culture. *Brain Res* 1999;816:276–285.
34. Olanow CW, Fahn S, Muenter M, et al. A multicenter double-blind placebo-controlled trial of pergolide as an adjunct to Sinemet in Parkinson's disease. *Mov Disord* 1994;9:40–47.
35. Calne DB, Burton K, Beckman J, et al. Dopamine agonists in Parkinson's disease. *Can J Neurol Sci* 1984; 11:221–224.
36. Saiardi A, Bozzi Y, Baik JH, et al. Antiproliferative role of dopamine: loss of D_2 receptors causes hormonal dysfunction and pituitary hyperplasia. *Neuron* 1997;19:115–126.
37. Kelly MA, Rubinstein M, Asa SL, et al. Pituitary lactotroph hyperplasia and chronic hyperprolactinemia in dopamine D_2 receptor–deficient mice. *Neuron* 1997; 19:103–113.
38. Ogawa N, Tanaka K, Asanuma M, et al. Bromocriptine protects mice against 6-hydroxydopamine and scavenges hydroxyl free radicals *in vitro. Brain Res* 1994; 657:207–213.
39. Yoshikawa T, Minamiyama Y, Naito Y, et al. Antioxidant properties of bromocriptine, a dopamine agonist. *J Neurochem* 1994;62:1034–1038.
40. Ubeda A, Montesinos C, Paya M, et al. Iron-reducing and free-radical–scavenging properties of apomorphine and some related benzylisoquinolines. *Free Radical Biol Med* 1993;15:159–167.
41. Sam EE, Verbeke N. Free radical scavenging properties of apomorphine enantiomers and dopamine: possible implication in their mechanism of action in parkinsonism. *J Neural Transm Parkinson Dis Dementia Sect* 1995;10:115–127.
42. Gassen M, Glinka Y, Pinchasi B, et al. Apomorphine is a highly potent free radical scavenger in rat brain mitochondrial fraction. *Eur J Pharmacol* 1996;308: 219–225.
43. Nishibayashi S, Asanuma M, Kohno M, et al. Scavenging effects of dopamine agonists on nitric oxide radicals. *J Neurochem* 1996;67:2208–2211.
44. Clow A, Freestone C, Lewis E, et al. The effect of pergolide and MDL 72974 on rat brain CuZn superoxide dismutase. *Neurosci Lett* 1993;164:41–43.
45. Linazasoro G. Subcutaneous apomorphine in the treatment of Parkinson's disease. *Neurologia* 1994;9:1–3.
46. Gassen M, Gross A, Youdim MB. Apomorphine enantiomers protect cultured pheochromocytoma (PC12) cells from oxidative stress induced by H_2O_2 and 6-hydroxydopamine. *Mov Disord* 1998;13:242–248.
47. Mena MA, Davila V, Bogaluvsky J, et al. A synergistic neurotrophic response to L-dihydroxyphenylalanine and nerve growth factor. *Mol Pharmacol* 1998;54: 678–686.
48. Fornai F, Battaglia G, Gesi M, et al. Dose-dependent protective effects of apomorphine against methamphetamine-induced nigrostriatal damage. *Brain Res* 2001;898:27–35.
49. Rakotoarison DA, Gressier B, Trotin F, et al. Antioxidant activities of polyphenolic extracts from flowers, *in vitro* callus and cell suspension cultures of Crataegus monogyna. *Pharmazie* 1997;52:60–64.
50. Williamson G, Faulkner K, Plumb GW. Glucosinolates and phenolics as antioxidants from plant foods. *Eur J Cancer Prev* 1998;7:17–21.
51. Calne DB, Teychenne PF, Claveria LE, et al. Bromocriptine in parkinsonism. *Br Med J* 1974;4: 442–444.
52. Kondo T, Ito T, Sugita Y. Bromocriptine scavenges methamphetamine-induced hydroxyl radicals and attenuates dopamine depletion in mouse striatum. *Ann NY Acad Sci* 1994;738:222–229.
53. Sawada H, Ibi M, Kihara T, et al. Dopamine D_2-type agonists protect mesencephalic neurons from glutamate neurotoxicity: mechanisms of neuroprotective treatment against oxidative stress. *Ann Neurol* 1998; 44:110–109.
54. Takashima H, Tsujihata M, Kishikawa M, et al. Bromocriptine protects dopaminergic neurons from levodopa-induced toxicity by stimulating D_2 receptors. *Exp Neurol* 1999;159:98–104.
55. Ogawa N, Tanaka K, Asanuma M. Bromocriptine markedly suppresses levodopa-induced abnormal increase of dopamine turnover in the parkinsonian striatum. *Neurochem Res* 2000;25:755–758.
56. Arai N, Isaji M, Miyata H, et al. Differential effects of three dopamine receptor agonists in MPTP-treated monkeys. *J Neural Transm Parkinson Dis Dementia Sect* 1995;10:55–62.
57. Gagnon C, Bedard PJ, Di Paolo T. Effect of chronic treatment of MPTP monkeys with dopamine D-1 and/or D-2 receptor agonists. *Eur J Pharmacol* 1990; 178:115–120.
58. Fredriksson A, Plaznik A, Sundström E, et al. Effects of D_1 and D_2 agonists on spontaneous motor activity in MPTP treated mice. *Pharmacol Toxicol* 1994;75: 36–41.
59. Colao A, Lombardi G, Annunziato L. Cabergoline. *Expert Opin Pharmacother* 2000;1:555–574.
60. Finotti N, Castagna L, Moretti A, et al. Reduction of

lipid peroxidation in different rat brain areas after cabergoline treatment. *Pharmacol Res* 2000;42: 287–291.
61. Nomoto M, Kita S, Iwata SI, et al. Effects of acute or prolonged administration of cabergoline on parkinsonism induced by MPTP in common marmosets. *Pharmacol Biochem Behav* 1998;59:717–721.
62. Hadj Tahar A, Gregoire L, Bangassoro E, et al. Sustained cabergoline treatment reverses levodopa-induced dyskinesias in parkinsonian monkeys. *Clin Neuropharmacol* 2000;23:195–202.
63. Markstein R. Dopamine receptor profile of co-dergocrine (Hydergine) and its components. *Eur J Pharmacol* 1982;86:145–155.
64. Canonico PL. D-2 dopamine receptor activation reduces free [^{3}H]arachidonate release induced by hypophysiotropic peptides in anterior pituitary cells. *Endocrinology* 1989;125:1180–1186.
65. Benzi G, Pastoris O, Marzatico F, et al. Influence of aging and drug treatment on the cerebral glutathione system. *Neurobiol Aging* 1988;9:371–375.
66. Bernocchi G, Gerzeli G, Scherini E, et al. Neuroprotective effects of alpha-dihydroergocryptine against damages in the substantia nigra caused by severe treatment with 1-methyl-4-phenyl-1,2,3,6-tetrahydropyridine. *Acta Neuropathol (Berlin)* 1993;85:404–413.
67. Marzatico F, Cafe C, Taborelli M, et al. Experimental Parkinson's disease in monkeys. Effect of ergot alkaloid derivative on lipid peroxidation in different brain areas. *Neurochem Res* 1993;18:1101–1106.
68. Favit A, Sortino MA, Aleppo G, et al. The inhibition of peroxide formation as a possible substrate for the neuroprotective action of dihydroergocryptine. *J Neural Transm* 1995;45[Suppl]:297–305.
69. Coppi G. Neuroprotective activity of alpha-dihydroergocryptine in animal models. *J Neural Transm* 1995; 45[Suppl]:307–318.
70. Goetz CG. Dopaminergic agonists in the treatment of Parkinson's disease. In: Olanow CW, Lieberman AN, eds. *The scientific basis for the treatment of Parkinson's disease.* Carnforth, UK: Parthenon Publishing Group, 1992:157–174.
71. Jankovic J, Orman J. Parallel double-blind study of pergolide in Parkinson's disease. *Adv Neurol* 1987;45: 551–554.
72. Gomez-Vargas M, Nishibayashi-Asanuma S, Asanuma M, et al. Pergolide scavenges both hydroxyl and nitric oxide free radicals *in vitro* and inhibits lipid peroxidation in different regions of the rat brain. *Brain Res* 1998;790:202–208.
73. Felten DL, Felten SY, Fuller RW, et al. Chronic dietary pergolide preserves nigrostriatal neuronal integrity in aged-Fischer-344 rats. *Neurobiol Aging* 1992;13: 339–351.
74. Asanuma M, Ogawa N, Nishibayashi S, et al. Protective effects of pergolide on dopamine levels in the 6-hydroxydopamine–lesioned mouse brain. *Arch Int Pharmacodyn Ther* 1995;329:221–230.
75. Hall ED, Andrus PK, Oostveen JA, et al. Neuroprotective effects of the dopamine D_2/D_3 agonist pramipexole against postischemic or methamphetamine-induced degeneration of nigrostriatal neurons. *Brain Res* 1996;742:80–88.
76. Ling ZD, Pieri SC, Carvey PM. Comparison of the neurotoxicity of dihydroxyphenylalanine stereoisomers in cultured dopamine neurons. *Clin Neuropharmacol* 1996;19:360–365.
77. Zou L, Xu J, Jankovic J, et al. Pramipexole inhibits lipid peroxidation and reduces injury in the substantia nigra induced by the dopaminergic neurotoxin 1-methyl-4-phenyl-1,2,3,6-tetrahydropyridine in C57BL/6 mice. *Neurosci Lett* 2000;281:167–170.
78. Cassarino DS, Fall CP, Smith TS, et al. Pramipexole reduces reactive oxygen species production *in vivo* and *in vitro* and inhibits the mitochondrial permeability transition produced by the parkinsonian neurotoxin methylpyridinium ion. *J Neurochem* 1998;71: 295–301.
79. Le WD, Jankovic J, Xie W, et al. Antioxidant property of pramipexole independent of dopamine receptor activation in neuroprotection. *J Neural Transm* 2000; 107:1165–1173.
80. Kitamura Y, Kohno Y, Nakazawa M, et al. Inhibitory effects of talipexole and pramipexole on MPTP-induced dopamine reduction in the striatum of C57BL/6N mice. *Jpn J Pharmacol* 1997;74:51–57.
81. Iida M, Miyazaki I, Tanaka K, et al. Dopamine D_2 receptor–mediated antioxidant and neuroprotective effects of ropinirole, a dopamine agonist. *Brain Res* 1999;838:51–59.
82. Johnston JP. Some observations upon a new inhibitor of monoamine oxidase in brain tissue. *Biochem Pharmacol* 1968;17:1285–1297.
83. Riederer P, Youdim MB, Rausch WD, et al. On the mode of action of L-deprenyl in the human central nervous system. *J Neural Transm* 1978;43:217–226.
84. Sonsalla PK, Golbe LI. Deprenyl as prophylaxis against Parkinson's disease? *Clin Neuropharmacol* 1988;11:500–511.
85. Riederer P, Sofic E, Rausch WD, et al. Transition metals, ferritin, glutathione, and ascorbic acid in parkinsonian brains. *J Neurochem* 1989;52:515–520.
86. Magyar K, Vizi ES, Ecseri Z, et al. Comparative pharmacological analysis of the optical isomers of phenyl-isopropyl-methyl-propinylamine (E-250). *Acta Physiol Acad Sci Hung* 1967;32:377–387.
87. Gerlach M, Youdim MB, Riederer P. Pharmacology of selegiline. *Neurology* 1996;47[Suppl]:S137–S145.
88. Cohen G, Spina MB. Deprenyl suppresses the oxidant stress associated with increased dopamine turnover. *Ann Neurol* 1989;26:689–690.
89. Oreland L, Gottfries CG. Brain and brain monoamine oxidase in aging and in dementia of Alzheimer's type. *Prog Neuropsychopharmacol Biol Psychiatry* 1986; 10:533–540.
90. Fowler CJ, Wiberg A, Oreland L, et al. The effect of age on the activity and molecular properties of human brain monoamine oxidase. *J Neural Transm* 1980;49: 1–20.
91. Glover V, Gibb C, Sandler M. The role of MAO in MPTP toxicity—a review. *J Neural Transm* 1986; 20[Suppl]:65–76.
92. Knoll J. The striatal dopamine dependency of life span in male rats. Longevity study with (–)deprenyl. *Mech Aging Dev* 1988;46:237–262.
93. Carrillo MC, Kanai S, Nokubo M, et al. (–) Deprenyl induces activities of both superoxide dismutase and catalase but not of glutathione peroxidase in the striatum of young male rats. *Life Sci* 1991;48:517–521.
94. Lai CT, Zuo DM, Yu PH. Is brain superoxide dismu-

tase activity increased following chronic treatment with L-deprenyl? *J Neural Transm* 1994;41[Suppl]: 221–229.
95. Langston JW. Selegiline as neuroprotective therapy in Parkinson's disease: concepts and controversies. *Neurology* 1990;40[Suppl]:1–6, 61–69.
96. Magyar K. Behaviour of (–)-deprenyl and its analogues. *J Neural Transm* 1994;41[Suppl]:167–175.
97. Chiba K, Trevor A, Castagnoli N Jr. Metabolism of the neurotoxic tertiary amine, MPTP, by brain monoamine oxidase. *Biochem Biophys Res Commun* 1984;120: 574–578.
98. Finnegan KT, Skratt JJ, Irwin I, et al. Protection against DSP-4–induced neurotoxicity by deprenyl is not related to its inhibition of MAO-B. *Eur J Pharmacol* 1990;184:119–126.
99. Wu RM, Murphy DL, Chiueh CC. Neuronal protective and rescue effects of deprenyl against MPP^+ dopaminergic toxicity. *J Neural Transm Gen Sect* 1995;100: 53–61.
100. Birkmayer W, Riederer P, Ambrozi L, et al. Implications of combined treatment with "Madopar" and L-deprenyl in Parkinson's disease. A long-term study. *Lancet* 1977;1:439–443.
101. Knoll J, Dallo J, Yen TT. Striatal dopamine, sexual activity and lifespan. Longevity of rats treated with (–) deprenyl. *Life Sci* 1989;45:525–531.
102. Carrillo MC, Kitani K, Kanai S, et al. (–)Deprenyl increases activities of superoxide dismutase and catalase in certain brain regions in old male mice. *Life Sci* 1994;54:975–981.
103. Mizuta I, Ohta M, Ohta K, et al. Selegiline and desmethylselegiline stimulate NGF, BDNF, and GDNF synthesis in cultured mouse astrocytes. *Biochem Biophys Res Commun* 2000;279:751–755.
104. Maruyama W, Naoi M. Neuroprotection by (–)-deprenyl and related compounds. *Mech Aging Dev* 1999; 111:189–200.
105. Kitani K, Kanai S, Sato Y, et al. Chronic treatment of (–)deprenyl prolongs the life span of male Fischer 344 rats. Further evidence. *Life Sci* 1993;52:281–288.
106. Parkinson Study Group. Effect of deprenyl on the progression of disability in early Parkinson's disease. *N Engl J Med* 1989;321:1364–1371.
107. Parkinson Study Group. Effects of tocopherol and deprenyl on the progression of disability in early Parkinson's disease. *N Engl J Med* 1993;328:176–183.
108. Parkinson Study Group. Cerebrospinal fluid homovanillic acid in the DATATOP study on Parkinson's disease. *Arch Neurol* 1995;52:237–245.
109. Mangoni A, Grassi MP, Frattola L, et al. Effects of a MAO-B inhibitor in the treatment of Alzheimer disease. *Eur Neurol* 1991;31:100–107.
110. Birkmayer W, Birkmayer GD. Effect of (–)deprenyl in long-term treatment of Parkinson's disease. A 10-years experience. *J Neural Transm* 1986;22[Suppl]: 219–225.
111. Tetrud JW, Langston JW. The effect of deprenyl (selegiline) on the natural history of Parkinson's disease. *Science* 1989;245:519–522.
112. Przuntek H, Conrad B, Dichgans J, et al. SELEDO: a 5-year long-term trial on the effect of selegiline in early parkinsonian patients treated with levodopa. *Eur J Neurol* 1999;6:141–150.
113. Youdim MB, Gross A, Finberg JP. Rasagiline [*N*-propargyl-1R(+)-aminoindan], a selective and potent inhibitor of mitochondrial monoamine oxidase B. *Br J Pharmacol* 2001;132:500–506.
114. Finberg JP, Lamensdorf I, Weinstock M, et al. Pharmacology of rasagiline (*N*-propargyl-1R-aminoindan). *Adv Neurol* 1999;80:495–499.
115. Finberg JP, Takeshima T, Johnston JM, et al. Increased survival of dopaminergic neurons by rasagiline, a monoamine oxidase-B inhibitor. *Neuroreport* 1998;9: 703–707.
116. Youdim MB, Wadia A, Tatton W, et al. The anti-parkinson drug rasagiline and its cholinesterase inhibitor derivatives exert neuroprotection unrelated to MAO inhibition in cell culture and *in vivo*. *Ann N Y Acad Sci* 2001;939:450–458.
117. Maruyama W, Yamamoto T, Kitani K, et al. Mechanism underlying anti-apoptotic activity of a (–) deprenyl–related propargylamine, rasagiline. *Mech Aging Dev* 2000;116:181–191.
118. Maruyama W, Akao Y, Youdim MB, et al. Neurotoxins induce apoptosis in dopamine neurons: protection by *N*-propargylamine-1(R)- and (S)-aminoindan, rasagiline and TV1022. *J Neural Transm* 2000;60: 171–186.
119. Huang W, Chen Y, Shohami E, et al. Neuroprotective effect of rasagiline, a selective monoamine oxidase-B inhibitor, against closed head injury in the mouse. *Eur J Pharmacol* 1999;366:127–135.
120. Carrillo MC, Minami C, Kitani K, et al. Enhancing effect of rasagiline on superoxide dismutase and catalase activities in the dopaminergic system in the rat. *Life Sci* 2000;67:577–585.
121. Goggi J, Theofilopoulos S, Riaz SS, et al. The neuronal survival effects of rasagiline and deprenyl on fetal human and rat ventral mesencephalic neurones in culture. *Neuroreport* 2000;11:3937–3941.
122. Kornhuber J, Mack-Burkhardt F, Kornhuber ME, et al. [^{3}H]MK-801 binding sites in post-mortem human frontal cortex. *Eur J Pharmacol* 1989;162:483–490.
123. Riederer P, Lange KW, Kornhuber J, et al. Glutamate receptor antagonism: neurotoxicity, anti-akinetic effects, and psychosis. *J Neural Transm* 1991;34[Suppl]: 203–210.
124. Carlsson M, Carlsson A. Interactions between glutamatergic and monoaminergic systems within the basal ganglia—implications for schizophrenia and Parkinson's disease. *Trends Neurosci* 1990;13:272–276.
125. Starr MS. Glutamate/dopamine D_1/D_2 balance in the basal ganglia and its relevance to Parkinson's disease. *Synapse* 1995;19:264–293.
126. Klockgether T, Turski L. Toward an understanding of the role of glutamate in experimental parkinsonism: agonist-sensitive sites in the basal ganglia. *Ann Neurol* 1993;34:585–593.
127. Choi DW. Excitotoxic cell death. *J Neurobiol* 1992;23: 1261–1276.
128. Small DL, Buchan AM. NMDA antagonists: their role in neuroprotection. *Int Rev Neurobiol* 1997;40: 137–171.
129. Schwab RS, England AC Jr, Poskanzer DC, et al. Amantadine in the treatment of Parkinson's disease. *JAMA* 1969;208:1168–1170.
130. Cochran KW, Maassab HF, Tsunoda A, et al. Studies on the antiviral activity of amantadine hydrochloride. *Ann N Y Acad Sci* 1965;130:432–439.

131. Nastuk WL, Su P, Doubilet P. Anticholinergic and membrane activities of amantadine in neuromuscular transmission. *Nature* 1976;264:76–79.
132. Gianutsos G, Chute S, Dunn JP. Pharmacological changes in dopaminergic systems induced by long-term administration of amantadine. *Eur J Pharmacol* 1985;110:357–361.
133. Chen HS, Pellegrini JW, Aggarwal SK, et al. Open-channel block of *N*-methyl-D-aspartate (NMDA) responses by memantine: therapeutic advantage against NMDA receptor-mediated neurotoxicity. *J Neurosci* 1992;12:4427–4436.
134. Lustig HS, Ahern KV, Greenberg DA. Antiparkinsonian drugs and *in vitro* excitotoxicity. *Brain Res* 1992; 597:148–150.
135. Rojas P, Altagracia M, Kravsov J, et al. Partially protective effect of amantadine in the MPTP model of Parkinson's disease. *Proc West Pharmacol Soc* 1992; 35:33–35.
136. Parkinson Study Group. DATATOP: a multicenter controlled clinical trial in early Parkinson's disease. *Arch Neurol* 1989;46:1052–1060.
137. Parkinson Study Group. Mortality in DATATOP: a multicenter trial in early Parkinson's disease. *Ann Neurol* 1998;43:318–325.
138. Przuntek H, Welzel D, Blumner E, et al. Bromocriptine lessens the incidence of mortality in L-dopa–treated parkinsonian patients: PRADO study discontinued. *Eur J Clin Pharmacol* 1992;43:357–363.
139. Przuntek H, Welzel D, Gerlach M, et al. Early institution of bromocriptine in Parkinson's disease inhibits the emergence of levodopa-associated motor side effects. Long-term results of the PRADO study. *J Neural Transm Gen Sect* 1996;103:699–715.
140. Lieberman A, Olanow CW, Sethi K, et al. A multicenter trial of ropinirole as adjunct treatment for Parkinson's disease. Ropinirole Study Group. *Neurology* 1998;51:1057–1062.
141. Sethi KD, O'Brien CF, Hammerstad JP, et al. Ropinirole for the treatment of early Parkinson disease: a 12-month experience. *Arch Neurol* 1998;55:1211–1216.
142. Korczyn AD, Brooks DJ, Brunt ER, et al. Ropinirole versus bromocriptine in the treatment of early Parkinson's disease: a 6-month interim report of a 3-year study. *Mov Disord* 1998;13:46–51.
143. Parkinson Study Group. A controlled trial of lazabemide (Ro 19-6327) in untreated Parkinson's disease. *Ann Neurol* 1993;33:350–356.
144. Parkinson Study Group. A controlled trial of lazabemide (Ro 19-6327) in levodopa-treated Parkinson's disease. *Arch Neurol* 1994;51:342–347.
145. Parkinson Study Group. Effect of lazabemide on the progression of disability in early Parkinson's disease. *Ann Neurol* 1996;40:99–107.
146. Larsen JP, Boas J, Erdal JE. Does selegiline modify the progression of early Parkinson's disease? Results from a five-year study. *Eur J Neurol* 1999;6:539–547.
147. Larsen JP, Boas J. The effects of early selegiline therapy on long-term levodopa treatment and parkinsonian disability: an interim analysis of a Norwegian—Danish 5-year study. *Mov Disord* 1997;12:175–182.
148. Ahlskog JE, Uitti RJ, O'Connor MK, et al. The effect of dopamine agonist therapy on dopamine transporter imaging in Parkinson's disease. *Mov Disord* 1999;14: 940–946.
149. Guttman M, Stewart D, Hussey D, et al. Influence of L-dopa and pramipexole on striatal dopamine transporter in early PD. *Neurology* 2001;56:1559–1564.
150. Linazasoro G, Obeso JA, Gomez JC, et al. Modification of dopamine D_2 receptor activity by pergolide in Parkinson's disease: an *in vivo* study by PET. *Clin Neuropharmacol* 1999;22:277–280.
151. Birkmayer W, Knoll J, Riederer P, et al. Increased life expectancy resulting from addition of L-deprenyl to Madopar treatment in Parkinson's disease: a longterm study. *J Neural Transm* 1985;64:113–127.
152. Gerlach M, Riederer P, Youdim MB. Molecular mechanisms for neurodegeneration. Synergism between reactive oxygen species, calcium, and excitotoxic amino acids. *Adv Neurol* 1996;69:177–194.
153. Szeleni I. *Inhibitors of monoamine oxidase B. Pharmacology and clinical use in neurodegenerative disorders.* Basel, Switzerland: Birkhauser, 1993.
154. Kushleika J, Checkoway H, Woods JS, et al. Selegiline and lymphocyte superoxide dismutase activities in Parkinson's disease. *Ann Neurol* 1996;39:378–381.
155. Gelowitz DL, Paterson IA. Neuronal sparing and behavioral effects of the antiapoptotic drug, (−)deprenyl, following kainic acid administration. *Pharmacol Biochem Behav* 1999;62:255–262.
156. Rinne JO. Nigral degeneration in Parkinson's disease in relation to clinical features. *Acta Neurol Scand* 1991;136[Suppl]:87–90.
157. Parkinson Study Group. Impact of deprenyl and tocopherol treatment on Parkinson's disease in DATATOP patients requiring levodopa. *Ann Neurol* 1996;39: 37–45.
158. Parkinson Study Group. Impact of deprenyl and tocopherol treatment on Parkinson's disease in DATATOP subjects not requiring levodopa. *Ann Neurol* 1996;39: 29–36.
159. Schulzer M, Mak E, Calne DB. The antiparkinson efficacy of deprenyl derives from transient improvement that is likely to be symptomatic. *Ann Neurol* 1992;32: 795–798.
160. Oakes D. Antiparkinson efficacy of deprenyl. DATATOP Steering Committee of Parkinson Study Group. *Ann Neurol* 1993;34:634.
161. Ward CD. Does selegiline delay progression of Parkinson's disease? A critical re-evaluation of the DATATOP study. *J Neurol Neurosurg Psychiatry* 1994;57:217–220.
162. Marsden CD. Parkinson's disease. *J Neurol Neurosurg Psychiatry* 1994;57:672–681.
163. LeWitt P, Oakes D, Cui L. The need for levodopa as an end point of Parkinson's disease progression in a clinical trial of selegiline and alpha-tocopherol. Parkinson Study Group. *Mov Disord* 1997;12:183–189.
164. Giladi N, McDermott MP, Fahn S, et al. Freezing of gait in PD: prospective assessment in the DATATOP cohort. *Neurology* 2001;56:1712–1721.
165. Lees AJ. Comparison of therapeutic effects and mortality data of levodopa and levodopa combined with selegiline in patients with early, mild Parkinson's disease. Parkinson's Disease Research Group of the United Kingdom. *BMJ* 1995;311:1602–1607.
166. Green AR, Mitchell BD, Tordoff AF, et al. Evidence for dopamine deamination by both type A and type B monoamine oxidase in rat brain *in vivo* and for the degree of inhibition of enzyme necessary for increased

functional activity of dopamine and 5-hydroxytryptamine. *Br J Pharmacol* 1977;60:343–349.
167. Fahn S. Is levodopa toxic? *Neurology* 1996;47[Suppl]: S184–S195.
168. Olanow C. A rationale for using dopamine agonists as primary symptomatic therapy in Parkinson's disease. In: CW CO, Obesco J, eds. *Dopamine agonists in early Parkinson's disease.* Kent, UK: Wells Medical Limited, 1997:37–52.
169. Olanow C, Jenner P, Brooks D. Dopamine agonists and neuroprotection in Parkinson's disease. In: Olanow C, Jenner P, eds. *Beyond the decade of the brain. Neuroprotection in Parkinson's disease,* vol 3. Kent, UK: Wells Medical Limited, 1998:331–340.
170. Parkinson Study Group. Pramipexole vs levodopa as initial treatment for Parkinson disease: a randomized controlled trial. *JAMA* 2000;284:1931–1938.
171. Lieberman A, Ranhosky A, Korts D. Clinical evaluation of pramipexole in advanced Parkinson's disease: results of a double-blind, placebo-controlled, parallel-group study. *Neurology* 1997;49:162–168.
172. Allain H, Destee A, Petit H, et al. Five-year follow-up of early lisuride and levodopa combination therapy versus levodopa monotherapy in de novo Parkinson's disease. The French Lisuride Study Group. *Eur Neurol* 2000;44:22–30.
173. Barone P, Bravi D, Bermejo-Pareja F, et al. Pergolide monotherapy in the treatment of early PD: a randomized, controlled study. *Neurology* 1999;53:573–579.
174. Bergamasco B, Frattola L, Muratorio A, et al. Alpha-dihydroergocryptine in the treatment of de novo parkinsonian patients: results of a multicentre, randomized, double-blind, placebo-controlled study. *Acta Neurol Scand* 2000;101:372–380.
175. Battistin L, Bardin PG, Ferro-Milone F, et al. Alpha-dihydroergocryptine in Parkinson's disease: a multicentre randomized double blind parallel group study. *Acta Neurol Scand* 1999;99:36–42.
176. Rinne UK, Bracco F, Chouza C, et al. Early treatment of Parkinson's disease with cabergoline delays the onset of motor complications. Results of a double-blind levodopa controlled trial. The PKDS009 Study Group. *Drugs* 1998;55:23–30.
177. Rinne UK. Combination therapy with lisuride and L-dopa in the early stages of Parkinson's disease decreases and delays the development of motor fluctuations. Long-term study over 10 years in comparison with L-dopa monotherapy. *Nervenarzt* 1999;70[Suppl]: S19–S25.
178. Brooks D, Rakshi J, Pavese N, et al. Relative rates of progression of early Parkinson's disease patients started on either a dopamine agonist (ropinirole) or levodopa: 2-year and 5-year follow-up [^{18}F]-Dopa PET findings. *Neurology* 2000;54[Suppl 3]:A113.
179. Marek K. β-CIT/SPECT assessments of progression of Parkinson's disease in subjects participating in the CALM PD study. *Neurology* 2000;54[Suppl 3]:A90.
179a. Whone AL, Remy P, Davis MR, et al. Slower progression in early Parkinson's disease treated with Ropinirole compared with L-Dopa. *Neurology* 2002;Suppl 7:58.
180. Fahn S. A pilot trial of high-dose alpha-tocopherol and ascorbate in early Parkinson's disease. *Ann Neurol* 1992;32:S128–S132.
181. Vatassery GT, Fahn S, Kuskowski MA. Alpha tocopherol in CSF of subjects taking high-dose vitamin E in the DATATOP study. *Neurology* 1998;50:1900–1902.
182. Schwab RS, Poskanzer DC, England AC Jr, et al. Amantadine in Parkinson's disease. Review of more than two years' experience. *JAMA* 1972;222:792–795.
183. Dallos V, Heathfield K, Stone P, et al. Use of amantadine in Parkinson's disease. Results of a double-blind trial. *Br Med J* 1970;4:24–26.
184. Mann DC, Pearce LA, Waterbury LD. Amantadine for Parkinson's disease. *Neurology* 1971;21:958–962.
185. Parkes JD, Baxter RC, Curzon G, et al. Treatment of Parkinson's disease with amantadine and levodopa. A one-year study. *Lancet* 1971;1:1083–1086.
186. Fahn S, Isgreen WP. Long-term evaluation of amantadine and levodopa combination in parkinsonism by double-blind crossover analyses. *Neurology* 1975;25: 695–700.
187. Savery F. Amantadine and a fixed combination of levodopa and carbidopa in the treatment of Parkinson's disease. *Dis Nerv Syst* 1977;38:605–608.
188. Luginger E, Wenning GK, Bosch S, et al. Beneficial effects of amantadine on L-dopa–induced dyskinesias in Parkinson's disease. *Mov Disord* 2000;15:873–878.
189. Snow BJ, Macdonald L, McAuley D, et al. The effect of amantadine on levodopa-induced dyskinesias in Parkinson's disease: a double-blind, placebo-controlled study. *Clin Neuropharmacol* 2000;23:82–85.
190. Del Dotto P, Pavese N, Gambaccini G, et al. Intravenous amantadine improves levodopa-induced dyskinesias: an acute double-blind placebo-controlled study. *Mov Disord* 2001;16:515–520.
191. Wilson JA, Farquhar DL, Primrose WR, et al. Long term amantadine treatment. The danger of withdrawal. *Scott Med J* 1987;32:135.
192. Danielczyk W. Therapy of akinetic crises. *Med Welt* 1973;24:1278–1282.
193. Kornhuber J, Weller M, Schoppmeyer K, et al. Amantadine and memantine are NMDA receptor antagonists with neuroprotective properties. *J Neural Transm* 1994;43[Suppl]:91–104.
194. Uitti RJ, Rajput AH, Ahlskog JE, et al. Amantadine treatment is an independent predictor of improved survival in Parkinson's disease. *Neurology* 1996;46:1551–1556.
195. Uitti RJ. More recent lessons from amantadine. *Neurology* 1999;52:676.
196. Heinonen EH, Savijärvi M, Kotila M, et al. Effects of monoamine oxidase inhibition by selegiline on concentrations of noradrenaline and monoamine metabolites in CSF of patients with Alzheimer's disease. *J Neural Transm Parkinson Dis Dementia Sect* 1993;5:193–202.
197. Fearnley JM, Lees AJ. Ageing and Parkinson's disease: substantia nigra regional selectivity. *Brain* 1991;114: 2283–301.
198. Gerlach M, Riederer PF. Time sequences of dopaminergic cell death in Parkinson's disease: indications for neuroprotective studies. *Adv Neurol* 1999;80:219–225.
199. Mörrish PK, Sawle GV, Brooks DJ. An [^{18}F]dopa-PET and clinical study of the rate of progression in Parkinson's disease. *Brain* 1996;119:585–591.
200. Louis ED, Tang MX, Cote L, et al. Progression of parkinsonian signs in Parkinson disease. *Arch Neurol* 1999;56:334–337.
201. Mössner R, Henneberg A, Schmitt A, et al. Allelic variation of serotonin transporter expression is associ-

ated with depression in Parkinson's disease. *Mol Psychiatry* 2001;6:350–352.
202. Mössner R, Schmitt A, Syagailo Y, et al. The serotonin transporter in Alzheimer's and Parkinson's disease. *J Neural Transm* 2000;[Suppl]:345–350.
203. Hughes AJ, Daniel SE, Kilford L, et al. Accuracy of clinical diagnosis of idiopathic Parkinson's disease: a clinico-pathological study of 100 cases. *J Neurol Neurosurg Psychiatry* 1992;55:181–184.
204. Fahn S, Elton R. Unified Parkinson's disease rating scale. In: Fahn S, Marsden C, Goldstein M, eds. *Recent developments in Parkinson's disease.* New York: Macmillan; 1987:153–167.
205. Vingerhoetz F, Schultzer M, Calne D, et al. Which clinical signs of Parkinson's disease best reflect the nigrostriatal lesion? *Ann Neurol* 1977;41:58–64.
206. Freedman B. Equipoise and the ethics of clinical research. *N Engl J Med* 1987;317:141–145.

Parkinson's Disease: Advances in Neurology, Vol. 91.
Edited by Ariel Gordin, Seppo Kaakkola, and Heikki Teräväinen
Lippincott Williams & Wilkins, Philadelphia © 2003

32

Sleep Disorders in Parkinson's Disease

Jan P. Larsen

Department of Neurology, Central Hospital of Rogaland, Stavanger, Norway

Insomnia is a frequent and important complaint of patients with Parkinson's disease (PD). Both the pathology of PD and the dopaminergic drugs may contribute to the much higher than expected frequency of sleep fragmentation and disrupted sleep among these patients. In addition, coexisting depression seems to be a major and frequent risk factor for insomnia in PD. Sleep disruption may be induced by increased dopaminergic drug treatment and should be avoided unless the patient's sleep is primarily disturbed by the motor manifestations of parkinsonism. Depression should be examined, and, if appropriate, be treated, in patients with PD with insomnia.

Patients with PD experience a wide range of parasomnias. Rapid eye movement (REM) sleep behavior disorder (RBD) is now a well-defined behavior in PD. RBD is effectively treated with clonazepam. Excessive daytime sleepiness (EDS) is common in PD, whereas sleep attacks seem to be rare manifestations of the disease or its treatment. EDS represents a pathological regulation of the sleep–wake cycle. The cerebral pathology of PD may show lesions in brain areas thought to be involved in this regulation. Significant EDS is found in 15% of the patients with PD, compared with 1% among healthy elderly, and seems to be primarily caused by the disease process of PD, and dopaminergic drugs may only provoke or worsen the symptom in predisposed patients with a more widespread cerebral pathology.

BACKGROUND

PD is a common neurodegenerative disorder, affecting more than 100 per 100,000 inhabitants (1). Patients with PD have a wide range of nonmotor problems that accompany the motor manifestations of parkinsonism. The nonmotor problems include cognitive impairment, autonomic dysfunction, psychiatric symptoms, and sleep disorders. These symptoms of the patients have received increasing interest and attention from physicians over recent years, and they may have a major influence on the lives of patients and their caregivers. Studies of health-related quality of life have shown that PD has a substantial impact on distress in patients (2) and that the variables that most strongly predict increased disease-related distress are symptoms of depression, insomnia, and impaired function (3).

The importance of sleep disorders in the management of PD has also been recognized by the possible impact of new dopaminergic drugs on daytime somnolence (4). This chapter discusses insomnia, parasomnias, and daytime sleeping problems in patients with PD. This information is important in the development of management plans for these patients.

SLEEP AND SLEEP DISORDERS IN PARKINSON'S DISEASE

Sleep is a special activity of the brain that is controlled by precise mechanisms that induce a specific sleep pattern and that results in restoration of body and mind (5). The normal sleep pattern consists of a succession of identifiable states that by polysomnography can be divided into five different stages. Sleep stages 1 through 4 include all stages of sleep from dozing (stage 1) to deep sleep (stages 3 and 4). These stages are characterized by an increasing amount of slow electroencephalogram (EEG) activity with low frequency (0.5 to 4.0 Hz) and high amplitude (delta activity). The fifth stage of sleep is REM sleep. REM sleep is associated with the EEG pattern seen in stage 1 sleep. At the same time, REMs are observed with an arousal and fluctuations in the functions of the nervous, respiratory, cardiovascular, sexual, and autonomic systems, whereas skeletal muscles are selectively inhibited. In contrast, non-REM sleep (stages 1 through 4) consists of a slowing down of all the previously mentioned functions.

The regulation of sleep–wake and the different stages of normal sleep are not fully understood. New concepts of sleep regulation have been developed (6), and the importance of precise anatomical structures, like the suprachiasmatic nucleus (7), has opened up for exciting perspectives in sleep research. The sleep cycle is modulated by a number of neurochemical systems, each of which appears to influence a specific stage of sleep. Slow-wave sleep depends, in part, on central serotonergic activity arising in cell bodies of the midline raphe nucleus of the pons (8). REM sleep depends, to some degree, on the integrity of the noradrenergic projections arising in the cell bodies of the locus ceruleus (9), and the timing of the initial REM cycle is partially dependent on cholinergic activity within the central nervous system (10). In addition, evidence suggests that various peptidergic systems influence sleep behavior. The complex interactions of these neurochemical systems appear to be under the control of a circadian "clock" that synchronizes the various systems involved in the regulation of sleep.

The neuropathology of PD is known to affect anatomical structures and central neurotransmitters that are involved in the modulation of the physiological sleep cycle, including abnormalities in the level of serotonin (11). Also, the treatment of PD includes agents that induce a number of alterations in central neurotransmitter systems and thus can cause sleep disturbances. In addition, there are both quantitative and qualitative changes of sleep with age (12). It is therefore expected that patients with PD who are in general elderly will have an increased risk for developing different types of sleep disorders.

Insomnia

Nocturnal problems in PD are more widespread than expected from the effect of aging alone. In 1982, a survey by Nausieda et al. (13) revealed prominent sleep complaints in 74 of 100 patients with PD. In 1988, Lees et al. (14) showed that 215 of 220 patients with PD experienced sleep disturbances. Insomnia is the most common symptom of sleep disturbance, both in the general population and among patients with PD. Insomnia can be separated into three different symptom complexes that may coexist or be present in isolation: sleep-initiation insomnia, sleep fragmentation, and early morning awakening.

Sleep disorders in PD have previously been studied in selected patient populations. These studies have demonstrated that sleep fragmentation is the most important problem for these patients. This finding has been confirmed in a study of a community-based population of patients with PD from the county of Rogaland, Norway (15). The study showed that 60% of this unselected group of patients reported a nocturnal sleeping problem. This was significantly more frequent than among patients with diabetes mellitus (46%) and healthy control subjects (33%) with comparable age and sex distribution. About a quarter (27%) of the patients with PD rated their overall nighttime problem as moderate to severe. The most common sleep disorders reported by the patients with PD were frequent awakening (sleep fragmentation) and early awakening. Sleep fragmentation was found in 39% of the patients, versus 12% among normal elderly controls. Problem with sleep initiation, or ability to fall

TABLE 32.1. *Number (percentage) of types of insomnia and use of sleeping pills in patients with Parkinson's disease and diabetes mellitus and healthy elderly control subjects*

	No. of patients	No. (%) with insomnia	No. (%) with frequent awakenings	No. (%) with difficulties falling asleep	No. (%) with early awakenings	No. (%) taking sleeping pills
Parkinson's disease	239	144 (60)	93 (39)	76 (32)	56 (23)	96 (40)
Diabetes mellitus	100	45 (45)*	21 (21)**	32 (32)	11 (11)*	35 (35)
Healthy elderly	100	33 (33)**	12 (12)**	22 (22)	11 (11)*	23 (23)**

Note: $*p < .05$, $**p < .01$ (Fischer's exact test, two-tailed; Parkinson's disease vs. diabetes mellitus and Parkinson's disease vs. healthy elderly).

asleep, was equally frequent among patients and controls. Of the patients with PD, 40% were using sleeping pills, compared with 23% of the healthy elderly (15) (Table 32.1).

The correlations between the presence of nocturnal sleeping problems and a wide range of clinical and demographic patient characteristics in this study population showed that the most important risk factor for developing insomnia in PD was coexisting symptoms of depression (15). In addition, a longer duration of levodopa treatment showed significant correlation with nocturnal sleep disorders.

Because insomnia is common and distressing in patients with PD, it is an important but difficult task for the physician to both recognize and develop management plans for insomnia in these patients. The primary step in the management of insomnia in patients with PD is to diagnose the type of insomnia and possible causes to the problem. In addition to parkinsonism itself, several possible sleep-disturbing factors must be considered (16). Motor manifestations of parkinsonism such as inability to move in bed, "stiffness," dystonic movements, and "cramps" may also disturb normal sleep. These complaints of PD may be improved by increased dopaminergic treatment. An increase in dopamimetic dosing may, however, disrupt the normal sleep architecture and adjustment of dopaminergic medication may have a different impact on sleep in different patients and situations. Stimulation with dopaminergic drugs is associated with arousal (17) and dopamine (DA) agonists produce arousal and suppress REM sleep (18,19). In some patients, dopaminergic medication will therefore induce fragmentation of sleep. In spite of this, treatment strategies with controlled-release formulations of levodopa and long-acting DA agonist are claimed to improve the overall nocturnal problems in patients with PD, if mobility is the issue (20,21). Van Hilten et al. (22) have evaluated the controversial effect of dopaminergic drugs on sleep by continuous activity monitoring during the night in 89 nondepressed patients with PD. The daily dose of levodopa or DA agonists, more than disease severity, was the strongest predictor of sleep disturbance. The authors concluded that dopaminergic drugs would cause sleep disruption in mild to moderate PD. In more seriously affected patients, the beneficial effect of dopaminergic drugs on disturbing nocturnal motor manifestations of parkinsonism will outweigh the adverse effects on sleep. A more aggressive dopaminergic treatment of nighttime problems in PD with long-acting DA agonists may therefore be indicated in a small and carefully selected group of patients. In most patients, this strategy will disrupt and disturb the sleep even further.

In addition to adjustment of dopaminergic medication, other nonmedical and medical strategies for improved nocturnal sleep may be considered. Depressive symptoms are frequent in patients with PD (23,24), and the presence of depression is the strongest predictor of disturbed sleep (15). It is mandatory to evaluate depression in any patient with PD with a nocturnal sleeping problem. Treatment with antidepressive medication may therefore be the most important drug strategy to overcome the insomnia in PD.

Parasomnias

Parasomnias include a variety of sleep-related behavioral phenomena. In patients with PD, the major disorders are vivid dreams, altered dream content, nightmares, night terrors with nocturnal vocalizations, RBD, nocturnal hallucinations, and somnambulism. Accurate estimates of the frequencies of these behaviors are not available, and the clinical differentiation between them is difficult. Some of these manifestations may also be different symptoms of the same pathological processes. Many of the parasomnias experienced by the patients with PD are only mildly disturbing for the patient. It is, however, important to also evaluate the distress and problems experienced by the spouse when considering possible drug therapies.

One distinct syndrome that has been clarified and fully described during the last years is RBD (25). Patients with this syndrome are executing excessive motor activity during dreaming, and they have lost the normal and expected skeletal muscle atonia of REM sleep. Among 93 consecutive patients with RBD (26), from the Mayo Sleep Disorder Center, 25 of them had idiopathic PD. Multiple system atrophy was diagnosed in 14 of the patients. Dementia with Lewy bodies is also associated with RBD. The syndrome was in these patients not associated with drugs such as levodopa, and RBD developed before parkinsonism in 52% of the patients with PD. Thirty-two percent of the patients had injured themselves, and 64% had assaulted their spouses. These situations are not uncommon among patients with PD, but their frequencies have not been formally studied.

The syndrome of RBD may both be disturbing to the spouse and also be of danger to the patient. Subdural hematomas occurred in two of the 93 patients described above (26). Other and more frequent injuries were related to falling out of bed or bumping into furniture or walls. For this syndrome, clonazepam has been shown to be highly effective in nearly 90% of the patients (27). It may be started at a dose of 0.5 mg in the evening and increased to 1.5 or 2.0 mg. Several of the other parasomnias experienced by patients with PD are drug related and are not discussed in this presentation.

Daytime Sleep Disorders

Sleep disorders during daytime in PD comprise EDS and so-called sleep attacks, or sudden onset of sleep, which were first associated with the use of the new DA agonists pramipexole and ropinirole.

Sleep architecture and regulation change with increasing age. The need for a short nap during the day is normal among older people. The daytime somnolence observed in some patients with PD is, however, far more pronounced and incapacitating. There is no universally accepted definition of the phenomenon of EDS, but EDS is defined, by some, as either 7 or more or 10 or more on the Epworth Sleepiness Scale (28). This scale measures the likelihood for dozing off or falling asleep in eight different situations of daily life and can give valuable information on somnolence in the routine examination of patients with PD. EDS represents, however, a somnolence that is related to pathology of general mechanisms of sleep–wake cycle and with the patient often at sleep for hours and frequently during the day. The patients may have a normal or prolonged nocturnal sleep as well. Sudden onset of sleep, or "sleep attacks," has been defined as a clinical phenomenon of an unavoidable and abrupt transition from wakefulness to sleep without somnolence before falling asleep (4). One of the major problems with this definition is that it requires another observer than the patient, as humans normally cannot remember what happened during the few last minutes before falling asleep. This topic is further discussed in Chapter 34.

There are few studies addressing EDS in PD. Factor et al. (29) found that 49% of patients with PD experienced daytime sleepiness with napping compared with 26% in control subjects. Van Hilten et al. (30) found no significant difference between patients and controls. In a community-based population of patients with PD, daytime somnolence was graded as *not present, mild somnolence,* and *EDS* (31). Patients with EDS fell asleep three times a day or more or the total sleeping time was more than 2 hours. In this study, mild somnolence was found in about 10% of both patients with PD and controls. In contrast, EDS was found in 15.5% of the patients and in only 1% of healthy elderly controls (Table 32.2). Compared with patients not reporting daytime somnolence, the patients with EDS had significantly higher staging of PD, were more disabled, and showed a higher frequency of cognitive decline and depressive symptoms. They had also been using levodopa for a longer time and had significantly more hallucinations than patients without EDS. These clinical correlates suggested that patients with PD with EDS have a more widespread and severe brain disease and that their sleepiness is caused by the cerebral pathology of PD. In contrast, it has previously been suggested that daytime somnolence resulted from nocturnal insomnia. In this study, the frequency of nocturnal sleeping problems were the same in patients with PD both with and without EDS, thereby emphasizing the importance of the postulated role played by intrinsic neurobiological factors.

Surviving patients in the above-mentioned community-based study of PD were reexamined in a follow-up study 4 years later (32). This study showed that EDS was still present at follow-up in all patients with moderate to severe somnolence at the baseline examination. In addition to the 10% of patients with EDS at baseline, 32 (20%) new patients developed EDS during the 4-year follow-up period. The patients who developed EDS showed a faster progression of cognitive impairment and an increase in severity of parkinsonism than the patients who remained without EDS. Neither a change in dose and type of dopaminergic medication, nor insomnia, seemed to have a major influence on the development of somnolence in patients with PD. The close correlation between development of moderate to severe somnolence and several other clinical features that indicate a more widespread cerebral pathology shows that in some patients, the disease process in PD is more extensive than in other patients, and that these patients are at special risk for developing somnolence. The well-known sedation or somnolence that are observed after acute or chronic medication with dopaminergic drugs (33) may therefore be more likely to occur or be particularly pronounced in predisposed patients with clinical or preclinical lesions in brain areas involved in regulation of the sleep–wake cycle.

There is no effective medical therapy for EDS. A reduction in dosage of dopaminergic drugs may relieve somnolence in some patients. In the management of patients with PD, it is important to recognize and diagnose the type and extent of somnolence because this problem may represent a risk factor in the patients' daily lives. Car driving is an activity that necessitates special concern in this context, and it is important to advise these pa-

TABLE 32.2. *Number (percentage) of patients with PD, DM, and healthy elderly with mild (MDS), moderate to severe (EDS), and all grades of excessive daytime sleepiness*

	No. of patients	Mean age in years (SD)	No. (%) with MDS	No. (%) with EDS	No. (%) of all patients with somnolence
Patients with PD	238	73.8 (8)	27 (11)	37 (16)	64 (27)
Patients with DM	100	72.7 (8)	9 (9)	4 (4)**	13 (13)**
Healthy elderly	100	72.8 (8)	9 (9)	1 (1)**	10 (10)**

Note: DM, diabetes mellitus; EDS, excessive daytime sleepiness; MDS, mild daytime sleepiness; PD, Parkinson's disease.

*$p < .05$, **$p < .01$ (Fischer's exact test, two-tailed; PD vs. DM and PD vs. healthy elderly).

tients on the hazards of car driving that are induced by daytime somnolence.

CONCLUSIONS

Insomnia has been shown to be more important than severity of parkinsonism for reduced quality of life in patients with PD. Insomnia, parasomnias, and daytime sleep disorders are all common in PD. These problems can be induced by the cerebral pathology of the disease process itself and by antiparkinsonian drugs. The management of sleep disorders in PD is based on recognizing the problem and giving a correct diagnosis to the cause of a sleep disorder experienced by the individual patient.

REFERENCES

1. Tandberg E, Larsen JP, Nessler EG, et al. The epidemiology of Parkinson's disease in the county of Rogaland, Norway. *Mov Disord* 1995;5:541–549.
2. Karlsen KH, Larsen JP, Tandberg E, et al. Quality of life measurements in patients with Parkinson's disease: a community-based study. *Eur J Neurol* 1998;5:443–450.
3. Karlsen KH, Larsen JP, Tandberg E, et al. The influence of clinical and demographic variables on quality of life in Parkinson's disease. *J Neurol Neurosurg Psychiatry* 1999;66:431–435.
4. Frucht S, Rogers JD, Greene PE, et al. Falling asleep at the wheel: motor vehicle mishaps in persons taking pramipexole and ropinirole. *Neurology* 1999;52: 1908–1910.
5. Hobson JA. *Sleep.* New York: Scientific American Library, 1989.
6. Sejnowski TJ, Destexhe A. Why do we sleep? *Brain Res* 2000;886:208–223.
7. Ibata Y, Okamura H, Tanaka M, et al. Functional morphology of the suprachiasmatic nucleus. *Front Neuroendocrinol* 1999;20:241–268.
8. Roussel B, Bouget A, Bobillier P, et al. Locus ceruleus, paradoxical sleep, and cerebral noradrenaline. *C R Seances Soc Biol Fil* 1967;161:2537–2541.
10. Hobson JA. Sleep and dreaming. *J Neurosci* 1990;10: 371–382.
11. Nauseida PA. Sleep disorders. In: Koller WC, eds. *Handbook of Parkinson's disease.* New York: Marcel Dekker Inc, 1987:371–380.
12. Swift CG, Shapiro CM. Sleep and sleep problems in elderly people. *Br Med J* 1993;306:1468–1471.
13. Nausieda PA, Weiner WJ, Kaplan LR, et al. Sleep disruption in the chronic levodopa therapy: an early feature of the levodopa psychosis. *Clin Neuropharmacol* 1982; 2:183–194.
14. Lees AJ, Blackburn NA, Campbell VL. The night time problems of Parkinson's disease. *Clin Neuropharmacol* 1988;6:512–519.
15. Tandberg E, Larsen JP, Karlsen K. A community-based study of sleep disorders in patients with Parkinson's disease. *Mov Disord* 1998;13:895–899.
16. Larsen JP, Tandberg E. Sleep disorders in patients with Parkinson's disease. Epidemiology and management. *CNS Drugs* 2001;15:267–275.
17. De Keyser J, Ebinger G, Vauquelin G. Evidence for a widespread dopaminergic innervation of the human cerebral neocortex. *Neurosci Lett* 1989;104:281–285.
18. Oningi E, Caporali MG, Massotti M. Stimulation of dopamine D-1 receptors by SKF 338393 includes EEG desynchronisaton and behavioral arousal. *Life Sci* 1985; 37:2327–2333.
19. Trampus M, Ferri N, Monopoli A, et al. The dopamine D_1 receptor is involved in the regulation of REM sleep in the rat. *Eur J Pharmacol* 1991;194:189–194.
20. Jansen ENH, Meerwaldt JD. Madopar HBS in parkinsonian patients with nocturnal akinesia. *Clin Neurol Neurosurg* 1988;90:35–39.
21. Lees AJ. A sustained-release formulation of L-dopa (Madopar HBS) in the treatment of nocturnal and early morning disabilities in Parkinson's disease. *Eur Neurol* 1987;27[Suppl 1]:126–134.
22. van Hilten B, Hoff JI, Middelkoop HAM, et al. Sleep disruption in Parkinson's disease. Assessment by continuous activity monitoring. *Arch Neurol* 1994;51: 922–928.
23. Cummings JL. Depression and Parkinson's disease: a review. *Am J Psychiatry* 1992;149:443–454.
24. Tandberg E, Larsen JP, Aarsland D, et al. The occurrence of depression in Parkinson's disease. A community-based study. *Arch Neurol* 1996;53:175–179.
25. Schenck CH, Mahowald MW. REM sleep parasomnias. *Neurol Clin* 1996;14:697–720.
26. Olson EJ, Boeve BF, Silber MH. Rapid eye movement sleep behaviour disorder: demographic, clinical and laboratory findings in 93 cases. *Brain* 2000;123:331–339.
27. Schenk CH, Mahowald MW. Polysomnographic, neurologic, psychiatric, and clinical outcome report on 70 consecutive cases with the REM sleep behavior disorder (RBD): sustained clonazepam efficacy in 89.5% of 57 treated patients. *Clev Clin J Med* 1990;57:10–24.
28. Johns MW. A new method for measuring daytime sleepiness: the Epworth Sleepiness Scale. *Sleep* 1991; 14:540–545.
29. Factor SA, McAlarny T, Sandchez-Ramos JR, et al. Sleep disorders and sleep effect in Parkinson's disease. *Mov Disord* 1990;5.280–285.
30. van Hilten JJ, Weggeman M, van der Velde EA, et al. Sleep, excessive daytime sleepiness and fatigue in Parkinson's disease. *J Neural Transm* 1993;5:235–244.
31. Tandberg E, Larsen JP, Karlsen K. Excessive daytime sleepiness and sleep benefit in Parkinson's disease. *Mov Disord* 1999;14:922–927.
32. Gjerstad MG, Aarsland D, Larsen JP. Development of daytime somnolence over time in Parkinson's disease. *Neurology* 2002;58:1544–1546.
33. Andreu N, Chalé JJ, Senard JM, et al. L-dopa-induced sedation: a double-blind cross-over controlled study versus triazolam and placebo in healthy volunteers. *Clin Neuropharm* 1999;22:15–23.

Parkinson's Disease: Advances in Neurology, Vol. 91.
Edited by Ariel Gordin, Seppo Kaakkola, and Heikki Teräväinen
Lippincott Williams & Wilkins, Philadelphia © 2003

33

Sleep Attacks—Facts and Fiction: A Critical Review

Carl Nikolaus Homann, Karoline Wenzel, Klaudia Suppan, Gerd Ivanic, Richard Crevenna, and Edwin Ott

Department of Neurology, Karl Franzens University, Graz, Austria

Recent publications (1–8) on sudden irresistible attacks of sleep (SIAS) in patients with Parkinson's disease (PD) had an enormous impact on patients and their families, on treating physicians, and on health authorities. Although having been on a continuous road of success for the past 40 years, antiparkinson medications have suffered some setbacks because of adverse medical reports. In 1998, selegiline was accused of causing reduced life expectancy (9), thereby prompting a marked reduction in selegiline prescriptions. After several cases of acute liver failure with death were published in 1998 (10), the catechol-*O*-methyltransferase (COMT) inhibitor tolcapone had to be withdrawn from the market in the European Union and other countries throughout the world (11). These two medications were considered adjunctive antiparkinson medications, so their replacement by other drugs did not pose a problem. In contrast to the recent reports that dopaminergic drugs induce SIAS possibly affect the most important class of PD medication and, thus, eventually all patients with PD, very important aspects of life, and the security of the general public as the most important of all. The 1999 SIAS reports were first met with skepticism on the part of PD experts and drug companies and by a seemingly overreaction on the part of national authorities. The following hypotheses were thus proposed: (a) SIAS do not exist, (b) SIAS do occur only with pramipexole or ropinirole, (c) SIAS can be prevented, (d) SIAS can be treated, and (e) patients taking pramipexole and ropinirole are unfit to drive. These views were put forward when the first reports on SIAS were issued and on the basis of insufficient preliminary data. But having been brought up by renowned opinion leaders in the field of movement disorders, as well as state authorities, they are still used as guidelines. Over the past 2 years, a huge body of data on SIAS has emerged, and it is now time to put these hypotheses to test and to identify the facts that are based on sound evidence.

SUDDEN IRRESISTIBLE ATTACKS OF SLEEP DO NOT EXIST?

Sleep Attacks as Side Effects Were Not Reported Before 1999

Sleep attacks have been described as events of overwhelming sleepiness without warning or with prodrome too short or overpowering to apply protective measures (12). Before 1999, no reports on SIAS or similar events can be found in the literature (13) or worldwide safety databases of manufacturers of dopaminergic medications (13).

Evidence, however, suggests that physicians before 1999 were reluctant to describe a new phenomenon for which a terminus technicus did not yet exist and for which they did not have a scientific explanation. Rather than saying that "there is something, but I don't know what it is," they lumped sleep attacks into the already existing terms: excessive daytime sleepiness (EDS), drowsiness, or somnolence. Hospital charts with detailed descriptions by unbiased physicians describing that patients with PD were suddenly and irresistibly falling asleep in inappropriate situations existed long before 1999 (5,14). These cases were retrospectively classified correctly as soon as the term for it existed.

Sleep Attacks Do Not Even Exist in Narcolepsy

The term sleep attack was historically first used in narcolepsy but later became obsolete as electrophysiological evidence suggested that electroencephalogram (EEG) changes indicative of drowsiness occur some time before the actual sudden loss of muscle tone (15). Due to this, sleep attacks are no longer a valid diagnosis of narcolepsy and are not included in the diagnostic manual for the international classification of sleep disorder diagnoses (3,16–18). If sleep attacks do not even exist in narcolepsy, then it would be highly unlikely that they exist as a side effect of dopamine (DA) agonists (3,15,19).

The only published electrophysiological study of true SIAS (8) seems to suggest that indeed just like in narcolepsy, there is no immediate change from wakening to sleeping states. However, polysomnography showed almost abrupt slowing of EEG background activity, occurrence of slow eye movements and K-complexes within 10 seconds, as well as sleep stage 2 within 60 seconds after stable wakefulness. The definition of SIAS is a clinical one and electrophysiological inaccuracy of a term is not a valid argument against the existence of a clinical entity. In view of this semantic dispute, it probably would have been wiser to call the phenomenon a narcolepsy-like event, rather than sleep attack. Whether these very short preceding electrophysiological changes of alertness can be used therapeutically has not yet been addressed. Biofeedback training sessions to recognize subclinical changes of alertness could possibly prevent SIAS. Constant EEG recordings with acoustic arousal tones could be beneficial in patients with frequent SIAS. Until such therapeutic interventions prove successful, the minute preceding electrophysiological changes that are clinically undetectable for either patient or environment remain irrelevant.

Sleep Attacks are but Episodes of Excessive Daytime Sleepiness

Several authors (3,19–21) questioned the clinical concept of sleep attacks, assuming that the initially reported road accidents were caused by a case of slowly dozing off. While five patients in the series by Frucht et al. (1) clearly speak of attacks without prior warning signs, the authors (3,19–21) accounted these events to the known sedative effect of pramipexole and ropinirole added to a known increased sleep propensity or EDS in patients with PD. Daytime somnolence was possibly further increased by reduced nighttime sleep and sleep disruption, which both occur in a high proportion of patients with PD (19,22). Wrong and hasty conclusions may have been drawn from retrospective reports of laypersons (patients or accompanying passengers), which have been based on interviews taken months after the event. As these interviews were capturing psychologically burdensome facts, reverse recall bias could also have played a significant role in inaccurately describing the events (23). One could therefore assume that these reports cannot really be considered reliable sources.

Although research has not found reduced reliability of delayed interviews in comparison to immediate interviews (24), it has been shown that expert witnesses are more accurate than lay witnesses (25). In this respect, two first-hand reports on patients falling asleep without prior signs of drowsiness given by a trained specialist are of particular value (5). The electrophysiological observation by Tracik and Ebersbach (8), which describes a normal background of wakefulness before the SIAS, provides additional evidence. These reports perfectly match the description of patients who experienced this periacute onset: "not like falling asleep but rather like a short circuit" (12). Other characteristic features of SIAS seem to be short duration, lack of arousability during the attack, and postictal full wakefulness and retrograde amnesia (5). These features seem to be quite distinct from descriptions of mere sleep events (19) on the basis of excessive daytime somnolence. Because these reports are but rare single observations, further investigations are needed.

SLEEP ATTACKS OCCUR WITH PRAMIPEXOLE AND ROPINIROLE ONLY

The first reports on SIAS, published in 1999, were all related to the non-ergot DA agonists pramipexole and ropinirole and occurred just months after they had first been put on the market. It was assumed that this side effect was restricted to the non-ergot subclass of dopaminergic medication. Time correlation seemed to make a strong case, and Frucht et al. (12) explicitly stated that "it is hard to imagine that an adverse event triggered by dopaminergic stimulation (a 'class effect') would be temporally linked in such a manner." The observation that switching from pramipexole or ropinirole to the ergot agonist pergolide resolved SIAS (12,26) also seems to favor the notion that SIAS are a side effect of non-ergots only.

As we have stated before, cases of SIAS were observed long before 1999 (5,19) but were reported as such only later. Although preliminary data seem to suggest that SIAS more frequently occur in non-ergot DA agonists, there are now abundant reports of SIAS caused by pergolide (2); levodopa (3,4); apomorphine (5); bromocriptine (6); piribedil (6); lisuride (7); and cabergoline (8)—that is, all available dopaminergic antiparkinsonian medications.

"SLEEP ATTACKS CAN BE PREVENTED"

Primary Prevention

Whether patients can be trained to recognize preceding sleepiness, as proposed by Lachenmayer (17), is not sure, because this has been done in healthy volunteers only, but not in patients with PD. If this technique proves successful, it could be applied for sleep events, but not for SIAS, because the latter are characterized by a lack of sufficient counteractable preceding clinical warning signs. It should be tested whether EEG-triggered therapeutic regimes, as suggested prior in this chapter, might possibly be helpful for SIAS.

Secondary Prevention

Screening for patients with PD at risk for developing SIAS was thought to be a feasible way of preventing some disastrous consequences of this phenomenon. One of the most frequently propagated tests (3) is the Epworth Sleepiness Scale (27), a questionnaire inquiring about various aspects of daytime sleepiness.

The Epworth Sleepiness Scale, however, was never formally validated for patients with PD (28). Currently available reports further suggest specificity to be low and sensitivity data to be contradictory. Pal et al. (29) found that 3 of 79 patients with pathological Epworth Sleepiness Scale scores had never had any SIAS. In one study of 200 patients with PD, this test proved a good predictor (97%) for those 29 patients who had a history of sleep events (38), but in another study of 638 patients with PD, sensitivity for predicting SIAS and their consequences was found to be less than 50% (30). Whether this discrepancy is due to different diagnostic criteria for SIAS remains to be shown because both studies exist in abstract form only.

Another test that was said to recognize patients at risk is the multiple sleep latency test (MSLT). Like the Epworth Sleepiness Scale, this test is not validated for patients with PD (28) but is also cumbersome and time consuming. Very few data are available on sensitivity and specificity. A small recent study suggests that a mean sleep latency score of less than 5 has a sensitivity of 50% only, a finding that speaks against a simple association of EDS and the quantity and quality of a prior night's sleep (31).

Very little is known whether risk factor exploration is of predictive value. The assumption that episodes of SIAS in inappropriate situations almost always precede SIAS with severe consequences (3) has not yet been backed up by sound evidence. Metaanalysis of all existing cases reported up to May 2001 (32) showed that recurrent SIAS were described in 20 of 123 cases only. The assumption that SIAS would occur with high doses only (3) has not been verified by case reports published over the past 2 years. SIAS were triggered by dopaminergic medication at the lower end of the normal therapeutic range, that is, with as low as 200 mg of levodopa, 2 mg of apomorphine, 0.75 mg of pramipexole, and 8 mg of ropinirole. A prospective study (7) showed that mean daily doses of antiparkinson drugs were not higher in patients with SIAS compared with those without SIAS. Age, disease duration, or time of exposure were not shown to have an important influence either. However, overrepresentation of male gender (ratio of 2.3:1) and a strong correlation with symptoms of dysautonomia (7) have been observed. Hopefully, in a future a combination of these and some other factors may provide ways of tracing out patients at particular risk of developing SIAS or provide hints about the still unknown pathophysiology.

SLEEP ATTACKS CAN BE TREATED?

Various treatment strategies have been attempted, primarily by altering the dose or the type of DA agonist, including two forms of active treatment, but most of these have not been performed in a controlled and prospective way.

The above-mentioned metaanalysis (32) reports that in 25 of 30 patients with sleep episodes in which treatment strategies were provided, the dose of the dopaminergic medication was either reduced (10 patients) or discontinued (15 patients). Mostly good results (88%) regarding cessation of sleep events were achieved. This strategy—at least on a longer perspective—however, will inevitably lead to a worsening of motor symptoms, counter to the primary aim of PD treatment. Switching from one DA agonist to another, particularly to one of a different molecular subtype, was attempted, but in two of three cases led to a recurrence of symptoms after a short-lasting remission (1) (Pirker W., *oral communication*, 2001) .

Active treatment was attempted with amantadine and modafinil, two agents with known psychostimulant properties. Amantadine, which is usually used for its antiparkinsonian effect, proved successful in one patient with possible SIAS. Other evidence that amantadine might prove a useful agent to treat SIAS was derived from a prospective study in which patients on amantadine were shown to have a reduced risk for developing SIAS (7). Modafinil proved effective in 21 patients with PD with EDS in a small prospective placebo-controlled crossover study (33). Whether this treatment will also be useful for true SIAS remains yet to be proven. Of all treatment attempts, psychostimulants seem to be the most promising strategy, but to date, an effective, meaningful, and evidence-based treatment for true SIAS has not yet been found.

PATIENTS TAKING PRAMIPEXOLE AND ROPINIROLE ARE UNFIT TO DRIVE?

If SIAS cannot be treated and their sometimes disastrous consequences that affect patients and environment alike cannot be prevented, then legal actions with the effect of banning patients on these medications from conducting dangerous activities such as driving seem to be justified. Therefore, patients treated with pramipexole, and until recently ropinirole, are prohibited from driving in Europe, often with major socioeconomic impact (34). Not only is driving considered a major factor for good quality of life, but it is also considered an individual right, particularly in Western countries (3). To justify a general restriction of this right for a large group of people irrespective of the individuals' specific risk, the phenomenon and its harmful consequences must occur sufficiently frequently.

Large differences exist in prevalence figures of SIAS. With a total of 1,987 examined patients, two retrospective (12,35) and seven prospective studies give prevalence figures of 0% to 30% (5,7,30,34,36–38) (Table 33.1). It is difficult to explain the discrepancies, except that the lower prevalence rates in some studies are most likely due to the use of more stringent diagnostic criteria and the inclusion of true SIAS only. Still, it must be taken into consideration that all these data were culled from movement disorder centers and prevalence rates of non-preselected patients with PD are still lacking.

Four studies (30,35,38,39) faced with the same limitation—that is, patients recruited from superspecialist centers—are available to provide data on sleep-related accidents. Prevalence rates for accidents for a total of 1,275 patients irrespective of accident outcome (almost all of them were indeed without bodily harm) were 2% (range, 0% to 4%). All three studies (40–42) that compared accident rates of patients with PD with those of the normal population showed that patients with PD caused fewer accidents.

On the basis of these data, it does not seem justified to generally ban all patients with PD from driving. Restrictions on driving should rather be done on an individual basis, depending on the patient's individual symptoms and degree of disability.

CONCLUSIONS

There is clear evidence that SIAS really do exist and are a class effect of all DA agonists. The few existing first-hand expert reports on the course of sleep events seem to suggest that SIAS occur suddenly without prodrome as entities distinct from sleep episodes, which are another type of irresistible sleep events characterized by slow onset and a prodrome of drowsiness. Contrary to mere sleep episodes in which modafinil seems to be successful, to date there is no specific treatment to counteract SIAS. Insufficient data are available to detect patients at risk or to provide other preventive strategies. Prospective studies are needed to test existing medications that proved successful in comparable conditions and to develop new agents. Large-scale population-based studies should provide insights on the prevalence of SIAS in the gen-

TABLE 33.1. *Studies on prevalence of SOS during waking hours*

Source	Reference type	Diagnosis	Recruitment	SOS	n	Prevalence
Hauser et al., 2000 (35)	Article	PD	MD center	SA	37	24%
Frucht et al., 2000 (12)	Article	PD	3 MD centers	SA	400	2%
Homann et al., 2000 (5)	Abstract	P-ism	MD center	SA	68	3%
Ferreira et al., 2000 (6)	Abstract	PD	MD center	SA	52	12%
Montastruc et al., 2001 (7)	Article	PD	MD center	SA	234	30%
Pal et al., 2001 (34)	Article	PD	MD center	SA	55	0%
Ondo et al., 2001 (37)	Article	PD	MD center	PDSA	303	23%
Lang et al., 2001 (30)	Abstract	PD	18 MD centers	DSA	638	0.7%
Stover et al., 2001 (38)	Abstract	PD	MD center	SA	200	14%
Total			28 MD centers		1,987	0–30%

DSA, driving-related sleep attack (with a clear definition as regarding the sudden onset without warning signs); PD, Parkinson's disease; P-ism, parkinsonism; SA, sleep attack; PDSA, possible driving-related sleep attack (for which a description on sleep onset is not provided); SOS, sudden onset of sleep.

eral population and possibly find new risk factors. But for any further research, it is crucial to form a consensus on a generally accepted definition of SIAS.

The most pressing issue, however, is that of road accidents; further studies should also lead in this direction. From the few existing reports, it is evident that patients taking pramipexole, ropinirole, and all other dopaminergic medications have caused accidents, but the incidence rate of these accidents is low, but particularly of that with relevant bodily harm. A general driving ban affecting all patients with PD on dopaminergic medication cannot be supported by sound evidence, and movement disorder specialists, together with PD self-help organizations, should address national authorities to reappraise their restrictive policies.

REFERENCES

1. Frucht SJ, Rogers JD, Greene PE, et al. Falling asleep at the wheel: motor vehicle mishaps in persons taking pramipexole and ropinirole. *Neurology* 1999;52: 1908–1910.
2. Arnold G. Comment on: Falling asleep at the wheel: motor vehicle mishaps in people taking pramipexole and ropinirole. *Neurology* 2000;54:275–276.
3. Olanow CW, Schapira A-HV, Roth T. Waking up to sleep episodes in Parkinson's disease. *Mov Disord* 2000; 15:212–215.
4. Ferreira JJ, Galitzky M, Brefel-Courbon C, et al. Sleep attacks as an adverse drug reaction of levodopa monotherapy. *Mov Disord* 2000;15A:129.
5. Homann CN, Suppan K, Wenzel K, et al. Sleep attacks with apomorphine. *Wien Klin Wochenschr* 2002;114: 430–431.
6. Ferreira JJ, Galitzky M, Montastruc JL, et al. Sleep attacks and Parkinson's disease treatment. *Lancet* 2000; 355:1333–1334.
7. Montastruc JL, Brefel-Courbon C, Senard JM, et al. Sleep attacks and antiparkinsonian drugs: a pilot prospective pharmacoepidemiologic study. *Clin Neuropharmacol* 2001;24:A181–A183.
8. Tracik F, Ebersbach G. Sudden daytime sleep onset in Parkinson's disease: polysomnographic recordings. *Mov Disord* 2001;16:500–506.
9. Ben-Shlomo Y, Churchyard A, Head J, et al. Investigation by Parkinson's Disease Research Group of United Kingdom into excess mortality seen with combined levodopa and selegiline treatment in patients with early, mild Parkinson's disease: further results of randomised trial and confidential inquiry. *Br Med J* 1998;316: 1191–1196.
10. Assal F, Spahr L, Hadengue A, et al. Tolcapone and fulminant hepatitis. *Lancet* 1998;352:958.
11. Kaakkola S. Clinical pharmacology, therapeutic use and potential of COMT inhibitors in Parkinson's disease. *Drugs* 2000;59:1233–1250.
12. Frucht SJ, Greene PE, Fahn S. Sleep episodes in Parkinson's disease: a wake-up call. *Mov Disord* 2000;15: 601–603.
13. Lledo M. Comment on: Falling asleep at the wheel: motor vehicle mishaps in people taking pramipexole and ropinirole. *Neurology* 2000;54:275.
14. Hoehn MM. Comment on: Falling asleep at the wheel: motor vehicle mishaps in people taking pramipexole and ropinirole. *Neurology* 2000;52:275.
15. Schafer D, Greulich W. Effects of parkinsonian medication on sleep. *J Neurol* 2000;247[Suppl 4]:24–27.
16. American Sleep Disorders Association. *International classification of sleep disorders revised: diagnostic and coding manual.* Rochester, MN: American Sleep Disorders Association, 1997.
17. Lachenmayer L. Parkinson's disease and the ability to drive. *J Neurol* 2000;247:28–30.
18. Olanow CW. Comment on: Falling asleep at the wheel: motor vehicle mishaps in people taking pramipexole and ropinirole. *Neurology* 2000;54:274.
19. Hoegl B, Poewe W. "Sudden sleep attacks" with pramipexole and ropinirole. *Neuropsychiatrie* 2000;14: 191–193.
20. Möller JC, Stiasny K, Cassel W, et al. "Sleep attacks" in Parkinson patients. A side effect of nonergoline dopamine agonists or a class effect of dopamine agonists? *Nervenarzt* 2000;71:670–676.
21. Clarenbach P. Parkinson's disease and sleep. *J Neurol* 2000;247[Suppl]:20–23.
22. Factor SA, McAlarney T, Sanchez R, et al. Sleep disorders and sleep effect in Parkinson's disease. *Mov Disord* 1990;5:280–285.
23. Weiner WJ. Comment on: Falling asleep at the wheel: motor vehicle mishaps in people taking pramipexole and ropinirole. *Neurology* 2000;54:274–275.
24. Swor RA, Jackson R, Chu K, et al. A preliminary study of the reliability of immediate vs. delayed interviews of cardiac arrest witnesses. *Prehosp Emerg Care* 1999;3: 110–114.
25. Lindholm T, Christianson SA, Karlsson I. Police officers and civilians as witnesses: intergroup biases and memory performance. *Appl Cogn Psychol* 1997;11: 431–444.
26. Pirker W, Happe S. Sleep attacks in Parkinson's disease. *Lancet* 2000;356:597–598.
27. Johns MW. A new method for measuring daytime sleepiness: the Epworth Sleepiness Scale. *Sleep* 1991; 14:540–545.
28. Ferreira JJ, Marques MA, Galitzky M, et al. Methodological problems to quantify excessive daytime sleepiness or the risk of sleep episodes in Parkinson's disease. *Mov Disord* 2000;15[Suppl A]:187–188.
29. Pal S, Bhattacharya C, Agapito C, et al. A comparative study of daytime sleepiness within Parkinson's disease patients treated with cabergoline, pramipexole and levodopa. *Mov Disord* 2000;[Suppl A]:110–111.
30. Lang AE, Hobson DE, Martin W, et al. Excessive daytime sleepiness and sudden onset sleep in Parkinson's disease: a survey from 18 Canadian movement disorders clinics. *Neurology* 2001;56[Suppl 3]:A13.
31. Rye DB, Bliwise DL, Dihenia B, et al. Daytime sleepiness in Parkinson's disease. *J Sleep Res* 2000;9:63–69.
32. Homann CN, Wenzel K, Suppan K, et al. Sleep attacks

in patients taking dopamine agonists: review. *BMJ* 2002; 324:1483–1487.

33. Adler CH, Caviness JN, Hentz JG, et al. Modafinil for the treatment of excessive daytime sleepiness in patients with Parkinson's disease. *Neurology* 2001;56[Suppl A]: S40.
34. Pal S, Bhattacharya C, Agapito C, et al. A study of excessive daytime sleepiness and its clinical significance in three groups of Parkinson's disease patients taking pramipexole, cabergoline and levodopa mono and combination therapy. *J Neural Transm* 2001;108:71–77.
35. Hauser RA, Gauger L, McDowell AW, et al. Pramipexole-induced somnolence and episodes of daytime sleep. *Mov Disord* 2000;15:658–663.
36. Ferreira JJ, Desboeuf K, Galitzky M, et al. Sleep attacks and Parkinson's disease: results of a questionnaire survey in a movement disorders outpatient clinic. *Mov Disord* 2000;15A:187.
37. Ondo WG, Dat Vuong K, Kahn H, et al. Daytime sleepiness and other sleep disorders in Parkinson's disease. *Neurology* 2001;57:1392–1396.
38. Stover NP, Okun MS, Watts RL. "Sleep attacks" and excessive daytime sleepiness (EDS) in Parkinson's disease: a survey of 200 consecutive patients. *Neurology* 2001;56[Suppl 3]:A213.
39. Frucht SJ, Greene PE, Fahn S. Sleep episodes in Parkinson's disease: a wake-up call. *Mov Disord* 2000;15: 601–603.
40. Ritter G, Steinberg H. Parkinsonism and driving fitness. *Munch Med Wochenschr* 1979;121:1329–1330.
41. Dubinsky RM, Gray C, Husted D, et al. Driving in Parkinson's disease. *Neurology* 1991;41:517–520.
42. Homann CN, Trummer M, Wenzel K, et al. Sleep attacks and severe road accidents in patients with Parkinson's disease—an infrequent finding. *Mov Disord* 2001; 16[Suppl A]:44.

Parkinson's Disease: Advances in Neurology, Vol. 91.
Edited by Ariel Gordin, Seppo Kaakkola, and Heikki Teräväinen
Lippincott Williams & Wilkins, Philadelphia © 2003

34

Dopamine Agonists, Sleep Disorders, and Driving in Parkinson's Disease

Ryan J. Uitti and Zbigniew K. Wszolek

Department of Neurology, Mayo Clinic Jacksonville, Jacksonville, Florida

Dopamine (DA) agonists represent a powerful class of pharmacological agents useful in the treatment of motor dysfunction in Parkinson's disease (PD). Increasing use of DA agonists during the course of illness, ranging from initial monotherapy to adjunctive therapy with other agents, requires consideration concerning potential effects of these agents on aspects other than merely motor function. Recent anecdotal reports have questioned whether DA agonists may lead to sudden irresistible sleep and potentially disastrous consequences. This chapter reviews issues relating to DA agonist pharmacotherapy and sleep effects in other movement disorders, sleep deprivation, and driving safety in the general population, as well as effects of DA agonists on sleep and driving in PD.

DOPAMINE AGONISTS AND SLEEP—ANATOMICAL AND ANIMAL STUDIES

The anatomical basis of sleep disturbances in PD may relate to DA depletion. The loss of dopaminergic neurons projecting from the ventral tegmental area to the cerebral cortex are normally thought to be associated with arousal mechanisms (1). Additionally, administration of high doses of apomorphine, a D_1/D_2 agonist, causes higher levels of motor activity and disturbed sleep, whereas low doses increase total nightly sleep time (2). The pedunculopontine nucleus (PPN) is also thought to be important in mediating inhibition of voluntary muscle activity during rapid eye movement (REM) sleep ("REM atonia"). Alternations of major input to the PPN from the internal segment of the globus pallidus and the subthalamic nucleus, in addition to neuronal cell loss within the PPN, may lead to increased motor activity in PD during sleep (3,4).

Although relatively few studies regarding sleep and DA agonists have been reported in animal experiments, it appears that D_3 agonists may be the most likely to influence sleep. Low doses of D_3 agonists, including pramipexole, tend to increase slow-wave and REM sleep and to reduce locomotion in rats. Higher doses of D_2/D_3 agonists, with consequent D_3 and D_2 activation, seem to offset the effects of predominantly D_3 activation and to improve locomotion without excessive sedation. Pramipexole (30 and 500 g/kg) did not significantly affect striatal DA release during the first 2 hours after drug administration, as measured by microdialysis (5), suggesting that effects on sleep may not be directly related to changes in auto-receptor function. In studies employing narcoleptic Doberman dogs, D_2/D_3 agonists delivered to the ventral tegmental area aggravate cataplexy and increase sleep. Conversely, D_2/D_3 antagonists reduced cataplexy (6).

DOPAMINE AGONISTS IN OTHER MOVEMENT DISORDERS: RESTLESS LEGS SYNDROME AND PERIODIC LIMB MOVEMENTS OF SLEEP

Restless legs syndrome (RLS) and periodic limb movements of sleep (PLMS) occur frequently with PD and have been evaluated regarding therapeutic effects of many DA agonists (7). For example, ropinirole increases total sleep time, sleep efficacy, and sleep staging in patients with RLS (8). Like levodopa, multiple DA agonists have been reported to be effective therapies for reducing symptoms and signs of RLS and PLMS in therapeutic trials (Table 34.1).

Generally speaking, few patients with RLS or PLMS report insomnia with DA agonists, in that these agents are routinely administered immediately before bedtime given the nocturnal exacerbation in the severity of these disorders. Some investigators have noted the absence of sudden unexpected sleep attacks in patients with RLS (n = 24 patients treated with pramipexole 0.37 mg per day) (9). The series reported is very small, but given the increased incidence of RLS and PLMS in PD, this type of observation is of interest.

SLEEP AND DRIVING IN SLEEP-DEPRIVED PERSONS

Although disruption of sleep is common in PD, occurring in most patients (10), it is also common in the general population. According to recent surveys, Americans living in the year 2000 sleep 7 hours per night in contrast to their counterparts in the 1900s who slept more than 9 hours per night (11). The National Sleep Foundation's 1998 Omnibus Sleep in America Poll suggests that large percentages of the American public are frequently sleep deprived (Table 34.2).

TABLE 34.1. *Dopamine agonists with therapeutic trials documenting benefit for restless legs syndrome and periodic limb movements of sleep*

Bromocriptine	D_2/D_1 agonist/antagonist (reference 41)
Cabergoline	D_2 agonist (reference 45)
Pergolide	D_2/D_1 agonist (reference 42)
Pramipexole	D_3/D_2 agonist (reference 7)
Ropinirole	D_2 agonist (references 8,43)
Talipexole	D_2 agonist (reference 44)

Although a myriad of repercussions relate to sleep deprivation, the potential for falling asleep while driving an automobile and consequent risk for causing injury or death to the driver and others is of particular importance. In the 1998 Omnibus Sleep Poll, 57% of those interviewed said that they had driven while drowsy in the past year and 23% indicated that they had actually fallen asleep at the wheel (12). Many countries have reported similar figures. In Great Britain, 29% of respondents to a mail survey reported that they "had felt close to falling asleep while driving" in the past year (13), and 10% of normal individuals indicated actually falling asleep while driving each year (14). In Norway, one of 12 drivers reported falling asleep while driving during the past year, with 5% of these episodes resulting in a crash (15).

The US National Highway Traffic Safety Administration estimates that 100,000 accidents and at least 1,500 deaths per year can be attributed to driver drowsiness in the United States. Drowsy-driving crashes or fall-asleep crashes represent only 1% to 3% of police-reported car crashes, whereas fall-asleep crashes represent 6% to 10% of all self-reported car crashes. Drowsy-driving or fall-asleep crashes generally have certain characteristics, as outlined in Table 34.3.

Interestingly, persons who fall asleep may not be good judges of how sleepy they are and how likely they are to fall asleep (16–18). A prospective study of long-haul truck drivers determined that 10% entered stage 1 sleep

TABLE 34.2. *Results of the 1998 Omnibus Sleep in America Poll (12)*

- 32% of American adults sleep 6 or less hours per night
- 64% sleep less than 8 hours per night
- 38% had excessive daytime sleepiness severe enough to interfere with their jobs

TABLE 34.3. *Characteristics of fall-asleep crashes*

- Usually occur late at night (12–7 a.m.) or in the mid-afternoon (2–4 p.m.)
- Usually involve a single vehicle running off the road
- Usually occur on high-speed roadways
- Driver is often alone
- Driver is often a young male, 16–25 years of age
- No skid marks or indication of braking

while driving during a 2-week period. Prodromal drowsiness was documented by videotape and electrophysiological monitoring, but not always appreciated by the subject (19). Itoi et al. (18) concluded that people's inability to judge sleep onset, and hence their susceptibility to sleep-related accidents, may be attributable to a scarcity of meaningful physiological warning signs in some individuals and to a failure to acknowledge the importance of meaningful physiological warning signs in others.

Even in the absence of falling asleep, sleep deprivation translates into less-than-normal motor control and judgment while driving. In one study, wakefulness of 17 hours decreased motor performance as much as a blood alcohol concentration of 0.05% (the legal limit in Finland, Norway, the Netherlands, and France) (20). Sleep-deprivation and driving-safety problems were also well documented in a survey of pediatric house-staff and faculty at Johns Hopkins University (21). Forty-four percent of the house-staff ("on call" one in four nights) reported falling asleep while stopped at a red light during their residency (1 to 3 years), compared with only 12.5% of the medical school faculty (no night "call") ($p <$ .001). Additionally, 25% of the house-staff had been in a sleep or drowsy-driving–related motor vehicle accident (MVA), fortunately without any serious injuries or fatalities. Forty-seven percent of the house-staff who had been involved in MVAs had a history of falling asleep at the wheel. House-staff had more traffic citations and were involved in more MVAs on their postcall days than on other workdays.

Other studies have evaluated factors leading to drowsy-driving crashes. A case–control study of drivers in police-reported crashes in the state of North Carolina identified drivers as either "asleep" or "fatigued" (n = 467) by the investigating officer and compared these with drivers in crashes who were not "asleep" or "fatigued" (n = 529) and a third sample of noncrash drivers (n = 407) (22). Work and sleep schedules were both strongly associated with involvement in a sleep-related crash. Drivers in sleep-related crashes were twice as likely to work more than one job and their primary job was much more likely to involve nonstandard hours. Working the nightshift increased the odds of a sleep-related crash by six times and the fewer hours slept directly correlated with greater odds for a sleep-related crash. Drivers in sleep- and fatigue-related crashes were more likely to have poor- or fair-quality sleep. Drivers in sleep-related crashes were also more than twice as likely to have elevated Epworth Sleepiness Scale (ESS) scores indicative of excessive daytime sleepiness (EDS) (23). On the day of their crash, sleep-related crashers reported being at the wheel significantly longer before their crash, having been awake for longer the day of their crash, and having slept fewer hours the night before. Half reported getting 6 or less hours of sleep the night before the crash, compared with less than 10% of the other drivers in crashes. One of five drivers reported sleeping fewer than 4 hours the night before the crash. Although most drivers agreed with the police officer's assessment of the role of sleepiness or fatigue in their crash, not all reported feeling drowsy before crashing. In fact, 44% of the sleep-related crash drivers and 51% of the fatigue-related crash drivers reported that they felt either "slightly" or "not at all" drowsy before their crash. These figures also suggest that the relative inability to recognize the true potential for falling asleep exists commonly in the general population.

Recent anecdotal reports of patients with PD describe rapid-onset irresistible episodes of sleep, so-called "sleep attacks" (24). The term sleep attack has been used in the literature on sleep solely in association with narcolepsy (25), apart from a paper authored by Matsunaga (26) in reference to idiopathic central nervous system (CNS) hypersomnolence. However, this author commented that none of the patients with idiopathic CNS hypersomnolence had "cataplexy, sleep paralysis, sleep attack, sleep apnea, or any other identifiable neurological disorders." Additionally, "sleep attacks" are not included as one of the 88 diagnostic classifications by the American Sleep Disorders Association (27).

Experts suggest that "sleepiness" is most simply defined as "the inclination to sleep." Roth et al. (28), in *Principles and Practice of Sleep Medicine,* observed that "heavy meals, warm rooms, boring lectures, and the monotony of long-distance automobile driving unmask the presence of physiological sleepiness but do not cause it." In conclusion, sleep deprivation in the general population is increasingly common and associated with episodes of falling asleep that increase risk dramatically for MVAs.

DOPAMINE AGONISTS, DRIVING, AND SLEEP EFFECTS IN PARKINSON'S DISEASE

Sleep disruption and increased motor activity during REM and non-REM sleep are a frequent finding in PD and multiple system atrophy (even in the untreated states) (10,29). Sleep and motor abilities may also affect one another. Patients who are severely immobile are more likely to have disturbed sleep than those with relatively good mobility. As well, "sleep benefit" or a lessened disability or feeling "on" after awakening occurs in approximately one of three patients with PD. Patients with such a sleep benefit tend to be younger, have a longer disease duration, take higher total daily doses of levodopa, have a longer duration of levodopa treatment, and exhibit less cognitive and physical disability (30).

Anecdotal reports regarding changes in sleep in patients with PD after use of DA agonists have occurred since the introduction of these agents. In 1978, Rabey et al. (31) reported nocturnal sleep patterns in six parkinsonian patients being treated with bromocriptine. There were no significant differences in sleep patterns in comparison with patients treated with levodopa. In the same year, Vardi et al. (32) reported six patients with PD who developed nocturnal myoclonic attacks after treatment with levodopa; these were recorded on electroencephalogram. The myoclonus persisted after substitution with bromocriptine. Somnolence is thought to occur more frequently with lisuride treatment than levodopa and bromocriptine (33). However, mere treatment of tremor in patients with PD does not appear to influence sleep. Specifically, treatment of tremor with thalamic stimulation (130 Hz, 2 to 3 V) did not alter sleep or sleep spindles or appear to cause sleep disruption (34).

Larger clinical trials report somnolence in 27% of patients with early PD treated with pramipexole (35) and 13% of patients treated with ropinirole (36).

Eight patients with PD taking pramipexole and one taking ropinirole were described who fell asleep while driving, causing MVAs (24). Five of the nine reported no warning of somnolence before falling asleep. The authors used the phrase "sudden irresistible attacks of sleep" to describe this scenario. The authors concluded that the two drugs were responsible for several reasons: All attacks occurred after the patients began taking pramipexole or ropinirole and stopped after the drugs were discontinued; no further MVAs occurred over several months (24). All eight patients were men. The average age was 65.1 years (54 to 83 years), and duration of illness was 6.4 years (2.5 to 13 years). The average dose of pramipexole (after 7 months) was 2.9 mg per day. After the MVA, pramipexole was discontinued in six and reduced in two patients. No further "sleep attacks" occurred. One patient who was subsequently treated with ropinirole (16 mg per day) experienced another "attack." Patients described sudden, irresistible overwhelming sleepiness without awareness of falling asleep. Similarly, another report described two patients receiving ropinirole and/or pramipexole who experienced sleep attacks and concluded that these were a class effect of non-ergot DA agonists (37).

These reports have led to major repercussions regarding the use and study of DA agonists as practitioners and institutional review boards consider whether patients prescribed DA agonists should be counseled to avoid driving motor vehicles while taking this class of medication (38). A few recent studies now provide more than anecdotal information.

In a study reported in the spring of 2001, 638 consecutive patients with PD were surveyed in 18 Canadian movement disorder group clinics (39). Antiparkinsonian medication use was as follows: 84.3% took levodopa, 46% took both levodopa and a DA agonist, 23% took pramipexole, 19% ropinirole, 11% pergolide, and 3% bromocriptine. The ESS score was 7 or greater in 55% of the 420 drivers. (Scores higher than 10 are generally strongly associated with EDS.) The ESS score was higher in patients treated with pramipexole than other DA agonists. EDS in normally alerting situations was more frequent with all DA agonists than levodopa alone. Falling asleep while driving occurred more in ropinirole-treated individuals than others. However, there were no statistically significant differences in falling asleep between non-ergot and ergot agonists; 16 patients (3.8%) fell asleep while driving ("sudden onset of sleep"); three of 16 did not report experiencing any preceding drowsiness or other warning.

The issue of falling asleep without apparent warning is of great importance. As pointed out earlier, it is well known that persons may be retrospectively unaware of somnolence that had preceded sleep because of the lack of memory associated with sleep onset and decreasing recognition of sedation over time (28). Sleep-monitoring studies, for instance, have repeatedly demonstrated that patients may fall asleep without recalling that they had a prodrome of somnolence despite clinical and electrophysiological signs of sleep and somnolence (19,20).

In perhaps the most informative study on the subject, Sanjiv et al. (40) reported a study employing ESS and a modification of this same scale in patients with PD receiving various medication regimens. The ESS modification was that the same ESS questions were asked regarding the likelihood of falling asleep during various activities with the added qualification: "How likely would you be to fall asleep without warning in a particular context?" Their study reported daytime somnolence in 160 patients with PD taking levodopa or levodopa with one of three different DA agonists (bromocriptine, ropinirole, or pramipexole), with 40 patients in each treatment regimen. They concluded that all these medications, taken at usual daily doses, could contribute to daytime sleepiness. Importantly, "dozing off" also correlated highly with "falling asleep without warning," as evidenced by the modified ESS correlating strongly with the ESS. They suggested that the ESS could serve as a marker for the modified ESS and increasing risk for falling asleep while driving and potential MVA risk. They also found that there was no significant difference among these antiparkinsonian medication regimens for causing daytime somnolence. In fact, on the basis of these data, the argument could be made that adjunctive use of DA agonists does not elevate the risk significantly above that of levodopa therapy alone.

CONCLUSIONS AND RECOMMENDATIONS

Sleep disorders commonly accompany motor disability in PD. The impact of pharmacological therapy directed at improving motor signs upon sleep is worthy of study for various reasons. Sleep improvements or disruption and increased daytime somnolence all influence quality of life and may do so even beyond impacts on motor function.

The bulk of information suggests that DA agonists produce some degree of somnolence in 10% to 25% of patients with PD. Because of recent anecdotal reports suggesting that

DA agonists may cause abrupt onset of sleep and increased risk for MVAs while driving, more systematic analysis of this topic is warranted. Data available to date suggest that (a) DA agonists and levodopa may increase somnolence, (b) no DA agonist is more likely than others to cause somnolence, (c) persons who fall asleep may not necessarily recall prodromal drowsiness, and (d) the risk for falling asleep while driving appears to be correlated with excessive daytime somnolence.

Consequently, patients with PD prescribed DA agonists should be warned about the potential for excessive daytime somnolence. Those developing excessive daytime somnolence should be warned about the potential for falling asleep and cautioned against driving. We believe there are no data at this time that dictate the need for routine restriction of driving privileges for patients taking DA agonists in whom there is no excessive daytime somnolence. Further study of this issue may provide rationale for more specific practice recommendations.

REFERENCES

1. De Keyser J, Ebinger G, Vauquelin G. Evidence for a widespread dopaminergic innervation of the human cerebral neocortex. *Neurosci Lett* 1989;104:281–285.
2. Cianchetti C. Dopamine agonists and sleep in man. In: Wauquier A, ed. *Sleep: neurotransmitters neuromodulators.* New York: Raven Press, 1985:121.
3. Rye DB, Bliwise DL. Movement disorders specific to sleep and the nocturnal manifestations of waking movement disorders. In: Watts RL, Koller WC, eds. *Movement disorders: neurologic principles and practice.* New York: McGraw-Hill Health Professions Division, 1997:687–714.
4. Zweig RM, Jankel WR, Hedreen JC, et al. The pedunculopontine nucleus in Parkinson's disease. *Ann Neurol* 1989;26:41–46.
5. Lagos P, Scorza C, Monti JM, et al. Effects of the D_3 preferring dopamine agonist pramipexole on sleep and waking, locomotor activity and striatal dopamine release in rats. *Eur Neuropsychopharmacol* 1998;8: 113–120.
6. Honda K, Riehl J, Mignot E, et al. Dopamine D_3 agonists into the substantia nigra aggravate cataplexy but do not modify sleep. *Neuroreport* 1999;10:3111–3118.
7. Montplaisir J, Godbout R, Poirier G, et al. Restless legs syndrome and periodic movements in sleep: physiopathology and treatment with L-dopa. *Clin Neuropharmacol* 1986;9:456–463.
8. Saletu B, Gruber G, Saletu M, et al. Sleep laboratory studies in restless legs syndrome patients as compared with normals and acute effects of ropinirole, I: findings on objective and subjective sleep and awakening quality. *Neuropsychobiology* 2000;41:181–189.
9. Stiasny K, Moller JC, Oertel WH. Safety of pramipexole in patients with restless legs syndrome. *Neurology* 2000;55:1589–1590.
10. Pal PK, Calne S, Samii A, et al. A review of normal sleep and its disturbances in Parkinson's disease. *Parkinsonism Related Disord* 1999;5:1–17.
11. Huang DY. The drowsy driver. *Jacksonville Med* 2001; 52:120–124.
12. Johnson EO. *Omnibus sleep in America poll.* Washington, DC: National Sleep Foundation, 1998.
13. Maycock G. Sleepiness and driving: the experience of U.K. car drivers. *Accid Anal Prev* 1997;29:453–462.
14. Horne JA, Reyner LA. Sleep related vehicle accidents. *Br Med J* 1995;310:565–567.
15. Sagberg F. Road accidents caused by drivers falling asleep. *Accid Anal Prev* 1999;31:639–649.
16. US Federal Highway Administration. *The driver fatigue and alertness study: a success story of partnerships, data and analysis.* Washington, DC: Federal Highway Administration, 1997:4.
17. Filliatrault DD, Cooper PJ, King DJ, et al. Efficiency of vehicle-based data to predict lane departure arising from loss of alertness due to fatigue. Paper presented at: the Association for the Advancement of Automotive Medicine; October 1996; Vancouver, British Columbia.
18. Itoi A, Cilveti R, Voth M, et al. *Can drivers avoid falling asleep at the wheel?* Washington, DC: AAA Foundation for Traffic Safety, 1993.
19. Mitler MM, Miller JC, Lipsitz JJ, et al. The sleep of long-haul truck drivers. *N Engl J Med* 1997;337: 755–761.
20. Dement WC. The perils of drowsy driving. *N Engl J Med* 1997;337:783–784.
21. Marcus CL, Loughlin GM. Effect of sleep deprivation on driving safety in housestaff. *Sleep* 1996;19:763–766.
22. Stutts JC, Wilkins JW, Vaughn BV. *Why do people have drowsy driving crashes? Input from drivers who just did.* AAA Foundation for Traffic Safety, 1999. Available at: www.aaafts.org/pdf/sleep.
23. Johns MW. A new method for measuring daytime sleepiness: the Epworth Sleepiness Scale. *Sleep* 1991; 14:540–545.
24. Frucht S, Rogers JD, Greene PE, et al. Falling asleep at the wheel: motor vehicle mishaps in persons taking pramipexole and ropinirole. *Neurology* 1999;52: 1908–1910.
25. Dement W, Rechtschaffen A, Gulevich G. The nature of the narcoleptic sleep attack. *Neurology* 1966;16:18–33.
26. Matsunaga H. Clinical study on idiopathic CNS hypersomnolence. *Jpn J Psychiatry Neurol* 1987;41: 637–644.
27. American Sleep Disorders Association. *International classification of sleep disorders revised: diagnostic and coding manual.* Rochester, MN: American Sleep Disorders Association, 1997.
28. Roth T, Roehrs EA, Traskadon MA. Daytime sleepiness and alertness. In: Kryger MH, Roth T, Dement WC, eds. *Principles and practice of sleep medicine,* 3rd ed. Philadelphia: WB Saunders, 2000:43–52.
29. Wetter TC, Collado-Seidel V, Pollmacher T, et al. Sleep and periodic leg movement patterns in drug-free pa-

tients with Parkinson's disease and multiple system atrophy. *Sleep* 2000;23:361–367.
30. Currie LJ, Bennett JP Jr, Harrison MB, et al. Clinical correlates of sleep benefit in Parkinson's disease. *Neurology* 1997;48:1115–1117.
31. Rabey J, Vardi J, Glaubman H, et al. EEG sleep study in parkinsonian patients under bromocriptine treatment. *Eur Neurol* 1978;17:345–350.
32. Vardi J, Glaubman H, Rabey JM, et al. Myoclonic attacks induced by L-dopa and bromocriptine in Parkinson patients: a sleep EEG study. *J Neurol* 1978;218:35–42.
33. Gopinathan G, Teräväinen H, Dambrosia JM, et al. Lisuride in parkinsonism. *Neurology* 1981;31:371–376.
34. Arnulf I, Bejjani BP, Garma L, et al. Effect of low and high frequency thalamic stimulation on sleep in patients with Parkinson's disease and essential tremor. *J Sleep Res* 2000;9:55–62.
35. Parkinson Study Group. Safety and efficacy of pramipexole in early Parkinson's disease. A randomized dose-ranging study. *JAMA* 1997;278:125–130.
36. Sethi KD, O'Brien CF, Hammerstad JP, et al. Ropinirole for the treatment of early Parkinson disease: a 12-month experience. Ropinirole Study Group. *Arch Neurol* 1998; 55:1211–1216.
37. Ryan M, Slevin JT, Wells A. Non-ergot dopamine agonist–induced sleep attacks. *Pharmacotherapy* 2000;20: 724–726.
38. Olanow CW, Schapira AH, Roth T. Waking up to sleep episodes in Parkinson's disease. *Mov Disord* 2000;15: 212–215.
39. Lang AE, Hobson DE, Martin W, et al. Excessive daytime sleepiness and sudden onset sleep in Parkinson's disease: a survey from 18 Canadian movement disorders clinics. *Neurology* 2001;56[Suppl]:A307.
40. Sanjiv CC, Schulzer M, Mak E, et al. Daytime somnolence in patients with Parkinson's disease. *Parkinsonism Relat D* 2001;7:283–286.
41. Becker PM, Jamieson AO, Brown WD. Dopaminergic agents in restless legs syndrome and periodic limb movements of sleep: response and complications of extended treatment in 49 cases. *Sleep* 1993;16:713–716.
42. Earley CJ, Yaffee JB, Allen RP. Randomized, double-blind, placebo-controlled trial of pergolide in restless legs syndrome. *Neurology* 1998;51:1599–1602.
43. Saletu M, Anderer P, Saletu B, et al. Sleep laboratory studies in restless legs syndrome patients as compared with normals and acute effects of ropinirole, II: findings on periodic leg movements, arousals and respiratory variables. *Neuropsychobiology* 2000;41:190–199.
44. Inoue Y, Mitani H, Nanba K, et al. Treatment of periodic leg movement disorder and restless leg syndrome with talipexole. *Psychiatry Clin Neurosci* 1999;53:283–285.
45. Stiasny K, Robbecke J, Schuler P, et al. Treatment of idiopathic restless legs syndrome (RLS) with the D_2-agonist cabergoline—an open clinical trial. *Sleep* 2000;23: 349–354.

Parkinson's Disease: Advances in Neurology, Vol. 91.
Edited by Ariel Gordin, Seppo Kaakkola, and Heikki Teräväinen
Lippincott Williams & Wilkins, Philadelphia © 2003

35

Dystonia in Parkinsonian Syndromes

Alberto Albanese

Instituto Nazionale Neurologico Carlo Besta, Universitá Cattolica del Sacro Cuore, Milano, Italy

It has long been assumed, with clinical observations dating back more to a century, that dystonia is an integral part of Parkinson's disease (PD) (1).

Dystonia associated with parkinsonism may also occur in various hereditary conditions involving the basal ganglia, such as Wilson's disease (2); Huntington's disease (3); Hallervorden–Spatz syndrome (4); corticobasal ganglionic degeneration (CBGD) (5); or progressive supranuclear palsy (6,7). Dystonia and parkinsonian signs are also key features of dopa-responsive dystonia (8); X-linked dystonia-parkinsonism (9); rapid-onset dystonia-parkinsonism (10,11); and hemiparkinsonian-hemiatrophy syndrome (12,13). Although dystonia and parkinsonism are commonly associated, their relationship is far from being understood. The main impediment for creating pathophysiological links between dystonia and the different parkinsonian syndromes has been the lack of diagnostic tests and the paucity of clinicopathological reports (6). The differential diagnosis of parkinsonian syndromes has been greatly improved in recent years, mainly after the introduction of validated diagnostic criteria and laboratory examinations, particularly genetic testing and brain imaging.

CLINICAL FEATURES OF DYSTONIA

Dystonia is currently defined as a syndrome of sustained muscle contractions, frequently causing twisting and repetitive movements or abnormal postures (14). This movement disorder is associated with a defect of cortical inhibition, resulting in inaccurate selection of movements, as well as with a disordered preparation for movement, resulting in inappropriate processing of sensory stimuli (15).

The most typical presentation is torsion dystonia, encompassing a combination of dystonic movements and dystonic postures (16,17). Dystonic movements have a twisting nature and a directional quality and are consistent and predictable (18). Dystonic postures are associated with a sensation of rigidity and traction and are primarily responsible for pain. In torsion dystonia patients, postures may appear some months or few years before dystonic movements are seen; the combination of these two clinical signs is a key feature for the clinical diagnosis of torsion dystonia. Fixed dystonia is the syndrome of dystonic postures without dystonic movements. As opposed to mobile (or torsion) dystonia, fixed dystonia is often secondary to other neurological disorders.

Dystonic movements and postures may be alleviated by a number of specific voluntary movements, which have been called "sensory tricks" or "*gestes antagonistes*" (19,20). They are thought to inhibit, at the central level, the cortical overflow that causes dystonia (21). Their finding is a clinical sign for the diagnosis of dystonia. Voluntary movements, particularly purposeful skilled actions, commonly aggravate dystonia, either mobile or fixed. Dystonic camptocormia is a focal form of fixed dystonia that is induced or aggravated by walking (22) and is typically relieved by the *geste antagoniste* of straightening the trunk by pushing against a cane or a wall. Dystonic camptocormia is occasionally reported as a primary disorder of the elderly and is commonly observed in PD.

CONTRACTURES IN PARKINSONIAN SYNDROMES

Deformities or contractures of the hands, and sometimes the feet, were recognized to occur in some parkinsonian patients in the pre-levodopa era. Charcot (23) pointed out that they were not dissimilar to those of rheumatoid arthritis, except that there was no swelling or stiffness in the joints. Similar observations were performed in the pre-levodopa era on clinically typical PD cases (24). It is difficult to be certain whether the cases described had idiopathic PD or other parkinsonian syndromes, such as post-encephalitic parkinsonism (25) or parkinsonism–dementia complex (26,27). Some of these hand deformities may have been due to contraction, rather than contracture because it has been observed that they could be corrected by stereotactic thalamotomy in severe cases of parkinsonism (28). The term contractures has also been occasionally used to indicate a fixed posture or deformity occurring in parkinsonian patients, some of whom have received a postmortem diagnosis of multiple system atrophy (MSA) (29–31). Therefore, the issue of whether contractures occurring in different parkinsonian syndromes have distinctive features has remained unsettled.

It is not established whether such contractures represent the consequence of longstanding fixed dystonic posturing (32) or whether they constitute a different pathophysiological entity. Several mechanisms are probably involved. Dystonia affecting the hands, either due to the disease itself or more commonly to drug use, gives rise to a slight ulnar deviation of the fingers, flexion of the metacarpophalangeal joint, and hyperextension of the interphalangeal joints (Fig. 35.1) (33). These deformities are initially intermittent and can be related to the timing of drugs but later become clenched-fist contractures. It is thought that hyperactivity of the small muscles of the hands is an important contributing factor in producing hand deformities in PD. It has been shown that blocking the ulnar nerve at the elbow with local anesthetic can reverse finger flexion deformities, whereas stimulation of the same nerve in normal hands can produce finger deformities similar to those observed in PD (28). The posture adopted by the patient, especially in cases with severe rigidity, also seems to be a contributing factor. The occurrence of hand deformities is related to the

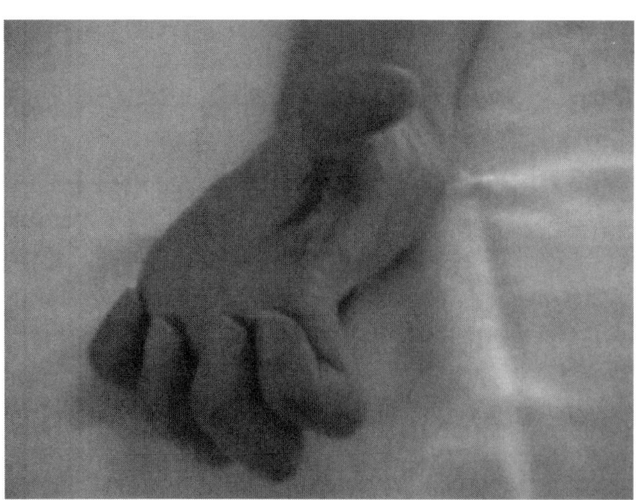

FIGURE 35.1. This patient with clinically typical Parkinson's disease dating for more than 10 years developed a fixed contracture of the left hand.

degree of muscular rigidity and is unrelated to the extent or duration of tremor (29).

The principal cause of contractures is a shortening of the length of muscle fibers due to a reduced number of sarcomeres, precipitated by prolonged immobilization of the muscles at short lengths during sustained muscle contraction. Additionally, changes in the physical properties (plasticity and viscoelasticity) of muscles, tendon, joint, and surrounding soft tissue occur, leading to atrophy and fibrosis (34). Contractures can develop quite rapidly and usually within 12 months (32).

The question of whether contractures represent an extremely severe form of fixed dystonia is also unsettled. Unlike fixed dystonia, contractures are not alleviated by *gestes antagonistes* and are not aggravated by performing voluntary or skilled movements.

DYSTONIA IN PARKINSON'S DISEASE

Dystonic manifestations now encountered in patients with PD are usually related to antiparkinsonian treatment. Dystonic foot response was recognized as an early parkinsonian feature well before the discovery of levodopa (1). Similar observations were performed in levodopa-treated patients, who developed "off"-related early morning foot dystonia after overnight medication withdrawal (35) or daytime foot dystonia (36). Dystonia is the most common early morning dyskinesia occurring in patients with PD (37). It has been readily established that dopaminergic medication could reverse foot dystonia in patients with PD (38). Attempts to correlate dystonia with plasma levodopa concentrations yielded inconsistent results (39,40), indicating that dystonia is not simply related to the pharmacokinetics of levodopa.

The distinction between dyskinesias occurring when adequate mobility is warranted by dopaminergic medication ("on" period) and those occurring in the "off" period (when medication has been withdrawn) provides the basis for the current classification. Because different forms of dystonia could be observed in the "on" and the "off" periods, the question has arisen about whether distinctive clinical features can be documented. Several forms of "off"-related dystonia (pretreatment, early morning, and "off"-period dystonia) have been recognized (41).

"Off"-period dystonia is the most common type of dystonia seen in PD. It is an often painful fixed dystonia occurring in the "off" periods, mainly affecting the limbs. Foot dystonia is the most common form. Typical "off"-period foot dystonia involves plantarflexion and inversion of the ankle, together with plantarflexion of the toes except for the big toe, which is frequently extended. Voluntary movement often aggravates fixed dystonia in PD, whereas action-foot dystonia may lead to recurrent spasms (38). Contractures, instead, often occur in the upper limb and are not aggravated by voluntary movement.

Although "on"-period dyskinesias were originally described as choreoathetoid (42), as opposed to pure dystonia in the "off" state, they are in fact choreodystonic. Mobile dystonia is commonly combined with chorea (or sometimes a different dyskinesia) in the "on" periods (43).

Interestingly, mobile dystonia has never been reported in PD "off" periods.

Clinical Features of "Off"-period Dystonia in PD

Charcot (23) was the first to draw attention to early dystonic foot posturing, and Purves-Stewart (1), a few years later, recognized similar foot posturing in five of his 28 cases. Numerous authors have since emphasized this clinical feature, making it the most common dystonic manifestation in untreated patients with alleged PD (36,41,44–46). Foot dystonia is often painful, it commonly occurs in the "off" period and may lead to "dystonic claudication" (38). Upper limb dystonia has also been recognized in classic (47) and more recent (36,41,44–46) descriptions of patients with PD.

Approximately one quarter to one third of the patients managed before the levodopa era may have eventually developed hand and foot dystonia (33). A wide variety of dystonic manifestations have recently been associated with PD, either coincident with its onset or up to 25 years before (49). These include cranial dystonia (44,45,48,49); cervical dystonia (44,45,48,49); axial dystonia with scoliosis (46,48); and various dystonic movement and posturing of both upper and lower limb, most often ipsilateral to the side most affected by parkinsonism (44–46, 48,49). Unilateral parkinsonism has also been observed in association with hemidystonia of the same body side (44–46,49).

Dystonia at disease onset and a progressive parkinsonism, with sustained response to low doses of levodopa and occurrence of "on"-period dyskinesias, is the classic presentation in patients with mutations of the parkin (*PARK2*) gene (50,51). Patients linking to the *PARK7* locus also present dystonia (52), but interestingly, dystonia is very rarely observed in patients linking to the *PARK6* locus (53). These data may indicate that genetic susceptibility to dystonia varies in different parkinsonian forms.

"Off"-period dystonia is more common than usually appreciated; increased blink rate in patients with PD may reveal "off"-period blepharospasm (54). A special focal form of "off"-period dystonia is the paradoxical contraction of the puborectalis muscle during straining for defecation, characterized by excessive recruitment of synergistic and antagonistic muscle groups during voluntary activity and lack of reciprocal inhibition (55). It has been observed that apomorphine can reverse acute constipation occurring as an "off"-related phenomenon soon after withdrawal of levodopa in patients with PD (56) and that this drug specifically improves anorectal dysfunction in PD (57). In our series, we observed that 13% of 120 patients with PD and chronic constipation could not defecate due to paradoxical puborectalis contraction at straining (58).

Clinical Features of "On"-period Dystonia in PD

In the first reports of chronic levodopa therapy, dyskinesias were recognized as a complication (59–64). It has been observed that the clinical features of levodopa-induced dyskinesias vary with the clinical fluctuation of parkinsonism, and that they possibly reflect changes of plasma concentrations of levodopa (65). Some descriptions of "on"-period dyskinesias have associated the time of dyskinesia onset with the motor improvement caused by levodopa (hence, levodopa-induced dyskinesia) and have described their clinical appearance (i.e., chorea, dystonia, myoclonus, and so on) (59,66). "On"-period dyskinesias are evidently related to the short-duration response to levodopa, starting from 15 minutes to 1 hour after a dose and disappearing after 1 to 3 hours (67). They can also be observed in relation to the short-duration response after the administration of dopamine agonists or as an aftermath of combined therapy in those patients taking multiple medications. "On"-period dyskinesias are not dependent on plasma levodopa concentrations (39,40), and the distinction between monophasic (or peak-dose) and biphasic (or beginning-of-dose and end-of-dose) dyskinesias is probably artificial (68). Dyskinesias related to medication have different clinical features from those induced by high-frequency stimulation of the subthalamic nucleus (69,70).

The most common clinical presentation of "on"-period dyskinesias is a combination of chorea and dystonia (43). In the earliest descriptions of levodopa-induced dyskinesias, their complex phenomenology was clearly recognized (59). A classic report on the pattern of "on"-period dyskinesias induced by levodopa clearly emphasized their dystonic nature (67), whereas more recent observations have reckoned that "on"-period dyskinesias are choreic in 70% of patients (71). In our experience, dystonic features are almost invariably present when dyskinesias affect the limbs, whereas isolated chorea is observed in dyskinesias of the face. Monophasic dyskinesias commonly present a combination of dystonia and chorea, whereas biphasic (beginning-of-dose and end-of-dose dyskinesias) mainly have dystonic features (Fig. 35.2). "On"-period chorea occurring in PD has the

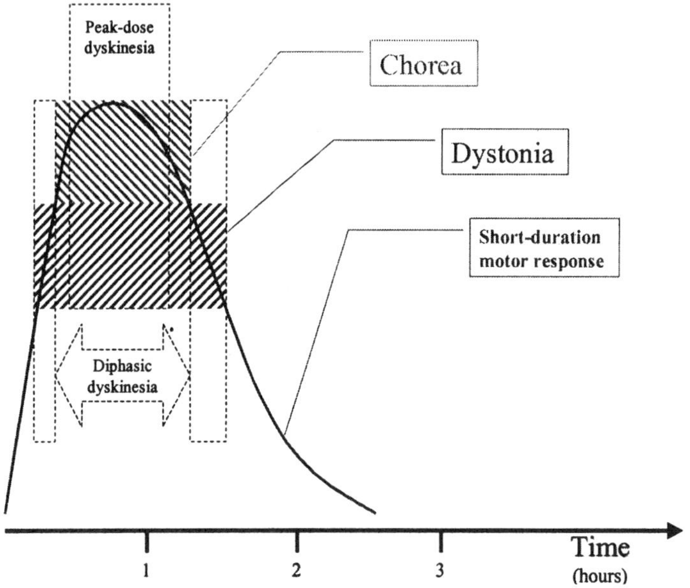

FIGURE 35.2. The clinical presentation of peak-dose dyskinesia is usually of a mixed type, choreic and dystonic, whereas diphasic dyskinesias are usually prevalently dystonic. This figure shows the time course of dystonia and chorea with reference to the short-duration motor response after a single acute administration of levodopa.

same neurophysiological features of degenerative chorea (72).

DYSTONIA IN PARKINSONIAN SYNDROMES

Although dystonia may occur in almost any of the parkinsonian syndromes, some have a particular tendency to associate with dystonia.

Degenerative Diseases with Parkinsonism and Dystonia

Nearly all reports of *CBGD* mention the presence of dystonia, but detailed characterization of the dystonic features is lacking (5,73,74). In a series of 66 patients with possible CBGD, 39 (59%) had dystonia (74). Of the four cases in this series who received a pathological confirmation of the diagnosis, three had dystonia during the course of the illness. Limb dystonia is the most common feature. Early asymmetrical limb dystonia commonly proceeds to fixed dystonic posturing (75). Typically, the arm is adducted at the shoulder, the elbows and wrists flexed, and the arm extending in front or behind the body. Axial dystonia is a less common feature (76).

A progressive nuchal dystonia leading to a permanent contracture was reported in the first description of *progressive supranuclear palsy* (7). Focal or segmental dystonia, for example, in the form of limb dystonia or blepharospasm is not uncommon (6,77,78). With disease progression, cranial and cervical dystonia lead to a progressive contracture that contracts the mandible to close the mouth and the neck into a characteristic extended posture. Contractures of the hands are not uncommon (Table 35.1).

Mobile dystonia is uncommon in *MSA*, although contractures and fixed dystonia have been reported as prominent features (79). The paradigmatic form of fixed dystonia in MSA is antecollis or head-drop not associated to trunk flexion or camptocormia (80). Figure 35.3 depicts a patient with severe fixed axial dystonia associated with a unilateral clenched

TABLE 35.1. *Paradigmatic features of "off"-period axial dystonia in three parkinsonian syndromes*

Disease	Clinical presentation of axial dystonia
Parkinson's disease	• Camptocormia
Progressive supranuclear palsy	• Extension cervical dystonia (retrocollis)
Multiple system atrophy	• Isolated flexion cervical dystonia (antecollis)
	• Same, combined with trunk flexion (disproportionate antecollis)

fist. Hand contractures have also been considered specific clinical markers, particularly if they are associated with local signs of dysautonomia (so-called "cold hands sign," Raynaud's phenomenon, and so on) (81).

Typically, *neurological Wilson's disease* presents insidiously with tremor, dystonia, rigidity, dysarthria, drooling, dysphagia, unsteady gait, and mental deterioration (82). Dystonia in the territory of the bulbar musculature is prominent; in one series, dystonia was more common than tremor as the initial feature (83). Cranial dystonia and pharyngeal dysmotility can be observed during the early disease stages (84). It may present as facial grimacing, blepharospasm, or lingual dystonia (85). A fixed "sardonic" smile with retracted lips and opened jaw, illustrated in Wilson's original report (82), is a highly typical feature. This fixed facial dystonia often progresses to impair closure of the mouth. Sustained dystonic postures are particularly common and, in addition to the bulbar region, can affect the trunk and limbs. The intensity of fixed dystonic postures can be so great as to require tendon release to relieve disability. Virtually, all untreated patients are affected by a progressive disturbance of speech. Lesser degrees of speech impairment include whispering dysphonia (86) and a characteristic inspiratory laugh, which "once heard is never forgotten" (87).

Post-encephalitic parkinsonism. In patients with encephalitis lethargica, various movement disorders were encountered during the acute encephalitic stage or during the post-en-

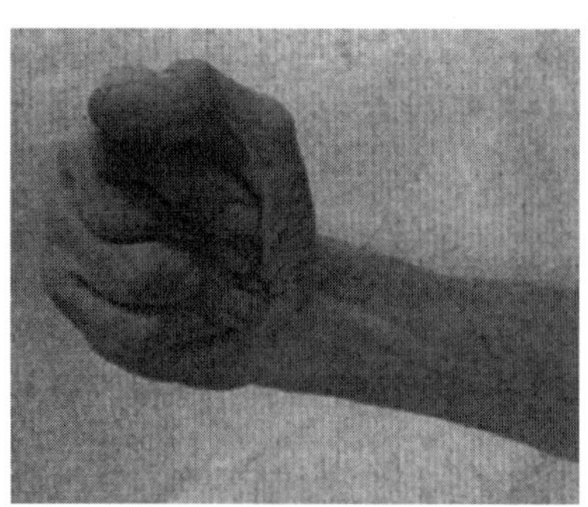

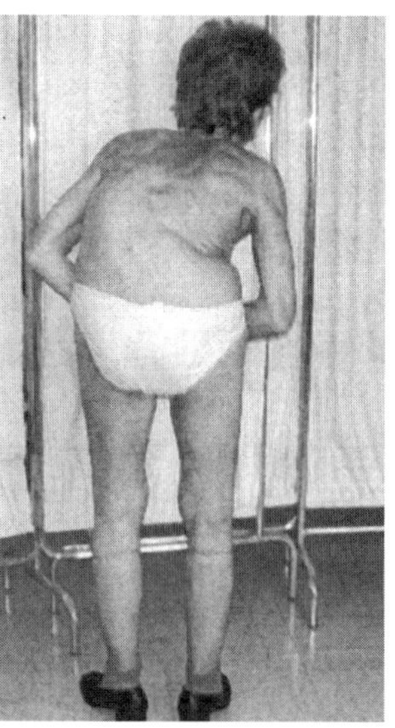

FIGURE 35.3. This patient has a 5-year history of multiple system atrophy and first developed a mobile dystonia of the right hand, in combination with a typical parkinsonian picture. **A:** The hand gradually turned into a fixed clenched fist. **B:** Camptocormia is associated with kyphosis and scoliosis of the spine.

cephalitic phase with or without parkinsonism (88–90). Dystonia was rarely described in post-encephalitic parkinsonism and usually had a cervical topography (90). It is likely that dystonia was largely unrecognized in the early reports if in a series of historical video segments on six post-encephalitic parkinsonism, five of the patients had dystonia (91).

Rapid-onset dystonia-parkinsonism is a rare autosomal-dominant movement disorder linked to chromosome 19q13 that is characterized by sudden onset of persistent primarily bulbar and upper limb dystonia and parkinsonism, generally during adolescence or early adulthood (10,92). Mild limb dystonia may occur years before the abrupt onset of combined dystonia-parkinsonism (93).

Different clinical types of *Hallervorden–Spatz syndrome* can be distinguished based on severity and age at disease onset. In early onset childhood types, the diagnosis is evident before 10 years of age; a rapidly progressive and a slowly progressive form have been described. In late-onset type, the diagnosis is evident after 10 years and before 18 years of age; it usually progresses slowly. The adult type of Hallervorden–Spatz syndrome also progresses slowly. In the early onset type, the motor disorder is characterized by dystonic postures, muscular rigidity, involuntary movements of choreoathetoid or tremulous type, and findings suggesting corticospinal tract dysfunction. Mental changes are indicative of dementia. The course, relentless and progressive, extends over several years, leading to death in early adulthood (94). The gene has been localized and recently identified (95).

Dopa-responsive dystonia is another genetic disorder associated with mutations of the guanosine triphosphate-cyclohydroxylase I gene on chromosome 14q (96). The classical phenotype presents in infancy or adolescence with postural abnormalities in the legs. Symptoms most often occur while walking and falls are common. Diurnal fluctuation of dystonia may be present, particularly in the form of "sleep benefit" (8), but because this is reported in 50% to 60% of cases, such an observation is not necessary for the diagnosis. Response to levodopa is sustained and dramatic; generalization occurs in untreated patients from 1 to 12 years after onset (97). Parkinsonian features usually occur later than dystonia; less common forms present at a later age with parkinsonian features (98). In a series of 86 patients, the following clinical features were reported as most common (99): abnormal gait, focal limb dystonia, scoliosis, rest or postural tremor, bradykinesia, rigidity, and diurnal fluctuations.

X-linked dystonia-parkinsonism (Lubag) is a rare disorder that mainly affects males of Filipino origin (9). Age at onset varies from adolescence to middle age; progression is to generalization. The patients have dystonia and associated parkinsonian signs in about one third of cases.

CONCLUSIONS

In conclusion, the number of diseases and syndromes in which parkinsonian features are associated with dystonia is so impressively high to impose the existence of links between these two conditions. Such links have not been fully elucidated. Efficacious symptomatic treatments only exist for PD, so a distinction between "on" and "off" periods is meaningless in other parkinsonian syndromes. However, it seems clear that "on"-period and "off"-period dystonia have different features in PD: Mobile dystonia occurs in the "on" period (when it is often combined with chorea), but not in the "off" period; the opposite is true for fixed dystonia. Untreatable parkinsonian syndromes must be compared to the "off" period in PD; still mobile dystonia is commonly observed in untreated parkinsonian syndromes (Table 35.2). This marks a clear difference with PD. Contractures occur in the "off" period in PD and in other parkinsonian syndromes; however, there are no clinical distinctive features.

The topography of dystonia is also a relevant clinical feature. It is proposed that orofacial and limb dystonia may be generated through different pathophysiological mechanisms. Limb or axial dystonia (which is a fea-

TABLE 35.2. *Presentation of different forms of dystonia in Parkinson's diseases compared with other parkinsonian syndromes*

Clinical feature	Parkinson's disease		Other parkinsonian syndromes	
	Off period	On period	Off period	On period[a]
Contractures	+	–	++	NA
Fixed dystonia	+++	–	++	NA
Mobile (torsion) dystonia	–	+++[b]	+++	–

Note: +, it may occur; ++, occurs often; +++, occurs very often; –, does not occur; NA, not available.
[a]On-period dystonia occurs in some, but not all, patients with a parkinsonian syndrome other than Parkinson's disease.
[b]It is often combined with chorea.

ture of a PD "off" period, of dopa-responsive dystonia, and others) may be caused by a state of reduced dopaminergic transmission. Orofacial dystonia (as observed in Hallervorden–Spatz syndrome) may be caused by pallidal dysfunction. Finally, combined forms may have a combined pathophysiology.

REFERENCES

1. Purves-Stewart J. Paralysis agitans with an account of a new symptom. *Lancet* 1898; 2:1258–1260.
2. Sternlieb I, Giblin DR, Scheinberg H. Wilson's disease. In: Marsden CD, Fahn S, eds. *Movement disorders,* 2nd ed. London: Butterworth, 1987:288–302.
3. Shoulson I. Huntington's disease. A decade of progress. *Neurol Clin* 1984;2:515–526.
4. Mourelatos Z, Golden JA. 24 year old female with progressive lower extremity dystonia, dysarthria, dysphagia and mental impairment. *Brain Pathol* 2000;10: 171–172.
5. Frucht S, Fahn S, Chin S, et al. Levodopa-induced dyskinesias in autopsy-proven cortical-basal ganglionic degeneration. *Mov Disord* 2000;15:340–343.
6. Rivest J, Quinn N, Marsden CD. Dystonia in Parkinson's disease, multiple system atrophy, and progressive supranuclear palsy. *Neurology* 1990;40:1571–1578.
7. Steele JC, Richardson JC, Olszewski J. Progressive supranuclear palsy. A heterogeneous degeneration involving the brain stem, basal ganglia and cerebellum with vertical gaze and pseudobulbar palsy, nuchal dystonia and dementia. *Arch Neurol* 1964;10:333–358.
8. Segawa M, Hosaka A, Miyagawa F, et al. Hereditary progressive dystonia with marked diurnal fluctuation. In: Eldridge R, Fahn S, eds. *Dystonia.* New York: Raven Press, 1976:215–233.
9. Wilhelmsen KC, Weeks DE, Nygaard TG, et al. Genetic mapping of "lubag" (X-linked dystonia-parkinsonism) in a Filipino kindred to the pericentromeric region of the X chromosome. *Ann Neurol* 1991;29:124–131.
10. Dobyns WB, Ozelius LJ, Kramer PL, et al. Rapid-onset dystonia-parkinsonism. *Neurology* 1993;43:2596–2602.
11. Brashear A, Butler IJ, Hyland K, et al. Cerebrospinal fluid homovanillic acid levels in rapid-onset dystonia-parkinsonism. *Ann Neurol* 1998;43:521–526.
12. Greene PE, Bressman SB, Ford B, et al. Parkinsonism, dystonia, and hemiatrophy. *Mov Disord* 2000;15: 537–541.
13. Nygaard TG, Duvoisin RG. Hereditary dystonia-parkinsonism syndrome of juvenile onset. *Neurology* 1986;36: 1424–1428.
14. Fahn S, Marsden CD, Calne DB. Classification and investigation of dystonia. In: Marsden CD, Fahn S, eds. *Movement disorders,* 2nd ed. London: Butterworth, 1987:332–358.
15. Hallett M. Disorder of movement preparation in dystonia. *Brain* 2000;123:1765–1766.
16. Albanese A. *I gangli motori e i disturbi del movimento. Neurobiologia clinica.* Padova: Piccin, 1991.
17. Ghika J, Albanese A. Dyskinesias. In: Fisher RS, Bogousslavsky J, eds. *Textbook of neurology.* Boston: Butterworth-Heinemann, 1998:247–254.
18. Bressman SB. Dystonia. *Curr Opin Neurol* 1998;11: 363–372.
19. Gomez-Wong E, Marti MJ, Cossu G, et al. The "geste antagonistique" induces transient modulation of the blink reflex in human patients with blepharospasm. *Neurosci Lett* 1998;251:125–128.
20. Greene PE, Bressman S. Exteroceptive and interoceptive stimuli in dystonia. *Mov Disord* 1998;13:549–551.
21. Hallett M. Is dystonia a sensory disorder? *Ann Neurol* 1995;38:139–140.
22. Djaldetti R, Mosberg-Galili R, Sroka H, et al. Camptocormia (bent spine) in patients with Parkinson's disease—characterization and possible pathogenesis of an unusual phenomenon. *Mov Disord* 1999;14:443–447.
23. Charcot JM. *Leçons sur les maladies du système nerveux.* Paris: A. Delahaye, 1872.
24. Reynolds F, Petropoulos G. Hand deformities in parkinsonism. *J Chronic Dis* 1965;18:593–595.
25. Martin JP. *The basal ganglia and posture.* London: Pitman, 1967.
26. Chan KM, Tsuji S, Gajdusek DC, et al. Studies on the natural history of parkinsonism-dementia of Guam, II: motor neuron involvement and postural deformities in advanced age. *Neurology* 1979;29:578.
27. Chen K-M, Chase TN. Parkinsonism-dementia. In: Vinken PJ, Bruyn GW, Klawans HL, eds. *Extrapyramidal disorders.* Amsterdam: Elsevier Science, 1986:167–173.
28. Gortvai P. Deformities of the hands and feet in parkinsonism and their reversibility by operation. *J Neurol Neurosurg Psychiatry* 1963;26:33–36.
29. Quinn NP, Ring H, Honavar M, et al. Contractures of

the extremities in parkinsonian subjects: a report of three cases with a possible association with bromocriptine treatment. *Clin Neuropharmacol* 1988;11:268–277.
30. Thomas A. Atrophie du cervelet et sclérose en plaques. *Rev Neurol Paris* 1903;3:121–131.
31. Trotter JL. Striatonigral degeneration: Alzheimer's disease and inflammatory changes. *Neurology* 1973;23: 1211–1216.
32. Kyriakides T, Hewer RL. Hand contractures in Parkinson's disease. *J Neurol Neurosurg Psychiatry* 1988;51: 1221–1223.
33. Marsden CD, Parkes JD, Quinn N. Fluctuations of disability in Parkinson's disease. Clinical aspects. In: Marsden CD, Fahn S, eds. *Movement disorders.* London: Butterworth, 1981:96–122.
34. O'Dwyer NJ, Ada L, Neilson PD. Spasticity and muscle contracture following stroke. *Brain* 1996;119: 1737–1749.
35. Melamed E. Early-morning dystonia: a late side effect of long term levodopa therapy in Parkinson's disease. *Arch Neurol* 1979;36:308–310.
36. Nausieda PA, Weiner WJ, Klawans HL. Dystonic foot response of parkinsonism. *Arch Neurol* 1980;37: 132–136.
37. Cubo E, Gracies JM, Benabou R, et al. Early morning "off" medication dyskinesias, dystonia, and choreic subtypes. *Arch Neurol* 2001;58:1379–1382.
38. Poewe W, Lees AJ, Stieger D, et al. Foot dystonia in Parkinson's disease: clinical phenomenology and neuropharmacology. *Adv Neurol* 1986;45:357–360.
39. McHale DM, Sage JI, Sonsalla PK, et al. Complex dystonia of Parkinson's disease: clinical features and relation to plasma levodopa profile. *Clin Neuropharmacol* 1990;13:164–170.
40. Zimmerman TR Jr, Sage JI, Lang AE, et al. Severe evening dyskinesias in advanced Parkinson's disease: clinical description, relation to plasma levodopa, and treatment. *Mov Disord* 1994;9:173–177.
41. Kidron D, Melamed E. Forms of dystonia in patients with Parkinson's disease. *Neurology* 1987;37: 1009–1011.
42. Lees AJ, Shaw KM, Stern GM. "Off period" dystonia and "on period" choreoathetosis in levodopa-treated patients with Parkinson's disease. *Lancet* 1977;2:1034.
43. Fahn S. The spectrum of levodopa-induced dyskinesias. *Ann Neurol* 2000;47[Suppl 1]:S2–S9.
44. LeWitt PA, Burns RS, Newman RP. Dystonia in untreated parkinsonism. *Clin Neuropharmacol* 1986;9: 293–297.
45. Poewe WH, Lees AJ, Stern GM. Dystonia in Parkinson's disease: clinical and pharmacological features. *Ann Neurol* 1988;23:73–78.
46. Quinn NP, Critchley P, Marsden CD. Young onset Parkinson's disease. *Mov Disord* 1987;2:73–91.
47. Souques MA. Rapport sur les syndromes parkinsoniens. *Rev Neurol (Paris)* 1921;37:534–573.
48. Katchen M, Duvoisin RC. Parkinsonism following dystonia in three patients. *Mov Disord* 1986;1:151–157.
49. Klawans HL, Paleologos N. Dystonia-Parkinson syndrome: differential effects of levodopa and dopamine agonists. *Clin Neuropharmacol* 1986;9:298–302.
50. Lucking CB, Durr A, Bonifati V, et al. Association between early-onset Parkinson's disease and mutations in the parkin gene. *N Engl J Med* 2000;342:1560–1567.
51. Tassin J, Durr A, Bonnet AM, et al. Levodopa-responsive dystonia. GTP cyclohydrolase I or parkin mutations? *Brain* 2000;123:1112–1121.
52. van Duijn CM, Dekker MC, Bonifati V, et al. Park7, a novel locus for autosomal recessive early-onset parkinsonism, on chromosome 1p36. *Am J Hum Genet* 2001; 69:629–634.
53. Valente EM, Bentivoglio AR, Dixon PH, et al. Localization of a novel locus for autosomal recessive early-onset parkinsonism, PARK6, on human chromosome 1p35-p36. *Am J Hum Genet* 2001;68:895–900.
54. Kimber TE, Thompson PD. Increased blink rate in advanced Parkinson's disease: a form of "off"-period dystonia? *Mov Disord* 2000;15:982–985.
55. Mathers SE, Kempster PA, Swash M, et al. Constipation and paradoxical puborectalis contraction in anismus and Parkinson's disease: a dystonic phenomenon? *J Neurol Neurosurg Psychiatry* 1988;51:1503–1507.
56. Merello M, Leiguarda R. Adynamic bowel syndrome in Parkinson's disease with dramatic response to apomorphine. *Clin Neuropharmacol* 1994;17:574–577.
57. Edwards LL, Quigley EM, Harned RK, et al. Defecatory function in Parkinson's disease: response to apomorphine. *Ann Neurol* 1993;33:490–493.
58. Bentivoglio AR, Maria G, Brisinda G, et al. Outlet type constipation in patients with Parkinson's disease treated with botulinum toxin. *Mov Disord* 2000;15[Suppl 3]: 124.
59. Barbeau A. L-Dopa therapy in Parkinson's disease: a critical review of nine years' experience. *Canad Med Assoc J* 1969;101:59–68.
60. Barbeau A. Long-term side-effects of levodopa. *Lancet* 1971;1:395.
61. Barbeau A. Diphasic dyskinesias during levodopa therapy. *Lancet* 1975;1:756.
62. Cotzias GC, Papavasiliou PS, Gellene R. Modification of parkinsonism. Chronic treatment with L-dopa. *N Engl J Med* 1969;280:337–345.
63. Cotzias GC, van Woert MH, Schiffer LM. Aromatic amino acids and modification of parkinsonism. *N Engl J Med* 1967; 276:374–379.
64. Yahr MD, Duvoisin RC, Shear MJ, et al. Treatment of parkinsonism with levodopa. *Arch Neurol* 1969;21: 343–354.
65. Fahn S. Fluctuations of disability in Parkinson's disease: pathophysiology. In: Marsden CD, Fahn S, eds. *Movement disorders.* London: Butterworth, 1982:123–145.
66. Duvoisin RC. Hyperkinetic reactions with L-dopa. *Current concepts in the treatment of parkinsonism.* New York: Raven Press, 1974:203–210.
67. Muenter MD, Sharpless NS, Tyce GM, et al. Patterns of dystonia ('I-D-I' and 'D-I-D') in response to L-dopa therapy for Parkinson's disease. *Mayo Clin Proc* 1977; 52:163–174.
68. Marconi R, Lefebvre-Caparros D, Bonnet AM, et al. Levodopa-induced dyskinesias in Parkinson's disease phenomenology and pathophysiology. *Mov Disord* 1994;9:2–12.
69. Krack P, Pollak P, Limousin P, et al. From off-period dystonia to peak-dose chorea. The clinical spectrum of varying subthalamic nucleus activity. *Brain* 1999;122: 1133–1146.
70. Moro E, Scerrati M, Romito LM, et al. Chronic subthalamic nucleus stimulation reduces medication requirements in Parkinson's disease. *Neurology* 1999;53: 85–90.

71. Luquin MR, Scipioni O, Vaamonde J, et al. Levodopa-induced dyskinesias in Parkinson's disease: clinical and pharmacological classification. *Mov Disord* 1992;7: 117–124.
72. Hashimoto T, Shindo M, Yanagisawa N. Enhanced associated movements in the contralateral limbs elicited by brisk voluntary contraction in choreic disorders. *Clin Neurophysiol* 2001;112:1612–1617.
73. Greene PE, Fahn S, Lang AE, et al. What is it? Case 1, 1990: progressive unilateral rigidity, bradykinesia, tremulousness, and apraxia, leading to fixed postural deformity of the involved limb. *Mov Disord* 1990;5: 341–351.
74. Vanek ZF, Jankovic J. Dystonia in corticobasal degeneration. *Adv Neurol* 2000;82:61–67.
75. Rinne JO, Lee MS, Thompson PD, et al. Corticobasal degeneration. A clinical study of 36 cases. *Brain* 1994; 117:1183–1196.
76. Wenning GK, Litvan I, Jankovic J, et al. Natural history and survival of 14 patients with corticobasal degeneration confirmed at postmortem examination. *J Neurol Neurosurg Psychiatry* 1998;64:184–189.
77. Barclay CL, Lang AE. Dystonia in progressive supranuclear palsy. *J Neurol Neurosurg Psychiatry* 1997;62: 352–356.
78. Rafal R, Friedman J. Limb dystonia in progressive supranuclear palsy. *Neurology* 1987;37:1546–1549.
79. Quinn N. Multiple system atrophy. In: Marsden CD, Fahn S, eds. *Movement disorders,* 3rd ed. London: Butterworth-Heinemann, 1994:262–281.
80. Quinn NJ. Disproportionate antecollis in multiple system atrophy. *Lancet* 1989;1:844.
81. Klein C, Brown R, Wenning G, et al. The "cold hands sign" in multiple system atrophy. *Mov Disord* 1997;12: 514–518.
82. Wilson SAK. Progressive lenticular degeneration: a familial nervous disease associated with cirrhosis of the liver. *Brain* 1912;34:295–309.
83. Starosta-Rubinstein S, Young AB, Kluin K, et al. Clinical assessment of 31 patients with Wilson's disease: correlations with structural changes on magnetic resonance imaging. *Arch Neurol* 1987;44:365–370.
84. Gulyas AE, Salazar-Grueso EF. Pharyngeal dysmotility in a patient with Wilson's disease. *Dysphagia* 1988;2: 230–234.
85. Liao KK, Wang SJ, Kwang SY, et al. Tongue dyskinesia as an early manifestation of Wilson's disease. *Brain Dev* 1995;13:451–453.
86. Parker N. Hereditary whispering dysphonia. *J Neurol Neurosurg Psychiatry* 1985;48:218–224.
87. Walshe JM, Yealland M. Wilson's disease: the problem of delayed diagnosis. *J Neurol Neurosurg Psychiatry* 1992;55:692–696.
88. Doyle JB. Clinical manifestations and treatment of epidemic encephalitis. *Calif West Med* 1924;28:1–13.
89. Economo C. Encephalitis lethargica. *Wien Klin Wochenschr* 1917;30:581–585.
90. Economo C. *Die encephalitis lethargica, ihre Nachkrankheiten und ihre Behandlung.* Berlin: Urban & Schwarzenberg, 1929.
91. Evidente BK, Gwinn KA, Ceviness JN, et al. Early cinematographic cases of post-encephalitic parkinsonism and other movement disorders. *Mov Disord* 1998;13: 167–169.
92. Kramer PL, Mineta M, Klein C, et al. Rapid-onset dystonia-parkinsonism: linkage to chromosome 19q13. *Ann Neurol* 1999;46:176–182.
93. Brashear A, Butler IJ, Ozelius LJ, et al. Rapid-onset dystonia-parkinsonism: a report of clinical, biochemical, and genetic studies in two families. *Adv Neurol* 1998;78:335–339.
94. Dooling EC, Schoene WC, Richardson EP. Hallervorden–Spatz syndrome. *Arch Neurol* 1974;30:70–83.
95. Zhou B, Westaway SK, Levinson B, et al. A novel pantothenate kinase gene (PANK2) is defective in Hallervorden–Spatz syndrome. *Nat Genet* 2001;28:345–349.
96. Ichinose H, Ohye T, Takahashi E, et al. Hereditary progressive dystonia with marked diurnal fluctuation caused by mutations in the GTP cyclohydrolase I gene. *Nat Genet* 1994;8:236–242.
97. Nygaard TG, Marsden CD, Fahn S. Dopa-responsive dystonia. Long-term treatment response and prognosis. *Neurology* 1991;41:174–181.
98. Bandmann O, Marsden CD, Wood NW. Atypical presentations of dopa-responsive dystonia. *Adv Neurol* 1998;78:283–290.
99. Nygaard TG, Marsden CD, Duvoisin RC. Dopa-responsive dystonia. In: Fahn S, Marsden CD, Calne DB, eds. *Dystonia,* 2nd ed. New York: Raven Press, 1988: 377–384.

Parkinson's Disease: Advances in Neurology, Vol. 91.
Edited by Ariel Gordin, Seppo Kaakkola, and Heikki Teräväinen
Lippincott Williams & Wilkins, Philadelphia © 2003

36

Treatment of Dystonia in Parkinson's Disease

Joseph King Ching Tsui

Neurodegenerative Disorders Centre, University of British Columbia, Vancouver, British Columbia, Canada

Dystonia is a well-described complication of Parkinson's disease (PD), either as a result of treatment with dopaminergic agents or as a part of the associated feature of the condition.

Dystonia may precede symptoms of idiopathic PD in some cases, and various regions of the body such as the neck, oromandibular region, upper limb, and foot may be affected (1,2). It is, however, a phenomenon more frequently observed in parkinsonian-plus syndromes. In a series of 66 patients, 59% had dystonia, most commonly presenting as asymmetrical dystonia of the arm or leg. More generalized dystonia occurred in 31% (3). Other focal dystonias, such as laryngeal dystonia, may be a feature of Shy–Drager syndrome or in Lubag X-linked dystonia-parkinsonism syndrome (4).

When associated with levodopa therapy, dystonia may occur in the early morning, end of dose, or peak dose. Early morning dystonia is present in 16% in a series of 383 patients. The common factors appeared to be longer disease duration and higher doses of levodopa. For those patients with dystonia before initiation of levodopa, there may be a higher chance of more peak-dose and diphasic dyskinesias (5). Foot dystonia may be extremely painful and difficult to manage (6). The mechanism of dystonia in PD remains debatable, but early morning dystonia may be dependent on the degree, rather than rate, of the decrease in levodopa (7).

Other unusual forms of dystonia include camptocormia (bent spine), which is typically worse during "off" periods and fatigue (8). Levodopa-associated hemifacial (9) and severe off-period facial dystonia in PD have been reported (10). Drug-induced dystonia and dysphonia (11) and belly dystonia in multiple systems (12) have been reported in isolated cases.

TREATMENT

Dystonia may be painful and disabling. It may occur by itself or as part of dyskinesia. Because in most instances, dystonia is a manifestation of long-term levodopa therapy, management consists mainly of manipulation of doses and frequency of dopaminergic drugs. Other medications may be added in an attempt to symptomatically improve the dystonia. Focal dystonias may be treated with botulinum toxin (BTX) injections. More recently, encouraging results have been published on the use of bilateral pallidal stimulation in generalized dystonia, which raises the possibility of its application in dystonia in PD.

Pharmacological Manipulation

Early morning dystonia is related to decreasing levels of levodopa and may be treated by adding a dose of a slow-release preparation of levodopa at bedtime. In the morning, a dose of standard preparation may help to boost drug levels. For other patterns of dystonia (e.g., end of dose and peak dose), the principle is to maintain a relatively stable drug level. This may be achieved by taking frequent small doses of levodopa, switching to controlled-release levodopa preparations, or adding a catechol-*O*-methyltransferase inhibitor. Use of liquid forms of levodopa and the reduction of protein intake in the daytime may also be considered in more resistant cases (13).

Addition of a dopamine (DA) agonists may reduce motor fluctuations including dystonia, but the efficacy is difficult to assess. In a recent review, eight double-blind clinical trials on the use of bromocriptine for reducing motor complications related to levodopa therapy were evaluated (14). Variations in duration of trials ranged from 4 to 40 weeks, and the inclusion criteria were not clearly defined. The threshold for using bromocriptine and titration schedules varied, and outcome measurements were not comparable among studies.

Other medications that have been used in the management of dystonia in PD include amantadine, anticholinergic drugs, Lioresal, clonazepam, lithium, and clozapine.

Botulinum Toxin Injections

BTX is useful in controlling focal dystonias in PD (15). Currently available preparations include type A toxins, Botox (Allergan) and Dysport (Speywood), and type B toxin, Myobloc (Elan). Most published reports were based on the use of Botox, and the suggested dosages in this chapter refer to this preparation.

Blepharospasm

Blepharospasm is more frequently associated with DA agonists but may occur with levodopa therapy or may be a part of the feature of the parkinsonian syndrome. In some cases, it may be difficult to differentiate blepharospasm from eyelid-opening apraxia. The latter is characterized by lack of spasms in the periorbital fibers of the orbicularis oculi and the association with hyperactive frontalis muscles. Injections of BTX into the orbicularis oculi bilaterally effectively control the symptoms of blepharospasm for 3 to 4 months. The total dosage per eye ranges from 25 to 50 mouse units (MU) (Botox), given in three to four divided doses, and sometimes, the pretarsal fibers would need to be injected as well.

Orofacial, Oromandibular, and Lingual Dystonia

Frequent facial grimacing and jaw opening or chewing movements, common in tardive dyskinesia, are also features of levodopa-induced dystonia. Lower facial muscles, such as the risorius, may be injected with 2.5 to 5 MU of Botox to alleviate the wide grinning that some patients might experience. Subcutaneous injections into the risorius are preferable to avoid inadvertent weakness induced in the buccinator, which would result in biting into the inside of the cheek.

For jaw-closing dystonia, injections of 50 to 75 MU of Botox into the masseters on each side are frequently effective without injecting the temporalis. Jaw-opening dystonia is more difficult to treat, although treating the lateral pterygoids (50 to 100 MU) may be useful in some cases. This may be performed transcutaneously over the mandibular notch, preferably with electromyographic guidance.

Lingual dystonia can be most distressing in some patients. Side-to-side movements or persistent tongue protrusion may affect patients' eating and talking. Delivery of 5 to 10 MU of Botox into the genioglossus on each side may be helpful. This may be performed percutaneously through the floor of the mouth, going through the mylohyoid muscle to reach the anterior part of the roof of the tongue, or it may be performed transorally. In any case, care must be taken to stay away from the posterior part of the root of the tongue to prevent it from falling back to obstruct the airway.

Cervical Dystonia

Levodopa-induced cervical dystonia frequently takes the form of retrocollis, although other patterns (laterocollis and anterocollis) may also be presenting. In progressive supranuclear palsy, retrocollis and severe neck rigidity may occur early in the course of illness. In many instances, walking is made more difficult because the patient is unable to look straight ahead. Eating may be affected with the neck hyperextended. Injections of 75 to 150 MU of Botox into the deep posterior neck muscle groups on each side may improve these symptoms significantly. When retrocollis is associated with tilting of the head to either side, unilateral injections into the splenius capitis may be necessary, in doses of 50 to 75 MU.

Laryngeal Dystonia

Laryngeal dystonia may be part of the presentation of parkinsonian-plus syndromes such as multiple system atrophy, Shy–Drager syndrome, and Lubag X-linked dystonia-parkinsonism syndrome (4,11). These patients have dysphonia, and occasionally, acute breathing laryngeal dystonia may cause distressing respiratory impairment. These symptoms do not respond to adjustment of oral medications, and injections of BTX into the cricoarytenoid muscles may be the only available treatment.

Limb Dystonia

Foot dystonia is more frequent than upper limb dystonia in PD. "Off" painful foot dystonia is one of the more common patterns found in PD. The foot is held in plantarflexion and inversion, frequently with toe curling and the great toe hyperextended. This causes the foot to drag when walking, and some patients may find it very uncomfortable to wear shoes. Pacchetti et al. (16) described treatment with BTX into the tibialis posterior, tibialis anterior, gastrocnemius, flexor digitorum longus, and extensor hallucis longus.

For a typical foot dystonia in PD, the tibialis posterior and the extensor hallucis longus are the most important muscles to treat. Doses of Botox range from 50 to 150 MU for the former and 20 to 50 for the latter.

Upper limb dystonia may be present in cases of PD-plus syndromes, particularly corticobasal ganglionic degeneration. Judicious use of BTX may improve hygienic care for a tightly clasped fist or improve the ease of dressing in upper limbs with tightly flexed wrists and elbows.

Truncal Dystonia

Truncal dystonia in PD commonly involves bending of the body forward. In most cases, truncal dystonia is resistant to all forms of treatment. Less common forms of extensor truncal dystonia in PD may be treated with injections of 300 to 400 MU of Botox into the paraspinal muscles at the back.

Stereotaxic Surgery

Pallidotomy, being effective in controlling dyskinesia contralateral to the side of operation, may also be helpful in reducing dystonic posturing (17). A more recent description of the improvement in three cases of generalized dystonia with bilateral pallidal stimulation (18) provides a basis for more exploration into its application in more generalized and resistant patterns of dystonia in PD and PD-plus syndromes.

CONCLUSIONS

Dystonia remains a therapeutic challenge and is one of the dose-limiting side effects in the treatment of PD. Most instances are related to dopaminergic therapy and may improve on manipulation of drug treatment. The use of BTX has been helpful in controlling focal dystonias and enables the inevitable increase in doses of dopaminergic drugs with increasing duration of disease. More studies on the use of deep brain stimulation should shed more light on the mechanism of dystonia in PD and may become another treatment option.

ACKNOWLEDGMENTS

The author wishes to acknowledge support from the Canadian Institute of Health Research and the Pacific Parkinson's Research Institute.

REFERENCES

1. Katchen M, Duvoisin RC. Parkinsonism following dystonia in three patients. *Mov Disord* 1986;1:151–157.
2. LeWitt PA, Burns RS, Newman RP. Dystonia in untreated parkinsonism. *Clin Neuropharmacol* 1986;9: 293–297.
3. Vanek Z, Jankovic J. Dystonia in corticobasal degeneration. *Mov Disord* 2001;16:252–257.
4. Lew MF, Shindo M, Moskowitz CB, et al. Adductor laryngeal breathing dystonia in a patient with Lubag (X-linked dystonia-parkinsonism syndrome). *Mov Disord* 1994;9:318–320.
5. Currie LJ, Harrison MB, Trugman JM, et al. Early morning dystonia in Parkinson's disease. *Neurology* 1998;51:283–295.
6. Kidron D, Melamed E. Forms of dystonia in patients with Parkinson's disease. *Neurology* 1987;37: 1009–1011.
7. McHale DM, Sage JI, Sonsalla PK, et al. Complex dystonia of Parkinson's disease: clinical features and relation to plasma levodopa profile. *Clin Neuropharmacol* 1990;13:164–170.
8. Djaldetti R, Mosberg-Galili R, Sroka H, et al. Camptocormia (bent spine) in patients with Parkinson's disease—characterization and possible pathogenesis of an unusual phenomenon. *Mov Disord* 1999;14:443–447.
9. Mark MH, Sage JI. Levodopa-associated hemifacial dystonia. *Mov Disord* 1991;6:383.
10. Miranda M, Chana P. Severe off-period facial dystonia in Parkinson's disease. *Mov Disord* 2000;15:163–164.
11. Negoro K, Morimatsu M, Nogaki H. Drug-induced dystonia and dysphonia in Parkinson's disease. *Mov Disord* 1998;13:978–979, and 1999;14:386.
12. Shan DE, Kwan SY, Ho HH, et al. Belly dystonia induced by levodopa and biperiden in a case of suspected multiple-system atrophy. *Mov Disord* 1996;11: 455–457.
13. Giron LT Jr, Koller WC. Methods of managing levodopa-induced dyskinesias. *Drug Safety* 1996;14: 365–374.
14. van Hilten JJ, Ramaker C, Van de Beek WJ, et al. Bromocriptine for levodopa-induced motor complications in Parkinson's disease. *Cochrane Database Syst Rev* 2000. CD001203.
15. Limousin P, Memin B, Pollak P. Treatment of dystonia occurring in parkinsonian syndromes by botulinum toxin. *Eur Neurol* 1997;37:66–67.
16. Pacchetti C, Albani G, Martignoni E, et al. "Off" painful dystonia in Parkinson's disease treated with botulinum toxin. *Mov Disord* 1995;10:333–336.
17. Vitek JL, Bakay RA. The role of pallidotomy in Parkinson's disease and dystonia. *Curr Opin Neurol* 1997;10: 332–339.
18. Tronnier VM, Fogel W. Pallidal stimulation for generalized dystonia. Report of three cases. *J Neurosurg* 2000; 92:453–456.

Parkinson's Disease: Advances in Neurology, Vol. 91.
Edited by Ariel Gordin, Seppo Kaakkola, and Heikki Teräväinen
Lippincott Williams & Wilkins, Philadelphia © 2003

37

Parkinson's Disease Is a Neuropsychiatric Disorder

*†‡Y. Agid, §I. Arnulf, **P. Bejjani, †F. Bloch, *†‡A. M. Bonnet, ¶P. Damier, ||B. Dubois, ‡C. François, *†‡J. L. Houeto, †D. Iacono, ‡C. Karachi, *†‡V. Mesnage, †O. Messouak, *‡M. Vidailhet, *†‡M. L. Welter, and ‡J. Yelnik

**Fédération de Neurologie; †Centre d'Investigation Clinique; ‡INSERM U289; §Service de Pneumologie; ||INSERM EPI 007, Hôpital de la Salpêtrière; ¶Service de Neurologie, CHU de Nantes, France; and **Parkinson & Movement Disorders Center, Hôpital Notre Dame des Secours, Beirut, Lebanon*

During the last century, Parkinson's disease (PD) was considered exclusively as a movement disorder. During the past 20 years, the complex characteristics of intellectual impairment of the disease were recognized. It is now time to accept that PD is also a psychiatric illness. Psychic disorders in patients with PD are well known to practitioners. Interestingly, they are not described in detail in textbooks of psychiatry, and they do not receive the attention they deserve in the training of movement disorder specialists.

At the onset of the disease, anxiety is a common symptom, and depression is found in at least 50% of patients, a figure that progressively increases during the course of the disease. Fluctuations in mood, emotional lability, lack of attention and motivation, bradyphrenia-related to frontal lobe–like symptomatology, and exaggeration of previous traits of personality are then observed in most patients (1). Psychic disturbances such as hypomania, hallucinations, and hypersexuality are observed in a few patients after several years of disease progression. Psychosis and delirium can be observed at the endstage of the disease, in particular in aged patients or when intellectual impairment is also associated. The respective roles of the antiparkinsonian treatment, including anticholinergics and dopamine (DA) receptor–stimulating agents, and the brain lesions characteristic of PD in the occurrence of psychic disturbances are difficult to evaluate because all the patients studied have undergone long-term treatment with levodopa and other antiparkinsonian adjuvants.

One way to approach the mechanisms of psychic disorders in PD is therefore to distinguish three interrelated components in patients: the premorbid personality, the mental disturbances associated with the natural history of the disease, and the adverse reactions to antiparkinsonian treatments. The premorbid personality includes psychological rigidity, adhesivity, obsessive behavior, and introversion (2). Whether these subtle personality traits are genetically associated with the propensity to develop PD or whether they correspond to the psychological consequences of an already present but incipient motor disability is still a matter of debate. Psychic disorders that are classically a part of the symptomatology of the disease are described in detail in Chapter 38. The most frequent are depression, anxiety, obsessive-compulsive behaviors, hallucinations and hallucinosis, and psychotic states (1). Fatigue and sleep disorders (insomnia, diurnal somnolence, and rapid eye movement sleep disorders) are often associated. The paradox is that the natural history of emotional and psychic disorders in PD is virtually unknown. In the past (i.e., before the era of levodopa), mental disturbances were very likely exaggerated (psychosis and hallucinations) because patients were overtreated with anticholinergic drugs. Nowadays, at least in industrialized countries, most if not all patients with PD are treated using substitutive therapy.

Psychic disorders such as those observed in PD are seen in patients with lesions affecting the limbic cortex. This area includes essentially the caudal orbitofrontal cortex, the amygdala and the retrosplenial cingulate complex, the hippocampal complex, the insula, and the septal area. These limbic regions are known to project toward subcortical areas within the brain, in particular the basal ganglia, and to project back to the cerebral cortex. These topographically organized segregated neuronal networks originating from limbic cortices and projecting back to them through the basal ganglia are scientifically well established (3). The precise routes used to transfer limbic information through the basal ganglia and the relationships between the limbic neuronal networks and the other parallel sensorimotor and associative cortical-subcortical-cortical loops are still a matter of debate, however. Within the basal ganglia, the main areas pertaining to the limbic system are the ventral striatum, the ventral part of the internal and external segments of the globus pallidus (GPi and GPe, respectively), the internal parts of the substantia nigra pars reticulata (SNpr), and of the subthalamic nucleus (STN), and the thalamus (including the centrum medianum and the parafascicular nucleus). It is highly probable that the dopaminergic neuronal systems originating in the ventral mesencephalon and projecting toward cortical structures (cerebral cortex, amygdala, septum) and the basal ganglia (principally, the striatum, but also the globus pallidus, STN, and thalamus) play an important role in controlling the functioning of cortical and subcortical limbic structures.

Assuming that the psychic symptoms are caused by a dysfunction of limbic neuronal networks, this chapter addresses two issues. Which psychiatric disorders are observed, in addition to motor symptomatology, in patients with lesions (including stroke, inflammation, tumors) of the basal ganglia? In PD, do psychic disorders result from the demodulation of limbic areas of the basal ganglia caused by the selective degeneration of dopaminergic neurons occurring in the ventral mesencephalon? In most sporadic forms of PD, the progressive accumulation of nondopaminergic brain lesions during the course of the disease leads to symptoms that are poorly responsive, or indeed unresponsive, to substitutive levodopa treatment. One may therefore ask whether these brain nondopaminergic lesions, which develop with time, contribute to the appearance of psychic disorders at the endstage of the disease.

BEHAVIORAL DISORDERS OBSERVED IN PATIENTS WITH LESIONS OF THE BASAL GANGLIA

The relationship between the psychiatric symptoms observed in patients with basal ganglia lesions and the localization and identity of the impaired neuronal networks implicated in these disorders are difficult to establish. In animals, experimental lesions can be restricted to confined areas of the basal ganglia, but the identification and description of psychic disorders remain necessarily limited. In contrast, in humans, mental disturbances can be exhaustively described, but in most cases, the localization and selectivity of the lesions cannot be ascertained. Either the limits of the damage are impossible to ascertain precisely (tumors), or the lesions are scattered in several brain areas (e.g., as in multiple sclerosis, stroke, and neurodegenerative disorders). Moreover, caution is needed in trying to interpret the data because most case reports are studied retrospectively, include few patients, and lack modern neuroimaging. Nevertheless, the accumulation of data related to behavioral disorders in basal ganglia diseases over the last few years has allowed several types of anatomic-clinical pictures to be identified (4). To illustrate this point, we will concentrate on three brain structures within the basal ganglia—the globus pallidus, the SNpr, and the STN—because a hyperactivity of these structures, resulting from the loss of dopaminergic neurons, is observed in patients with PD (3).

Psychic Disorders in Patients with Dysfunction of the Pallidum

When examining a patient with bilateral lesions of the globus pallidus, one is confronted with four possible situations: absence of symptoms, akinesia, frontal lobe–like symptomatology, and autoactivation deficit. Patients with autoactivation deficit (5) look inert, expressing nothing spontaneously. In severe cases, patients are unable to think spontaneously (e.g., when asked, "what are you thinking about," the patient responds, "nothing")—what Laplane et al. (5) called "consciousness without content." This odd clinical picture is characterized by three main features: It disappears when the subject is stimulated by the environment (loss of psychic autoactivation), which distinguishes this syndrome from schizophrenia; affectivity is usually flattened, but intellectual capacities are relatively preserved, unlike in the case of dementia; psychic disturbances, in particular stereotypies and obsessive-compulsive–like behaviors, are associated in several patients. Although the lesions responsible for psychic autoactivation deficit are confined to both pallidal regions, in particular the GPi, other lesions not necessarily detected on neuroimaging are very likely associated as the causes are of the general type (anoxia, carbon monoxide intoxication, encephalitis). Why pallidal lesions result in either parkinsonism, frontal lobe symptomatology, or autoactivation deficit is unknown. These clinical pictures could be caused by the selective dysfunction of the sensorimotor, associative, and limbic parts of the pallidal circuitry, but this remains to be demonstrated. It may be hypothesized that symptoms such as stereotypies, compulsions, and arithmomania, which are observed in patients with bilateral pallidal lesions, result at least partly from dysfunction of the limbic territories of the globus pallidus.

Psychic Disturbances and Dysfunction of the Substantia Nigra Pars Reticulata

In addition to the globus pallidus, the SNpr, located on the output pathways of the basal ganglia, is also metabolically hyperactive in patients with PD. No specific neurodegenerative disorder is known to affect selectively the SNpr, which is a small elongated structure located at the anterior and superior border of the substantia nigra pars compacta (SNpc), which gives rise to nigrostriatal dopaminergic neurons. We have, nevertheless, had the opportunity to observe a patient with a restrictive and selective dysfunction of the SNpr, resulting in a major reversible depression (6). This 65-year-old woman, with a 30-year history of PD and no previous history of psychiatric disorders, was severely disabled by levodopa-induced motor complications. She was therefore treated by bilateral continuous high-frequency stimulation of the STN. Neurosurgical treatment was so effective that drug therapy could be completely withdrawn. During the postoperative evaluation, the effects of stimulation through the different electrodes of the implanted leads were tested to identify the optimal therapeutic target. When stimulation was applied through one of the electrodes that was not located within the therapeutic target (i.e., the STN) but within the SNpc and the SNpr, the patient started to cry and express feelings of sadness, guilt, uselessness, and hopelessness. This transient acute depressive state disappeared about 1 minute after stimulation was stopped and was followed by a mildly hypomanic state. The patient gave her consent to participate in a positron emission tomography study using $H_2{}^{15}O$. A significant increase in blood flow was detected in the right parietal lobe, orbitofrontal cortex, globus pallidus, left amygdala, and anterior thalamus on the left side (ipsilateral to the nigral stimulation). This result was consistent with an activation of the nigrothalamic neuronal system, extending to limbic structures such as the amygdala and the orbitofrontal cortex. Two conclusions were drawn from this clinical observation: (a) The major depression observed in this patient very likely resulted from inactivation of the limbic territories within the nigral-thalamic-orbital-frontal neuronal network, thus confirming the important role of topographically organized limbic systems within the basal ganglia, the dysfunction of which can result in highly specific and well-identified psychiatric symptoms and (b) the fact that an acute depressive state can be triggered by a restricted manipulation of the upper brainstem suggests that psychic disturbances can be caused by the dysfunction not only of the cortical mesencephalic structures but also of the most inferior parts of the basal ganglia. This may explain why psychic symptoms such as depression can respond so dramatically to drugs known to interact with the metabolism of various neurotransmitters known to be abundant within the basal ganglia.

Behavioral Disorders and Dysfunction of the Subthalamic Nucleus

To our knowledge, the question of psychiatric disorders observed in patients with selective lesions of the STN has not yet been directly addressed, other than in a few isolated case reports (4). The STN has recently received much attention due to the major improvement in motor disability obtained in patients with PD treated by continuous bilateral high-frequency stimulation of the STN (see previous discussion). The method currently used improves motor disability by 50% to 90%, improves motor fluctuations and levodopa-induced dyskinesia by 60% to 90%, and permits a 50% to 80% reduction in doses of antiparkinsonian medication compared with the preoperative state. The neurosurgical intervention has little or no effect on cognitive functions (7). However, several investigators have been intrigued by the observation of unexpected psychic changes that counteract the advantages of neurosurgery-induced motor improvement. For instance, despite major postoperative clinical improvement, some patients remain unsatisfied or somewhat apathetic. Others exhibit social maladjustment, such as a deterioration in conjugal relationships and difficulty in integrating a new sociofamilial environment after many years of severe motor disability. Such psychological difficulties can reasonably be attributed to difficulty in social and familial adjustment as a consequence of the remarkable postoperative improvement in motor disability. In a retrospective examination of 24 parkinsonian patients successfully treated by bilateral STN stimulation, several other types of behavioral disorders were distinguished (8). (a) The amplification or decompensation of preexisting disorders that had passed unnoticed, such as depression, and severe behavioral disorders with drug dependence were observed in a few patients. We hypothesized that the psychiatric symptoms were no longer apparent in highly disabled patients during the course of PD before surgery but were fully expressed thereafter—that is, at a time when patients returned to an almost normal life. (b) Increased anxiety and emotional hyperreactivity was found in a large proportion of patients. The results indicate that STN stimulation–induced improvement in parkinsonian motor disability is not necessarily accompanied by a marked amelioration of psychic functions and quality of life. The appearance of personality disorders and decompensation of previous psychiatric disorders in a few patients after the operation suggest that a careful psychological and psychiatric interview must be performed before inclusion for surgery. The mechanism by which stimulation of the STN contributed to psychic disturbances in these patients has yet to be established. That a picture of thymoaffective disinhibition has been described after lesion of the STN (9) and that stimulation-induced laughing was reported in patients treated by bilateral STN stimulation (10) suggests that stimulation-induced STN dysfunction may play a role of its own in the observed emotional processes. It may reasonably be assumed that these psychiatric disturbances were triggered, at least partly, by the selective dysfunction of the limbic nigral output toward the corticolimbic cortex, although this still remains to be demonstrated.

ANATOMIC-FUNCTIONAL BASES OF PSYCHIC DISORDERS IN PARKINSON'S DISEASE

Dopaminergic Neuronal Dysfunction and Psychic Disorders

As previously stated, we have concentrated on the psychiatric clinical picture associated with lesions of each of these three structures (globus pallidus, SNpr, and STN) because dysfunction of these territories is known to occur in PD. Hyperactivity of these nuclei has been observed in monkeys rendered parkinsonian with methylphenyltetrahydropyridine and in postmortem material from patients with PD (3), resulting from the decreased dopaminergic transmission caused by the degeneration of the nigrostriatal dopaminergic system. We therefore assume that the observed hyperactivity of limbic territories within the overactive globus pallidus, SNpr, and STN can result in emotional disorders, in much the same way as akinesia, rigidity, and tremor result from a hyperactivity of the sensorimotor part of these nuclei. In other words, the deafferentation of the striatum provoked by the selective degeneration of the nigrostriatal dopaminergic system is assumed to contribute to psychic disorders as a result of the demodulation of the limbic part of the cortical-subcortical-cortical loop.

Dopaminergic neurons originating in the ventral mesencephalon also project to regions of the basal ganglia other than the striatum (e.g., the globus pallidus and the STN), including their limbic territories. The partial degeneration of these extrastriatal dopaminergic pathways very likely also contributes to the emotional disorders characteristic of patients with PD via the partial demodulation of the limbic neuronal circuitry of the basal ganglia. Finally, dopaminergic neurons originating in the internal part of the mesencephalon (i.e., the ventral tegmental area) are known to project directly toward limbic and cortical regions of the brain. It has been claimed that the partial degeneration of the dopaminergic subcortical-cortical neuronal systems described in patients with PD plays a role in depression (11). It is easily understandable that when patients with PD undergo long-term treatment or overtreatment with levodopa and related compounds, the reestablishment of normal or increased DA transmission can lead to the appearance of hypomanic states and delirium, due the hypersensitivity of postsynaptic DA receptors resulting at the presynaptic level from the loss of dopaminergic innervation in limbic territories. This can be expressed by the adage, "Levodopa-induced psychic disorders are to the dysfunction of the mesial-cortical-limbic dopaminergic system what levodopa-induced abnormal involuntary movements are to the dysfunction of the nigrostriatal dopaminergic system."

In brief, in patients with PD, the characteristic degeneration of dopaminergic neurons projecting toward the various limbic territories of the basal ganglia and cerebral cortex very likely play a role in the occurrence of behavioral disorders, through the demodulation of limbic cortical-subcortical-cortical circuits.

Nondopaminergic Neuronal Dysfunction and Psychic Disorders

In addition to this "DA-dependent" mental clinical picture, the psychic functions of patients with PD can be affected by lesions involving both specific (which are part of the pathological picture of PD) and nonspecific (additional nonparkinsonian lesions) neuronal losses.

Nondopaminergic lesions in PD can be schematically separated into subcortical-cortical and subcortical lesions. The partial degeneration of subcortical-cortical neuronal systems, such as the noradrenergic, serotonergic, and cholinergic neurons originating in the locus ceruleus, raphe nuclei, and substantia innominata and projecting toward the amygdala, cingular area, and orbitofrontal cortex, very likely also contribute to the emotional disorders observed in patients with PD. The role of the dysfunction of these aminergic and cholinergic neurons in cognitive defects (decreased attention, vigilance, motivation, and memory; frontal lobe–like symptomatology) is widely accepted. Because these neuronal pathways also project to limbic areas within the cerebral cortex, it can reasonably be concluded that the demodulation of the cerebral cortex by these aminergic and cholinergic neurons can also result in symptoms such as depression, anxiety, and emotional hyperactivity, which are commonly seen in patients with PD.

Several other nondopaminergic lesions are also observed in patients with PD, depending on the form of the disease, its duration, and the age of the patient. These lesions are found in subcortical brain regions, but few of them have been described (nucleus vagus, pedunculopontine nucleus, hypothalamus). Lewy bodies and Alzheimer's disease histopathological changes indicative of neuronal loss are found in the cerebral cortex of patients with mental disorders, in particular during old age and after a long duration of the disease. These widely distributed lesions within the cerebral cortex are known to contribute to intellectual impairment and dementia in patients with PD. They also very likely play a major role in the appearance of psychiatric symptoms such as hallucinations, delirium, and psychosis. When these neurodegenerative lesions characteristic of PD occur in patients, they are often associated with vascular lesions (infarcts, lacunae, microvasculopathy). Depending on the localization of these additional nonspecific lesions, they logically also contribute to the intellectual and behavioral impairment seen in elderly patients with PD.

CONCLUSIONS

It is now time to recognize that in addition to motor and intellectual symptoms, PD is also characterized by a large constellation of psychic disorders, the severity of which is variable depending on the category of PD (the term *Parkinson's diseases* should be used instead of Parkinson's disease), the age of patients, and the duration of the disease. These psychiatric symptoms are known to play a major role in the problems that patients experience in reintegrating their sociofamilial environment. Whatever their semiologic pattern, these behavioral disorders result from the reversible (dopaminergic demodulation of neuronal pathways) or irreversible (loss of neurons) dysfunction of limbic territories within subcortical and cortical areas of the brain of patients with PD. PD is, thus, a neuropsychiatric disorder.

REFERENCES

1. de Ajuriaguerra J. Etude psychopathologique des parkinsoniens. In: de Ajuriaguerra J, ed. *Monoamine noyaux gris centraux et syndrome de Parkinson.* Paris: Masson, 1970:327–351.
2. Menza MA, Golbe LI, Cody RA, et al. Dopamine-related personality traits in Parkinson's disease. *Neurology* 1993;43:505–508.
3. Obeso JA, Rodriguez-Oroz MC, Rodriguez M, et al. Pathophysiology of the basal ganglia in Parkinson's disease. *Trends Neurosci* 2000;23[Suppl 10]:S8–S19.
4. Ghika J. Mood and behavior in disorders of the basal ganglia. In: Bogousslavsky J, Cummings JL, eds. *Behavior and mood disorders in focal brain lesions.* Cambridge: Cambridge University Press, 2000:122–201.
5. Laplane D, Baulac M, Widlocher D, et al. Pure psychic akinesia with bilateral lesions of basal ganglia. *J Neurol Neurosurg Psychiatry* 1984;47:377–385.
6. Bejjani BP, Damier P, Arnulf I, et al. Transient acute depression induced by high-frequency deep-brain stimulation. *N Engl J Med* 1999;340:1476–1480.
7. Ardouin C, Pillon B, Peiffer E, et al. Bilateral subthalamic or pallidal stimulation for Parkinson's disease affects neither memory nor executive functions: a consecutive series of 62 patients. *Ann Neurol* 1999;46: 217–223.
8. Houeto JL, Mesnage V, Mallet L, et al. Behavioural disorders, Parkinson's disease and subthalamic stimulation. *J Neurol Neurosurg Psychiatry* 2002;72:701–707.
9. Trillet M, Vighetto A, Croisile B, et al. Hemiballismus with logorrhea and thymo-affective disinhibition caused by hematoma of the left subthalamic nucleus. *Rev Neurol (Paris)* 1995;151:416–419.
10. Krack P, Kumar R, Ardouin C, et al. Mirthful laughter induced by subthalamic nucleus stimulation. *Mov Disord* 2001;16:867–875.
11. Agid Y, Ruberg M, Dubois B, et al. Biochemical substrates of mental disturbances in Parkinson's disease. In: Hassler RG, Christ JF, eds. *Advances in Neurology: Parkinson-specific motor and mental disorders. Role of the pallidum: pathophysiological, biochemical, and therapeutic,* vol 40. New York: Raven Press, 1983: 211–218.

Parkinson's Disease: Advances in Neurology, Vol. 91.
Edited by Ariel Gordin, Seppo Kaakkola, and Heikki Teräväinen
Lippincott Williams & Wilkins, Philadelphia © 2003

38

Depression in Parkinson's Disease

D. Brandstädter and W. H. Oertel

Department of Neurology, Philipps-University of Marburg, Marburg, Germany

This chapter is an update of an earlier manuscript presented in *Advances of Neurology* series (1); we particularly focus on recent studies published between 1998 and 2001 and review treatment options of depression in Parkinson's disease (PD) according to the evidence-based medicine criteria shown in Table 38.1.

CHARACTERISTICS

Depression represents the most important nonmotor feature of idiopathic PD and appears to have a greater impact on quality of life in idiopathic PD than central motor symptoms (2,3). The main symptoms of depression in PD are loss of self-esteem, hopelessness, worthlessness, pessimism about the future, and sadness (without guilt or self-approach) (4,5). Depressed parkinsonian patients often have suicidal ideation; however, the suicide rate is low in these patients. Stenager et al. (6) investigated the cause of death in 458 patients with idiopathic PD compared with that in the general population and found no increased risk for suicide in these patients.

Anxiety symptoms and panic attacks are frequently seen in patients with idiopathic PD with depression and can often precede motor symptoms (7,8), indicating a special relationship between anxiety and depression in PD. The types of anxiety found in idiopathic PD are generalized anxiety disorders, panic disorders, social phobias, phobic disorders, agoraphobias, obsessive-compulsive disorders, and anxiety disorders not otherwise specified (9). Menza et al. (10) showed that 92% of patients with idiopathic PD who had a diagnosis of having an anxiety disorder also had depressive disorders or symptoms and that 67% of patients with a depressive disorder had a diagnosis of having an anxiety disorder. Walsh and Bennett (9) proposed that anxiety in idiopathic PD, in combination with depression, may represent a specific depressive subtype.

An important problem is the differential diagnosis between depression and dementia in PD (11). Depression and dementia have complex relations, and depression may clinically present as dementia ("pseudodementia"). Furthermore, depression may possibly precede dementia in PD (12), although according to a recently published community-based prospective study of Aarsland et al. (13), depression appears to be no independent risk factor for dementia. Other population-based investigations proposed a frequent coexistence of depression and dementia in idiopathic PD (14,15), suggesting a common underlying mechanism.

In a population-based study, Schrag et al. (16) assessed factors contributing to depression according to the World Health Organization model of impairment, disability, and handicap (17). They found that the patients' perception of handicap seemed to be more important than the severity of symptomatic impairment. This observation shows the im-

TABLE 38.1. *Definitions for the classification of evidence and levels of recommendations*

Class I: Evidence provided by one or more well-designed randomized, controlled clinical trials, including overviews (metaanalysis) of such trials.
Standard: Principle for patient management that reflects a high degree of clinical certainty (usually this requires class I evidence that directly addresses the clinical question or overwhelming class II evidence when circumstances preclude randomized clinical trials).
Class II: Evidence provided by well-designed observational studies with concurrent controls (e.g., case–control or cohort studies).
Guideline: Recommendation for patient management that reflects moderate clinical certainty (usually this requires class II evidence or a strong consenus of class III evidence).
Class III: Evidence provided by expert opinion, case series, and case reports, as well as studies with historical controls.
Practice option: Strategy for patient management for which the clinical utility is uncertain (inconclusive or conflicting evidence or opinion).

portance of addressing social and personal circumstances of depressed patients with idiopathic PD and underlines the strategy to treat depression in PD independently of management of motor symptoms.

PREVALENCE AND RISK FACTORS

In a "MEDLINE" search, Slaughter et al. (18) analyzed all English-language articles published between 1922 and 1998 for prevalence of depression in PD. The reported occurrence of depression in these studies ranged from 7% to 70%, due to different definitions of depression and assessment techniques. In a further step, the authors focused on articles that specifically used *Diagnostic and Statistical Manual of Mental Disorders,* Third Edition, and *Diagnostic and Statistical Manual of Mental Disorders,* Third Edition-Revised, criteria. Dysthymia was present in 22.5% of the patients, minor depression was diagnosed in 36.6% of the evaluated patients, and major depression was found in 24.8% of the patients. Depression as a combination of these different categories—minor depression, major depression, and dysthymic disorder—was reported in 42.4% of the patients.

Celesia and Wanamaker (19) found in a longitudinal study of parkinsonian patients evidence of depression in 37% of the patients. However, the prevalence of depression was not related to the stage of the illness. Depression was most common in stages I (38%), III (42%), and IV (50%), but less frequent in stages II (18%) and V (22%). A nearly similar pattern of results was published by Starkstein et al. (20). The data from these two studies failed to show a linear increase of depression with the severity of PD. Santamaria et al. (21) found a significant association between depression and duration of illness in patients with early onset PD, but not in those with late-onset PD. However, the number of depressed parkinsonian patients in this study was limited (n = 11). A study of Starkstein et al. (22) supported this observation and there appears to be growing evidence that different subgroups of parkinsonian patients may be more vulnerable to depression than others.

A relationship between the kind of motor deficits and the depressive syndromes has been frequently discussed (20,23–26). Bradykinesia, rigidity, and postural changes are suggested to be more prominent in depressed patients with idiopathic PD than in nondepressed patients (27,28).

The studies assessing the influence of family history in idiopathic PD (29,30) found no higher rate for psychiatric illness in depressed patients with idiopathic PD. However, a past history of depression has been proposed to be a risk factor for developing depression in PD (29,30).

Furthermore, female gender has been suggested to be a risk factor for depression in idiopathic PD (19,26,31); however, because others (32–35) have failed to identify this association, further studies are necessary for consensus.

ETIOLOGY OF DEPRESSION

Genetic factors are known to play an important role in predisposition to depression in the elderly population. Recently, Menza et al. (36) investigated a polymorphism in the regulatory region of the serotonin transporter, which has been previously linked to anxiety, in 32 patients with idiopathic PD. The short allele of this polymorphism leads to less efficient transcription, resulting in less serotonin uptake. The authors found that the patients with the short allele of this polymorphism had significant higher scores on the Hamilton Depression Scale (HAMD) and the Hamilton Anxiety Scale (HAMA). The authors proposed that the short allele of the serotonin transporter appears to be a risk factor for anxiety and depression in idiopathic PD.

Several authors (25,26,37,38) proposed that patients with idiopathic PD probably suffer from a greater degree of depression than patients with other diseases, indicating a relation to the neuropathology of PD. Depression in idiopathic PD has been linked to degeneration of dopaminergic, noradrenergic, serotonergic, and cholinergic nuclei. Particularly, changes in serotonergic transmitter pathways have been proposed to be associated with depression in PD. Several studies found decreased levels of the serotonin metabolite 5-hydroxyindoleacetic acid (5-HIAA) in the cerebrospinal fluid (CSF) of depressed parkinsonian patients compared with parkinsonian patients without depression and normal controls (39,40). In a study of Mayeux et al. (40) including patients with PD with depression and dementia, a significant reduction in CSF 5-HIAA concentration was found in patients with dementia and/or depression compared with those without dementia or depression. Patients with PD with depression and dementia had the lowest levels of 5-HIAA in the CSF, suggesting that dementia and depression not only may coexist but also may share a common biological mechanism. Paulus and Jellinger (41) found a more severe reduction of serotonergic neurons in the dorsal raphe nucleus in depressed patients with PD than in nondepressed patients with PD. Chan-Palay and Asan (42) noted a correlation of cell loss in locus coeruleus with "atypical" depression, suggesting a possible role of norepinephrine in the etiology of depression in idiopathic PD. Torrack and Morris (43) found severe degeneration of ventral tegmental dopaminergic neurons and proposed that a selective disruption of ventral tegmental afferents of the cortex may be responsible for the behavioral symptoms in PD.

Data from functional imaging studies, using fluorodeoxyglucose positron emission tomography (PET) showed relative hypometabolism involving the caudate and orbital inferior area of the frontal lobe in patients with idiopathic PD with depression compared with nondepressed patients and normal controls (44,45). In addition, the magnitude of hypometabolism correlated with the severity of depression. Because dopaminergic projections from the ventral tegmental area show regional specificity for the orbitofrontal cortex, Mayberg et al. (46) proposed that a degeneration of the mesial-cortical-limbic dopaminergic system in parkinsonian patients may secondarily cause a metabolic dysfunction in the orbitofrontal region of the cortex. Recently, Kennedy et al. (47) assessed the effect of treatment with paroxetine on regional glucose metabolism measured with PET in patients with major depression. After treatment with paroxetine, elevated levels of glucose metabolism in several frontal regions, including the dorsolateral prefrontal cortex, medial and ventral areas, and anterior cingulate and inferior parietal cortices, could be measured, whereas in some untreated patients, a hypometabolism in these regions could be observed. After 8 weeks of treatment with fluoxetine (20 to 40 mg per day) in depressed patients with idiopathic PD, an increased glucose metabolism, mainly in the left prefrontal regions and the orbitofrontal and the anterior and posterior cingulate cortices, could be measured in treatment responders compared with baseline (48). Further data in depressed patients with idiopathic PD are necessary to confirm these results.

In summary, the etiology of depression in PD still remains unknown; however endogenous, reactive, or both mechanisms are discussed (1).

PHARMACOLOGICAL TREATMENT

Levodopa and Dopamine Agonists

Many studies showed an improvement of depressive syndromes in idiopathic PD after controlling motor symptoms with antiparkinsonian drugs. Improvement of depression and anxiety with levodopa and dopamine (DA) agonists has been described (49–52). In an open-label trial, Jouvent et al. (49) investigated the effect of high-dose bromocriptine treatment (range, 85 to 220 mg per day) on depressive and motor symptoms in ten patients with idiopathic PD, showing significant improvement of both symptoms after treatment. In a randomized double-blind study of eight patients with idiopathic PD and motor fluctuations, Maricle et al. (51) found a significant mood elevation and anxiety reduction after levodopa infusion (0 to 1 mg/kg per hour). However, these studies have often been criticized, because of the possibility that improvement may be secondary to optimization of motor symptoms and the lack of class I evidence trials.

Recently, preliminary data of a randomized uncontrolled 8-month open-label study regarding the efficacy of the DA agonists pramipexole and pergolide for the treatment of mild and moderate depression in PD have been published (53). Depression was quantified using the Zung Self Rating Depression Scale and the Montgomery–Asberg Depression Rating Scale (MADRS), motor impairment was assessed with the Unified Parkinson's Disease Rating Scale Part III (UPDRS-III) and Part IV. The authors observed a statistically significant decrease in the total Zung Self Rating Depression Scale score in both treatment groups compared with baseline, whereas the decrease of the total MADRS score reached only statistical significance in the pramipexole group. However, in the pergolide group, the MADRS scores at baseline appeared to be very low, suggesting very mild depression. This fact could be a probable reason for insufficient statistical significance in the MADRS scores of the pergolide group after treatment compared with baseline. However, the authors emphasized that the preliminary data need further statistical analysis.

We conclude that class II and class III studies show that DA-replenishing strategies are useful and seem to be efficacious for the treatment of depression probably secondary to optimization of antimotor-antiparkinsonian treatment.

Monoamine Oxidase Inhibitors

Monoamine oxidase (MAO) inhibitors have been proposed to improve depressive symptoms in PD. DA is a substrate for both isoforms of MAO. The subtype MAO-A primarily deaminates serotonin and noradrenaline, the MAO-B subtype is relatively selective for DA metabolism. Moclobemide (a reversible competitive inhibitor of MAO-A) and selegiline (an irreversible noncompetitive inhibitor of MAO-B; in high doses also with MAO-A inhibitory activity) have been investigated for antidepressant efficacy in PD.

In a randomized study, Jansen Steur and Ballering (54) assessed the effect of moclobemide alone (600 mg per day) and moclobemide in combination with selegiline (10 mg per day) in ten patients with idiopathic PD and major depression for 6 weeks. The HAMD was used for quantification of depression 1 week before and 6 weeks after treatment. The authors reported improvement in both groups after treatment. The authors did not mention whether the improvement in the moclobemide group after treatment was statistically significant. However, the improvement in the group receiving moclobemide alone was significantly less ($p < .0029$) than that seen in the combined moclobemide and selegiline group.

In a double-blind placebo-controlled study, Lees et al. (55) investigated the effect of selegiline (10 mg per day) in 41 patients with fluctuating and nonfluctuating PD for 1 month. Depression was quantified with the Zung Self Rating Depression Scale and 15 of the patients were found to be depressed. After treatment with selegiline, the authors did not find a statistically significant improvement of depression compared with placebo.

Our conclusion is that current available evidence of class II and class III studies supports the efficacy of moclobemide in combination with selegiline in the treatment of depression in patients with idiopathic PD; however, selegiline or moclobemide monotherapy appears to be unlikely to ameliorate depression in patients with PD.

Tricyclic Antidepressants

Tricyclic antidepressants (TCAs) represent a traditionally available group of medication for the treatment of depression in PD. However, in the elderly, TCAs must be used with caution. The anticholinergic side effects of TCAs can cause urinary retention, paralytic ileus, acute glaucoma, decrease of cognitive function, and severe postural hypotension (4). Furthermore, in cognitively impaired patients, delusion can be induced (56).

Several clinical studies with TCAs indicate an improvement of depression in PD. In 1969, Laitinen (57) showed in a randomized placebo-controlled trial the efficacy of 100 mg of desipramine per day for the treatment of 39 depressed parkinsonian patients. One patient had hereditary parkinsonism, six had had encephalitis, and 32 patients had PD of unknown etiology. Interestingly, 16 patients had been operated, 4 of them in both thalami. After increasing desipramine over approximately 6 days, a daily dose of 100 mg of desipramine was maintained for 3 weeks. The listed side effects in the desipramine group were mental confusion, nausea, and giddiness. In the desipramine group, 16 patients of 20 completed the trial, 10 of them (63%) with a " good improvement." Despite the double-blind randomized design, this study is of limited value, because no criteria for the quantification of depression and motor symptoms were given and not all included patients suffered from idiopathic PD. In another, double-blind placebo-controlled study (58), imipramine was proposed to be efficacious for the treatment of depression in PD; however, because of methodologic limits, this study is not mentioned in detail.

In a randomized, double-blind crossover study, Anderson et al. (59) assessed the effect of nortriptyline (25 to 150 mg per day) on 22 parkinsonian patients. The patients were randomly allocated to group I, receiving first placebo for 4 weeks and then nortriptyline for 4 weeks, or group II, receiving first nortriptyline and then placebo. Unfortunately, the etiology of parkinsonism or primary objectives of this study were not given. Depression was quantified using a depression rating scale designed by Anderson himself (59), which was not validated or generally accepted. Motor signs were measured with a rating scale for posture (0 to 4 points). Akinesia, rigidity, and tremor were rated by a 0- to 3-point scale, with a possible maximum of 21 points for each symptom. Furthermore, the gait was analyzed with a rating of 0 for complete normality and 20 for maximal disability, and time tests for general movement and finer movements were practiced. The median depression score was statistically significantly reduced ($p < .001$) in the nortriptyline group compared with baseline and the placebo group. There was no worsening of motor signs according to the given rating scales. Three patients dropped out of the study, two because of severe orthostatic hypotension and one patient wished to stop the study after crossover to the placebo period.

We conclude that currently available evidence suggests TCAs to be efficacious for the treatment of depression in PD; however, the study designs of the published placebo-controlled trials with TCAs are insufficient. Furthermore, during treatment with TCAs the anticholinergic side effects, particularly in parkinsonian patients with dementia, should be considered.

Selective Serotonin Reuptake Inhibitors

The more recently introduced selective serotonin reuptake inhibitors (SSRIs) have equal antidepressant efficacy to TCAs; however, they appear to have a favorable side-effect profile, particularly in the elderly (5,18). One side effect that may be of concern is that SSRIs are metabolized in the liver by the cytochrome P450 enzyme system and can increase the risk of toxicity of other drugs that are metabolized by this system (60). Furthermore, SSRIs either alone or in combination with selegiline can cause the "serotonin syndrome" (61). The criteria for this diagnosis include the presence of at least three of the following symptoms: tremor, diarrhea, myoclonus, hyperreflexia, fever, shivering, incoordination, and mental status changes (4,5). A study of published cases suggested that 0.24% of the patients taking both an SSRI or a TCA and selegiline reported symptoms that are possibly consistent with the "serotonin syndrome" (66). Only 0.04% of these cases were estimated as serious. However, it is generally recommended that a combination of an SSRI or a TCA with selegiline should be avoided.

So far, there have been no randomized controlled trials of any SSRIs for the treatment of depression in PD.

Ceravolo et al. (63) assessed the effect of paroxetine on motor and depressive symptoms in 33 patients with PD in a 6-month open-label trial. Depression was diagnosed according to *DSM-IV* criteria (dysthymia in 19, major depression in 14). Motor function was assessed by the UPDRS-III. Depression was quantified before and after 1, 3, and 6 months using the Beck Depression Inventory (BDI) and the HAMD. Paroxetine was gradually increased up to 20 mg per day. During the trial, no change of levodopa or DA agonists doses was allowed. The measured scores on BDI and HAMD improved after treatment of depression but were not highly significant ($p < .05$). Paroxetine did not aggravate parkinsonian symptoms, although increased tremor in one patient was observed.

In a larger open-label study with paroxetine, Tesei et al. (64) measured the effect of 20 mg of paroxetine in 65 patients with idiopathic PD and depression according to *DSM-IV* criteria and a HAMD score of more than 16. There was no change in antiparkinsonian medication during the study. In the 52 patients who completed the study, a significant improvement in the HAMD score, mainly in anxiety- and sleep-related symptoms, could be observed. However, 13 patients stopped paroxetine in the first month of treatment, two of them because of increased "off" time and tremor, the others because of anxiety (n = 4), nausea (n = 4), agitation (n = 1), confusion (n = 1), and headache (n = 1).

In an 7-week open-label trial, Hauser and Zesiewicz (65) investigated the effect of sertraline in 15 patients with PD and depression. Sertraline was titrated from 25 mg to a predetermined maximum of 50 mg per day. Depression was assessed with the BDI, motor symptoms were measured with the UPDRS, and a 1- to 10-point scale for "energy levels." BDI scores significantly improved in ten patients, whereas scores worsened in four and remained unchanged in one. Worsening of UPDRS scores or of individual energy levels could not be observed.

Recently, Dell' Agnello et al. (66) assessed the effect of different SSRIs in depressed patients with idiopathic PD in a 6-month open-label study. In this study, 62 nondemented patients were included in four treatment groups (15 patients received citalopram, 16 fluoxetine, 16 fluvoxamine, and 15 sertraline). Depression was quantified using the BDI and HAMD at baseline and after 1, 3, and 6 months. The results indicated high improvement in depression scores ($p < .05$) compared with baseline with all SSRIs. There was no significant decline in motor scores measured with the UPDRS during treatment.

In agreement with these studies, others also reported the efficacy of SSRIs in the treatment of depression in patients with idiopathic PD (67,68), and in addition to the few mentioned patients with worsening of extrapyramidal symptoms during treatment with SSRIs, several case reports described increased motor disability after the use of fluoxetine (69); fluvoxamine (70); and paroxetine (71,72).

Because of the absence of class I studies, we conclude that a benefit of SSRIs for the treatment of depression in patients with idiopathic PD has not definitively been established. However, the available evidence supports a level of "guideline" recommendation. Thus, we conclude that SSRIs are safe and seem to be effective in improving depression in patients with idiopathic PD.

Other Drugs

Goetz et al. (73) proposed bupropion to alleviate depression in patients with idiopathic PD. The authors investigated the effect of bupropion in 11 men and nine women with idiopathic PD and depression. Fourteen patients were enrolled according to a double-blind parallel protocol, 12 patients received bupropion in an open-label fashion (six patients as crossover from the double-blind placebo group). After 9-week of treatment with bupropion (450 mg per day), significant improvement of extrapyramidal symptoms quantified with the New York University Parkinson's Disease Scale (NYUPDS) and the Northwestern University Disability Scale (NUDS) could be measured. Depression was estimated using a global impression scale. Improvement of depression could be observed in five of the 12 depressed patients. In summary, the study is limited because of a small sample of patients and invalid depression rating. Furthermore, bupropion should be used with caution regarding its dopaminergic effects and the potential to cause seizures (74,75). Recently, the effect of *S*-adenosyl-L-methionine (SAM) has been investigated in 13 depressed patients with PD, showing at least a 50% improvement in 10 patients measured with the HAMD (76). The mean HAMD score before treatment was 27.09 (±6.04) and 9.55 (±7.29) after SAM treatment.

We conclude that current class III studies on bupropion and SAM are insufficient to recommend these drugs for therapy for depression in PD.

In clinical studies for the treatment of major depression, novel antidepressant drugs like reboxetine, nefazodone, venlafaxine, and mirtazapine were considered to be as effective as TCAs and SSRIs (77–81). As yet, only case reports (82–84), but no sufficient trials, have been published describing the use of these drugs in PD. Further studies are needed to investigate the effect of these novel drugs on depressive symptoms in PD.

NONPHARMACOLOGICAL TREATMENT

Psychotherapy

In our experience, psychotherapy, particularly at the time of diagnosis, and psychoeducational support of the patient's family and other caregivers (85) can be very helpful; however, the usefulness remains uncertain because controlled trial applications in idiopathic PD are missing.

Electroconvulsive Therapy

Electroconvulsive therapy (ECT) has been used as treatment of depression in PD, particularly in patients without a treatment response to antidepressants. The mechanisms of ECT remain unclear. Various neurotransmitter changes have been found in animal studies after electroconvulsive shock including increased DA concentrations (86,87).

Interestingly, a marked improvement on parkinsonian symptoms could be temporarily observed in some studies after ECT treatment including parkinsonian patients with psychiatric comorbidity (88). Anderson et al. (89) showed in a double-blind controlled study in parkinsonian patients without psychiatric comorbidity an increased "on" time after ECT treatment from 32% to 71%, whereas the percentage of "on" time in the sham group remained unchanged. Several authors observed a high incidence of ECT-induced delirium in patients with PD. Figiel (90) compared the incidence of delirium in 20 depressed patients with a history of cerebrovascular accident with 20 age-matched depressed patients with PD. An interictal ECT-induced delirium occurred in 25% of the patients with cerebrovascular accidents compared with 85% of patients with PD. The period of delirium was reversible but varied between 7 days and 3 months after completion of ECT. In another study (91), delirium after ECT treatment in 11 depressed patients with PD was so severe that ECT had to be discontinued in 6 patients.

Despite a wide range of articles, mostly case reports, there are no published randomized controlled studies on the efficacy and clinical benefit of ECT treatment in patients with PD and depression.

In a retrospective study, Moellentine et al. (92) compared the outcome of 25 patients with parkinsonism after ECT treatment to 25 psychiatric control patients. Patients were given three ECT treatments per week unless transient delirium resulted in postponement or discontinuation of treatment. Several rating scales including the HAMA and HAMD and the Brief Psychiatric Rating Scale (BPRS) were performed before and after a medium number of six ECT treatments. Extrapyramidal symptoms improved subjectively in 14 patients and worsened in one patient. The authors noted a significant improvement in the HAMD and BPRS scores after ECT treatment; however, mean depression scores before and after treatment were not given.

Douyon et al. (93) investigated the effect of ECT (seven bilateral sessions) in seven patients with idiopathic PD. The NYUPDS was used for quantification of motor function, and depression was assessed using the HAMD. Depression and motor function were quantified at baseline, 24 hours after the second, fourth, and the last ECT treatment and 72 hours after the last treatment. The authors found significant improvement in motor function after each treatment and increased dyskinesia in two patients after the last ECT session. Only in four of the seven patients, HAMD scores were given at baseline and after treatment, with a reduction in the HAMD scores between 27% to 80%.

Based on the evidence of class III studies, we conclude that ECT seems to be efficacious for the treatment of depression in PD; however, currently available data are insufficient to recommend ECT treatment in routine care of depressed patients with idiopathic PD.

CONCLUSION AND RECOMMENDATIONS

There are no adequately controlled trials (class I) demonstrating pharmacological efficacy for any agent in depressed patients with idiopathic PD.

TCAs and SSRIs should be considered for the treatment of depression in patients with idiopathic PD with side-effect profiles guiding the choice of agent (Guideline).

So far, there is insufficient evidence to support the use of new antidepressants to treat depression in idiopathic PD (Practice Option).

DA-replenishing strategies with levodopa or DA agonists are recommended as probably useful for amelioration of depression in idiopathic PD (Guideline).

A combination of selegiline and moclobemide seems to be efficacious for the treatment of depression in idiopathic PD, despite a lack of available evidence (Guideline).

Available evidence is insufficient to recommend selegiline (10 mg per day) or moclobemide (600 mg per day) monotherapy for the treatment of depression in idiopathic PD (Guideline).

There is insufficient evidence to recommend bupropion or SAM for treatment of depression in patients with idiopathic PD (Practice Option).

Some depressed patients with PD may benefit from psychotherapy or ECT treatment, but class I or class II data are lacking (Practice Option).

REFERENCES

1. Oertel WH, Hoeglinger GU, Eichhorn T, et al. Depression in Parkinson's disease: an update. *Adv Neurol* 2001;86:373–383.
2. Kuopio AM, Martilla RJ, Helenius H, et al. The quality of life in Parkinson's disease. *Mov Disord* 2000;15: 216–223.
3. Schrag A, Jahanshahi M, Quinn N. What contributes to quality of life in Parkinson's disease? *J Neurol Neurosurg Psychiatry* 2000;69:308–312.
4. Cummings JL, Masterman DL. Depression in patients with Parkinson's disease. *Int J Geriatr Psychiatry* 1999; 14:711–718.
5. Zesiewicz TA, Gold M, Chari C, et al. Current issues in depression in Parkinson's disease. *Am J Geriatr Psychiatry* 1999;7:110–118.
6. Stenager EN, Wermuth L, Senager E, et al. Suicide in patients with Parkinson's disease: epidemiological studies. *Acta Psychiatr Scand* 1994;90:70–72.
7. Stein M, Heuser IJ, Juncos JL, et al. Anxiety disorders in patients with Parkinson's disease. *Am J Psychiatry* 1990;147:217–220.
8. Poewe W, Luginger E. Depression in Parkinson's disease. *Neurology* 1999;52[Suppl 3]:S2–S6.
9. Walsh K, Bennett G. Parkinson's disease and anxiety. *Postgrad Med J* 2001;77:89–93.
10. Menza MA, Robertson-Hoffmann DE, Bonapace AS. Parkinson's disease and anxiety: comorbidity with depression. *Biol Psychiatry* 1993;34:465–470.
11. Derix MMA, Gilhuis HJ, Hoogendijk W. Depressive syndrome in Parkinson's disease: diagnostic pitfalls. In: Wolters EC, Scheltens P, eds. *Mental dysfunction in Parkinson's disease.* Amsterdam: IOS Press, 1993: 325–333.
12. Kral VA, Emery O. Long term follow-up of depressive pseudodementia. *Can J Psychiatry* 1989;34:445–447.
13. Aarsland D, Andersen K, Larsen JP, et al. Risk of dementia in Parkinson's disease. *Neurology* 2001;56: 730–736.
14. Sano M, Stern Y, Williams J, et al. Coexisting dementia and depression in Parkinson's disease. *Arch Neurol* 1989;46:1284–1286.
15. Tröster AI, Paolo AM, Lyons KE, et al. The influence of depression on cognition in Parkinson's disease: a pattern of impairment distinguishable from Alzheimer's disease. *Neurology* 1995;45:672–676.
16. Schrag A, Jahanshahi M, Quinn P. What contributes to depression in Parkinson's disease? *Psychol Med* 2001; 31:65–73.
17. World Health Organization. *International classification of impairments, disabilities and handicaps. A manual of classification relating to the consequences of disease.* Geneva: World Health Organization, 1980.
18. Slaughter JR, Slaughter KA, Nichols D, et al. Prevalence, clinical manifestations, etiology and treatment of depression in Parkinson's disease.*J Neuropsychol Clin Neurosci* 201;13:187–196.
19. Celesia GG, Wanamaker WM. Psychiatric disturbances in Parkinson's disease.*Dis Nerv Syst* 1972;33:577–583.
20. Starkstein SE, Mayberg HS, Leiguarda R, et al. A prospective longitudinal study of depression, cognitive decline and physical impairment in patients with Parkinson's disease. *J Neurol Neurosurg Psychiatry* 1992;55:377–382.
21. Santamaria J, Tolosa E, Valles A. Parkinson's disease with depression: a possible subgroup of idiopathic parkinsonism. *Neurology* 1986;36:1130–1133.
22. Starkstein SE, Berthier ML, Bolduc PL, et al. Depression in patients with early versus later onset of Parkinson's disease. *Neurology* 1989;39:1141–1145.
23. Brown RG, Mac Carthy B, Gotham AM, et al. Depression and disability in Parkinson's disease: a follow-up study of 132 cases. *Psychol Med* 1988;18:49–55.
24. Mindham RHS, Marsden CD, Parkes JD. Psychiatric symptoms during levodopa therapy for Parkinson's disease and their relationship to physical disability. *Psychol Med* 1976;6:23–33.
25. Ehmann TS, Beninger RJ, Gawel MJ, et al. Depressive symptoms in Parkinson's disease: a comparison with disabled control subjects. *J Geriatr Psychiatry Neurol* 1990;3:3–9.
26. Gotham AM, Brown RG, Marsden CD. Depression in Parkinson's disease: a quantitative and qualitative analysis. *J Neurol Neurosurg Psychiatry* 1986;49:381–389.
27. Kuzis G, Sabe L, Tiberti C, et al. Cognitive functions in major depression and in Parkinson's disease. *Arch Neurol* 1997;54:982–986.
28. Starkstein SE, Petracca G, Chemerinski E, et al. Depression in classic versus akinetic-rigid Parkinson's disease. *Mov Disord* 1998;13:29–33.
29. Mayeux R, Stern Y, Rosen J, et al. Depression, intellectual impairment and Parkinson's disease. *Neurology* 1981;31:645–650.
30. Starkstein SE, Preziosi TJ, Bolduc PL, et al. Depression in Parkinson's disease. *J Nerv Ment Dis* 1990;178: 27–31.
31. Warburton JW. Depressive symptoms in Parkinson patients referred for thalamotomy. *J Neurol Neurosurg Psychiatry* 1967;30:368–370.
32. Brown GL, Wilson WP. Parkinsonism and depression. *South Med J* 1972;65:540–545.
33. Huber SJ, Freidenberg DL, Paulson GW, et al. The pattern of depressive symptoms in Parkinson's disease. *J Neurol Neurosurg Psychiatry* 1990;53:275–278.
34. Robins AH. Depression in patients with parkinsonism. *Br J Psychiatry* 1976;128:141–145.
35. Singer E. The effect of treatment with levodopa on Parkinson patients' social functioning and outlook on life. *J Chronic Dis* 1974;27:581–594.
36. Menza MA, Palermo B, DiPaola R, et al. Depression and anxiety in Parkinson's disease. Possible effect of genetic variation in the serotonin transporter. *J Geriatr Psychiatry Neurol* 1999;12:49–52.
37. Brown R, Jahanshahi M. Depression in Parkinson's disease: a psychosocial viewpoint. *Adv Neurol* 1995;65: 61–84.
38. Horn S. Some psychological factors in parkinsonism. *J Neurol Neurosurg Psychiatry* 1974;37:27–31.
39. Kostic VS, Djuricic BM, Covickovic-Sternic N, et al. Depression and Parkinson's disease: a possible role of serotonergic mechanisms. *J Neurol* 1987;234: 94–96.
40. Mayeux R, Stern Y, Cote L, et al. Altered serotonin me-

tabolism in depressed patients with Parkinson's disease. *Neurology* 1984;34:642–646.

41. Paulus W, Jellinger, K. The neuropathologic basis of different clinical subgroups of Parkinson's disease. *J Neuropathol Exp Neurol* 1991;50:339–342.
42. Chan-Palay V, Asan E. Quantitation of catecholamine neurons of the locus coeruleus in senile dementia of the Alzheimer's type and in Parkinson's disease with and without dementia and depression. *J Comp Neurol* 1989; 287:373–392.
43. Torrack RM, Morris JC. The association of ventral tegmental area histopathology with adult dementia. *Arch Neurol* 1988;45:211–218.
44. Ring HA, Bench CJ, Trimble MR, et al. Depression in Parkinson's disease. A positron emission study. *Br J Psychiatry* 1994;165:333–339.
45. Paulus W, Trenkwalder C. Imaging of nonmotor symptoms in Parkinson-syndromes. *Clin Neurosci* 1998;5: 115–120.
46. Mayberg SH, Starkstein SE, Sadzot B, et al. Selective hypometabolism in the frontal lobe in depressed patients with Parkinson's disease. *Ann Neurol* 1990;8: 57–64.
47. Kennedy HS, Kenneth RE, Krüger S, et al. Changes in regional brain glucose metabolism measured with positron emission tomography after paroxetine treatment of major depression. *Am J Psychiatry* 2001;158: 899–905.
48. Stefurak TL, New P, Mahurin RK, et al. Response specific regional metabolic changes with fluoxetine treatment in depressed Parkinson's patients. *Mov Disord* 2001;16[Suppl 1]:S39.
49. Jouvent R, Abensour P, Bonnet AM, et al. Antiparkinsonian and antidepressant effects of high doses of bromocriptine. *J Affect Disord* 1983;5:141–145.
50. Barbeau A. L-dopa therapy in Parkinson's disease: a critical review of nine years' experience. *J Can Med Assoc* 1969;101:791–800.
51. Maricle RA, Nutt JG, Valentine RJ, et al. Dose response relationship of levodopa with mood and anxiety in fluctuating Parkinson's disease: a double-blind, placebo-controlled study. *Neurology* 1995;45:1757–1760.
52. Sporn J, Ghaemi SN, Sambur MR, et al. Pramipexole augmentation in the treatment of unipolar and bipolar depression: a retrospective chart review. *Ann Clin Psychol* 2000;12:137–140.
53. Rektorova I, Rektor I, Bares M, et al. Depression in Parkinson's disease: an eight-month, randomized, open-label, national, multi-centre comparative study of pramipexole and pergolide. *Mov Disord* 2001;16[Suppl 1]:S32.
54. Steur EN, Ballering LA. Moclobemide and selegiline in the treatment of depression in Parkinson's disease. *J Neurol Neurosurg Psychiatry* 1997;63:547.
55. Lees AJ, Shaw KM, Kohout LH, et al. Deprenyl in Parkinson's disease. *Lancet* 1977;15:791–795.
56. Drevets WC. Geriatric depression: brain imaging correlates and pharmacologic considerations. *J Clin Psychiatry* 1994;5[Suppl A]:71–81.
57. Laitinen L. Desipramine in treatment of Parkinson's disease. *Acta Neurol Scand* 1969;45:109–113.
58. Strang RR. Imipramine in the treatment of Parkinson's disease: a double-blind placebo study. *Br Med J* 1965;2: 33–34.
59. Anderson J, Aabro E, Gulmannm N, et al. Antidepressive treatment in Parkinson's disease: a controlled trial of the effect of nortriptyline in patients with Parkinson's disease treated with L-dopa. *Acta Neurol Scand* 1980; 62:210–219.
60. Stoudemire A. New antidepressant drugs and the treatment of depression in the medically ill patient. *Psychiatr Clin North Am* 1996;19:495–514.
61. Ritter JL, Alexander B. Retrospective study of selegiline-antidepressant drug interactions and review of the literature. *Ann Clin Psychiatry* 1997;9:7–13.
62. Richard IH, Kurlan R, Tanner C, et al. Serotonin syndrome and the combined use of deprenyl and an antidepressant in Parkinson's disease. Parkinson Study Group. *Neurology* 1997;48:1070–1077.
63. Ceravolo R, Nuti A, Piccinni A, et al. Paroxetine in Parkinson's disease: effects on motor and depressive symptoms. *Neurology* 2000;55:1216–1218.
64. Tesei S, Antonini A, Canesi M, et al. Tolerability of paroxetine in Parkinson's disease. A prospective study. *Mov Disord* 2000;15:986–989.
65. Hauser RA, Zesiewicz TA. Sertraline for the treatment of depression in Parkinson's disease. *Brain Res* 1997; 12:756–757.
66. Dell'Agnello G, Ceravolo R, Nuti A, et al. SSRIs do not worsen Parkinson's disease: evidence from an open-label, prospective study. *Clin Neuropharmacol* 2001;24: 221–227.
67. Simons JA. Fluoxetine in Parkinson's disease. *Mov Disord* 1996;11:581–582.
68. Meara RJ, Bhowmick BK, Hobson JP. An open uncontrolled study of the use of sertraline in the treatment of depression in Parkinson's disease. *J Serotonin Res* 1996;4:243–249.
69. Steur E. Increase of Parkinson disability after fluoxetine medication. *Neurology* 1993;43:211–213.
70. Wils V. Extrapyramidal symptoms in a patient treated with fluvoxamine. *J Neurol Neurosurg Psychiatry* 1992; 55:330–331.
71. Wittgens W, Donath O, Trenckmann U. Treatment of depressive syndromes in Parkinson's disease with paroxetine. *Mov Disord* 1997;12:128.
72. Jimenez-Jimenez FJ, Tejeiro J, Martinez-Juncuera G, et al. Parkinsonism exacerbated by paroxetine. *Neurology* 1994;44:2406.
73. Goetz CG, Tanner CM, Klawans HL. Bupropion in Parkinson's disease. *Neurology* 1984;34:1092-1094.
74. Tom T, Cummings JL. Depression in Parkinson's disease: pharmacological characteristics and treatment. *Drugs Aging* 1998;12:55–74.
75. Fonda D. Parkinson's disease in the elderly: psychiatric manifestations. *Geriatrics* 1985;40:109–114.
76. Di Rocco A, Rogers JD, Brown R, et al. *S*-Adenosyl-methionine improves depression in patients with Parkinson's disease in an open-label clinical trial. *Mov Disord* 2000;15:1225–1229.
77. Montgomery SA. Reboxetine: additional benefits to the depressed patient. *J Psychopharmacol* 1997;11[Suppl 4]:S9–S15.
78. Montgomery SA, Reimitz PE, Zivkov M. Mirtazapine versus amitriptyline in the long-term, treatment of depression: a double-blind placebo-controlled study. *Int Clin Psychopharmacol* 1998;13:63–73.
79. Hirschfeld RM. Efficacy of SSRIs and newer antidepressants in severe depression: comparison with TCAs. *J Clin Psychiatry* 1999;60:326–335.

80. Fontaine R, Ontineros A, Eli R, et al. A double-blind comparison of nefazodone, imipramine and placebo in major depression. *J Clin Psychiatry* 1994;55:234–241.
81. Benkert O, Szegedi A, Kohnen R. Mirtazapine compared with paroxetine in major depression. *J Clin Psychiatry* 2000;61:656–663.
82. Lemke MR. Reboxetine treatment of depression in Parkinson's disease. *J Clin Psychiatry* 2000;61:872.
83. Benazzi F. Parkinson's disease worsened by nefazodone. *Int J Geriatr Psychiatry* 1997;12:1195.
84. Norman C, Hesslinger B, Frauenknecht S, et al. Psychosis during chronic levodopa triggered by the new antidepressive drug mirtazapine. *Pharmacopsychiatry* 1997;30:263–265.
85. Ellgring JH. Depression, psychosis and dementia: impact on the family. *Neurology* 1999;52[Suppl 3]: S17–S20.
86. Sackheim HA, Devanand DP, Nobler MS. Electroconvulsive therapy. In: Bloom FE, Kupfer DJ, eds. *Psychopharmacology. The fourth generation in progress.* Philadelphia: Lippincott Williams and Wilkins, 1995:1123–1141.
87. Nutt DJ, Glue P. The neurobiology of ECT: animal studies. In: Coffey CE, ed. *The clinical science of electroconvulsive therapy.* Washington: American Psychiatric Press, 1993:213–234.
88. Faber R, Trimble MR. Electroconvulsive therapy in Parkinson's disease and other movement disorders. *Mov Disord* 1991;6:293–303.
89. Anderson K, Balldin J, Gottfries CG, et al. A double-blind evaluation of electroconvulsive therapy in Parkinson's disease with "on-off" phenomena. *Acta Neurol Scand* 1987;76:191–199.
90. Figiel GS. ECT and delirium in Parkinson's disease. *Am J Psychiatry* 1992;149:1759–1760.
91. Oh JJ, Rummans TA, O'Connor MK, et al. Cognitive impairment after ECT in patients with Parkinson's disease and psychiatric illness. *Am J Psychiatry* 1992;149: 271.
92. Moellentine C, Rummans T, Ahlskog JE, et al. T. Effectiveness of ECT in patients with parkinsonism. *J Neuropsychiatry* 1998;10:187–193.
93. Douyon R, Serby M, Klutchko B, et al. ECT and Parkinson's disease revisited: a "naturalistic" study. *Am J Psychiatry* 1989;146:1451–1455.

Parkinson's Disease: Advances in Neurology, Vol. 91.
Edited by Ariel Gordin, Seppo Kaakkola, and Heikki Teräväinen
Lippincott Williams & Wilkins, Philadelphia © 2003

39

Differential Diagnosis of Parkinsonism

Alicia G. Facca and William C. Koller

Department of Neurology, University of Miami, School of Medicine, Miami, Florida

The neurodegenerative diseases with parkinsonian features are conditions that resemble Parkinson's disease (PD) clinically but have a presumed different pathophysiology, histological findings, prognosis, and response to therapy. Even for the experienced clinician, a relative high rate of diagnostic error has been shown in these rigid akinetic syndromes when comparing clinical with autopsy data (1–10).

PD is a heterogenic disease regarding age at onset, symptoms, and rate of progression. The recognized classic motor abnormalities associated with PD are tremor (resting, postural); bradykinesia; rigidity; postural instability; hypomimia; dysarthria; hypophonia; sialorrhea; loss of associated movements; shuffling and festinating gait; freezing; micrographia; stooped posture; and dystonia (2, 3,11–13). The neurobehavioral manifestations associated with PD include depression, bradyphrenia, dementia, apathy, fearfulness, anxiety, emotional lability, social withdrawn, and difficulty with executive functions and task completion (2,3,11–18). The autonomic dysfunction associated with PD includes orthostasis, constipation, impaired thermal regulation, urinary problems, sexual dysfunction, and seborrhea. Sensory disturbances associated with PD include pain, paresthesias, and dysesthesias. Sleep disturbances associated with PD include rapid eye movement (REM) sleep behavior disorder, fragmented sleep, difficulty falling asleep, and periodic leg movements of sleep. As PD progresses, the patients commonly develop functional disabilities including difficulty with writing, turning in bed, buttoning, talking, slowness, difficulty in performing activities of daily living (ADL), and gait difficulty (12). The clinical findings that were shown to increase the accuracy of the correct diagnosis of PD include presence of resting tremor, unilateral onset, masked facies, and dramatic and sustained response to levodopa treatment (12,13, 19–27).

The diagnostic criteria for PD published by Calne et al. (4) are divided in clinically possible, clinically probable, and clinically definite. For clinically possible PD, the diagnostic criteria require the presence of any one of the salient features: tremor, rigidity, or bradykinesia. Impairment of postural reflexes is not included because it is too specific. The tremor must be of recent onset but may be postural or resting. For clinically probable PD, the diagnostic criteria require the presence of any two of the cardinal features: resting tremor, rigidity, or bradykinesia and impairment of postural reflexes. Alternatively, asymmetrical resting tremor, asymmetrical rigidity, or asymmetrical bradykinesia are sufficient. For clinically definite PD, the diagnostic criteria require the combination of the features: resting tremor, rigidity, or bradykinesia and impairment of postural reflexes. Alternatives sufficient are two of these features, with asymmetry present in one of the first three features (13).

More recently, peripheral sympathetic function has been studied in patients with PD without autonomic failure. One study used ^{123}I-labeled metaiodobenzylguanidine (MIBG) scintillography. In the early phase of the disease, only cardiac MIBG uptake was severely reduced. In patients with PD without dysautonomia, both the early and delayed reduction in MIBG uptake (27) occurred selectively in the heart of patients with PD in stages I to III in the Hoehn–Yahr scale. This is considered to be specific in PD and useful in the differential diagnosis of the parkinsonian syndromes (27).

The neuropathological findings are substantial nerve cell depletion, with accompanying gliosis in the substantia nigra, the presence of Lewy bodies (LB) in the substantia nigra. LB can also be present in the locus ceruleus, nucleus basalis of Meynert, dorsal motor nucleus of the vagus nerve, and hypothalamus (13,19).

ATYPICAL PARKINSONIAN FEATURES

The possibility of the diagnosis of a parkinsonian syndrome other than PD can be suggested by the appearance of signs and symptoms that are distinctly unusual in PD, such as early and severe autonomic dysfunction, supranuclear gaze palsy, early dementia, early gait instability, isolated gait instability, early and severe bulbar signs, profound asymmetry of corticospinal or motor signs, symmetrical and bilateral involvement from onset, lack of response to levodopa, recent exposure to dopamine-blocking agents, recent toxic metabolic encephalopathy, trauma, hydrocephalus, and cerebrovascular disease. It is important to mention that these "atypical signs" do not exclude the diagnosis of PD but may suggest other neurodegenerative disorders with parkinsonian features such as progressive supranuclear palsy (PSP), multiple system atrophy (MSA), corticobasal degeneration (CBD), dementia with LB (DLB), or other syndromes (2,13).

A variety of parkinsonian syndromes can present with one or more of the same parkinsonian features as PD and can cause considerably diagnostic confusion. Clinically, a careful analysis of the time at onset, sequence of symptoms' presentation, presence of atypical features, progression of disease, response to therapy, and nature of disability can increase the chances of a correct clinical diagnosis of idiopathic PD from the atypical neurodegenerative rigid akinetic parkinsonian syndromes. Routine laboratory evaluation is usually not helpful. Evaluation of autonomic nervous system function using measures of cardiovascular reflex control during controlled deep breathing, heart rate variability (HRV), orthostatic blood pressure, external anal sphincter electromyography (EMG), urethral EMG, postganglionic cardiac adrenergic neurons, and MIBG uptake have been shown to be helpful in the differential diagnosis between the different neurodegenerative syndromes with parkinsonism, particularly PD and MSA (26–29). Neuroimaging techniques may sometimes show specific abnormalities seen in the non-PD parkinsonian syndromes. Distinct neuropathological findings have been found in many atypical parkinsonian syndromes (33).

Individual clinical presentations, findings, signs, and symptoms that are usually specific and increase the accuracy of the diagnosis of the different entities are reviewed.

DEMENTIA WITH LEWY BODIES

Frederick Lewy first described LB in 1914, as cytoplasmic inclusions found in cells of the substantia nigra in patients with PD. In the 1960s, a DLB in the neocortex was described. However, such cases were thought to be very rare, until the 1980s when sensitive immunohistochemistry became available. DLB was then recognized as a common entity and currently is the second most common degenerative dementia after Alzheimer's disease (AD) in older patients (36). DLB is slightly more common in women when compared with AD

(37). Autopsy studies suggest that DLB accounts for 10% to 20% of dementia cases. Up to 40% of patients with AD have concomitant DLB. Onset of cognitive decline to death was found to be 7.7 years (SD = 3.0) in one study (36–38). Several nomenclatures have been used to describe this syndrome, including LB dementia, diffuse LB disease, LB disease, senile dementia of the LB type, and LB variant of AD. A consortium meeting recommended the term DLB in 1996 (39).

DLB is defined as a progressive degenerative DLB localized to the cortex and associated with early variable extrapyramidal disorder. Characteristic symptoms include fluctuating cognitive impairment consistent with dementia (these typically are pronounced variations in alertness with bouts of confusion that can vary in duration from minutes to weeks), deficits in executive function (complex attention) and visuospatial skills, mild anterograde memory loss, memory retrieval more impaired than memory storage, early psychotic features such as well-formed and complex visual hallucinations, delusions, unexplained syncope, REM sleep disorder, parkinsonian features, gait disorder, and hypersensitivity to neuroleptic drugs. Spontaneous parkinsonism is the final core feature of DLB and often the one that leads to the diagnosis being considered (40–43). On retrospective brain bank studies, more than 50% of the patients did not have parkinsonian symptoms on initial presentation (42–44,48). In retrospective studies comparing DLB with PD, the absence of resting tremor, the presence of myoclonus, the symmetry of extrapyramidal symptoms, and the lack of response to levodopa were more likely features of DLB than PD (42,45). Patients with DLB are at greater risk of neuroleptic hypersensitivity, defined as deterioration in parkinsonism, irreversible cognitive decline, delirium, or neuroleptic malignant syndrome. These adverse effects have been reported in these patients with the use of atypical neuroleptics and with low-dose treatment regimens (47).

The consensus criteria for the clinical diagnosis of DLB (39) include the development of progressive cognitive decline sufficient to interfere with social or occupational function. The clinical diagnostic criteria for probable DLB requires two core features for the clinical diagnosis and only one core feature for the diagnosis of possible DLB. The essential core features include a cognitive state that fluctuates significantly in terms of alertness and attention, recurrent (especially detailed) visual hallucinations, and spontaneous motor features of parkinsonism. The supportive diagnostic features are frequent falls, syncope, transient loss of consciousness, neuroleptic hypersensitivity, systematized delusions, and nonvisual hallucinations. The presence or evidence of other physical or neurological illness sufficient to explain the clinical features goes against the diagnosis of DLB. In 1999, the above criteria were revised (49). The specificity of a clinical and pathological diagnosis of probable DLB using the above consensus was considered high (more than 85%). The additional supportive features for the clinical diagnosis of DLB added to the consensus are depression and REM sleep behavior disorder. Anti-ubiquitin is the method of choice in routine immunohistochemistry for detection of LB in both clinical diagnosis and research purposes. The use of α-synuclein antibodies to label LB and Lewy's neurites are likely to be more useful in research laboratories, particularly for clinicopathological correlative studies (49).

The distinct neuropsychological profile emerges early in DLB (36). The typical early profile is one of disproportional involvement of domains such as attention, executive function, and visuospatial function (51). Visual deficits affect perceptual, spatial, and constructive abilities; when matched patients with DLB with PD for degree of dementia, memory function was superior to that seen in AD (52). Clock drawing demonstrates the visuoconstructive deficit, and patients with CBD fail to improve their performance when asked to copy the drawing (45). Patients with DLB performed significantly worse than patients with AD on forward digit span, sustained attention, Stroop's test, and the Wisconsin Card Sorting Test consistent with attention and executive deficits, when compared with matched patients with AD for age, education, and Mini-Mental State Examination scores (53). The same pattern was observed on the fragmented letters, object decision, and cube analysis subtests of the visual object and space perception battery consistent with visuoperceptual dysfunction. Letter fluency and test results of semantic memory (including category fluency) were similarly impaired in both groups, but the AD group showed significantly worse performance on delayed story recall (a test of episodic memory) (40).

Interestingly, a retrospective study of patients with AD, in which pathology was divided into those with and those without superimposed LB, reported similar findings (55); using subtests of the Mattis Dementia Rating Scale and the Folstein Mini-Mental State Examination, subjects with dual pathology (AD/DLB) showed worse initiation and registration ability, with relatively preserved delayed recall, when compared with the AD group. Disruption of the corticostriatal connections in the frontal lobe is most likely associated with these symptoms. As with other neurodegenerative dementias, the trend over time is for the development of global impairment.

The pathological hallmark is the presence of ubiquitin-positive LB in the cortex and brainstem. Nonpyramidal cells in layers V and VI of the neocortex may contain LBs. Cortical LB density correlates with age at disease onset. There is also a significant interaction between the density of limbic cortical LB and the development of dementia. Apolipoprotein E4 allele is increased twofold to threefold in DLB (as in AD), and the production of β-amyloid occurs in most of the cases. An extensive cholinergic deficit in the neocortex has been identified (56).

Neuroimaging has not demonstrated any specific structural diagnostic pattern in DLB. Nevertheless, preservation of mesial temporal structures, when present in a patient with a clinical profile consistent with DLB, has been shown to be a useful sign of DLB (57). However, due to the common coexistence of AD pathology, atrophy in this region is often the case and, if seen, should not discourage one *per se* from the diagnosis.

PROGRESSIVE SUPRANUCLEAR PALSY

In 1964, Steele et al. (58) described PSP as a clinical diagnosis, although a few descriptions had been previously reported. PSP is the most common parkinsonian syndrome after PD. In a study performed in Olmsted County, Minnesota (59), the average annual incidence of PSP was estimated to be 5.3 per 100,000 per year for ages 50 to 99, being higher in men. The incidence increases with age from 1.7 (ages 50 to 59 years) to 14.7 (ages 80 to 99 years). A large population study in the United Kingdom found an age-adjusted prevalence rate of 6.4 per 100,000 (60). The prognosis and survival of PSP is around 5 to 6 years from the onset of clinical symptoms.

The clinical presentation of PSP includes symmetrical bradykinesia or rigidity (proximal more than distal), abnormal neck posture, especially retrocollis, early dysarthria and dysphagia, early onset and severe postural instability, gait difficulty, supranuclear gaze palsy, especially of vertical downgaze, and early onset of cognitive impairment or dementia. Cognitive impairment should include at least two of the following: apathy, impairment in abstract thoughts, decreased verbal fluency, and use of behavioral or frontal release signs (61–65). The NINDS-SPSP proposed clinical diagnostic criteria of PSP based on neuropathological proven cases include an inclusion and exclusion criteria for clinically possible and probable PSP (66). The mandatory exclusion criteria for both probable and possible PSP include histology compatible with encephalitis, presence of alien-hand syndrome, cortical sensory deficits, focal frontal or temporoparietal atrophy, hallucinations or delusions unrelated to dopaminergic therapy, cortical dementia of Alzheimer's type (with severe amnesia, aphasia, or agnosia), prominent early cerebellar symptoms, prominent early and unexplained dysautonomia (urinary incontinence, impotence, or symptomatic postural hypotension), severe asymmetrical parkinsonian signs (bradykinesia), neuroradiological evidence of relevant structural abnormalities (basal ganglia or brainstem infarcts, lobar atrophy), and Whipple's disease (confirmed by polymerase chain reaction [PCR] if indicated). The mandatory inclusion criteria for clinically probable PSP include a gradually progressive disorder, onset at an age older than 40 years, vertical supranuclear ophthalmoparesis (either upward- or downward-gaze abnormalities), and prominent postural instability with falls in the first year of symptom onset. The mandatory inclusion criteria for clinically possible PSP include a gradually progressive disorder, onset after the age of 40 years, either vertical supranuclear ophthalmoparesis (upward or downward gaze) or slowing of vertical saccades, and prominent postural instability with falls within 1 year of symptom onset. Definite PSP includes clinically probable or possible PSP and histological findings typical of PSP.

In the NINDS series, the above criteria for *probable* were 100% specific but only 50% sensitive, and those for *possible* were 83% sensitive and 93% specific. More recently, different clinical investigators (63,66) using an independent study sample confirmed a high specificity and positive predictive value for both positive and probable NINDS-SPSP criteria.

The neuropathological features of PSP are characterized by abundant neurofibrillary tangles, neuronal loss, and gliosis affecting the striatum, pallidum, subthalamic nucleus, substantia nigra, oculomotor complex, periaqueductal gray, superior colliculi, basis pontis, dentate nucleus, and prefrontal cortex. In PSP, tau is composed by filamentous aggregates with four-repeat isoform (E10+) that accumulate in the cells and glia in the cortical and subcortical areas. The NINDS neuropathological adopted inclusion criteria for typical PSP include a high density of neurofibrillary tangles and neuropil threads in at least three of the following areas: pallidum, subthalamic nucleus, substantia nigra, or pons; and a low to high density of neurofibrillary tangles or neuropil threads in at least three of the following: striatum, oculomotor complex, medulla, or dentate nucleus; and clinical history compatible with PSP. Also, it requires the presence of a high density of neurofibrillary tangles and neuropil threads in at least three of the following areas: pallidum, subthalamic nucleus, substantia nigra, or pons; and a low to high density of neurofibrillary tangles or neuropil threads in the least three of the following areas: striatum, oculomotor complex, medulla, or dentate nucleus, and clinical history compatible with PSP. The NINDS neuropathological adopted exclusion criteria for PSP include a large or numerous infarcts; marked diffuse or focal atrophy; LB; changes diagnostic of AD, oligodendroglial argyrophilic inclusions; Pick's bodies; diffuse spongiosis; prion p-positive amyloid plaques (67–71).

Routine laboratory study results in serum, urine, and cerebrospinal fluid (CSF) are normal. Neuroradiologic findings in computed tomography (CT) and magnetic resonance imaging (MRI) scans of the brain are usually of little help in establishing the diagnosis of PSP, but they can be helpful to exclude other parkinsonian syndromes. Due to significant technical difficulties with bone artifact in the posterior fossa, focal midbrain abnormalities are better seen on MRI scan. More than 50% of the patients with PSP will have definite atrophy of the midbrain and the region around the third ventricle (72,73). On MRI sagittal images, a thinning of the superior part of the quadrigeminal plate can be seen. Proton-density MRI sequences may demonstrate minimal signal changes in the periaqueductal region. Magnetic resonance spectroscopy on patients with PSP has shown decrease in Na/Cre ratio in brainstem, centrum semiovale, frontal cortex, and precentral cortex. Also a decrease in Na/Cho ratio has been seen in the lentiform nucleus (74). Blood-flow studies using fluorodeoxyglucose positron emission tomography (PET) and IMP single-photon emission CT (SPECT) had shown nonspecific findings including marked decrease of blood flow and metabolism in frontal and striatal areas. PET scan studies using fluorodopa had shown hypometabolism of glucose in frontal cortex and decreased fluorodopa uptake in presynaptic nigrostriatal dopaminergic system. PET scan studies using BR-bromospiperone or C-raclopride had shown decreased striatal D_2 receptor density (75–77).

The degree of abnormalities in the autonomic nervous system function in PSP using reflex control of heart rate, HRV, and orthostatic blood pressure remains controversial (32). Higher (78) and lower (79,80) degrees of dysautonomia in PSP when compared with PD have been reported.

MULTIPLE SYSTEM ATROPHY

MSA is a sporadic progressive neurodegenerative disorder of unknown etiology. Clinically, it presents with parkinsonian features, cerebellar ataxia, autonomic failure, and pyramidal signs. The parkinsonism is typically poorly responsive to levodopa or dopamine agonists (82,83). MSA represents a group of three diseases with overlapping clinical and pathological findings: olivopontocerebellar atrophy (OPCA), striatonigral degeneration (SND), and Shy–Drager syndrome (SDS).

Dejerine and Thomas (83) first used the term OPCA in 1900 when they described two patients with a degenerative disorder leading to progressive cerebellar dysfunction and parkinsonism. In 1960, Van de Eecken et al. (84) reported three patients with SND with atrophy of the caudate nucleus and putamen. Also, in 1960, Shy and Drager (85) described a neurological syndrome of orthostatic hypotension in patients who also demonstrated parkinsonian features, which they named SDS. In 1969, Graham and Oppenheimer noted that the clinical and pathological findings of OPCA, SND, and SDS significantly overlapped. They named these disorders as MSA to describe patients with these disorders. Recent neurobiological research has justified the grouping of these conditions under a common pathophysiological definition. A consensus conference in 1998 developed diagnostic criteria for MSA based on four clinical presentations (86). These diagnostic findings were subdivided into four categories depending on the most prevalent neurosystem involved: autonomic dysfunction, cerebellar dysfunction, corticospinal dysfunction, and parkinsonism. The patients with predominant parkinsonism were named MSA-P (which would replace the term SND). Patients with predominant cerebellar features were named MDA-C (which would replace the term OPCA). The term SDS was abandoned by this conference because autonomic dysfunction appears in all forms of MSA (82,83,87–89).

Patients with MSA-P present with parkinsonian features, typically asymmetrical tremor, bradykinesia, rigidity, and postural instability, which are unresponsive to levodopa or dopamine agonist therapy. The tremor tends to be postural and irregular, unlike the typical resting "pill-rolling" tremor of PD. A significant number of these patients (41% to 66%) will eventually develop autonomic dysfunction. Hypokinetic dysarthria develops in some patients. Patients with MSA-C present with predominant cerebellar features, including gait and limb ataxia, ataxia dysarthria, sustained gaze-evoked nystagmus, and autonomic dysfunction. They develop breakdown of the smooth pursuit (saccadic pursuit movements). Patients with predominantly autonomic failure develop urinary dysfunction (urinary frequency, urgency, incontinence, or urinary retention) or orthostatic hypotension, which are seen early in the presentation. Erectile dysfunction or impotence is observed in nearly all men with MSA. Patients with corticospinal tract dysfunction present with extensor plantar responses and hyperreflexia. In one study, initial symptoms were orthostatic hypotension (68%), parkinsonism (46%), autonomic symptoms (41%), and cerebellar signs and symptoms (5%). Respiratory stridor is observed in 33% of the patients though rarely requires tracheostomy. Cognitive dysfunction is much less common than in the other parkinsonian syndromes discussed here (88–93).

Incidence is not clearly known due to diagnostic confusion between MSA, PD, PSP with cerebellar features, and DLB associated with orthostatic hypotension. Prevalences of 16.4 per 100,000 have been reported. A Minnesota study estimated an annual incidence rate of MSA to be on average three cases per 100,000 population. A rural Bavaria study found a prevalence of MSA of 0.31% of the general population older than 65 years and 0.71% of the PD population older than 65 years. Some authors estimate that 3% to 10% of patients diagnosed with PD will actually have MSA-P. In the differential diagnosis of MSA, autonomic insufficiency and cerebellar signs are the most helpful features. MSA has a male predominance in several studies (83).

MSA is a progressive disease that eventually leads to disability and death. The median survival in one study was 6.2 years (range, between 0.5 and 24 years). The patients with the cerebellar subtype of MSA have a better prognosis.

Autonomic function testing using HRV during forced inspiration was found to be significantly reduced in MSA. Hypotensive response during orthostatic provocation was significant in both patients with MSA and patients with PD. On an individual basis, decreased HRV and severe hypotensive responses were seen in MSA regardless of age and disease duration, whereas patients with PD demonstrated this combination of abnormalities in autonomic function only at advanced age and long duration of disease (32).

Neuroimaging in MSA usually correlates with the abnormal neuronal subsystem. Atrophy of the brainstem and cerebellum is predominantly seen in MSA-C. Atrophy of the putamen and caudate nucleus appears to be more involved in patients presenting with MSA-P. The globus pallidus is usually spared in MSA. Hyperintensities are seen on T2-weighted and proton-density MRI sequences within the pons, middle cerebellar peduncle, and cerebellum. Correlations between these MRI findings and histopathological studies support the theory that iron deposition, microgliosis, astrocytosis, and severe neuronal loss appear to contribute to these abnormalities in putaminal atrophy, hyperintensities in the rim of the putamen and infratentorial changes. Alteration of the volume of the inferior olivary nucleus and putaminal hypodensity relative to the globus pallidus was not found to be useful. PET scan has demonstrated reduced metabolic activity in the putamen and decreased dopaminergic function within the nigrostriatal system has been demonstrated in patients with MSA; however, these findings are also seen in patients with PD. In patients with MSA-C, a reduced metabolic activity in the cerebellum has been found (94–96).

The macroscopic pathological findings of patients with MSA correlate with the neuroimaging and clinical findings. Each subtype of MSA demonstrates a different degree of atrophy in the extrapyramidal system, spinocerebellar system, pyramidal system, and autonomic nervous system. To a certain extend, all MSA subtypes will have some depigmentation of the substantia nigra and locus ceruleus. The intermediolateral cell column in the spinal cord is preferentially involved. Atrophy of the motor and premotor cortices has been noted. Patients with MSA-P primarily develop atrophy of the extrapyramidal system (the posterolateral putamen and ventrolateral substantia nigra appear atrophic and pallid). Patients with MSA-C develop atrophy of the cerebellum, middle cerebellar peduncles, inferior olives, and basis pontis (97).

Histopathological findings include neuronal loss, gliosis, and microvacuolization within the involved neuronal system. Iron and ferritin levels appear to be increased within the substantia nigra and striatum. Oligodendroglial and microglial cells are predominantly involved. Neurons and astrocytes are relatively spared. Iron levels have been found to be five times higher than reference range values in MSA. Iron was also found to be associated with coarse electron-dense granules and fine granular and fibrillary material in lamellated structures. This excessive iron accumulation was found to correlate with the abnormal signal voids noted in these locations on MRI scans. Iron has been associated not only with oxidative stress, but also with the formation of fibril formation from α-synuclein that may be responsible for the formation of glial cytoplasmic inclusions (GCIs) (98,99).

Microscopic findings of patients with MSA are distinctive for the cytoplasmic inclusions found in the oligodendroglial cells, as well as neuronal loss, astrocytosis, and loss of myelin. These lesions are located predominately within the substantia nigra, locus ceruleus, putamen, inferior olives, pontine nuclei, Purkinje's cells, and the intermediolateral columns of the spinal cord. The caudate nucleus, globus pallidus, dentate nucleus, corticospinal tracts, anterior horn cells of the spinal cord, and vestibular nuclei are relatively spared. In 1989, GCIs were described in MSA. GCIs are argyrophilic inclusions localized within the cytoplasm. They have variable size and shape. The distributions of GCIs follow suprasegmental motor system, supraspinal autonomic system, and their targets. These include the primary and secondary motor cortices, pyramidal and extrapyramidal tracts, and the corticocerebellar system. The density of GCIs correlates with the severity of MSA. The distribution of the GCIs correlates with the subtype (98,100–110).

CORTICOBASAL DEGENERATION

CBD was first described by Rebeiz et al. (111) and Wenning et al. (112) in 1967 and 1968. The initial description included three patients with abnormally slow voluntary limb movement, tremor, dystonic posturing, rigidity, decreased dexterity, and numbness of the affected limb. The symptoms progressed gradually to involve a gait disorder, limb rigidity, and impairment of sensory modalities. Cognitive function was described as being intact (113–115). Postmortem pathological evaluation revealed asymmetrical frontoparietal cortical atrophy and neuronal loss with gliosis. The neuronal cell bodies lacked Nissl's substance, which was described as "achromatic." Considerable loss of pigmented neurons in the substantia nigra was found in all three patients. Subcortical neuronal involvement was variable and secondary corticospinal tract degeneration was also found. On preparations with hematoxylin and eosin, the pyramidal neurons in the third and fifth cortical layers were swollen with an eosinophilic and hyaline appearance (117).

Currently, CBG is an increasingly recognized neurodegenerative disease with parkinsonian features presenting clinically with progressive motor and cognitive symptoms (118). It usually presents in mid to late adult life with a mean onset of symptoms at age 63 years (SD = 7.7). The youngest case with pathological confirmation was at age 45 years. Both men and women are affected. Some authors have observed a female predominance (114–117). Family histories of exposure to toxic or infectious agents of affected patients are usually negative. Current understanding suggests that CBD is a sporadic disease; however, some authors have suggested that a specific genetic background may predispose to the development of the disease (119). The progression of the symptoms leads to death in usually 5 to 10 years after the onset of symptoms. Shorter survival is associated with early onset of symptoms such as bilateral parkinsonism and frontal subcortical dysfunction.

The most common initial motor symptom in CBD, reported in half of the patients on initial visit, has been limb clumsiness with or without rigidity (120). During the course of the disease, the patient usually develops an asymmetrical akinetic-rigid parkinsonism; irregular and fast (6 to 8 Hz) action and postural tremor; asymmetrical limb dystonia (most commonly in the upper extremity); postural instability; reflex myoclonus on the affected limb; higher cortical signs (cortical sensory loss, apraxia, and alien limb phenomenon); gait disorder with postural instability; speech impairment (dysarthria, dysphasia, dysphonia, echolalia, palilalia, and slowness of speech production); dysphagia; orofacial dyspraxia; loss of facial expression; unilateral painful paresthesias; corticospinal tract signs; and behavioral problems. These symptoms have an insidious onset and a gradual progression. A characteristic feature of this atypical parkinsonian syndrome is a poor response to levodopa treatment. Eye movement abnormalities are common in CBD and may be helpful in the early differential diagnosis. Vertical saccades are usually normal. Extraocular movements have a breakdown of the smooth pursuit and a decreased velocity. Horizontal saccades are hypometric and have significant increased latency. Blepharospasm and eyelid-opening apraxia have been reported. Cortical dysfunction including apraxia, dementia, cortical sensory loss, ideomotor, and limb kinetic apraxia (deceased dexterity and fine movements) usually become evident after the first year of disease. Initial onset of abnormalities in two-point discrimination and somatosensory extinction to double simultaneous stimulation presenting several years before apraxia or parkinsonism has been reported (121). Different types of apraxia can be seen depending on the initial affected areas and pattern of disease progression. The degree of cognitive impairment has been strongly correlated to the degree of callosal atrophy and ventricular dilatation, which are both secondary to the cortical atrophy (122). The speech problems are present in most patients and, in advanced stages, may evolve to include paraphrasic errors, aphasia, anarthria, and aphonia. Swallowing abnormalities are also common in advanced stages. In advanced stages, focal myoclonus may be superimposed on the tremor (116).

Cognitive and neuropsychological profiles in clinically diagnosed CBG show difficulties with executive function, complex attention, impairment with timing, sequencing, immediate recall, naming praxis, and spatial orientation. Recognition memory may be preserved, but encoding and delayed recall may be impaired. A frontal-subcortical dysfunction pattern or dementia is very suggestive of CBG (123). Neuropsychiatric features include depression, apathy, irritability, agitation, anxiety, disinhibition, delusions, and obsessive-compulsive behavior (124). Right hemisphere involvement presents with symptoms such as increased disinhibition, apathy, irritability, and lower depression scores.

A proposed diagnostic criterion (125) includes an initial presentation with predominance if either basal ganglia dysfunction or cortical signs. This proposed criterion for the clinical diagnosis of CBD includes the presence of limb rigidity and at least one cortical sign (alien-limb phenomenon, apraxia, or cortical sensory loss) or alternatively rigidity, limb dystonia, and focal reflex myoclonus (125).

Routine laboratory study results in serum, urine, and CSF are normal. Ceruloplasmin, serum copper, and heavy-metal toxic urine screen results are also normal. Some patients will have decreased levels of somatostatin in CSF (126).

Neuropathological gross findings include superior frontoparietal cortical atrophy, which is often asymmetrical and involves the perirolandic cortex. The middle and inferior frontal cortical gyri and the cingular and insular cortices may also be involved. The temporal cortex is usually unaffected unless concomitant pathology is present. Cerebellar and occipital cortices are affected. There is a variable severity of involvement in the subcortical nuclei. The head of the caudate may have a flattened appearance and the thalamus tends to be smaller. Severe loss of neuromelanin pigment is seen in the substantia nigra; however, it is preserved in the locus ceruleus. There is attenuation of the subcortical white matter adjacent to the affected areas. Attenuation and degeneration of the corticobulbar and corticospinal fibers may be seen in the cerebral peduncles. Neuronal loss may result in secondary hydrocephalus *ex vacuo,* aqueduct of Sylvius dilatation, and atrophy of the corpus callosum (117,122,127). Microscopic findings include cortical and subcortical neuronal loss and gliosis. An astrocytic gliosis is more pronounced in the superficial layers of the cortex and at the gray matter–white matter junction. In the white matter, there is loss of myelin and axons with gliosis along the corticostriatal and corticobulbar in areas adjacent to the involved cortex. The substantia nigra had moderate to severe neuronal loss with neuromelanin visualized within phagocytes. A variable degree of involvement may be seen in the basal ganglia, thalamus, periaqueductal gray matter, red nucleus, subthalamic nucleus, dentate nucleus, and inferior olivary nucleus (116,117). A characteristic neuropathological feature of CBD is the presence of ballooned and achromatic neurons, which are eosinophilic on hematoxylin and eosin stain, lack Nissl's substance, and are usually vacuolar. They are most commonly seen in the degenerated deep layers of the frontoparietal cortex but can also be found in other cortical and subcortical structures (such as the insular cortex, anterior cingulate gyrus, amygdala, and claustrum). The ballooned neurons sometimes are positive for ubiquitin immunocytochemical staining (but not for the epitopes specific for AD) (112,116,127–129). Using immunocytochemistry, ballooned neurons do not stain positive for α-synuclein, which is a specific and sensitive marker for LB. Pick's bodies are rarely observed in CBG. Tau, a microtubule-associated phosphoprotein that promotes tubulin polymerization and stabilization of microtubules, is present in CBD in axons and is expressed in glial cells (134). Tau in CBD is generated from transcripts in exon-10 on chromosome 17 (119). Pathological tau has abnormal phosphorylation and solubility and forms abnormal filamentous structures. Focal tau is identified on silver stain preparations, and tau immunohistochemistry within cortical neurons, underlying white matter, globus pallidus, caudate, putamen, subthalamic nucleus, red nucleus, and brainstem nucleus. Focal tau immunoreactivity is found in ballooned neurons, neurofibrillary tangles, neuropil threads, grains, glia, and neuronal inclusions (69,129). The locus ceruleus, raphe nuclei, tegmental gray matter, and substantial nigra frequently have neurofibrillary lesions that are tau immunoreactive. In glial cells, the most common tau-immunoreactive astrocytic lesion in CBD is a grainlike process that resembles a neuritic plaque of AD (69). Tau-positive astrocytic glial plaques are argyrophilic structures, which were thought to be characteristic of CBD but have also been found in PSP. The plaques in CBD do not contain amyloid (129).

Electroencephalogram (EEG) results are usually normal on presentation. With disease progression, the EEG may demonstrate symmetrical slowing, being more prominent over the affected hemisphere (115,116). In advanced stages, the EEG may show nonspecific bilateral slowing. An electrophysiological study of myoclonus in patients with CBD demonstrates absence of preceding cortical discharge, making it a reflex myoclonus. EMG and nerve conduction studies (NCS) may show subclinical focal or generalized neuropathies.

In early stages of the disease, brain CT and MRI results are usually normal. With disease progression, asymmetrical atrophy localized to the posterior frontal and parietal cortices becomes evident with secondary dilatation of the lateral ventricle on the side of the atrophy. Most patients will have asymmetrical frontal cortex atrophy. In more advanced stages, bilateral cortical atrophy might be present. Cortical abnormalities are better seen on MRI using fluid-attenuated inversion recovery sequences. With progressive cortical atrophy, abnormal signal attenuation might be present in the underlying white mater and corpus callosum. Fluorodeoxyglucose PET studies in patients with CBG have shown a global reduction of oxygen and glucose metabolism, most prominent in the cerebral hemisphere contralateral to the most affected limb (130). SPECT scans have shown reduction in cerebral blood flow in the frontoparietal, medial frontal, and temporal cortical regions (131–133). The only subcortical structure that shows asymmetrical decreased metabolism was the thalamus (130). Nigrostriatal dopaminergic dysfunction has been documented by decreased fluorodopa uptake with PET scan in the striatum (up to 25%) (133) and reduced postsynaptic striatal D_2 receptor binding of ^{123}I-iodobenzamide on SPECT scan. The caudate and putamen have symmetrically decreased fluorodopa uptake with PET scan. Dopamine-transporting labeling using 2-β-carboxymethoxy, 3-beta (4-odophenyl)-trioane [^{123}I]-β-CIT on SPECT scanning has demonstrated symmetrical striatal reduction in clinically diagnosed CBD. In a patient with a clinical diagnosis of probable CBG, the combination of finding such as asymmetrically reduced frontoparietal glucose utilization and/or cerebral blood flow, in addition to bilateral reduction of fluorodopa uptake in the caudate and putamen nucleus, can not only provide information about the pattern of brain dysfunction but also provide a strong supportive evidence for the diagnosis of CBD (118).

REFERENCES

1. Hughes AJ. Clinicopathological aspects of Parkinson's disease. *Eur Neurol* 1997;39[Suppl 2]:13–20.
2. Hughes AJ, Ben-Shlomo Y, Daniel SE, et al. What features improve the accuracy of clinical diagnosis in Parkinson's disease. A clinicopathologic study. *Neurology* 1992;42:1142–1146.
3. Hughes AJ, Ben-Shlomo Y, Daniel SE, et al. Diagnosis of Parkinson's disease. *Neurology* 1993;43:1630.
4. Calne DB, Snow BJ, Lee C. Criteria for diagnosing Parkinson's disease. *Ann Neurol* 1992;32[Suppl]: S125–S127.
5. Larsen JP, Dupont E, Tandberg E. Clinical diagnosis of Parkinson's disease: proposal of diagnostic subgroups classified at different levels of confidence. *Acta Neurol Scand* 1994;89:242–251.
6. Ward CD, Gibb WR. Research diagnostic criteria for Parkinson's disease. *Adv Neurol* 1990;53:245–249.
7. Rajput AH, Rozdilsky B, Rajput A, et al. Levodopa efficacy and the pathological basis of Parkinson's syndrome. *Clin Neuropharmacol* 1990;13:553–558.
8. Colosimo C, Albanese A, Hughes AJ, et al. Some specific clinical features differentiate multiple system atrophy (striatonigral variety) from Parkinson's disease. *Arch Neurol* 1995;52:294–298.
9. Louis ED, Klatka LA, Lio Y, et al. Comparison of extrapyramidal features in 31 pathologically confirmed cases of diffuse Lewy body disease and 34 pathological confirmed of Parkinson's disease. *Neurology* 1997; 48:376–380.
10. Rajput AH, Rozdisky B, Ang L. Occurrence of resting tremor in Parkinson's disease. *Arch Neurol* 1995;52: 294–298.
11. Hoehn MM, Yahr MD. Parkinsonism: onset, progression and mortality. *Neurology* 1967;17:427–442.
12. Watts RL, Koller WC. *Movement disorders: neurologic principles and practice.* Philadelphia: McGraw-Hill, 1997.
13. Gelb DJ, Olever E, Gilmas S. Diagnostic criteria for Parkinson's disease. *Arch Neurol* 1999;56:33–39.
14. Mayeux R. The mental state in Parkinson's disease. In: Koller WC, ed. *Handbook of Parkinson's disease,* 2nd ed. New York, NY: Marcel Dekker Inc, 1992:159–184.
15. Tandberg E, Larsen JP, Aarsland D, et al. The occurrence of depression in Parkinson's disease: a community-based study. *Arch Neurol* 1996;53:175–179.
16. Cummings JL. Neuropsychiatric complications of drug treatment of Parkinson's disease. In: Huber SJ, Cummings JL, eds. *Parkinson's disease: neurobehavioral aspects.* New York, NY: Oxford University Press, 1992:313–327.
17. Celesia GG, Wanamaker WM. Psychiatric disturbances in Parkinson's disease. *Dis Nerv Syst* 1972;33:577–583.
18. Bell K, Dooneief G, Marder K, et al. Non-drug-induced psychosis in Parkinson's disease. *Neurology* 1991;41[Suppl 1]:191.
19. Gibb WRG. Accuracy in the clinical diagnosis of parkinsonian syndromes. *Postgrad Med J* 1988;64: 345–351.
20. Rajput AH, Rozdilsky B, Rajput A. Accuracy of clinical diagnosis in parkinsonism—a prospective study. *Can J Neurol Sci* 1991;18:275–278.
21. Hughes AJ, Daniel SE, Kilford L, et al. Accuracy of clinical diagnosis of idiopathic Parkinson's disease: a clinico-pathological study of 100 cases. *J Neurol Neurosurg Psychiatry* 1992;55:181–184.
22. Hughes AJ, Daniel SE, Lees AJ. The clinical features of Parkinson's disease in 100 histologically proven cases. *Adv Neurol* 1993;60:595–599.
23. Koller WC, Montgomery EB. Issues in the early diagnosis of Parkinson's disease. *Neurology* 1997; 49[Suppl 1]:S10–S25.
24. Rajput AH, Jankovic J, McDermott M, and the Parkinson Study Group. Diagnostic accuracy in early Parkinson's disease. *Neurology* 1997;48[Suppl]:A369.
25. Rajput AH. Clinical features of tremor in extrapyramidal syndromes. In: Findley LJ, Koller WC, eds. *Handbook of tremor disorders.* New York, NY: Marcel Dekker Inc, 1995:275–291.
26. Martin WE, Loewenson RB, Resch JA, et al. Parkinson's disease: clinical analysis of 100 patients. *Neurology* 1973;23:783–790.
27. Taki J, Nakajma K, Hwang EH, et al. Peripheral sympathetic dysfunction in patients with Parkinson's disease without autonomic failure is heart selective and disease specific. *Eur J Nucl Med* 2000;27:566–573.
28. Sandroni P, Ahlskog JE, Fearly RD, et al. Autonomic involvement in extrapyramidal and cerebellar disorders. *Clin Auton Res* 1991;1:147–155.
29. Bordet R, Benhadjali J, Destee A, et al. Sympathetic skin response and R-R interval variability in multiple system atrophy and idiopathic Parkinson's disease. *Mov Disord* 1996;11:268–272.
30. Tanner CM, Goetz CG, Klawans HL. Autonomic nervous system disorders in Parkinson's disease. In: Koller WC, ed. *Handbook of Parkinson's disease,* 2nd ed. New York, NY: Marcel Dekker Inc, 1992:185–215.
31. Mathias CJ. Disorders affecting autonomic function in parkinsonian patients. *Adv Neurol* 1996;69:383–391.
32. Holmberg B, Kallio M, Johnels B, et al. Cardiovascular reflex testing contributes to clinical evaluation and differential diagnosis of parkinsonian syndromes. *Mov Disord* 2001;16:217–225.
33. Jellinger KA. The neuropathologic diagnosis of secondary parkinsonian syndromes. *Adv Neurol* 1996;69: 293–303.

34. Gibb WRG. The neuropathology of parkinsonian disorders. In: Jankovic J, Tolosa E, eds. *Parkinson's disease and movement disorders,* 2nd ed. Baltimore, MD: Williams & Wilkins, 1993:253–270.
35. Forno LS. Neuropathology of Parkinson's disease. *J Neuropathol Exp Neurol* 1996;55:259–272.
36. Nestor P, Hodges J. Non-Alzheimer dementias. *Semin Neurol* 2000;20:439–446.
37. Imamura T, Hirono N, Hashimoto M. Clinical diagnosis of dementia with Lewy bodies in a Japanese dementia registry. *Dementia Geriatr Cogn Disord* 1999; 10:210–216.
38. Olichney JM, Galasko D, Salmon DP. Cognitive decline is faster in Lewy body variant than in Alzheimer's disease. *Neurology* 1998;51:351–357.
39. McKeith IG, Galasko D, Kosaka K. Consensus guidelines for the clinical and pathologic diagnosis of dementia with Lewy bodies (DLB): report of the consortium on DLB international workshop. *Neurology* 1996;47:1113–1124.
40. Mesulam M-M. *Principles of behavioral neurology.* Oxford Press, 2000.
41. Ballard C, McKeith I, Harrison R. A detailed phenomenological comparison of complex visual hallucinations in dementia with Lewy bodies and Alzheimer's disease. *Int Psychogeriatr* 1997;9:381–388.
42. Louis ED, Klatka LA, Liu Y, et al. Comparison of extrapyramidal features in 31 pathologically confirmed cases of diffuse Lewy body disease and 34 pathologically confirmed cases of Parkinson's disease. *Neurology* 1997;48:376–380.
43. Ferman TJ, Boeve BF, Smith GE. REM sleep behavior disorder and dementia: cognitive differences when compared with AD. *Neurology* 1999;52:951–957.
44. Ala TA, Yang KH, Sung JH, et al. Hallucinations and signs of parkinsonism help distinguish patients with dementia and cortical Lewy bodies from patients with Alzheimer's disease at presentation: a clinicopathological study. *J Neurol Neurosurg Psychiatry* 1997;62: 16–21.
45. Gnanalingham KK, Byrne EJ, Thornton A, et al. Motor and cognitive function in Lewy body dementia: comparison with Alzheimer's and Parkinson's diseases. *J Neurol Neurosurg Psychiatry* 1997;62:243–252.
46. Papka M, Rubio A, Schiffer RB. A review of Lewy body disease , an emerging concept of cortical dementia. *J Neuropsych Clin Neurosci* 1998;10:267–279.
47. Ballard C, Grace J, McKeith I, et al. Neuroleptic sensitivity in dementia with Lewy bodies and Alzheimer's disease. *Lancet* 1998;351:1032–1033.
48. Boeve BF, Silber MH, Ferman TJ. REM sleep behavior disorder and degenerative dementia: an association likely reflecting Lewy body disease. *Neurology* 1998; 51:363–370.
49. McKeith IG, Perry EK, Perry RH. Report of the second dementia with Lewy body international workshop: diagnosis and treatment. Consortium on dementia with Lewy bodies. *Neurology* 1999:53:902–905.
50. Ballard C, McKeith IG. Psychiatric features in diffuse Lewy body disease. *Neurology* 1998;50:573–573.
51. Hansen L, Salmon D, Galasko D. The Lewy body variant of Alzheimer's disease: a clinical and pathologic entity. *Neurology* 1990;40:1–8.
52. Shimomura T, Mori E, Yamashita H. Cognitive loss in dementia with Lewy bodies and Alzheimer's disease. *Arch Neurol* 1998;55:1547–1552.
53. Calderon J, Perry RJ, Erzinclioglu SW, et al. Perception, attention, and working memory are disproportionately impaired in dementia with Lewy body (DLB) compared to Alzheimer's disease. *J Neurol Neurosurg Psychiatry* 2001;70:157–164.
54. Warrington EK, James M. *The visual object and space perception battery.* Bury St. Edmunds, UK: Thames Valley Test Company, 1991.
55. Connor DJ, Salmon DP, Sandy TJ, et al. Cognitive profiles of autopsy-confirmed Lewy body variant vs. pure Alzheimer's disease [published erratum in *Arch Neurol* 1998;55:1352]. *Arch Neurol* 1998;55:994–1000.
56. Perry R, McKeith I, Perry E. Lewy body dementia—clinical, pathological and neurochemical interconnections. *J Neurol Trans* 1997;51[Suppl]:95–109.
57. Barber R, Gholkar A, Scheltens P, et al. Medial temporal lobe atrophy on MRI in dementia with Lewy bodies. *Neurology* 1999;52:1153–1158.
58. Steele JC, Richardson JC, Olszewski J. Progressive supranuclear palsy. A heterogenous degeneration involving the brain stem, basal ganglia and cerebellum with vertical gaze and pseudobulbar palsy, nuchal dystonia and dementia. *Arch Neurol* 1964;10:333–359.
59. Bower JH, Maraganore M, Shannon K, et al. Incidence of progressive supranuclear palsy and multiple system atrophy in Olmsted County, Minnesota, 1976 to 1990. *Neurology* 1997;49:1284–1288.
60. Nath U, Ben-Shlomo Y, Thomson RG, et al. The prevalence of progressive supranuclear palsy (Steele–Richardson–Olszewski syndrome) in the UK. *Brain* 2001;24:1438–1449.
61. Litvan I. Diagnosis and management of progressive supranuclear palsy. *Semin Neurol* 2001;21:41–48.
62. Litvan I, Agid Y, Jankovic J, et al. Accuracy of clinical criteria for the diagnosis of progressive supranuclear palsy (Steele–Richardson–Olszewski syndrome). *Neurology* 1996;46:922–930.
63. Lopez OL, Litvan I, Catt KE, et al. Accuracy of four clinical diagnostic criteria for the diagnosis of neurodegenerative dementias. *Neurology* 1999;53: 1292–1299.
64. Litvan I. Progressive supranuclear palsy revisited. *Acta Neurol Scand* 1998,98:73–84.
65. Litvan I, Agid Y, Calne D, et al. Clinical research criteria for Richardson–Olszewski syndrome). Report of the NINDS-SPSP International Workshop. *Neurology* 1996;47:1–9.
66. Hauw JJ, Daniel SE, Dickson D, et al. Preliminary NINDS neuropathologic criteria for Steele–Richardson–Olszewski syndrome (progressive supranuclear palsy). *Neurology* 1994;44:2015–2019.
67. Goedert M. Filamentous nerve cell inclusions in neurodegenerative diseases: tauopathies and alpha-synucleinopathies. *Philos Trans R Soc Lond B Biol Sci* 1999;354:1101–1118.
68. Sergeant N, Wattez A, Delacourte A. Neurofibrillary degeneration in progressive supranuclear palsy and corticobasal degeneration: tau pathologies with exclusively "exon 10" isoforms. *J Neurochem* 1999;72:1243–1249.
69. Feany MB, Dickson D. Neurodegenerative disorders with extensive tau pathology: a comparative study and review. *Ann Neurol* 1996;40:139–148.
70. Collins SJ, Ahlskog JE, Parisi JE, et al. Progressive supranuclear palsy: neuropathologically based diagnostic clinical criteria. *J Neurol Neurosurg Psychiatry* 1995;58:167–173.

71. Daniel SE, de Bruin VMS, Lees AJ. The clinical and pathologic spectrum of Steele–Richardson–Olszewski syndrome (progressive supranuclear palsy): a reappraisal. *Brain* 1995;118:759–770.
72. Savoiardo M, Girotti F, Strada I, et al. Magnetic resonance imaging in progressive supranuclear palsy and other parkinsonian disorders. *J Neural Transm* 1994; 42(Suppl.):93–110.
73. Schrag A, Good CD, Miszkiel K, et al. Differentiation of atypical parkinsonian syndromes with routine MRI. *Neurology* 2000;54:697–702.
74. Tedeschi G, Litvan I, Bonavita S, et al. Proton magnetic resonance spectroscopic imaging in progressive supranuclear palsy, Parkinson's disease and corticobasal degeneration. *Brain* 1997;120:1541–1552.
75. D'Antona R, Baron JC, Samson Y, et al. Subcortical dementia. Frontal cortex hypermetabolism detected by positron tomography in patients with progressive supranuclear palsy. *Brain* 1985;108:785–799.
76. Foster NL, Gilman S, Berent S, et al. Cerebral hypometabolism in progressive supranuclear palsy studied with positron emission tomography. *Ann Neurol* 1988;24:399–406.
77. Blin J, Baron JC, Dubios B, et al. Positron emission tomography study in progressive supranuclear palsy: brain hypometabolic pattern and clinicometabolic correlations. *Arch Neurol* 1990;47:747–752.
78. Van Dirk JG, Haan J, Koenderik M, et al. Autonomic nervous function in progressive supranuclear palsy. *Arch Neurol* 1991;48:1083–1084.
79. Gutrecht JA. Autonomic cardiovascular reflexes in progressive supranuclear palsy. *J Auton Nerv Syst* 1992;39:29–35.
80. Kimber J, Mathias CJ, Lees AJ, et al. Physiological, pharmacological and neurohormonal assessment of autonomic function in progressive supranuclear palsy. *Brain* 2000;123:1422–1430.
81. Wenning GK, Sholomo YB, Magalhães M, et al. Clinical features and natural history of multiple system atrophy: an analysis of 100 cases. *Brain* 1994;117: 835–845.
82. Wenning GK, Seppi K, Scherfler C, et al. Multiple system atrophy. *Semin Neurol* 2001;21:33–40.
83. Dejerine J, Thomas A. L'atrophie olivo-ponto-cerebelleuse. *Nouv Iconog Salpetriere* 1900;13:330–370.
84. Adams R, van Bogaert L, van der Eecken H. Degenerescenes nigro-striees et cerebello-nigro-striees. *Phychiatr Neurol* 1967;14:2219–2259.
85. Shy GM, Drager GA. A neurological syndrome associated with orthostatic hypotension. *Arch Neurol* 1960; 2:511–527.
86. Gilman S, Low PA, Quinn N. Consensus statement on the diagnosis of multiple system atrophy. *J Auton Nerv Syst* 1998;74:189–192.
87. Wenning GK, Tison F, Ben Shlomo Y, et al. Multiple system atrophy: a review of 203 pathologically proven cases. *Mov Disord* 1997;12:133–147.
88. Quinn N. Multiple system atrophy: the nature of the beast. *J Neurol Neurosurg Psychiatry* 1989:78–89.
89. Litvan I, Booth V, Wenning GK. Retrospective application of a set of clinical diagnostic criteria for the diagnosis of multiple system atrophy. *J Neural Transm* 1998;105:217–227.
90. Wenning GK, Scherfler C, Granata R. Time course of symptomatic orthostatic hypotension and urinary incontinence in patients with postmortem confirmed parkinsonian syndromes: a clinicopathological study. *J Neurol Neurosurg Psychiatry* 1999;67:620–623.
91. Quinn N. Multiple system atrophy. In: Marsden CD, Fahn S, eds. *Movement disorders,* 3rd ed. London: Butterworth-Heinemann, 1994:262–281.
92. Beck RO, Betts CD, Fowler CJ. Genitourinary dysfunction in multiple system atrophy: clinical features and treatment in 62 cases. *J Urol* 1994;151: 1336–1341.
93. Schulz JB, Skalej M, Wedekind D. Magnetic resonance imaging-based volumetry differentiates idiopathic Parkinson's syndrome from multiple system atrophy and progressive supranuclear palsy. *Ann Neurol* 1999;45:65–74.
94. Schrag A, Kingsley D, Phatouros C. Clinical usefulness of magnetic resonance imaging in multiple system atrophy. *J Neurol Neurosurg Psychiatry* 1998;65: 65–71.
95. Davie CA, Wenning GK, Barker GJ. Differentiation of multiple system atrophy from idiopathic Parkinson's disease using proton magnetic resonance spectroscopy. *Ann Neurol* 1995;37:204–210.
96. Schwarz J, Weis S, Kraft E. Signal changes on MRI and increases in reactive microgliosis, astrogliosis, and iron in the putamen of two patients with multiple system atrophy. *J Neurol Neurosurg Psychiatry* 1996;60: 98–101.
97. Daniel SE. The neuropathology and neurochemistry of multiple system atrophy. In: Bannister R, Mathias C, eds. *A textbook of clinical disorders of autonomic nervous system,* 3rd ed. Oxford: Oxford University Press, 1992:564.
98. Papp MI, Lantos PL. Accumulation of tubular structures in oligodendroglial and neuronal cells as the basic alteration in multiple system atrophy. *J Neurol Sci* 1992;107:172–182.
99. Lantos PL. The definition of multiple system atrophy: a review of recent developments. *J Neuropathol Exp Neurol* 1998;57:1099–1111.
100. Papp MI, Lantos PL. The distribution of oligodendroglial inclusions in multiple system atrophy and its relevance to clinical symptomatology. *Brain* 1994;117: 235–243.
101. Papp MI, Kahn JE, Lantos PL. Glial cytoplasmic inclusions in the CNS of patients with multiple system atrophy (striatonigral degeneration olivo-pontocerebellar atrophy and Shy–Drager syndrome). *J Neurol Sci* 1989;94:79–100.
102. Cairns NJ, Atkinson PF, Hanger DP, et al. Tau protein in the glial cytoplasmic inclusions of multiple system atrophy can be distinguished from abnormal tau in Alzheimer's disease. *Neurosci Lett* 1997;230:49–52.
103. Spillantini MG, Crowther RA, Jakes R, et al. Filamentous alpha-synuclein inclusions link multiple system atrophy with Parkinson's disease and dementia with Lewy bodies. *Neurosci Lett* 1998;251:205–208.
104. Takeda A, Arai N, Komori T, et al. Tau immunoreactivity in glial cytoplasmic inclusions in multiple system atrophy. *Neurosci Lett* 1997;234:63–66.
105. Goedert M, Spillantini MG. Lewy body diseases and multiple system atrophy as alpha-synucleinopathies. *Mol Psychiatry* 1998;3:462–465.
106. Wakabayashi K, Yoshimoto M, Tsuji S, et al. Alpha-synuclein immunoreactivity in glial cytoplasmic inclusions in multiple system atrophy. *Neurosci Lett* 1998; 249:180–182.

107. Arima K, Ueda K, Sunohara N. NACP/alpha-synuclein immunoreactivity in fibrillary components of neuronal and oligodendroglial cytoplasmic inclusions in the pontine nuclei in multiple system atrophy. *Acta Neuropathol (Berlin)* 1998;96:439–444.
108. Tu P, Galvin JE, Baba M. Glial cytoplasmic inclusions in white matter oligodendrocytes of multiple system atrophy brains contain insoluble α-synuclein. *Ann Neurol* 1998;44:415–422.
109. Dickson DW, Liu W, Hardy J. Widespread alterations of alpha-synuclein in multiple system atrophy. *Am J Pathol* 1999;155:1241–1251.
110. Rebeiz JJ, Kolodny EH, Richardson EP. Corticodentatonigral degeneration with neuronal achromasia: a progressive disorder of late adult life. *Trans Am Neurol Assoc* 1967;92:23–26.
111. Rebeiz JJ, Kolodny EH, Richardson EP. Corticodentatonigral degeneration with neuronal achromasia. *Arch Neurol* 1968;18:20–33.
112. Wenning GK, Litvan I, Jankovic J, et al. Natural history and survival of 14 patients with corticobasal degeneration confirmed at postmortem examination. *J Neurol Neurosurg Psychiatry* 1998;64:184–189.
113. Rinne JO, Lee MS, Thompson PD, et al. Corticobasal degeneration: a clinical study of 36 cases. *Brain* 1994; 117:1183–1196.
114. Watts RL, Mirra SS, Richardson EP. Corticobasal ganglionic degeneration. In: Marsden CD, Fahn S, eds. *Movement disorders,* 3rd ed. London: Butterworth, 1994:282–299.
115. Watts R, Brewer RP, Schneider JA, et al. Corticobasal degeneration. In: Watts RL, Koller WC, eds. *Movement disorders: neurologic principles and practice.* New York: McGraw Hill, Inc, 1997:611–621.
116. Schneider JA, Watts RL, Gearing M, et al. Corticobasal degeneration: neuropathological and clinical heterogeneity. *Neurology* 1994;48:959–989.
117. Stover N, Watts RL. Corticobasal degeneration. *Semin Neurol* 2001;21:49–58.
118. Di Maria E, Tabaton M, Vigo T, et al. Corticobasal degeneration shares a common genetic background with progressive supranuclear palsy. *Ann Neurol* 2000;47: 374–377.
119. Kumar R, Bergeron C, Pöllanen MS, et al. Cortical basal ganglionic degeneration. In: Jankovic J, Tolosa E, eds. *Parkinson's disease and movement disorders.* Baltimore: Williams & Wilkins, 1998:297–316.
120. Otsuki M, Soma Y, Yoshimura N, et al. Slowly progressive limb-kinetic apraxia. *Eur Neurol* 1997;37: 100–103.
121. Yamauchi H, Fukuyama H, Nagahama Y, et al. Atrophy of the corpus callosum, cortical hypometabolism, and cognitive impairment in corticobasal degeneration. *Arch Neurol* 1998;55:609–614.
122. Lerner A, Friedland R, Riley D, et al. Dementia with pathological findings of corticobasal ganglionic degeneration. *Ann Neurol* 1992;32:271.
123. Cummings JL, Litvan I. Corticobasal degeneration. Neuropsychiatric aspects of corticobasal degeneration. *Adv Neurol* 2000;82:147–152.
124. Riley D, Lang A. Corticobasal degeneration. clinical diagnostic criteria. *Adv Neurol* 2000;82:29–34.
125. Watts RL, William RS, Growdon JH, et al. Corticobasal ganglionic degeneration. *Neurology* 1985; 35[Suppl 1]:178.
126. Watts RL, Mirra SS, Young RR, et al. Corticobasal ganglionic degeneration (CBD) with neuronal achromasia: clinical pathological study of two cases. *Neurology* 1989;39[Suppl 1]:140.
127. Smith TW, Lippa CF, de Girolama U. Immunocytochemical study of ballooned neurons in cortical degeneration with neuronal achromasia. *Clin Neuropathol* 1992;11:28–35.
128. Dickson DW. Neuropathologic differentiation of progressive supranuclear palsy and corticobasal degeneration. *J Neurol* 1999;246[Suppl 2]:6–15.
129. Brooks DJ. Corticobasal degeneration. Functional imaging studies in corticobasal degeneration. *Adv Neurol* 2000;82:209–215.
130. Okuda B, Tachibana H, Kawabata K, et al. Cerebral blood flow correlates of higher brain dysfunctions in corticobasal degeneration. *J Geriatr Psychiatry Neurol* 1999;12:189–193.
131. Laureys S, Salmon E, Garraux G, et al. Fluorodopa uptake and glucose metabolism in early stages of corticobasal degeneration. *J Neurol* 1999;246:1151–1158.
132. Sawle GV, Brooks DJ, Marsden CD, et al. Corticobasal degeneration. A unique pattern of regional cortical oxygen hypometabolism and striatal fluorodopa uptake demonstrated by positron emission tomography. *Brain* 1991;114:541–556.
133. Delacourte A, Buee L. Normal and pathological tau proteins as factors for microtubule assembly. *Int Rev Cytol* 1997:167–224.

Parkinson's Disease: Advances in Neurology, Vol. 91.
Edited by Ariel Gordin, Seppo Kaakkola, and Heikki Teräväinen
Lippincott Williams & Wilkins, Philadelphia © 2003

40

Essential Tremor and Parkinsonism

Alex Rajput and Michele Rajput

University of Saskatchewan, Royal University Hospital, Saskatoon, Saskatchewan, Canada

Essential tremor (ET) is the most common pathological tremor (1). Reported prevalence is 0.35% to 4.0% in the general population (2), 0.35% to 6.6% in those older than 40 years (2), and 12.6% to 14.0% in those 65 years or older (3). Parkinson's syndrome (PS) is less prevalent than ET but is common in the elderly. In Western countries, 0.3% of the general population (4) and 1.8% of those 65 and older have Parkinson's disease (PD) (5). Given the frequency of each of these disorders, it is not surprising that a number of patients have both ET and PS. After identifying this subgroup of patients, the primary question is one of the significance of the overlap.

COMPARISON OF CLINICAL FEATURES

PS is a clinical diagnosis that requires two of the following three criteria: bradykinesia, rigidity, and resting tremor (RT) (6). Because postural instability is present in about 70% of the general population age 70 years and older, it is not a reliable symptom. Bradykinesia is the most reliable differentiator while "cogwheeling" in patients with ET may be mistaken for the cogwheel rigidity of PS (7,8). The tremor observed in ET is typically postural and kinetic tremor, although late in the course of ET, patients may have RT (7,8). The evolution of tremor also varies—amplitude increases and frequency decreases with disease progression in ET, whereas PS tremor peaks and then has decreasing amplitude and may subside entirely. Although uncommon, patients with PS may have onset with RT in the lower limbs, but this is never so in ET. Head tremor and vocal cord tremor may be seen in ET but are absent in PS.

Other features are also useful in the differential diagnosis. The posture in PS is often flexed compared with typical age-related postural changes in ET. Gait is affected in all patients with PS eventually, with diminished arm swing, shuffling gait, difficulty changing directions, and freezing. As a rule, gait is not affected in ET. Handwriting becomes smaller (micrographic) in patients with PS and may be tremulous in ET. Facial expression is reduced (hypomimia) in PS but is not affected in ET.

Patients with ET usually have a longer history of symptoms before seeking medical attention. There is frequently a positive family history in ET with an autosomal-dominant pattern of inheritance. In contrast, parkinsonian patients present earlier because they are more disabled by the symptoms, particularly bradykinesia. Family history is often negative, and the role of genetics in most PS cases is uncertain.

TIMING OF OVERLAP

There are three possible scenarios for the sequence of ET/PD overlap: (a) ET diagnosed first followed by PS, (b) PS diagnosed first, followed by ET, and (c) both ET and PS diagnosed simultaneously.

The first situation is the most common and the easiest to recognize. The diagnosis of PS in a person with existing ET requires that all three of the criteria previously listed (bradykinesia, rigidity, and RT) be met. In the other two situations, it is difficult to classify clinically that two different disorders coexist. If a patient already has PS, tremor is typically less prominent with time, so a worsening postural/kinetic tremor in late PS indicates a positive diagnosis of ET.

RELATIONSHIP BETWEEN ESSENTIAL TREMOR AND PARKINSONISM

Most studies of a possible association between ET and PD have been epidemiological. Although some past studies found an increased risk of idiopathic PD in patients with ET (9–13), other studies reported only average risk of PD in ET (14–18). A primary reason for differences in reported risks of PD in ET is the misdiagnosis of PD based on RT and cogwheeling in patients with ET (6). Presence of all three PS criteria allows for a more accurate diagnosis of PS in patients with ET, and bradykinesia is the most reliable feature of PS in these patients.

PATHOLOGY AND BIOCHEMISTRY OF THE BRAIN

ET is not associated with the same pathological and biochemical changes that are associated with parkinsonism.

The gross pathology of idiopathic PD shows neuronal loss and gliosis of the substantia nigra with Lewy bodies. Similar changes are also noted in the locus ceruleus. In contrast, the gross pathology of ET is normal.

In 1960, Ehringer and Hornykiewicz (19) reported dopamine deficiency of the substantia nigra and its striatal projections in PD. One year later, Brickmayer and Hornykiewicz reported clinical improvement in patients with PD after intravenous levodopa, a precursor of dopamine (20).

In the first report of a biochemical abnormality in ET, Rajput et al. (21) compared three ET brains and three control brains. The levels of norepinephrine (NE) in the locus ceruleus, dentate nucleus, inferior olive, and cerebellar cortex were significantly higher in the ET group. The levels of NE in the red nucleus, however, were not significantly different. In contrast, NE levels in autopsy-verified PD brains were significantly lower compared with those in controls (22).

ESSENTIAL TREMOR, RESTING TREMOR, AND PARKINSONISM

In 1993, we reported findings of nine ET autopsies (6). Of the nine, three had only ET, and three had ET plus RT without other features of PS. The remaining three had ET and PS with all three cardinal features: bradykinesia, rigidity, and RT. Of those with ET and PS, two had a history of neuroleptic use, and one had an infarct in the basal ganglia. None of our nine patients had substantia nigra neuronal loss or Lewy bodies.

By 2001, we completed 20 ET autopsies, including the nine described above. Of the 20, eight had only ET, six had ET plus RT without other PS features, and six had ET and PS with all three features of PS. Three of these six patients have already been discussed above. Two others had ET and progressive supranuclear palsy (PSP); however, neither had ophthalmoplegia during life and the PSP diagnosis was made at autopsy. Only one of the 20 patients had both ET and PD with Lewy bodies in the substantia nigra.

CONCLUSIONS

ET and PD are different disorders. The clinical features, biochemistry, gross pathology, and pharmacotherapy of ET and PD are different. Any overlap between ET and PS is incidental (9,12,13). Some patients with ET develop RT as a natural evolution of the disease (6). Overlap of these conditions is seen more often in specialty movement disorder clinics due to referral of patients who are difficult to diagnosis and treat. There are no biological markers for either disorder, so diagnoses are clinical.

REFERENCES

1. Larsen TA, Calne DB. Essential tremor. *Clin Neuropharmacol* 1983;6:185–206.
2. Findley LJ. Epidemiology and genetics of essential tremor. *Neurology* 2000;54[Suppl 4]:S8–S13.
3. Moghal S, Rajput AH, D'Arcy C, et al. Prevalence of movement disorders in elderly community residents. *Neuroepidemiology* 1994;13:175–178.
4. Schoenberg BS, Anderson DW, Haerer AF. Prevalence of Parkinson's disease in the biracial population of Copiah County, Mississippi. *Neurology* 1985;35:841–845.
5. de Rijk MC, Launer LJ, Berger K, et al. Prevalence of Parkinson's disease in Europe: a collaborative study of population based cohorts. *Neurology* 2000;54[Suppl 5]: S21–S23.
6. Rajput AH, Rozdilsky B, Ang L, et al. Significance of parkinsonian manifestations in essential tremor. *Can J Neurol Sci* 1993;20:114–117.
7. Findley LJ, Gresty MA, Halmagyi GM. Tremor and cogwheel phenomena and clonus in Parkinson's disease. *J Neurol Neurosurg Psychiatry* 1981;44:534–546.
8. Salisachs P, Findley LJ. Problems in the differential diagnosis of essential tremor. In: Finley LJ, Capildeo R, eds. *Movement disorders: tremor.* London: MacMillan Press Ltd, 1984:219–224.
9. Geraghty JJ, Jankovic J, Zetusky WJ. Association between essential tremor and Parkinson's disease. *Ann Neurol* 1985;17:329–333.
10. Hornabrook RW, Nagurney JT. Essential tremor in Papua, New Guinea. *Brain* 1976;99:659–672.
11. Lang AE, Kierans C, Blair RDG. Association between familial tremor and Parkinson's disease. *Ann Neurol* 1986;19:306–307.
12. Roy M, Boyer L, Barbeau A. A prospective study of 50 cases of familial Parkinson's disease. *Can J Neurol Sci* 1983;10:37–42.
13. Marttila RJ, Rinne UK. Parkinson's disease and essential tremor in families of patients with early-onset Parkinson's disease. *J Neurol Neurosurg Psychiatry* 1988;51:429–431.
14. Rajput AH, Offord KP, Beard CM, et al. Essential tremor in Rochester, Minnesota: a 45-year study. *J Neurol Neurosurg Psychiatry* 1984;47:466–470.
15. Cleeves L, Findley LJ, Koller W. Lack of association between essential tremor and Parkinson's disease. *Ann Neurol* 1988;24:23–26.
16. Martilla RJ, Rautakorpi I, Rinne UK. The relation of essential tremor to Parkinson's disease. *J Neurol Neurosurg Psychiatry* 1984;47:734–735.
17. Bain PG, Findley LJ, Thompson PD, et al. a study of hereditary essential tremor. *Brain* 1994;117:805–824.
18. Pahwa R, Koller WC. Is there a relationship between Parkinson's disease and essential tremor? *Clin Neuropharmacol* 1993;16:30–35.
19. Ehringer H, Hornykiewicz O. Verteilung von Noradrenalin und dopamine (3-hydroxytyramin) im gehirn des menschen und ihr verhalten bei erkrangungen des extrapyramidalen systems. *Klin Wochenschr* 1960;38: 1236–1239.
20. Birkmayer W, Hornykiewicz O. Der 1-3,4,Dioxyphenylalanin (=DOPA) effekt bei der Parkinson Akinese. *Wien Klin Wochenschr* 1961;73:787–788.
21. Rajput AH, Hornykiewicz O, Deng Y, et al. Increased noradrenaline levels in essential tremor brain. *Neurology* 2001;56[Suppl 3]:A302.
22. Kish SJ, Shannak KS, Rajput AH, et al. Cerebellar norepinephrine in patients with Parkinson's disease and control subjects. *Arch Neurol* 1984;41(6):612–614.

Parkinson's Disease: Advances in Neurology, Vol. 91.
Edited by Ariel Gordin, Seppo Kaakkola, and Heikki Teräväinen
Lippincott Williams & Wilkins, Philadelphia © 2003

41

Genetics and Biochemistry of Dopa-responsive Dystonia: Significance of Striatal Tyrosine Hydroxylase Protein Loss

Yoshiaki Furukawa

Movement Disorders Research Laboratory, Centre for Addiction and Mental Health-Clarke Division, Toronto, Ontario, Canada

Dopa-responsive dystonia (DRD) is a syndrome characterized by childhood-onset dystonia and a dramatic and sustained response to relatively low doses of levodopa (1–3). This clinical syndrome typically presents with gait disturbance due to foot dystonia, later development of some parkinsonian features, and worsening of symptoms and signs toward the evening (diurnal fluctuation). There are two known causative genes for DRD: (a) the gene (*GCH1*) coding for guanosine triphosphate (GTP) cyclohydrolase I (GTPCH), the enzyme in the biosynthetic pathway of tetrahydrobiopterin (BH4; the essential cofactor for tyrosine hydroxylase [TH]); and (b) the human TH gene (*TH*) (3–5). Many patients with DRD, including apparently sporadic cases, have dominantly inherited *GCH1* mutations (4,6–19). In contrast, only several patients with DRD have shown recessively inherited *TH* mutations (the mild form of TH deficiency) (5,20–22). There have been two autopsied patients with GTPCH-deficient DRD, but no reports of autopsied cases with TH-deficient DRD (15,23). In both autopsied patients with DRD, although loss of enzyme protein was reasonably considered to be limited to GTPCH, TH protein concentrations were decreased in the striatum. This chapter summarizes recent advances in the genetics and biochemistry of DRD, with a special emphasis on the importance of striatal TH protein reduction in GTPCH-deficient DRD.

GENETIC ASPECTS

Autosomal-dominant GTPCH-deficient DRD

The enzyme GTPCH catalyzes the first step in the biosynthesis of BH4, the natural cofactor for TH, tryptophan hydroxylase, and phenylalanine hydroxylase (PAH). The atomic structure of GTPCH from *Escherichia coli* has demonstrated that this enzyme is a homodecamer formed by a face-to-face association of two pentamers (24). Patients with recessively inherited GTPCH deficiency (usually homozygotes) develop BH4-dependent hyperphenylalaninemia (HPA) in the first 6 months of life and severe neurological dysfunction (e.g., convulsions, mental retardation, developmental motor delay, truncal hypotonia, and limb hypertonia) (25–27). By contrast, patients with autosomal-dominant GTPCH-deficient DRD (usually heterozygotes) never develop HPA, whereas a subclinical defect in phenylalanine metabolism is often detected by the phenylalanine loading test (28). Recently, a novel phenotype of GTPCH deficiency (dystonia with motor delay), which is clinically and biochemically intermediate between GTPCH-deficient DRD (mild) and GTPCH-deficient HPA (severe), has been reported (29). Patients with this phenotype (compound heterozygotes) have generalized dystonia, developmental motor delay, and no overt HPA in infancy. The different susceptibility to a BH4-deficient condition among the three hydroxylases may be related to differences in Km values for BH4 and in the degree of possible regulatory effects of BH4 on stability/expression of the hydroxylase proteins (3) (see below).

In patients with these GTPCH deficiencies, more than 85 different mutations have been identified in the coding region (including the splice sites) of *GCH1* (19). The reason there are many independent mutations throughout all of the six exons of *GCH1* (missense and nonsense mutations, small deletions and insertions, splice site mutations) is unknown. Approximately 70% of them are missense or nonsense mutations. In reports on DRD, in which a relatively large number of pedigrees was genetically examined by five groups, no mutations in either the coding region or the splice sites of *GCH1* were found in 21% to 51% (as a whole, 44%) of families, using conventional genomic DNA sequencing of this gene (4,6,7,10,11,15–19). Because "coding region mutation-negative" pedigrees include families having an apparently sporadic patient or only a few affected siblings, some of these families may have autosomal-recessive TH-deficient DRD. In fact, we have found a compound heterozygote for *TH* mutations in one of our *GCH1* mutation–negative DRD pedigrees (22). For coding region mutation-negative DRD families, in which positive linkage to the *GCH1* locus or biochemical dysfunction of GTPCH has been identified, possible explanations are the following: (a) a mutation in noncoding regulatory regions of *GCH1;* (b) a large genomic deletion of one or more exons of *GCH1;* (c) an intragenic duplication or inversion of *GCH1;* and (d) a mutation in, as yet undefined, regulatory genes (having an influence on *GCH1* expression) or other genes (which products interact with GTPCH and can modify the enzyme function). Recently, point mutations in the 5'-untranslated region of *GCH1,* decreased *GCH1* messenger RNA (mRNA) expression from one allele with no coding region mutation, and a large genomic deletion in *GCH1* (which is undetectable by the usual genomic DNA sequence analysis of this gene) have been reported (10,16,18,30). Although Tassin et al. (18) found *parkin* mutations in some of their patients, whose symptoms were similar to those in DRD (clinical differentiation between early onset parkinsonism and DRD is sometimes difficult) (8,31), detailed clinical and/or biochemical (see below) data have not suggested mutations of this gene in our DRD families with no detectable *GCH1* mutations (Yoshiaki Furukawa, 2000).

Advances in the molecular genetics of DRD have extended the clinical phenotype of this treatable syndrome to include adult-onset "benign" parkinsonism, various types of focal dystonia, DRD simulating cerebral palsy or spastic paraplegia, dystonia with a relapsing-remitting course, and so forth (3,7,10,14,18, 22,32). However, no clear correlations between specific clinical features and types of mutations in *GCH1* are established, and isolated scoliosis and pure writer's cramp in members of DRD families were not always associated with *GCH1* mutations identified in the probands with the classic phenotype (33, and Yoshiaki Furukawa, 1999). In coexpression studies, it has been demonstrated that GTPCH protein with dominantly inherited but not recessively inherited mutations of *GCH1* inactivated the normal enzyme, suggesting a critical role of this dominant negative effect in the phenotypical heterogeneity (9,12,34). In this case, the more mutant peptides interacting with the wild-type peptides, the greater the opportunity to form nonfunctional multimers. Nevertheless, Suzuki et al. (35) have suggested that in GTPCH-deficient DRD, (a) the dominant negative effect through the formation of chimeric GTPCH protein is unlikely as a cause of decreased enzyme activity, but (b) low GTPCH protein content, which was observed in phytohemagglutinin (PHA)-stimulated mononuclear blood cells (MBCs) of some DRD patients, may have a role in the mechanism of dominant inheritance.

It is important to note that approximately 30% to 50% of patients with DRD have no family history of dystonia (2,36). Some of these apparently sporadic patients can be explained by gender-related incomplete penetrance of *GCH1* mutations, independent *de novo* mutations in *GCH1* (suggesting a relatively high spontaneous mutation rate in this gene) and recessively inherited *TH* mutations (11,22). In genetically confirmed patients with the autosomal-dominant form of DRD, the penetrance was much higher in women (87%) than in men (38%) (11). Ichinose et al. (4) originally reported that activity levels of GTPCH in PHA-stimulated MBCs were lower in women than in men. In a recent report from the same group, however, there was no difference of GTPCH activity levels in PHA-stimulated MBCs between women and men (37). In autopsied human brain, there was also no obvious sex-related difference of striatal biopterin levels in healthy children (38). Other genetic and/or environmental factors relating to gender may modulate the outcome of a *GCH1* mutation in GTPCH-deficient DRD.

Autosomal-recessive TH-deficient DRD

The enzyme TH, a BH4-dependent monooxygenase, catalyzes the rate-limiting step (the formation of dopa from tyrosine) in the biosynthesis of catecholamines. The native TH enzyme is a tetramer of four identical subunits (39). According to Bartholomé and Lüdecke (40), TH-deficient DRD is characterized by leg dystonia (onset approximately at age 4 years), diurnal fluctuation of symptoms, and a good response to levodopa therapy. By July 2001, 13 different *TH* mutations (10 missense mutations, two small deletions, one branch-site mutation) have been reported in 14 patients with TH deficiency (homozygotes or compound heterozygotes) from 12 unrelated families. Clinical features of four families were similar to those of GTPCH-deficient DRD pedigrees (5,20–22,40–42). A sustained response to low doses of levodopa and no motor adverse effects during chronic levodopa treatment (for more than 30 years) have been confirmed in two brothers (onset at ages 2 and 5 years), who were clinically diagnosed as DRD (41,42) and in one patient (onset at age 20 months) with the clinical diagnosis of hypokinetic rigid syndrome (family A and family B in reference 21). However, symptoms and signs of patients in eight other families were much more severe than those of autosomal-dominant DRD cases with partial GTPCH deficiency (43–51). All of these patients with the severe form of TH deficiency (onset at younger than 6 months) had developmental motor delay, truncal hypotonia, rigidity of extremities, and hypokinesia.

In a family with DRD due to a homozygous missense mutation in *TH* (the mild form of TH deficiency), the mutated recombinant enzyme showed about 15% of specific activity compared with the wild type in a coupled *in vitro* transcription-translation assay system (5,20). The same group also reported a parkinsonian patient with the severe form of TH deficiency caused by another missense mutation (43). In this patient, the mutant TH revealed 0.3% to 16% of wild-type enzyme activity in three complementary expression systems. Recently, two compound heterozygotes for *TH* mutations have been reported: one with the mild form (having a missense mutation in the tetramerization domain and a deletion) (22) and the other with the severe form of TH deficiency (having a missense mutation in the catalytic domain and a deletion) (44,47,49) (Table 41.1). Both *TH* deletions found in these patients shift the translational reading frame and predict the same premature termination codon by chance. Thus, a comparison between the compound heterozygotes suggests that an effect on TH activity *in vivo* of a missense mutation in the

TABLE 41.1. *Clinical features of compound heterozygotes for mutations in the human tyrosine hydroxylase (TH) gene: the mild form vs. the severe form of TH deficiency*

	Sex	Age at onset	Mutations	Symptoms and signs
Patient with the mild form (22)	M	13 months	296delT in exon-3 (premature termination at T^{338} AA)[a] Asp498Gly in exon-14[b]	No developmental motor delay Dopa-responsive dystonia simulating spastic paraplegia Fine postural tremor of both hands Stiffness and fatigue after exercise
Patient with the severe form (44,47,49)	M	4 months	291delC in exon-3 (premature termination at T^{338} AA)[a] Arg233His in exon-6[b,c]	Severe motor retardation Truncal hypotonia, rigidity of the limbs Severe hypokinesia No diurnal fluctuation

Numbering of nucleotide or amino acid is based on human *TH* mRNA type 4 (reference 52).

[a]Note that both *TH* deletions shift the translational reading frame and predict the same premature stop codon (T^{338} AA) by chance.

[b]The missense mutations (Asp498Gly and Arg233His) are located in the tetramerization and catalytic domains, respectively (reference 39).

[c]The mutation (Arg233His) has been identified in four other families with the severe form of TH deficiency (references 44,45,47,49,51).

tetramerization domain may be milder than that in the catalytic domain of this enzyme.

Conclusions of Genetic Aspects

Because not all patients with DRD have mutations in the coding region (including the splice sites) of *GCH1* or *TH,* the present DNA testing for DRD is not suitable for routine clinical practice. However, because positive results of molecular genetic studies can provide information on prognosis (i.e., DRD vs. more severe metabolic disorders or progressive neurodegenerative diseases), an effort to find mutations in patients with this treatable syndrome is indispensable.

BIOCHEMICAL ASPECTS

Autopsied Patients

The clinical details of the two autopsied patients with DRD are described elsewhere (8,15,23,53). In brief, case 1 (an apparently sporadic patient) started walking on tiptoes at 5 years of age. On examination at age 8, case 1 had flexion inversion of the feet (right-side predominant) while walking and intermittent dystonia of the right arm. Her dystonic symptoms were well controlled by 250 mg levodopa three times a day for 11 years until her death due to an automobile accident at 19 years of age. Case 2 developed inversion of the right foot and gait disturbance when she was 12 years old. At approximately age 20 years, dystonia of the left hand was apparent. Her gait disturbance and loss of hand dexterity progressed after 45 years of age. On examination at age 57 (while taking levodopa at 250 mg once a day), case 2 had dystonia of her right foot and left hand, postural tremor, hypomimia, diminished arm swing, increased muscle tone in the right leg, postural instability, and hyperreflexia in the lower extremities. After a 7-day levodopa holiday, she had a greater impairment of motor function and a resting tremor in the hands. Case 2 was then successfully treated (she became functionally normal) with 100 mg of levodopa with a decarboxylase inhibitor once a day for more than a decade. She died of breast cancer at age 68. Fluorodopa PET demonstrated normal results in case 2 as well as in her affected identical twin and daughter (54). Neuropathological studies showed no Lewy bodies and a normal population of cells with reduced melanin in the substantia nigra of cases 1 and 2 (15,23). There were no degenerative changes also in other brain areas of both patients.

GCH1 Mutations

On one allele, case 1 had a G-to-T transversion in exon-1 of *GCH1* (at nucleotide position 193), resulting in a substitution of the glutamic acid residue with a termination codon (Glu65Ter) (15). In addition, this patient had a C-to-T transition in exon-1 (at nucleotide position 68) on the other allele, causing a proline to leucine amino acid change at codon-23 (Pro23Leu), whereas she developed the classic phenotype of DRD (without any motor delay and HPA). Functional analysis of the mutated recombinant GTPCH protein with the Pro23Leu substitution revealed that catalytic activity of this mutant protein was not affected compared with that of the wild-type protein in a prokaryotic expression system. Unlike other missense mutation sites reported in GTPCH deficiencies, proline at codon-23 is not conserved across human, rat, and mouse species and is located at the N-terminal periphery of the enzyme (24,55). Kinetic parameters of purified recombinant human GTPCH expressed in *E. coli* were not markedly changed, even after truncating its N-terminal 45 residues (35). These findings suggest that the Pro23Leu substitution has no considerable effect on GTPCH activity. In fact, this amino acid change has recently been reported to be a polymorphism that occurs in 3% of the healthy Swiss population (56). In contrast to case 1, no significant *GCH1* mutation has been identified in case 2. However, biochemical findings clearly demonstrated GTPCH dysfunction in brain of case 2 (see later discussion).

Brain Biopterin and Neopterin

An allele having a significant *GCH1* mutation produces dysfunctional GTPCH protein and consequently results in reduced total biopterin (BP) and total neopterin (NP). BP includes BH4, quinonoid dihydrobiopterin, dihydrobiopterin, as well as (oxidized) biopterin, and most brain BP exists as BH4 (57). NP consists of degradation products of dihydroneopterin triphosphate (the first intermediate in the biosynthesis of BH4), which is synthesized from GTP by GTPCH. Reduced NP levels in cerebrospinal fluid (CSF) have been found in genetically confirmed patients with GTPCH-deficient DRD, dystonia with motor delay, and GTPCH-deficient HPA, but not in patients with other BH4-deficient disorders (8,26,27,29,58). Patients with GTPCH-deficient HPA had no detectable NP in CSF and no measurable GTPCH activity in liver biopsy specimens (25,26). Thus, NP (the byproducts of the GTPCH reaction) is generally considered to reflect GTPCH activity.

In the two autopsied patients with DRD, brain BP concentrations were substantially reduced (putamen, −84% [mean]; caudate, −86%; frontal cortex, −62%) compared with age-matched normal controls (15) (Fig. 41.1). The patients with DRD also had substantially decreased brain NP levels (putamen, −62%; caudate, more than −62%; frontal cortex, more than −64%) (15) (Fig. 41.1). Recently, reduced concentrations of BP and NP in DRD case 2 have been confirmed in five other brain areas (internal segment of the globus pallidus, external segment of the globus pallidus, red nucleus, occipital cortex, and cerebellar cortex) (Yoshiaki Furukawa and Stephen J. Kish, 2000). These pterin results can be explained by congenital partial GTPCH deficiency. In two conditions characterized by degeneration of nigrostriatal dopaminergic neurons—Parkinson's disease (PD) and methylphenyltetrahydropyridine (MPTP)-treated primate model—BP levels in the striatum were significantly decreased, whereas BP concentrations in the frontal cortex were normal (15). Levels of NP both in the striatum

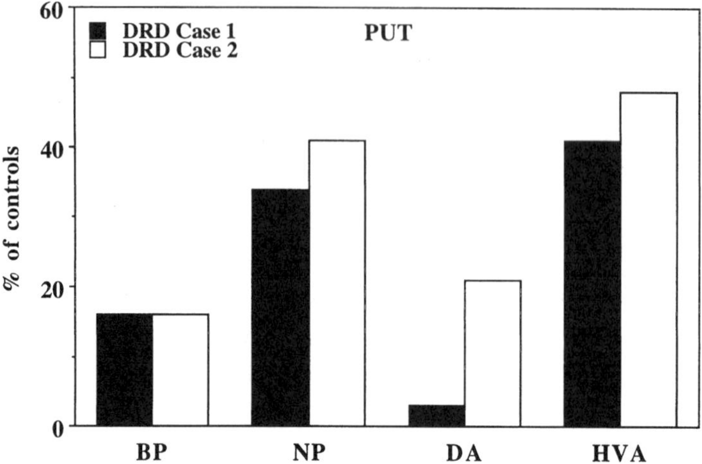

FIGURE 41.1. Total biopterin (BP), total neopterin (NP), dopamine (DA), and homovanillic acid (HVA) levels in the putamen (PUT) of two dopa-responsive dystonia (DRD) patients with guanosine triphosphate cyclohydrolase I dysfunction (case 1, 19 years; case 2, 68 years) expressed as percentages of age-matched control means. BP and NP concentrations were measured in the intermediate subregion (15), and DA and HVA levels were determined in the caudal subregion of the PUT (15,23).

and in the frontal cortex were preserved in patients with PD and MPTP-treated monkeys. The brain findings provide additional support for the use of CSF BP and NP in the differential diagnoses of the following disorders responsive to levodopa: (a) GTPCH-deficient DRD (reduced BP and NP); (b) PD and early onset parkinsonism, including the autosomal-recessive form caused by *parkin* mutations (decreased BP associated with normal NP); and (c) normal BP and NP in TH-deficient DRD (3,8,31,44,47).

Striatal Dopamine and Homovanillic Acid

Subregional dopamine (DA) data in the striatum pointed to an involvement of the putamen and, in particular, the caudal portion of the putamen, as the striatal subdivision that was most affected by DA loss (–88%) in the patients with GTPCH-deficient DRD (15,23) (Fig. 41.1). In this caudal putamen of both patients, concentrations of homovanillic acid (HVA) were also reduced (–55%) and the molar ratios of HVA to DA were shifted in favor of HVA, indicating upregulation of DA turnover (15,23) (Fig. 41.1). In contrast to these patients with DRD, DA and HVA levels in the caudal subregion of the putamen were normal in an autopsied patient with primary torsion dystonia having a GAG deletion in the *TOR1A* (*DYT1*) gene (59). The caudal portion of the putamen is known to be most affected by DA depletion (–99%) in patients with PD (60,61).

The development of parkinsonism in DRD case 2, who initially presented with dystonia, could be explained by the overlap of age-related decreases of striatal BP and DA during adulthood on a congenital partial BP deficit (38,62). In the putamen of human brain, the magnitude of a significant decline of BP from adolescence to senescence (–53%, 26-years group vs. 85 years) is comparable to that of DA during aging (–60%, 22-years group vs. 84 years). These data also suggest that the age-related decline of brain BP could contribute to adult-onset parkinsonian patients without preceding dystonia in GTPCH-deficient DRD families (38).

Striatal TH Protein and Other DA Nerve Terminal Markers

Striatal levels of dopa decarboxylase (DDC; a DA biosynthetic enzyme that does not use BH4 as a cofactor) protein, the DA transporter (^{3}H-WIN 35428 binding), and the vesicular monoamine transporter (^{3}H-dihydrotetrabenazine binding) are all markedly decreased in patients with PD (63,64). These DA nerve terminal markers in the striatum were normal in cases 1 and 2, indicating that nigrostriatal dopaminergic terminals are preserved in GTPCH-deficient DRD (15) (Fig. 41.2). This observation in the autopsied patients is in agreement with *in vivo* findings in fluorodopa positron emission tomography and single-photon emission computed tomography studies on DRD, including the report of normal striatal fluorodopa uptake (which depends on DDC activity) in case 2 (13,54). Unexpectedly, however, TH protein concentrations were reduced in the striatum, particularly in the putamen (more than –97%), of both patients with DRD (15) (Fig. 41.2). These data suggest that striatal DA reduction in GTPCH-deficient DRD is caused by decreased TH activity, resulting from low cofactor level and actual loss of TH protein. The human data are supported by findings of decreased TH protein but normal DDC activity in the striatum of the GTPCH-deficient *hph-1* mouse (65). Thus, the two abnormal gene products identified so far in DRD are related to TH molecules.

We previously speculated that striatal TH protein loss in GTPCH-deficient DRD is caused by a diminished regulatory effect of BH4 on the steady-state level (stability/expression) of TH molecules (15). This speculation is supported by recent gene transfer data, suggesting that coexpression of GTPCH with TH stabilizes TH protein *in vivo* (66), and by the discovery of BH4 responsiveness in a novel subtype of PAH deficiency probably due to stabilization of some mutant PAH molecules by the cofactor BH4 (67). Because TH protein levels in the substantia nigra, where

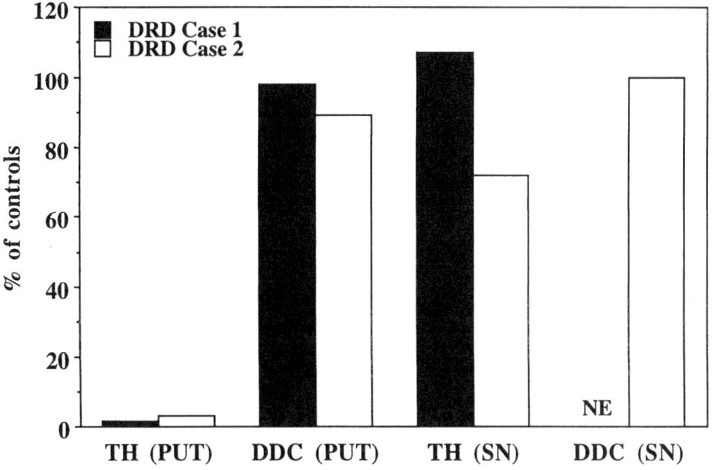

FIGURE 41.2. Tyrosine hydroxylase (TH) protein and dopa decarboxylase (DDC) protein levels in the putamen (PUT) and substantia nigra (SN) of two dopa-responsive dystonia (DRD) patients with guanosine triphosphate cyclohydrolase I dysfunction (case 1, 19 years; case 2, 68 years) expressed as percentages of age-matched control means. TH and DDC protein concentrations were measured in the caudal subregion of the PUT (15) and in the substantia nigra pars compacta (15,23). The TH protein level in the caudal PUT of case 1 was less than 2% of the control mean. The DDC concentration in the substantia nigra of case 1 was not determined. (NE, not examined.)

striatal TH molecules are synthesized, were preserved in the two patients with GTPCH-deficient DRD, BH4 could have a regulatory effect on stability, rather than on expression, of this enzyme protein (15,23) (Fig. 41.2). Alternatively, there might be a dysfunction of TH protein transport from the substantia nigra to the striatum due to congenital BH4 deficiency. A significant BP increase in the human striatum during early postnatal period suggests a contribution of BH4 to maturation of the nigrostriatal DA biosynthetic system (38). Finally, our recent finding of only a modest reduction (−52%) of TH protein in the putamen of an asymptomatic *GCH1* mutation carrier in a DRD pedigree suggests that the extent of striatal TH protein loss may play an important role in determining the symptomatic state of GTPCH-deficient DRD (68).

Conclusions of Biochemical Aspects

Postmortem brain data suggest that DA loss in the striatum, especially in the putamen, of patients with GTPCH-deficient DRD is caused by reduced TH activity due not only to low concentration of its cofactor BH4 but also to loss of TH protein. The TH protein reduction in the striatum but not in the substantia nigra could be explained by a diminished regulatory effect of BH4 on stability of TH molecules in the autosomal-dominant form of DRD.

SUMMARY

Notwithstanding the discovery of *GCH1* and *TH* mutations in autosomal-dominant and autosomal-recessive DRD, respectively, a therapeutic trial with levodopa is still the most practical approach to the diagnosis of DRD. The trial needs to be considered in all children with dystonic and/or parkinsonian symptoms or with unexplained gait disorders. Further accumulation of patients with TH-

deficient DRD (the mild form of TH deficiency) is necessary to establish the clinical characteristics of this disorder. Regarding GTPCH-deficient DRD, there remain important unresolved issues, including questions of incomplete penetrance of *GCH1* mutations, female predominance of affected subjects, and intrafamilial phenotypic variation. A clarification of the mechanism of striatal TH protein loss in GTPCH-deficient DRD may provide a new clue to the pathogenesis of this major form of DRD.

REFERENCES

1. Nygaard TG. Dopa-responsive dystonia: delineation of the clinical syndrome and clues to pathogenesis. *Adv Neurol* 1993;60:577–585.
2. Segawa M, Nomura Y. Hereditary progressive dystonia with marked diurnal fluctuation. In: Segawa M, ed. *Hereditary progressive dystonia with marked diurnal fluctuation.* New York: Parthenon Publishing, 1993: 3–19.
3. Furukawa Y, Kish SJ. Dopa-responsive dystonia: recent advances and remaining issues to be addressed. *Mov Disord* 1999;14:709–715.
4. Ichinose H, Ohye T, Takahashi E, et al. Hereditary progressive dystonia with marked diurnal fluctuation caused by mutations in the GTP cyclohydrolase I gene. *Nat Genet* 1994;8:236–242.
5. Lüdecke B, Dworniczak B, Bartholomé K. A point mutation in the tyrosine hydroxylase gene associated with Segawa's syndrome. *Hum Genet* 1995;95:123–125.
6. Ichinose H, Ohye T, Segawa M, et al. GTP cyclohydrolase I gene in hereditary progressive dystonia with marked diurnal fluctuation. *Neurosci Lett* 1995;196:5–8.
7. Bandmann O, Nygaard TG, Surtees R, et al. Dopa-responsive dystonia in British patients: new mutations of the GTP-cyclohydrolase I gene and evidence for genetic heterogeneity. *Hum Mol Genet* 1996;5:403–406.
8. Furukawa Y, Shimadzu M, Rajput AH, et al. GTP-cyclohydrolase I gene mutations in hereditary progressive and dopa-responsive dystonia. *Ann Neurol* 1996;39: 609–617.
9. Hirano M, Tamaru Y, Ito H, et al. Mutant GTP cyclohydrolase I mRNA levels contribute to dopa-responsive dystonia onset. *Ann Neurol* 1996;40:796–798.
10. Bandmann O, Valente EM, Holmans P, et al. Dopa-responsive dystonia: a clinical and molecular genetic study. *Ann Neurol* 1998;44:649–656.
11. Furukawa Y, Lang AE, Trugman JM, et al. Gender-related penetrance and *de novo* GTP-cyclohydrolase I gene mutations in dopa-responsive dystonia. *Neurology* 1998;50:1015–1020.
12. Hirano M, Yanagihara T, Ueno S. Dominant negative effect of GTP cyclohydrolase I mutations in dopa-responsive hereditary progressive dystonia. *Ann Neurol* 1998; 44:365–371.
13. Jeon BS, Jeong J-M, Park S-S, et al. Dopamine transporter density measured by [^{123}I]-CIT single-photon emission computed tomography is normal in dopa-responsive dystonia. *Ann Neurol* 1998;43:792–800.
14. Steinberger D, Weber Y, Korinthenberg R, et al. High penetrance and pronounced variation in expressivity of *GCH1* mutations in five families with dopa-responsive dystonia. *Ann Neurol* 1998;43:634–639.
15. Furukawa Y, Nygaard TG, Gütlich M, et al. Striatal

biopterin and tyrosine hydroxylase protein reduction in dopa-responsive dystonia. *Neurology* 1999:53; 1032–1041.

16. Furukawa Y, Guttman M, Sparagana SP, et al. Dopa-responsive dystonia due to a large deletion in the GTP cyclohydrolase I gene. *Ann Neurol* 2000;47:517–520.
17. Steinberger D, Korinthenberg R, Topka H, et al. Dopa-responsive dystonia: mutation analysis of *GCH1* and analysis of therapeutic doses of L-dopa. *Neurology* 2000;55:1735–1737.
18. Tassin J, Dürr A, Bonnet A-M, et al. Levodopa-responsive dystonia: GTP cyclohydrolase I or parkin mutations? *Brain* 2000;123:1112–1121.
19. Furukawa Y. Dopa-responsive dystonia. In: GeneReveiws at GeneTests-GeneClinics (database online). Seattle: University of Washington, 2002. Available at: www.geneclinics.org.
20. Knappskog PM, Flatmark T, Mallet J, et al. Recessively inherited L-DOPA–responsive dystonia caused by a point mutation (Q381K) in the tyrosine hydroxylase gene. *Hum Mol Genet* 1995;4:1209–1212.
21. Swaans RJM, Rondot P, Renier WO, et al. Four novel mutations in the tyrosine hydroxylase gene in patients with infantile parkinsonism. *Ann Hum Genet* 2000;64: 25–31.
22. Furukawa Y, Graf WD, Wong H, et al. Dopa-responsive dystonia simulating spastic paraplegia due to tyrosine hydroxylase (TH) gene mutations. *Neurology* 2001;56: 260–263.
23. Rajput AH, Gibb WRG, Zhong XH, et al. Dopa-responsive dystonia: pathological and biochemical observations in a case. *Ann Neurol* 1994;35:396–402.
24. Nar H, Huber R, Meining W, et al. Atomic structure of GTP cyclohydrolase I. *Structure* 1995;3:459–466.
25. Niederwieser A, Blau N, Wang M, et al. GTP cyclohydrolase I deficiency, a new enzyme defect causing hyperphenylalaninemia with neopterin, biopterin, dopamine, and serotonin deficiencies and muscular hypotonia. *Eur J Pediatr* 1984;141:208–214.
26. Ichinose H, Ohye T, Matsuda Y, et al. Characterization of mouse and human GTP cyclohydrolase I genes: mutations in patients with GTP cyclohydrolase I deficiency. *J Biol Chem* 1995;270:10062–10071.
27. Blau N, Barnes I, Dhondt JL. International database of tetrahydrobiopterin deficiencies. *J Inherit Metab Dis* 1996;19:8–14.
28. Hyland K, Fryburg JS, Wilson WG, et al. Oral phenylalanine loading in dopa-responsive dystonia: a possible diagnostic test. *Neurology* 1997;48:1290–1297.
29. Furukawa Y, Kish SJ, Bebin EM, et al. Dystonia with motor delay in compound heterozygotes for GTP-cyclohydrolase I gene mutations. *Ann Neurol* 1998;44:10–16.
30. Inagaki H, Ohye T, Suzuki T, et al. Decrease in GTP cyclohydrolase I gene expression caused by inactivation of one allele in hereditary progressive dystonia with marked diurnal fluctuation. *Biochem Biophys Res Commun* 1999;260:747–751.
31. Furukawa Y, Mizuno Y, Narabayashi H. Early-onset parkinsonism with dystonia: clinical and biochemical differences from hereditary progressive dystonia or DOPA-responsive dystonia. *Adv Neurol* 1996;69:327–337.
32. Nygaard TG, Wilhelmsen KC, Risch NJ, et al. Linkage mapping of dopa-responsive dystonia (DRD) to chromosome 14q. *Nat Genet* 1993;5:386–391.
33. Furukawa Y, Kish SJ, Lang AE. Scoliosis in a dopa-responsive dystonia family with a mutation of the GTP cyclohydrolase I gene. *Neurology* 2000;54:2187.
34. Hirano M, Ueno S. Mutant GTP cyclohydrolase I in autosomal dominant dystonia and recessive hyperphenylalaninemia. *Neurology* 1999;52:182–184.
35. Suzuki T, Ohye T, Inagaki H, et al. Characterization of wild-type and mutants of recombinant human GTP cyclohydrolase I: relationship to etiology of dopa-responsive dystonia. *J Neurochem* 1999;73:2510–2516.
36. Nygaard TG, Snow BJ, Fahn S, et al. Dopa-responsive dystonia: clinical characteristics and definition. In: Segawa M, ed. *Hereditary progressive dystonia with marked diurnal fluctuation.* New York: Parthenon Publishing, 1993:21–35.
37. Hibiya M, Ichinose H, Ozaki N, et al. Normal values and age-dependent changes in GTP cyclohydrolase I activity in stimulated mononuclear blood cells measured by high-performance liquid chromatography. *J Chromatogr B* 2000;740:35–42.
38. Furukawa Y, Kish SJ. Influence of development and aging on brain biopterin: implications for dopa-responsive dystonia onset. *Neurology* 1998;51:632–634.
39. Goodwill KE, Sabatier C, Marks C, et al. Crystal structure of tyrosine hydroxylase at 2.3 Å and its implications for inherited neurodegenerative diseases. *Nat Struct Biol* 1997;4:578–585.
40. Bartholomé K, Lüdecke B. Mutations in the tyrosine hydroxylase gene cause various forms of L-dopa–responsive dystonia. *Adv Pharmacol* 1998;42:48–49.
41. Rondot P, Ziegler M. Dystonia–L-dopa responsive or juvenile parkinsonism? *J Neurol Transm* 1983;Suppl19: 273–281.
42. Rondot P, Aicardi J, Goutières F, et al. Dystonies dopasensibles. *Rev Neurol* 1992;148:680–686.
43. Lüdecke B, Knappskog PM, Clayton PT, et al. Recessively inherited L-DOPA–responsive parkinsonism in infancy caused by a point mutation (L205P) in the tyrosine hydroxylase gene. *Hum Mol Genet* 1996;5:1023–1028.
44. Bräutigam C, Wevers RA, Jansen RJT, et al. Biochemical hallmarks of tyrosine hydroxylase deficiency. *Clin Chem* 1998;44:1897–1904.
45. van den Heuvel LPWJ, Luiten B, Smeitink JAM, et al. A common point mutation in the tyrosine hydroxylase gene in autosomal recessive L-DOPA–responsive dystonia in the Dutch population. *Hum Genet* 1998;102: 644–646.
46. Bräutigam C, Steenbergen-Spanjers GCH, Hoffmann GF, et al. Biochemical and molecular genetic characteristics of the severe form of tyrosine hydroxylase deficiency. *Clin Chem* 1999;45:2073–2078.
47. Wevers RA, de Ruk-van Andel JF, Bräutigam C, et al. A review of biochemical and molecular genetic aspects of tyrosine hydroxylase deficiency including a novel mutation (291delC). *J Inher Metab Dis* 1999;22: 364–373.
48. de Lonlay P, Nassogne MC, van Gennip AH, et al. Tyrosine hydroxylase deficiency unresponsive to L-dopa treatment with unusual clinical and biochemical presentation. *J Inherit Metab Dis* 2000;23:819–825.
49. de Rijk-van Andel JF, Gabreëls FJM, Geurtz B, et al. L-dopa–responsive infantile hypokinetic rigid parkinsonism due to tyrosine hydroxylase deficiency. *Neurology* 2000;55:1926–1928.
50. Dionisi-Vici C, Hoffmann GF, Leuzzi V, et al. Tyrosine hydroxylase deficiency with severe clinical course:

clinical and biochemical investigations and optimization of therapy. *J Pediatr* 2000;136:560–562.
51. Janssen RJRJ, Wevers RA, Häussler M, et al. A branch site mutation leading to aberrant splicing of the human tyrosine hydroxylase gene in a child with a severe extrapyramidal movement disorder. *Ann Hum Genet* 2000; 64:375–382.
52. Nagatsu T, Ichinose H. Comparative studies on the structure of human tyrosine hydroxylase with those of the enzyme of various mammals. *Comp Biochem Physiol* 1991;98:203–210.
53. Nygaard TG, Duvoisin RC. Hereditary dystonia-parkinsonism syndrome of juvenile onset. *Neurology* 1986;36: 1424–1428.
54. Snow BJ, Nygaard TG, Takahashi H, et al. Positron emission tomographic studies of dopa-responsive dystonia and early-onset idiopathic parkinsonism. *Ann Neurol* 1993;34:733–738.
55. Nomura T, Ichinose H, Sumi-Ichinose C, et al. Cloning and sequencing of cDNA encoding mouse GTP cyclohydrolase I. *Biochem Biophys Res Commun* 1993;191: 523–527.
56. Hauf M, Cousin P, Solida A, et al. A family with segmental dystonia: evidence for polymorphism in GTP cyclohydrolase I gene (GCH I). *Mov Disord* 2000; 15[Suppl 3]:154–155.
57. Furukawa Y, Shimadzu M, Hornykiewicz O, et al. Molecular and biochemical aspects of hereditary progressive and dopa-responsive dystonia. *Adv Neurol* 1998; 78:267–282.
58. Furukawa Y, Nishi K, Kondo T, et al. CSF biopterin levels and clinical features of patients with juvenile parkinsonism. *Adv Neurol* 1993;60:562–567.
59. Furukawa Y, Hornykiewicz O, Fahn S, Kish SJ. Striatal dopamine in early-onset primary torsion dystonia with the *DYT1* mutation. *Neurology* 2000;54:1193–1195.
60. Kish SJ, Shannak K, Hornykiewicz O. Uneven pattern of dopamine loss in the striatum of patients with idiopathic Parkinson's disease: pathophysiologic and clinical implications. *N Engl J Med* 1988;318:876–880.
61. Hornykiewicz O. Biochemical aspects of Parkinson's disease. *Neurology* 1998;51[Suppl 2]:S2–S9.
62. Kish SJ, Shannak K, Rajput A, et al. Aging produces a specific pattern of striatal dopamine loss: implications for the etiology of idiopathic Parkinson's disease. *J Neurochem* 1992;58:642–648.
63. Zhong X-H, Haycock JW, Shannak K, et al. Striatal dihydroxyphenylalanine decarboxylase and tyrosine hydroxylase protein in idiopathic Parkinson's disease and dominantly inherited olivopontocerebellar atrophy. *Mov Disord* 1995;10:10–17.
64. Wilson JM, Levey AI, Rajput A, et al. Differential changes in neurochemical markers of striatal dopamine nerve terminals in idiopathic Parkinson's disease. *Neurology* 1996;47:718–726.
65. Hyland K, Gunasekera RS, Engle T, et al. Tetrahydrobiopterin and biogenic amine metabolism in the *hph-1* mouse. *J Neurochem* 1996;67:752–759.
66. Leff SE, Rendahl KG, Spratt SK, et al. *In vivo* L-DOPA production by genetically modified primary rat fibroblast or 9L gliosarcoma cell grafts via coexpression of GTP cyclohydrolase I with tyrosine hydroxylase. *Exp Neurol* 1998;151:249–264.
67. Lindner M, Haas D, Zschocke J, et al. Tetrahydrobiopterin responsiveness in phenylketonuria differs between patients with the same genotype. *Mol Genet Metab* 2001;73:104–106.
68. Furukawa Y, Nygaard T, Wong H, et al. Striatal tyrosine hydroxylase protein and dopamine levels in an asymptomatic carrier of a GCH1 mutation in a DRD family. *Mov Disord* 2000;15[Suppl 3]:138.

Parkinson's Disease: Advances in Neurology, Vol. 91.
Edited by Ariel Gordin, Seppo Kaakkola, and Heikki Teräväinen
Lippincott Williams & Wilkins, Philadelphia © 2003

42

Differential Diagnosis between Early Parkinson's Disease and Dementia with Lewy Bodies

Raimo Sulkava

Department of Public Health and General Practice, University of Kuopio, Kuopio, Finland

Estimates of the prevalence proportion of dementia with Lewy bodies (DLB), based on neuropathological series and on registers of research centers, range from 15% to 35% of all demented subjects (1,2). In our own population-based Kuopio 75+ study, the proportion of probable DLB was 15% and that of possible DLB 22%. The clinical diagnostic criteria of DLB by McKeith et al. (3) have been demonstrated to have a sensitivity of 0.22 to 0.83 and a specificity of 0.85 to 1.00 based on a neuropathological diagnosis. The accuracy of clinical diagnosis in a specialist clinic compared with the neuropathological diagnosis was 0.88 (4).

The prevalence of Parkinson's disease (PD) rises from 0.9% to 5.1% from the age-group 65 to 69 years to the age-group 85 to 89 years, respectively (5). The accuracy of clinical PD has recently been reported to be 0.90, with most of the misdiagnosed being cases of multiple system atrophy (MSA) (6).

Table 42.1 shows the most generally used clinical criteria for DLB based on the International Consensus criteria (3). One of the three core features in the criteria is spontaneous motor features of parkinsonism, which are present in approximately two thirds of patients with DLB at presentation (7). Thus, it is common that early DLB is diagnosed as PD, particularly if the clear-cut visual hallucinations are not present or the patient does not tell about these symptoms to other people.

Often, in the early stages of DLB, no prominent and permanent memory impairment occurs and the criteria of the dementia syndrome of the *Diagnostic and Statistical Manual of Mental Disorders,* Fourth Edition, classification are not fulfilled. Therefore, the suggested term "dementia with Lewy bodies" is not a very good one for the purposes of clinicians who make the diagnosis. Furthermore, the patient and the relatives are often not willing to accept the dementia diagnosis, if they can see that the patient is capable to remember and to take care of him or herself. However, to make the diagnosis of DLB, there have to be some symptoms of cognitive decline at least in the patient history.

It is important to make the differential diagnosis between PD and DLB as early as possible because the prospects for treatment are partially different in these conditions. Table 42.2 shows clinically relevant clinical and neuropsychological features at the time of presentation in PD and DLB (7). In addition to the clinical consensus criteria of DLB, these features can be used to help the early differential diagnosis between PD and DLB.

PD is quite often associated with neuropsychiatric features, including visual hallucinations, which is one of the core features in DLB. However, in PD visual hallucinations and other neuropsychiatric symptoms, like delusions, come generally late in the course of

TABLE 42.1. *Consensus criteria for the clinical diagnosis of probable and possible dementia with Lewy bodies (DLB) (see reference 3)*

1. The central feature for a diagnosis of DLB is progressive cognitive decline. *Prominent or persistent memory impairment may not necessarily occur in the early stages but is usually evident with progression.* Deficits on tests of attention and of frontal-subcortical skills and visuospatial ability may be especially prominent
2. Two of the following core features are essential for the diagnosis of probable DLB, and one is essential for possible DLB
   a. Fluctuating cognition with pronounced variation in attention and alertness
   b. Recurrent visual hallucinations that are typically well formed and detailed
   c. Spontaneous motor features of parkinsonism
3. Features supportive of the diagnosis are
   a. Repeated falls
   b. Syncope
   c. Transient loss of consciousness
   d. Neuroleptic sensitivity
   e. Systematized delusions
   f. Hallucinations in other modalities
4. A diagnosis of DLB is less likely in the presence of
   a. Stroke disease, evident as focal neurological signs or on brain imaging brain disorder sufficient to account for the clinical picture
   b. Evidence of physical examination and investigation of any physical illness or other brain disorder

disease and often with high doses of levodopa. Patients with DLB often have a history of episodes of neuropsychiatric symptoms, though not necessarily just at the time of presentation. However, neuropsychological examinations often reveal mild cognitive deficits also in early PD (8). Depression, however, is common both in PD and DLB.

Typical fluctuations of particular cognitive symptoms are seen in more than half of the cases in DLB at the time of presentation. Attention and alertness can vary even during the examination. Episodes of syncopal attacks or unresponsiveness are not rare, even in early DLB, but are not seen in early PD. Patients with these symptoms have often been examined earlier by a cardiologist because of suspected cardiac arrhythmias.

Contrary to PD, in more than half of the patients with DLB, the treatment with levodopa is a failure (9). On the other hand, treatment with acetylcholine esterase inhibitors may be successful, particularly in deteriorated attention and behavioral symptoms (10).

The most widely used brain imaging techniques, including computed tomography, magnetic resonance imaging, single-photon emission computed tomography (SPECT),

TABLE 42.2. *Features that are helpful in the differential diagnosis between early Parkinson's disease (PD) and dementia with Lewy bodies (DLB) at the time of presentation*

	PD	DLB
Impairment of psychomotor functions	Mild	More marked
Executive dysfunction	Often	Often
Visuospatial impairment	Seldom	Often
Visual hallucinations	No	Often
Other hallucinations, eg. auditory	No	Sometimes
Extrapyramidal symptoms	Always	Often
Effect of levodopa	Good	Variable
Fluctuations of symptoms	Not marked	Marked
Symptoms of depression	Often	Often
Delusions	No	Often
Absence of rest tremor	Sometimes	Often
Syncopal attacks	No	Sometimes
Episodes of unresponsiveness	No	Sometimes
Balance disorders	Sometimes	Seldom

and positron emission tomography (PET), can be used in the diagnosis of Alzheimer's disease, vascular dementia, and frontotemporal dementia, but they are not useful in the differential diagnosis between early PD and DLB (11). These conditions share the same type of pathology that produces the same type of metabolic lesions on SPECT and PET, at least in the early stages of disease.

CONCLUSIONS

In conclusion, a differential diagnosis between PD and DLB is in most cases possible even at the time of presentation. A careful clinical neurological examination and a good history by the patient and by a close relative are needed. A neuropsychological investigation is often needed to reveal subtle cognitive deficits. Treatment with levodopa and an acetylcholine esterase inhibitor and follow-up add information are needed for the correct diagnosis.

REFERENCES

1. Hansen L, Salmon D, Galasko D, et al. The Lewy body variant of Alzheimer's disease: a clinical and pathological entity. *Neurology* 1990;40:1–8.
2. Perry RH, Irving D, Blessed G, et al. Senile dementia of Lewy body type: a clinically and neuropathologically distinct form of Lewy body dementia in the elderly. *J Neurol Sci* 1990;95:119–139.
3. McKeith IG, Galasko D, Kosaka K, et al. Consensus guideline for the clinical and pathologic diagnosis of dementia with Lewy bodies (DLB): report of the consortium on DLB international workshop. *Neurology* 1996;47:1113-1124.
4. McKeith IG, Ballard CG, Perry RH, et al. Prospective validation of consensus criteria for the diagnosis of dementia with Lewy bodies. *Neurology* 2000;54: 1050–1058.
5. De Rijk MC, Tzourio C, Breteler MM, et al. Prevalence of parkinsonism and Parkinson's disease in Europe: the EUROPARKINSON Collaborative Study. European community concerted action on the epidemiology of Parkinson's disease. *J Neurol Neurosurg Psychiatry* 1997;62:10–15.
6. Hughes AJ, Daniel SE, Lees AJ. Improved accuracy of clinical diagnosis of Lewy body Parkinson's disease. *Neurology* 2001;57:1497–1499.
7. McKeith IG, Burn D. Spectrum of Parkinson's disease, Parkinson's dementia, and Lewy body dementia. *Neurol Clin* 2000;18:865–883.
8. Hietanen M, Teräväinen H. Cognitive performance in early Parkinson's disease. *Acta Neurol Scand* 1986;73: 151–159.
9. Louis ED, Klatka LA, Liu Y, et al. Comparison of extrapyramidal features in 31 pathologically confirmed cases of diffuse Lewy body disease and 34 pathologically confirmed cases of Parkinson's disease. *Neurology* 1997;48:376–380.
10. McKeith IG, Grace JB, Walker Z, et al. Rivastigmine in the treatment of dementia with Lewy bodies. *Int J Geriatr Psychiatr* 2000;15:387–392.
11. Jagust WJ. Neuroimaging in dementia. *Neurol Clin* 2000;18:885–901.

Subject Index

Page numbers followed by 'f' indicate figures. Page numbers followed by 't' indicate tables

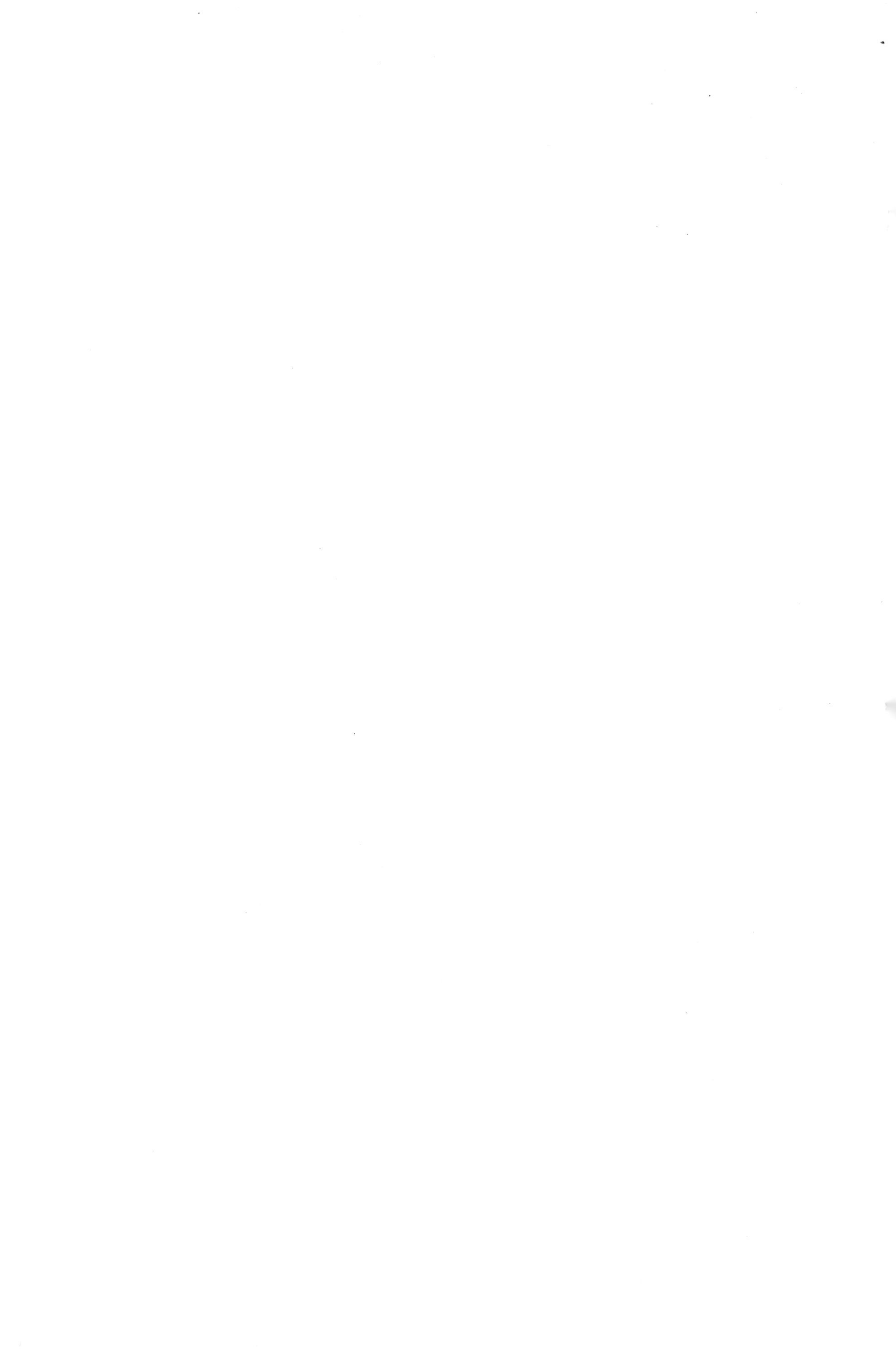